RENEWALS 691-4574

DATE DUE

AUG 0 6			
MAR 13			

Demco, Inc. 38-293

Cerebrovascular Disorders

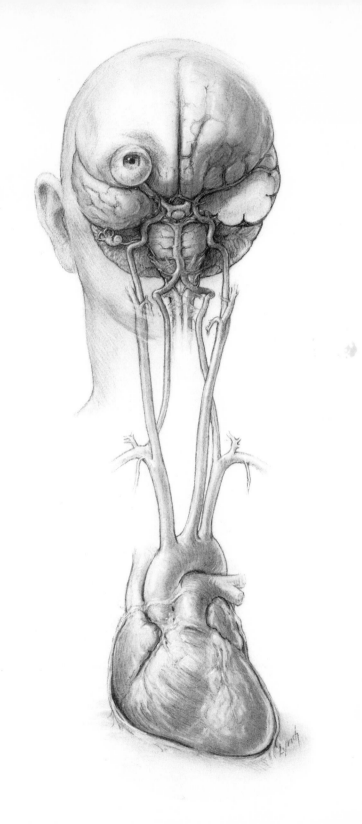

CEREBROVASCULAR DISORDERS

SECOND EDITION

With Chapters on Applied Embryology, Vascular Anatomy,
and Physiology of the Brain and Spinal Cord

JAMES F. TOOLE, M.D.

The Walter C. Teagle Professor of Neurology
Chairman of the Department of Neurology
Bowman Gray School of Medicine
Wake Forest University
Winston-Salem, North Carolina

ANEEL N. PATEL, M.D. (Bombay)
M.R.C.P. (Edinburgh)
F.R.C.P. (Canada)

Associate Professor of Neurology
Albany Medical College of Union University
Albany, New York

A Blakiston Publication

New York St. Louis San Francisco Düsseldorf Johannesburg
Kuala Lumpur London Mexico Montreal New Delhi
Panama Rio de Janeiro Singapore Sydney Toronto

CEREBROVASCULAR
DISORDERS

234567890   VHVH   7987654

This book was set in Times Roman by Rocappi, Inc.
The editors were Paul K. Schneider and Sally Barhydt Mobley;
the designer was Anne Canevari Green;
and the production supervisor was Leroy A. Young.
The printer and binder was Von Hoffman Press, Inc.

Library of Congress Cataloging in Publication Data

Toole, James F
    Cerebrovascular disorders.

    Includes bibliographies.
    1.   Cerebrovascular disease.   I.   Patel, Aneel N.,
joint author.   II.   Title.   [DNLM: 1.   Cerebrovascular
disorders.   WL355 T671c 1975]
RC388.5.T6   1974   616.8'1   73-8957
ISBN   0-07-064970-7

The first edition of this book was dedicated to the taxpayers of the United States. Their annual sacrifice channeled through the National Institutes of Health of the U.S. Public Health Service has supported us in our neurologic training and research. We hope that for many of them this volume will result in the prevention of disability and in better medical care.

This edition is dedicated to Louis Pasteur, who at age 46 had a vascular episode which left him with a left hemiparesis. Despite this, he made scientific contributions which changed the course of humanity.

Writing a book was an adventure. To begin with it was a toy, an amusement; then it became a mistress, and then a master, and then a tyrant.

Winston S. Churchill

Contents

Preface

Strokes kill more than 275,000 and disable another 300,000 Americans every year, making it a leading cause of death and long-term disability. Of the 2½ million stroke victims alive in the United States at any one time, a third are younger than 65 years of age and 10 percent require institutional care. The resulting grief cannot be calculated, but the annual expense—estimated at 1.2 billion dollars for medical care and over 3 billion dollars in lost earnings—can be. Despite this toll, many physicians have only a limited knowledge of the cerebral circulation and its diseases; consequently, the care received by many of their patients is not optimal.

We have written our book for clinicians, and our emphasis is on the diagnosis and management of common problems. Beginning with background information on the embryology, anatomy, and physiology of the cerebral circulation, the discussion progresses to an in-depth consideration of all forms of cerebrovascular disease, with emphasis on atherosclerosis.

Although much of the material presented in the first edition has been retained, the new features of this second edition include a chapter on brain infarction, an expanded chapter on physiology of the cerebral circulation, a new chapter on applied embryology, and a chapter on rare and unusual forms of cerebrovascular disease.

Our book does not attempt to be encyclopedic, but it does provide a thorough treatment of the subject. For those who may wish to pursue these topics further, the authors have compiled an extensive bibliography which follows each chapter.

Acknowledgments

This book could not have been completed without the help of many people, whom we gratefully acknowledge. Miss Suzanne Pickett typed and edited the manuscript and coordinated our efforts. Mrs. Edward Jackson did the reediting and polished our syntax. The artwork was supervised by Mr. George Lynch, Department of Medical Illustrations, Bowman Gray School of Medicine.

Unless otherwise specified, the radiographs and brain scans have been taken from the files of the Department of Radiology and the pathologic specimens from the Department of Pathology, Bowman Gray School of Medicine. Dr. Frank Farrell selected many of the radiographs.

Although several chapters were reviewed by physicians who are authorities in their respective fields, we alone are responsible for any errors or omissions which exist in the following pages. The following people have been particularly helpful: Dr. Lois A. Gillilan, Department of Anatomy, University of Kentucky Medical Center, Lexington, Kentucky; Dr. Abraham T. Lu, Neuropathologist, Rancho Los Amigos Hospital, Associate Clinical Professor of Pathology and Neurology, University of Southern California School of Medicine, Downey, Calif., for the chapter on embryology; Dr. John Moossy, Professor of Pathology and Neurology, University of Pittsburgh, Pittsburgh, Pa.; Dr. David L. Kelly, Section of Neurosurgery, Bowman Gray School of Medicine, Winston-Salem, N.C., for his review of the chapters dealing with intracranial hemorrhage; Dr. G. J. Poole, Department of Radiology, Section on Neuroradiology, for the chapters on embryology and anatomy; Dr. Lawrence McHenry for the chapters on physiology and brain infarction; and Anne, Jimmy, Bill, and Sean, who cut and pasted.

James F. Toole
Aneel N. Patel

Cerebrovascular Disorders

Applied Embryology

And surely we are all out of the computation of our age, and every man is some months older than he bethinks him; for we live, move, have a being, and are subject to the actions of the elements and the malice of disease, in that other world, the truest microcosm, the Womb of our Mother.

Sir Thomas Browne
Religio Medici, 1642

We begin our book on cerebrovascular disorders with life's beginning because the embryonal development of the vascular supply to the brain determines the outcome of many diseases in adult life. For example, unusual configurations of the circle of Willis, arteriovenous malformations, congenital saccular aneurysms, and hypoplasia or agenesis of normal vascular channels are abnormalities which result from defective embryogenesis of the neurovascular system. How the vessels differentiate and what may go awry in the process are the subjects of this chapter.

Concomitant with the development of the neural groove, angioblasts appear in the mesoderm—first as solid cords and then as tubes which proliferate into plexuses through which plasma begins to flow.

As the neural groove evolves into a tube, capillary plexuses proliferate around and within it. Some capillaries become the preferential ones and enlarge into arteries and veins. In this early

1

stage each somite of the tube has circumferentially oriented arteries and veins, but with cephalization some channels anastomose with others to form longitudinal vessels. One of these, the internal carotid system, supplies all the blood to the brain in the embryo. A caudal branch of the internal carotid (the primitive trigeminal arterial plexus) joins with the longitudinal neural arterial plexus (the future basilar artery) to supply the entire hindbrain. The segmental arteries continue to supply the spinal cord; only later do their branches unite to form longitudinal arteries such as the vertebral and the anterior median spinal artery. After this union occurs, involution of the longitudinal arterial plexus begins; and when the vertebral arteries have established continuity with the basilar artery, the primitive trigeminal artery disappears altogether.

DEVELOPMENT OF THE AORTOCRANIAL ARTERIES

Aortic Arch

During embryogenesis the paired ventral and dorsal aortae are connected to each other by six pairs of aortic arches. Dorsal segments of the first and second pairs of arches involute, and their ventral portions become the external carotid arteries. Dorsal portions of the third and fourth arches disappear next, leaving only the proximal segment of the third to form part of the internal carotid. The right fourth aortic arch, together with a part of the right dorsal aorta, forms the proximal portion of the right subclavian artery. The left fourth aortic arch takes part in the formation of the arch of the aorta. The fifth pair of arches involutes and disappears, while the distal portion of the left sixth aortic arch forms the ductus arteriosus.

Clinical Correlation

1 In approximately 70 percent of people the brachiocephalic, left common carotid, and left subclavian arteries originate separately from the aortic arch. In about 20 percent of the Caucasian population and 35 percent of the Negro population in the United States, the brachiocephalic and left common carotid arteries share a common origin located on the right side of the aortic arch. In about 8 percent of the population, the left common carotid artery arises as a *branch* of the brachiocephalic artery (Fig. 1-1).

2 Anomalies of the aortic arch can cause disturbances in patterns of blood flow with resultant turbulence. This leads to trauma to the vessel wall and possibly the development of atherosclerosis.

Vertebral Arteries

The vertebral arteries develop from longitudinal anastomoses between segmental arteries which originate from the paired dorsal aortae and the hypoglossal arteries. The upper five segmental arteries eventually disappear, leaving the seventh to form the junction between the subclavian and vertebral arteries.

Clinical Correlation

1 In rare cases in which the vertebral arteries do not join the basilar artery, the embryonal arrangement of brainstem blood supply from the carotid arterial system persists.

2 In about 5 percent of the population the left vertebral artery originates from the aortic arch between the left common carotid and the left subclavian arteries. In such cases it will not fill with contrast material during left subclavian or left brachial artery angiography.

3 Maldevelopment of the cranium and vertebral column may be associated with anomalies of the arterial tree. In both platybasia and occipitocervical synostosis, for example, there may be atresia of one vertebral artery or a failure of both vertebrals to join the basilar artery (Fig. 1-2A and B).

4 In rare instances the vertebral artery arises from the common or the external carotid artery.

5 If the intersegmental anastomoses are atypical, the vertebral artery may not travel

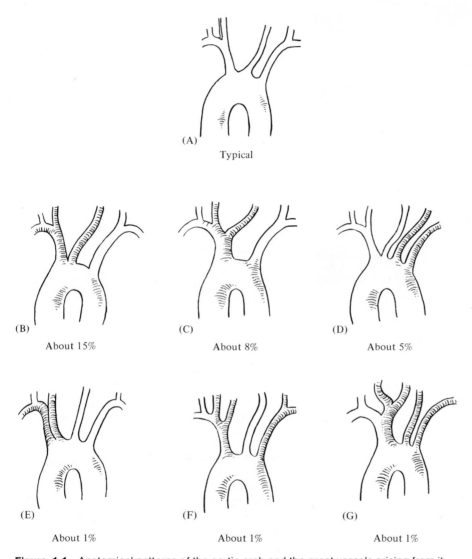

Figure 1-1 Anatomical patterns of the aortic arch and the great vessels arising from it.

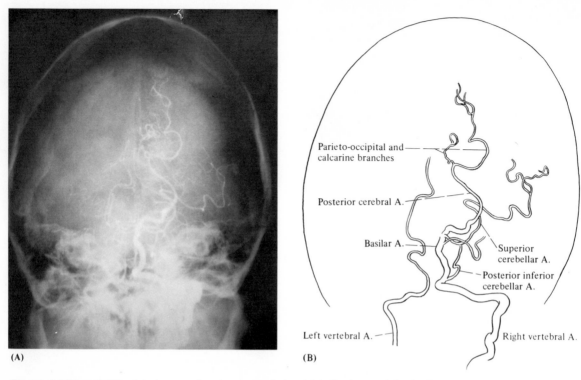

(A)

(B)

Figure 1-2(A) and (B) Arteriogram showing anomaly in which the two vertebral arteries do not join to form the basilar artery; the right ends as the posterior inferior cerebellar artery.

through its canal within the cervical transverse processes before entering the posterior cranial fossa, or it may be bifid, with one branch running within and the other outside the canal.

Subclavian Arteries

The proximal portion of the right subclavian artery is formed from a segment of the right fourth aortic arch, the dorsal aorta, and the seventh segmental artery. The left subclavian artery develops from the seventh intersegmental artery. As the embryo lengthens and the limbs move caudally, both subclavian arteries migrate along the dorsal aorta to a more caudal position.

Clinical Correlation If the right third aortic arch does not involute, the right subclavian artery may arise from the descending aorta distal

to the ductus arteriosus, a condition called aberrant right subclavian artery. In such cases the arch of the aorta will not be visualized in right brachial arteriograms (Fig. 1-3).

Internal Carotid Arteries

At the end of 4 weeks' gestation, when the embryo is approximately 5 mm long, the first two aortic arches (the mandibular and hyoid arteries) begin to regress. At this stage the internal carotid arteries originate from the third aortic arch. Each forms an anterior division which travels toward Rathke's pouch and a posterior division, or primitive trigeminal artery, which travels dorsally to join the longitudinal neural plexus lying on the ventral surface of the brainstem. A plexiform anastomosis forms between

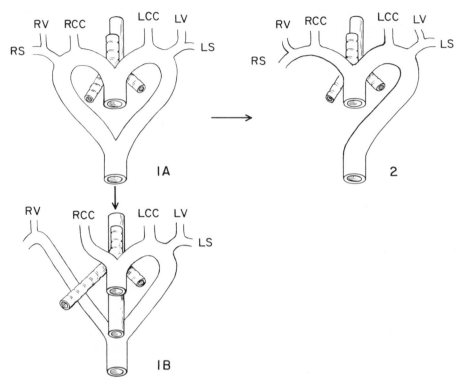

Figure 1-3 1A: Embryonal form of the aortic arch. 1B: Persistent right subclavian artery. 2: Usual adult pattern.

the two anterior divisions. The otic and hypoglossal connections between the developing carotid arteries and the paired longitudinal neural plexuses are present at this stage.

When the embryo measures about 8 mm, the two internal carotid arteries are better defined and the mandibular arteries have been reduced to remnants. Following anastomosis of the internal carotids, the longitudinal neural plexus fuses to form the basilar artery, and the trigeminal arteries involute.

Clinical Correlation

1 The common carotid arteries usually bifurcate at the level of the upper border of the thyroid cartilage (opposite the C_4-C_5 disk). In unusual cases, however, the bifurcation occurs at levels varying from C_1 to T_2.

2 The internal carotid artery may show anomalous loops, coilings, and tortuosities. Although these usually cause no symptoms, they may be responsible for injury to the artery during the course of tonsillectomies or myringotomies.

3 Hypoplasia of the internal carotid artery may be confused with arterial stenosis secondary to disease. In cases of hypoplasia, x-rays of the base of the skull will reveal a small or absent carotid canal.

DEVELOPMENT OF INTRACRANIAL ARTERIES

The differentiation of the vascular system from the mesoderm leads to the formation of a vascular plexus which soon evolves into a network of endothelial tubes. At first all the channels in this network look alike; later they acquire muscular and adventitial coats of varying thickness and become arteries, capillaries, and veins. The cerebral arteries, however, do not develop the medial coat and internal elastic lamina to the same degree as arteries in other parts of the body, and their adventitia consists of a fragile arachnoid membrane.

When the embryo reaches a length of 12 mm (about 32 days), the internal carotids give off to the telencephalon several small branches which are the forerunners of the anterior choroidal and the anterior, middle, and posterior cerebral arteries. The basilar artery is in the process of forming, and branches begin to arise at the level of each cranial nerve. The cerebellum is forming, and the superior cerebellar arteries are prominent. The vertebral arteries are still developing and do not yet connect with the basilar artery; the carotid arteries, therefore, must supply not only the forebrain but also the brainstem and cerebellum.

At the 12- to 14-mm stage (32 to 40 days) the stapedial and ventral pharyngeal arteries give rise to branches of the external carotid artery. The common carotid artery is formed after obliteration of the anastomosis between the third and fourth aortic arches. The anterior choroidal, anterior cerebral, and middle cerebral arteries are well developed, and the homologue of the anterior communicating artery is seen as a plexiform anastomosis.

At the 15-mm stage (40 days) the circulation in the scalp, dura, and pia mater begins to differentiate. Shortly thereafter, when the embryo is 16 to 19 mm long, the stems of the anterior and posterior inferior cerebellar arteries appear. At the 20- to 24-mm stage (44 to 45 days) the circle of Willis can be recognized. The dorsal division of the stapedial artery develops into the middle meningeal artery; the ventral division becomes the ophthalmic artery. The recurrent artery of Heubner arises from the primitive olfactory artery. When the embryo reaches a

length of 40 mm (at about 52 days), nearly all the intracranial arteries which remain throughout life have formed. However, there continues to be an increase in the number of venous anastomoses and in the proliferation of capillaries in the neocortex.

Clinical Correlation

1 In most cases, variations of the cerebral arteries are explained by the persistence or hyperinvolution of anastomotic vessels normally found in the embryo (rete mirabile).

2 Immature branchings or incomplete involution of embryonal vessels which cause defects in the media in the adult are thought to represent a persistence of the primordial plexus of angioblastic tissue.

3 Ocular, facial, or parietooccipital angiomata (which may coexist in the Sturge-Weber-Dimitri syndrome) represent a persistence of the anterior vascular plexus that drains the forebrain and eye during the early stages of development.

4 Maturational arrest prior to complete differentiation of dural and cranial arteries leads to cirsoid angiomata involving the scalp, epidural space, dura, and pia mater.

5 Persistence of the primitive trigeminal artery interconnecting the internal carotid with the basilar artery is known in adult life as caroticobasilar anastomosis. In some instances only a remnant of the primitive trigeminal artery persists, causing an aneurysm or point of weakness in the internal carotid or basilar arteries.

6 Failure of the two longitudinal neural plexuses to fuse properly results in a double, fenestrated, or sacculated basilar artery.

7 Variations of the circle of Willis—for example, a stringlike anterior or posterior communicating artery—may jeopardize its role as the potential collateral channel and lead to an increase in the incidence of brain infarction (Fig. 1-4).

8 The incidence of congenital saccular aneurysms is increased in individuals who have an unusual configuration of the circle of Willis.

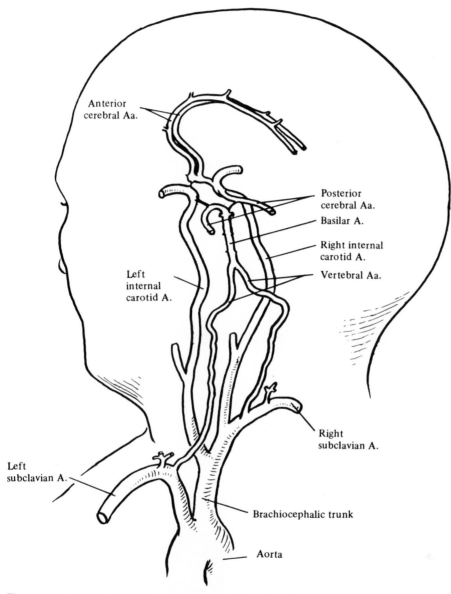

Figure 1-4 Arterial anatomy of a 54-year-old man who died of a massive brain infarction resulting from occlusion of his right internal carotid artery at the carotid sinus. The configuration of his circle of Willis was such that both anterior cerebrals, right middle cerebral, and right posterior cerebral arteries were supplied by the right carotid. Because of the very small caliber of his posterior communicating and left anterior cerebral arteries, there was no collateral supply from the vertebral-basilar or left internal carotid arteries through the circle of Willis. An incidental finding at autopsy was a brachiocephalic trunk.

Persistent Anastomotic Channels

Embryonic channels which may persist into adult life are:

1 The primitive trigeminal artery connecting the carotid and the basilar arteries proximal to the posterior communicating artery (Fig. 1-5)

2 The primitive otic artery connecting internal carotid and basilar arterial systems

3 The primitive hypoglossal artery connecting internal carotid and basilar arterial systems

4 The primitive stapedial artery connecting internal carotid and middle meningeal arteries

5 The primitive ophthalmic artery connecting the lacrimal branch of the ophthalmic artery with the middle meningeal artery

6 The anastomotic channels between the two vertebral arteries

7 The anastomotic channels between the ophthalmic and meningeal arteries

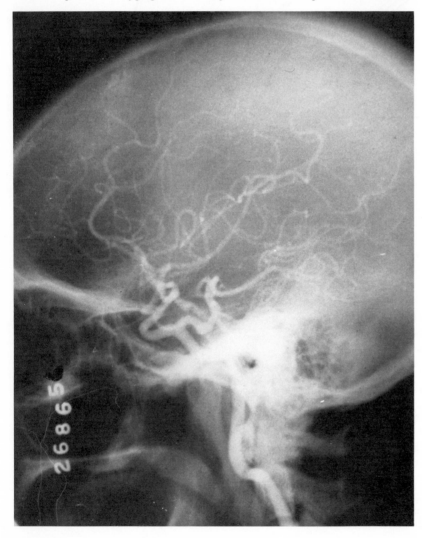

Figure 1-5 Persistent primitive trigeminal artery joining the internal carotid artery to the basilar artery (caroticobasilar anastomosis).

Clinical Correlation

1 In most cases these persistent embryonic anastomoses are asymptomatic and are detected only by angiography or at necropsy.

2 Occasionally they may harbor an aneurysm or compress a cranial nerve.

3 Some of these channels serve as sources of collateral circulation in patients with occlusive cerebrovascular disease.

4 Ophthalmodynamometry readings will not reflect the true pressure in the internal carotid artery in instances in which the ophthalmic artery receives its major blood supply from the meningeal arteries via an accessory ophthalmic artery or in cases of caroticobasilar anastomosis.

DEVELOPMENT OF INTRACRANIAL VEINS

When the embryo is 2 to 3 mm long, drainage of the dorsal aspect of the neural tube takes place through a single hindbrain channel which is continuous with the anterior cardinal vein. By the 5- to 8-mm stage (about 24 to 32 days of gestation) the hindbrain channel has been replaced by the primary head sinus, which lies intradurally. The three dural plexuses that feed into the primary head sinus (anterior, middle, and posterior) drain the prosencephalon-mesencephalon, the metencephalon, and the myeloencephalon, respectively. Within the next 2 or 3 days, when the embryo is 8 to 12 mm in length, the primitive telencephalic and diencephalic veins appear. The rostral end of the anterior dural plexus gives rise to the primitive marginal sinuses, and the posterior dural plexus joins the anterior cardinal veins to form the jugular veins.

At the 12- to 16-mm stage (32 to 40 days) the dura mater differentiates from the pia mater, a plexiform channel interconnects the three dural plexuses, and anastomotic channels appear between the mesencephalic and diencephalic veins. Shortly thereafter, the primary head sinus begins to involute. The channel interconnecting the middle and posterior dural plexuses becomes the forerunner of the sigmoid sinus. The primitive transverse sinus is formed from a portion of the marginal sinuses and the interconnection between the anterior and middle dural plexuses. Within 2 or 3 days the primary head sinus has almost disappeared and the prootic sinus drains the supraorbital and maxillary veins. Telencephalic and ventral diencephalic veins form the tentorial sinus caudoventral to the cerebral hemispheres.

By the time the embryo has reached a length of 40 mm (after 52 days) the arterial tree closely resembles the postnatal configuration, but the venous pattern is still lagging behind. The marginal sinuses are just fusing together to form the midline sagittal sinus. The inferior choroidal vein drains the choroidal plexus into the tentorial sinus.

In the 12-week-old fetus, which measures 60 to 80 mm, the expanding cerebral hemispheres are growing caudally over the midbrain and the primitive cerebellar hemispheres. By the end of the 80-mm stage most of the adult veins can be recognized, the tentorial plexus has been converted into the confluens sinuum (torcular Herophili), and most of the cerebral hemispheres drain into it. The internal cerebral veins receive blood from the basal ganglia. Longitudinal pial anastomoses between the telencephalic and diencephalic veins form the basal veins of Rosenthal.

After the third month the anterior and posterior cerebellar veins are identifiable, the central area of the cerebellar hemisphere drains into the great cerebral vein, and the superior surface of the cerebellar hemisphere drains into either the transverse, the superior petrosal sinus, or the great cerebral vein.

SUGGESTED READINGS

General

du Boulay, G. H.: "The Evolution of the Cerebral Arterial Tree," in Background to Migraine, R. Smith, (ed.), Springer Verlag, New York, 1967, Chap. 5.

Girard, P. F., and Devic, M.: "Malformations vasculaires cerebrales et cardiopathies congenitales," in Proceedings of the First International Congress of Neuropathology, Rome, 1952, Vol. 3, Rosenberg & Sellier, Torino, 1954, pp. 280-285.

Jollie, M.: Chordate Morphology, Reinhold Publishing Corporation, New York, 1962, pp. 347-366.

Kaplan, H. A., and Ford, D. H.: The Brain Vascular System, Elsevier Publishing Company, Amsterdam, 1966.

Moffat, D. B.: The embryology of the arteries of the brain, *Ann. Roy. Coll. Surg. Engl.,* **30**:368, 1962.

Manterola, A., Towbin, A., and Yakovlev, P. I.: Cerebral infarction in the human fetus near term, *J. Neuropathol. Exptl. Neurol.,* **25**:479, 1966.

Rudolph, A. H.: The changes in the circulation after birth; their importance in congenital heart disease, *Circulation,* **41**:343, 1970.

von Bonin, G.: "Embryology of the cerebral circulation," in Transactions of the First Princeton Conference, E. H. Luckey (ed.), Grune & Stratton, Inc., New York, 1955, pp. 8-14.

Wierdis, T., Giannini, V., and Iaia, E.: Foetal and neonatal cerebrovascular disease. Early results of post-mortem carotid angiography, *Panminerva Medica,* **7**:325, 1965.

Development of the Aortocranial Arteries

Vertebral Arteries

Bernini, F. P., Bravaccio, F., Colucci D'Amato, C., and Smaltino, F.: Malformazioni della cerniera occipito-vertebrale associate ad anomalie dell arteria vertebrale (Considerazioni Clinico-Pathogeneticke), *Acta Neurol. (Napoli),* **22**:762, 1967.

Flynn, R. E.: External origin of the dominant vertebral artery, *J. Neurosurg.,* **29**:300, 1968.

Mizukami, M., Tomita, T., Mine, T., and Mihara, H.: Bypass anomaly of the vertebral artery associated with cerebral aneurysm and arteriovenous malformation, *J. Neurosurg.,* **37**:204, 1972.

Singh, S., and Singh, S. P.: Atresia of the vertebral artery and its clinical significance, *Neurology (India),* **19**:172, 1971.

Wackenheim, A., and Babin, E.: Excursion extratransversaire de l'artère vertébrale, une anomalie peu connue, susceptible de pertuber diverses épreuves de compression cervicale, *Presse med.,* **77**(35):1213, 1969.

Internal Carotid Arteries

Goldman, N. C., Singleton, G. T., and Holly, E. H.: Aberrant internal carotid artery. Presenting as a mass in the middle ear, *Arch. Otolaryngol.,* **94**:268, 1971.

Hills, J., and Sament, S.: Bilateral agenesis of the internal carotid artery associated with cardiac and other anomalies. Case report, *Neurology,* **18**:142, 1968.

Lhermitte, F., Gautier, J. C., Poirier, J., and Tyrer, J. H.: Hypoplasia of the internal carotid artery, *Neurology,* **18**:439, 1968.

Lie, T. A.: Congenital Anomalies of the Carotid Arteries, Excerpta Medica Foundation, The Williams & Wilkins Company, Baltimore, 1968.

McAfee, D. K., Anson, B. J., and McDonald, J. J.: Variation in the point of bifurcation of the common carotid artery, *Quart. Bull. Northwestern Univ. Med. School,* **27**:226, 1953.

Newton, T. H., and Young, D. A.: Anomalous origin of the occipital artery from the internal carotid artery, *Radiology,* **90**:550, 1968.

Smith, K. R., Jr., Nelson, J. S., and Dooley, J. M., Jr.: Bilateral "hypoplasia" of the internal carotid arteries, *Neurology,* **18**:1149, 1969.

Smith, R. R., Kees, C. J., and Hogg, I. D.: Agenesis of the internal carotid artery with an unusual primitive collateral; case report, *J. Neurosurg.,* **37**:460, 1972.

Weibel, J., and Fields, W. S.: Tortuosity, coiling, and kinking of the internal carotid artery. I. Relationship of morphological variation to cerebrovascular insufficiency, *Neurology,* **15**:462, 1965.

Development of Intracranial Arteries

Abbie, A. A.: The morphology of the fore-brain arteries, with especial reference to the evolution of the basal ganglia, *J. Anat.,* **78**:433, 1933/34.

Brucher, J.: Origin of the ophthalmic artery from the middle meningeal artery, *Radiology,* **93**:51, 1969.

Gillilan, L. A.: The collateral circulation of the human orbit, *Arch. Ophthalmol.,* **65**:684, 1961.

Handa, J., Teraura, T., Imai, T., and Handa, H.: Agenesis of the corpus callosum associated with multiple developmental anomalies of the cerebral arteries, *Radiology*, **92**:1301, 1969.

LeMay, M., and Gooding, C. A.: The clinical significance of the azygos anterior cerebral artery (A.C.A.), *Am. J. Roentgenol.*, **98**:602, 1966.

McCormick, W. F.: A unique anomaly of the intracranial arteries of man, *Neurology*, **19**:77, 1969.

Occleshaw, J. V., and Garland, P.: Bilateral rete carotidis, *Brit. J. Radiol.*, **42**:851, 1969.

Rockett, J. F., and Johnson, T. H., Jr.: Bilateral rete mirabile intracranial (vascular) anastomosis in man. A case report, *Radiology*, **90**:46, 1968.

Scharrer, E.: The blood vessels of the nervous tissue, *Quart. Rev. Biol.*, **19**:308, 1944.

Weidner, W., Hanafee, W., and Markham, C. H.: Intracranial collateral circulation via leptomeningeal and rete mirabile anastomoses, *Neurology*, **15**:39, 1965.

Circle of Willis

Battacharji, S. K., Hutchinson, E. C., and McCall, A. J.: The circle of Willis—The incidence of developmental abnormalities in normal and infarcted brains, *Brain*, **90**:947, 1967.

Berk, M. E.: Some anomalies of the circle of Willis, *Brit. J. Radiol.*, **34**:221, 1961.

Fisher, C. M.: The circle of Willis: Anatomical variations, *Vascular Diseases*, **2**:99, 1965.

Persistent Anastomotic Channels

Bingham, W. G., Jr., and Hayes, G. J.: Persistent carotid-basilar anastomosis. Report of two cases, *J. Neurosurg.*, **18**:398, 1961.

Blain, J. G., and Logothetis, J.: The persistent hypoglossal artery, *J. Neurol. Neurosurg. Psychiat.*, **29**:346, 1966.

Campbell, R. L., and Dyken, M. L.: Four cases of carotid-basilar anastomosis associated with central nervous system dysfunction, *J. Neurol. Neurosurg. Psychiat.*, **24**:250, 1961.

Dickmann, G. H., Pardal, C., Amezua, L., and Zamboni, O.: Persistencia de la arteria trigeminal (7 casos), *Acta neurochir.*, **17**:205, 1967.

Kempe, L. G., and Smith, D. R.: Trigeminal neuralgia, facial spasm, intermedius and glossopharyngeal neuralgia with persistent carotid basilar anastomosis, *J. Neurosurg.*, **31**:445, 1969.

Rath, S., Mathai, K. V., and Chandy, J.: Persistent trigeminal artery, *Arch. Neurol.*, **19**:121, 1968.

Renier, W.O., and Hommes, O. R.: On the clinical significance of the primitive trigeminal artery. A study of seven cases, *Europ. Neurol.*, **5**:34, 1971.

Wollschlaeger, G., and Wollschlaeger, P. B.: The primitive trigeminal artery as seen angiographically and at postmortem examination, *Am. J. Roentgenol.*, **92**:761, 1964.

Development of Intracranial Veins

Padget, D. H.: The cranial venous system in man in reference to development, adult configuration, and relation to the arteries, *Am. J. Anat.*, **98**:307, 1956.

————: The development of the cranial venous system in man, from the viewpoint of comparative anatomy, *Contrib. Embryol. Carnegie Inst.*, **36**(247):81, 1957.

Streeter, G. L.: The development of the venous sinuses of the dura mater in the human embryo, *Am. J. Anat.*, **18**:145, 1915.

Additional References

Barnett, C. H., and Marsden, C. D.: Functions of mammalian carotid rete mirabile, *Nature*, **191**:88, 1961.

Gillilan, L. A., and Markesbery, W. R.: Arteriovenous shunts in the blood supply to the brains of some common laboratory animals, with special attention to the *rete mirabile conjugatum* in the cat, *J. Comp. Neurol.*, **121**:305, 1963.

Applied Anatomy of the Brain Arteries

Those who have dissected or inspected many bodies have at least learned to doubt; when others, who are ignorant of anatomy and do not take the trouble to attend to it, are in no doubt at all.

Morgagni

AORTIC ARCH

The brain receives blood from the heart by way of the aortic arch, which gives rise to the brachiocephalic (innominate), left common carotid, and left subclavian arteries. Arising behind the manubrium sterni, the brachiocephalic ascends to the level of the sternoclavicular notch, where it divides into the right common carotid and the right subclavian arteries. The left common carotid usually arises from the aortic arch just to the left of the brachiocephalic, but it may spring from the brachiocephalic itself. The subclavian

arteries give rise to the vertebral arteries. Paired vertebral and carotid arteries ascend through the neck and penetrate the skull to supply the brain (Fig. 2–1).

Clinical Correlation Once known as the "girdle of venus" because of the frequent involvement of its ascending portion by acquired syphilis, the aortic arch is now more often the site of atherosclerotic degeneration. Atheromatous plaques may stenose or occlude the ostia of the great vessels supplying the brain, or degeneration may cause rupture of the intima, with dis-

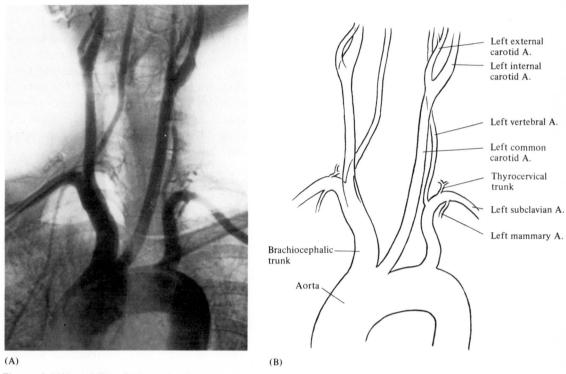

(A)   (B)

Figure 2-1(A) and (B) Catheter is placed in aortic arch from femoral artery. Injection of contrast material causes simultaneous opacification of aortocervical arteries.

section of the arch and occlusion of its branches. Inflammatory angiopathy (Takayasu's disease) also involves arteries arising from the aortic arch. All these conditions can impair cerebral circulation and produce neurologic deficits.

The brain is divided by the tentorium cerebelli into supra- and infratentorial structures. Those above the tentorium receive blood from the internal carotid and the posterior cerebral artery, which usually is the termination of the vertebral-basilar system; those below it are supplied through the vertebral and basilar arteries. The carotid system supplies the eyes, the basal ganglia, most of the hypothalamus, and the frontal and parietal lobes as well as most of the temporal lobes. The vertebral-basilar system nourishes portions of the temporal lobe, the entire occipital lobe, most of the thalamus, and the midbrain, pons, medulla oblongata, cerebellum, inner ear, and upper part of the spinal cord.

TYPES OF ARTERIES SUPPLYING THE BRAIN

The pattern of arterial supply is basically the same for the entire brain and is dependent on three types of vessels.

1 Long circumferential branches of the parent arteries course around the ventral and lateral aspects of the neural structures to the dorsal surface, where they anastomose with distal surface branches of other long circumferential vessels. They conduct blood for long distances over the surface of the hemispheres or brainstem, while giving off innumerable unnamed perforating branches which penetrate the substance of the brain.

2 Short circumferential or lateral perforating branches arise from the parent artery and travel for shorter distances before plunging through the surface of the brain to supply gray and white matter.

3 Paramedian or medial perforating arteries spring from the parent vessel and penetrate the brain on either side of the midline as soon as they arise. The paramedian branches supply central nuclear areas close to the midline, and the short circumferentials supply a zone immediately between those nourished by the paramedian and the long circumferential branches. Unlike the long circumferentials, the other two types of vessels have very limited anastomoses.

Clinical Correlation In cerebral angiograms only the long circumferential conducting arteries are shown consistently. Occasionally the largest of the short circumferential branches can be seen; but the unnamed perforators from all these types of vessels are never visible. For this reason, only about 10 percent of intracranial arteries can be demonstrated by angiography.

CAROTID SYSTEM

Carotid System in the Neck

Common and Internal Carotid Arteries The two common carotid arteries with their adventitial sympathetic nerves lie adjacent to the internal jugular veins, the vagus nerves, and the cervical sympathetic nerve plexuses. They ascend alongside the trachea, behind the sternocleidomastoid muscle, approximately to the upper border of the thyroid cartilage just below the angle of the mandible, where each divides into external and internal carotid arteries. Just distal to the bifurcation, the internal carotid artery has a bulbous expansion, the carotid sinus. This is richly supplied with receptors innervated by the glossopharyngeal nerve, and it helps to regulate cardiac action. The carotid body is

similarly innervated and lies adjacent to the sinus.

At their point of origin, the internal and external carotid arteries lie closely related to each other, and the external carotid usually lies somewhat medial to the internal carotid for a short distance before they separate. The internal carotid artery ascends behind the faucial tonsil and lateral to it. Just above the tonsil, it lies anterior to the transverse processes of the upper three cervical vertebrae.

Clinical Correlation

1 The common carotid on each side is normally easy to palpate unless, as sometimes happens, it is tortuous and lies buried behind the trachea on one side. Such a situation can give the false impression of common carotid occlusion.

2 In occasional patients inflammation of the artery may cause neck pain (carotidynia) and tenderness on palpation of the vessel.

3 The portions of the common and internal carotid arteries which pass through the neck are sometimes tortuous, and the resultant looping and kinking may suggest aneurysmal dilatation to the palpating fingers. Some physicians believe that the kinks and loops cause artery insufficiency and advocate surgical procedures to correct them.

4 In about half of patients the common carotid bifurcation is located at C_4 just below the angle of the jaw. In another 30 percent it is above this level, and in the remainder it is below C_4. These variations sometimes make it difficult to massage or compress the sinus, and they pose problems for the surgeon who attempts reconstruction of the internal carotid artery near its bifurcation.

5 The region of the carotid bifurcation and the carotid sinus is a common site for the deposition of atherosclerotic plaques, possibly because eddy currents can develop in the bloodstream at orifices and angulations of arteries.

6 Hypersensitivity of the carotid sinus may be responsible for transient loss of consciousness.

7 By involving sympathetic fibers in the wall of the internal carotid artery, diseases such as atherosclerosis as well as trauma from angiography or ligation may cause Horner's syndrome.

8 By displacing the lateral mass of the atlas forward against the posterior surface of the internal carotid, rotation of the head can compress the artery and at times initiate episodes of cerebral vascular insufficiency.

9 Cervical adenitis or herpetic ulcers of the pharynx can inflame the adjacent artery to produce a substrate causing a clot to form. This clot may occlude the artery or may cause septic embolism to the brain.

10 Palpation for the internal carotid pulse in the oropharynx posterolateral to the palatine tonsil may be more helpful than external palpation below the angle of the jaw; in the latter location, accompanying pulsations from the external carotid may be confusing.

11 Aneurysm of the internal carotid artery near its origin may present as a pharyngeal mass.

External Carotids At its origin the external carotid artery lies anterior and usually somewhat medial to the internal carotid. In contrast to the internal carotid, which almost always ascends from its origin in the neck into the skull without a single branch, the external carotid artery begins to branch into the superior thyroid, facial, ascending pharyngeal, lingual, posterior auricular, and occipital arteries. It terminates by dividing into the superficial temporal and maxillary arteries.

Ethmoidal and lacrimal branches of the ophthalmic artery, the ascending pharyngeal, maxillary, and occipital arteries supply the dura mater. The most important branch is the middle meningeal artery, which arises from the maxillary and provides the bulk of the meningeal circulation. It penetrates the base of the skull through the foramen spinosum of the sphenoid bone and runs forward and laterally in a groove or canal on the greater wing of the sphenoid, giving off branches to the dura of the convexity.

Clinical Correlation

1 Pulsation of branches of the external carotid gives clues to the patency of the internal as well as the external carotid system. Most important for this purpose are the facial artery, which can be palpated beneath the angle of the jaw; the superficial temporal artery, which can be felt anterior to the tragus of the ear; and the posterior auricular and occipital arteries, which can be palpated in the occipital region.

2 The external carotid can act as a source of collateral supply to the brain when the internal carotid is occluded.

3 Cranial arteritis frequently affects these arteries.

4 Fractures of the skull, particularly those in the region of the pterion, may sever the middle meningeal artery, causing an epidural hematoma.

5 Meningiomas and some arteriovenous malformations in the middle and anterior cranial fossae are supplied, at least in part, by branches of the middle meningeal artery; with such lesions, dilatation of the artery or exiting venous plexus may cause enlargement of the foramen spinosum.

6 Aneurysms and arteriovenous fistulae of the meningeal vessels are generally traumatic in origin and manifest themselves as extradural hemorrhage of late or "subacute" onset.

7 Arteriovenous shunt between an external carotid extracranial branch and an intracranial dural sinus is the result of an anomalous emissary vein leading from a main scalp artery directly into a large dural sinus. The rise of intracranial venous pressure will produce signs of raised intracranial pressure. Unless a bruit is listened for on the scalp and an external carotid angiogram is carried out, the cause of such intracranial raised pressure will be missed.

8 Intracranial angiomatous malformations supplied by extracranial external carotid branches are rare.

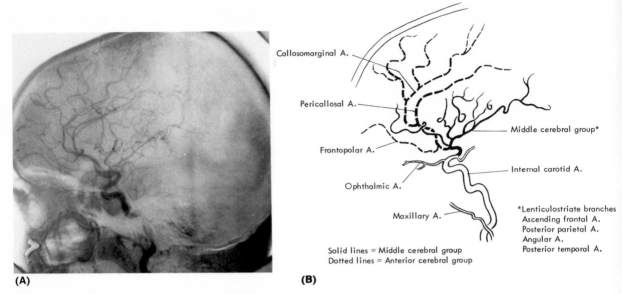

(A)

(B)

Callosomarginal A.

Pericallosal A.

Frontopolar A.

Ophthalmic A.

Maxillary A.

Middle cerebral group*

Internal carotid A.

*Lenticulostriate branches
Ascending frontal A.
Posterior parietal A.
Angular A.
Posterior temporal A.

Solid lines = Middle cerebral group
Dotted lines = Anterior cerebral group

Figure 2-2(A) and (B) Arteriographic appearance of the branches of the internal carotid artery in lateral projection.

9 Extracranial angiomatous malformations communicating with cerebral vessels are not uncommon.

Carotid System in the Head

The internal carotid artery penetrates the base of the skull through the carotid canal in the petrous portion of the temporal bone. It is separated from air cells in the middle ear by a bony wall, which may be thin in youth and partially absorbed in later life. After running through the canal for almost 1 cm, the carotid enters the cranium between the layers of the dura mater; here it lies just beneath the Gasserian ganglion of the trigeminal nerve, which it supplies with small branches. The internal carotid then ascends abruptly along the posterolateral aspect of the sella turcica to enter the cavernous sinus. Within this venous plexus the artery curves forward, then upward to a position medial to the anterior clinoid process. Then the carotid doubles back to form the upper portion of the sinuous curve which has been named the *carotid si-*

phon. Hypophyseal arteries from this portion of the carotid perfuse the pituitary gland. The paired superior and inferior hypophyseal arteries divide into capillary loops, which then form the pituitary portal system. The portal veins in turn drain into the venous sinuses around the gland.

Closely related to the lateral side of the artery are the cranial nerves that lie in the lateral wall of the cavernous sinus (the oculomotor, trochlear, and abducens, as well as the first two divisions of the trigeminal).

The internal carotid artery begins its subarachnoid course by perforating the dura mater medial to the anterior clinoid process and passing above the oculomotor and below the optic nerve. At this level the clinically important branches of the internal carotid artery begin to arise in quick succession. These are, in their usual order of appearance, the *ophthalmic, posterior communicating, anterior choroidal,* and *anterior* and *middle cerebral arteries* (Fig. 2-2A and B).

Clinical Correlation

1 Because of the proximity of the carotid artery to the middle ear, carotid murmurs can sometimes be heard by the patient throughout his waking hours and may cause him great distress.

2 Middle-ear infection sometimes extends into the carotid canal, causing carotid periarteritis.

3 Dilatation of the carotid artery where it lies beneath the Gasserian ganglion is thought by some to be a cause of trigeminal neuralgia.

4 An aneurysm of the carotid artery within the cavernous sinus may compress ocular and trigeminal nerves, producing paralysis of extraocular movement and supraorbital pain.

5 The internal carotid artery is the only artery in the body within a venous plexus. Rupture in this location may produce an arteriovenous (caroticocavernous) fistula.

Ophthalmic Artery This vessel arises from the anterior portion of the carotid siphon and passes through the optic foramen into the orbital cavity with the optic nerve; there it divides into multiple branches that supply the orbital contents and anastomose with branches of the external carotid artery. Its most important branch, the central artery of the retina, perforates the globe at the optic disk to divide into the branches that supply the retina. These are the arteries seen with the ophthalmoscope.

Clinical Correlation

1 Because the ophthalmic artery is a branch of the internal carotid, an indication of blood pressure within the carotid can be obtained by measuring ophthalmic artery pressures (ophthalmodynamometry).

2 Abnormalities of the retinal arterioles can be a clue to disease of the cerebral arterioles, since both are terminal branches of the internal carotid artery.

3 Temporary loss of vision in one eye (amaurosis fugax) accompanied by symptoms or signs involving the opposite side of the body suggests disease of the common or internal carotid arte-

ries, because the carotid supplies both the globe and the homolateral cerebral hemisphere.

4 Because branches of the ophthalmic artery anastomose with external carotid branches, the ophthalmic can be a channel for collateral circulation when the internal carotid is occluded.

5 Supraorbital branches of the ophthalmic artery supply the skin of the medial aspect of the forehead, and abnormalities in the pulsation, pressure, flow, and skin temperature can be clues to disease of the internal carotid artery.

Posterior Communicating Artery The posterior communicating artery arises as the internal carotid artery sweeps backward above the sella turcica. It passes horizontally backward and slightly medially to join the posterior cerebral artery, which is the terminal branch of the basilar artery. From the embryologic standpoint, the posterior communicating and posterior cerebral arteries are branches of the carotid, but blood reaching the posterior cerebral arteries is usually derived from the vertebral-basilar system. The posterior communicating arteries vary greatly in caliber from person to person, and often one of them is much smaller than the other. Occasionally both are threadlike, forming a tenuous link between the carotid and vertebral-basilar systems, and rarely both are absent.

Perforating branches spring in great profusion from the side of the artery adjacent to the brain. The anterior group supplies the hypothalamus and ventral thalamus, the anterior third of the optic tract, and the posterior limb of the internal capsule. Those arising posteriorly penetrate the interpeduncular space to supply the subthalamic nucleus (body of Luys). These paramedian (ganglionic) arteries do not anastomose with one another; hence occlusion of any one of them will produce infarction in the area deprived of its blood supply.

Clinical Correlation

1 When sufficiently large, the posterior communicating arteries act as channels which equilibrate pressure between the carotid and the vertebral-basilar system, but blood in the two normally does not mix. If pressure is reduced in one, large volumes of blood may shunt between the carotid and the vertebral-basilar system.

2 The posterior communicating artery travels above the oculomotor nerve. Because of this proximity, aneurysms on the artery may cause oculomotor nerve paresis or palsy.

3 Obstruction of penetrating branches supplying the body of Luys leads to contralateral hemiballism.

Anterior Choroidal Artery The anterior choroidal artery usually arises from the internal carotid just above the origin of the posterior communicating artery. At times it originates from the posterior communicating or middle cerebral artery. It runs posteriorly, crossing beneath the optic tract and along its inner surface to the level of the anterior part of the lateral geniculate body. Here it turns laterally and breaks into a number of branches, many of which enter the temporal horn of the lateral ventricle to supply the choroid plexus. It supplies the portions of the posterior limb of the internal capsule which contain the auditory and optic radiations. It also supplies the globus pallidus and gives off twigs that supply the optic tract and the lateral geniculate body. Like the ganglionic branches of the posterior communicating artery and those of the anterior and middle cerebral arteries, the perforating branches of the anterior choroidal artery are end arteries which penetrate the brain individually as a bank of vessels and ramify as a capillary network.

Clinical Correlation

1 Vascular occlusions usually produce neurologic deficit. However, some patients with parkinsonism show improvement after ligation of the anterior choroidal arteries.

2 It has been postulated that compression of the branches of the anterior choroidal artery against the free edge of the tentorium cerebelli at birth is responsible for the sclerotic lesions of the uncus and hippocampus sometimes found in individuals with temporal lobe epilepsy.

3 Occlusion of this artery is rare and apparently is sometimes asymptomatic. It may cause contralateral hemianopia, hemiplegia, and hemihypalgesia.

Anterior Cerebral Artery This branch of the internal carotid arises close to the Sylvian fissure. It proceeds anteromedially in a horizontal plane, crossing the optic nerve and the anterior perforated substance of the frontal lobe. Numerous unnamed but highly important ganglionic branches penetrate the brain at this site. One vessel is of sufficient size to be named. The medial striate artery (recurrent artery of Heubner) arises from the anterior cerebral artery just proximal or just distal to the anterior communicating and takes a recurrent course laterally over the anterior perforated substance after giving off a few branches to the orbital cortex. It dips into the anterior perforated space to supply the anterior portion of the caudate nucleus and adjacent portions of the basal ganglia and anterior limb of the internal capsule.

The two anterior cerebral arteries run a parallel course around the genu of the corpus callosum onto its upper aspect. Distal to the anterior communicating artery, small anastomoses between the anterior cerebral arteries occur at variable intervals, and these arteries become progressively smaller as they travel along the corpus callosum to its splenium. There they anastomose with distal branches of the *posterior cerebral arteries,* forming another interconnection between the carotid and vertebral-basilar system (Fig. 2–3).

Somewhat distal to Heubner's artery the anterior cerebral gives off the frontopolar artery which supplies the anterior portion of the frontal lobe on its medial side, and the callosomarginal artery which runs in the cingulate sulcus to

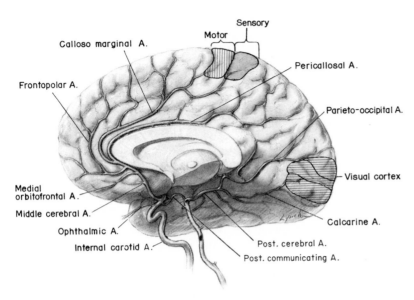

Figure 2-3 Arterial supply of the medial and inferior surfaces of the cerebral hemisphere. Arteries normally lie buried in the sulci.

the paracentral lobule. Consequently, the cingulum is bounded inferiorly by the anterior cerebral artery and superiorly by its callosomarginal branch. Branches of the callosomarginal artery ascend the medial aspect of the frontal lobe deep in the sulci, then loop over the superior margin of the hemisphere onto its lateral surface. They anastomose freely with the terminal branches of the middle cerebral artery, which ascends on the lateral surface of the hemisphere from the Sylvian fissure. All these large named arteries branch and rebranch to form an extensive superficial network of surface vessels which ramify and anastomose with one another. From these surface vessels perforating arteries, which function for all intents and purposes as end arteries, penetrate the brain.

Anterior Communicating Artery When the two anterior cerebral arteries reach the midline just above the optic chiasm at the base of the brain, they are joined together by the anterior communicating artery. This communication, which may be single, paired, trebled, or absent,

is a highly important anastomosis between the two carotid circulations. Along with the two posterior communicating arteries and the basilar artery, it completes the polygonal circle of Willis.

Clinical Correlation

1 The syndrome resulting from occlusion of the anterior cerebral artery depends on the point at which occlusion occurs and the patency of anastomotic channels.
  a Obstruction of the terminal portions of the anterior cerebral artery distal to the origin of the callosomarginal artery does not cause symptoms which can be recognized clinically.
  b If the callosomarginal artery itself is obstructed and if adequate anastomoses between it and the middle cerebral artery do not exist, infarction of the paracentral lobule occurs, leading to paralysis of the contralateral leg, with associated cortical sensory loss and sometimes bladder and bowel incontinence. In such instances the face, arm, and torso will be spared, since their

cortical area of representation is supplied by the middle cerebral artery. Hemiplegia and aphasia do not occur.

c Obstruction of the anterior cerebral artery proximal to its callosomarginal branch but distal to the anterior communicating artery may cause infarction of a large segment of the medial surface of the frontal lobe with resulting paralysis of the opposite lower limb, grasp reflex, incontinence, intellectual deterioration, sucking reflex, apraxia, and sometimes aphasia.

d An occlusion proximal to the origin of the recurrent artery of Heubner may produce no deficit whatsoever if the anterior communicating artery allows ample collateral supply from the opposite anterior cerebral artery. However, if the anterior communicating artery is small or nonexistent, all the above-described changes plus infarction of the anterior limb of the internal capsules results, causing so-called frontal ataxia because of involvement of the frontoponto-cerebellar projections.

e In occasional patients the distal portions of both anterior cerebral arteries arise from one stem. If the stem is obstructed in such patients, or if both vessels are occluded, akinetic mutism results. The patient appears to be alert, with eyes open, but does not respond to stimuli. A similar state may also be seen with lesions of the brainstem.

2 The anterior cerebral artery is easily seen on angiograms. Displacement from its normal midline position suggests pressure or traction on one cerebral hemisphere (Fig. 2-4A and B).

3 Displacement of the frontopolar artery may be the only radiographic sign of tumor in the frontal lobe.

4 Occlusion of Heubner's end artery produces infarction in the anterior limb of the internal capsule, with consequent frontal lobe ataxia and possibly some intellectual impairment if the occlusion is on the dominant side.

5 Stretching of the pericallosal branch of the anterior cerebral artery suggests enlarged lateral ventricles or a tumor of the corpus callosum.

Middle Cerebral Artery After giving off the anterior cerebral artery, the internal carotid becomes the middle cerebral artery by undergoing a change of name. It turns laterally into the Sylvian fissure, where it is encased by the base of the frontal lobe above and the superior surface of the temporal lobe below. The numerous paramedian or ganglionic branches which it gives off into the anterior perforated substance supply the putamen, the head of the caudate, the globus pallidus, and the genu and posterior limbs of the internal capsule. The most prominent of these perforating end arteries are the lenticulostriates, which once were said to be the arteries of cerebral hemorrhage. These arteries are long and relatively unbranched in their course into the ganglion. They do not anastomose with one another as do the surface conducting arteries.

In the Sylvian fissure, on the lateral surface of the insula, the middle cerebral divides into a bank of branches which travel in the sulci of the frontal, parietal, and superior surfaces of the temporal lobe (Fig. 2-5). These are the *ascending frontal*, the *anterior* and *posterior temporal*, the *posterior parietal*, and the *angular arteries*. They soon begin to give off a series of unnamed branches which ramify with one another over the surface of the brain. This network gives off perforators which, acting as end arteries, nourish the brain. The site at which the main stem of the middle cerebral artery divides into the branches varies from person to person. In addition to this the exact course of its branches varies greatly. However, the area supplied by all is rather constant, so that the clinician can identify the individual branches angiographically.

The *anterior temporal artery*, arising just distal to the origin of the lenticulostriate arteries, supplies the pole of the temporal lobe. The *ascending frontal*, or *orbital frontal*, *artery* is the largest

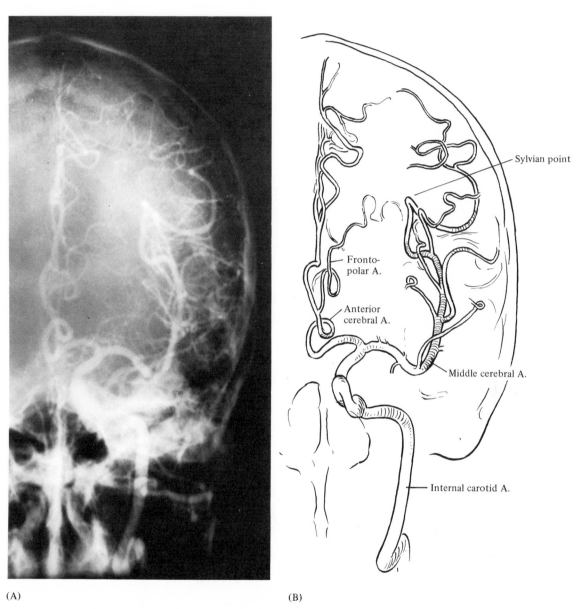

(A)

(B)

Figure 2-4(A) and (B) Arteriogram of the internal carotid artery and its branches. Displacement of the anterior cerebral artery from its normal midline position is best seen in this projection.

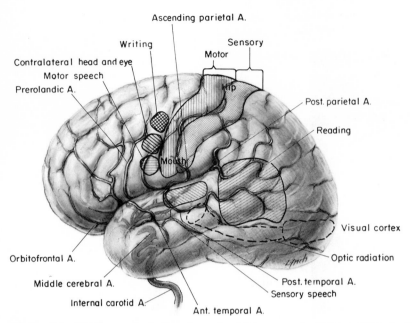

Figure 2-5 Middle cerebral area of supply of the convexity of the cerebrum. Arteries normally lie buried in the sulci.

and most complex branch of the middle cerebral artery. Its branches pass deep in the sulci anteriorly and laterally, then ascend the convexity of the frontal lobe to anastomose terminally with branches of the callosomarginal artery coming over the lip of the hemisphere. The *posterior temporal artery* supplies the superior and lateral aspects of the temporal lobe. The *posterior parietal artery* proceeds laterally and posteriorly up through the Sylvian fissure; in most persons it gives off a major branch, the *angular artery,* which helps it to supply the lateral surface of the parietal lobe and superior portions of the temporal lobe of the brain. The terminal portions of these arteries anastomose with branches of the anterior and posterior cerebral arteries (Fig. 2-6).

Clinical Correlation

1 The middle cerebral artery supplies a much larger area than either the anterior or the posterior arteries and carries about 80 percent of the blood received by the cerebral hemispheres.

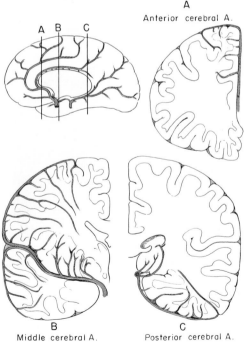

Figure 2-6

2 The middle cerebral and its branches are occluded by thrombus or embolism more often than any other intracranial artery.

3 The middle cerebral artery supplies the insula, part of the orbital portion of the frontal lobe, the inferior and middle frontal gyri, portions of the precentral and postcentral gyri on the lateral surface of the brain, the superior and inferior parietal lobules, the superior and middle temporal gyri of the temporal lobe, and portions of the parietal lobe. Consequently, the clinical syndromes produced by occlusion of this artery or of one of its branches vary widely, depending upon which branches are occluded and whether or not anastomotic channels are open.

4 Because the lenticulostriate branches of this artery do not anastomose with one another, occlusion of any one results in infarction of the tissue it supplies.

5 In the dominant hemisphere this artery has been called "the artery of aphasia."

6 Proximal obstruction of this artery leads to contralateral hemiplegia (most severe in the arm), hemihypalgesia, homonymous hemianopia, and signs of parietal lobe dysfunction.

THE VERTEBRAL-BASILAR ARTERIAL SYSTEM

The right subclavian artery stems from the brachiocephalic artery behind the sternoclavicular joint and lies wholly in the root of the neck; the left subclavian, arising from the aortic arch in the superior mediastinum, has an intrathoracic course as well. Usually the vertebral arteries are the first branches of the subclavian arteries. Originating in the root of the neck, the vertebrals ascend in the osseous canal of the transverse processes of the cervical vertebrae to the base of the skull, which they enter through the foramen magnum (Fig. 2–7). They join each other intracranially to form the basilar artery. The subclavian, vertebral, and basilar arteries act as a unit in supplying the posterior circulation. The system is unique, for nowhere else in the body do two major arteries (the vertebrals)

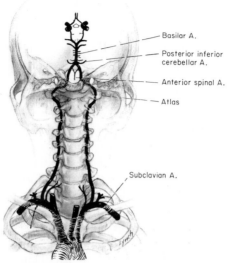

Basilar A.

Posterior inferior cerebellar A.

Anterior spinal A.

Atlas

Subclavian A.

Figure 2-7

normally join to form a single one (the basilar). The blood which this system carries is the most vital in the brain, for into the brainstem, which it supplies, are crowded all the ascending and descending tracts, most of the cranial nerves, and the centers which maintain consciousness and homeostasis.

Vertebral Arteries

In 1 percent of individuals, the left vertebral artery arises directly from the arch of the aorta between the common carotid and the left subclavian arteries. Almost always one of the vertebral arteries is larger than the other, but when one is small, the other is likely to be unusually large, so that the amount of blood supplied to the posterior circulation remains constant. Occasionally one is so hypoplastic that it carries very little blood, and rarely one may be absent altogether.

After the vertebral artery arises from the subclavian, it ascends for a short distance through the root of the neck just medial to the scalenus anterior muscle until it enters a foramen in one of the transverse processes—usually that of the sixth cervical vertebra. Less frequently it may enter at C_7 or C_5, and in rare cases it may travel to C_4 before entering the canal.

The vertebral artery then travels through the bony tunnel formed by the adjacent transverse processes and ligaments of the cervical vertebrae 6 up to 1 (the atlas). In this tunnel it is accompanied by a plexus of veins and a very dense plexus of sympathetic nerves that interconnect with cervical ganglia. Abutting the artery at each level are cervical nerves and the joint spaces of the vertebrae. Twigs given off by the vertebral artery supply the cervical nerves, the vertebrae and their joints, and large muscular branches which exit through the vertebral foramina to supply the posterior muscles of the neck. Other branches of the vertebral artery enter the spinal canal along with the cervical nerves, to supply the spinal cord. Particularly important is a large, rather constant branch which enters the canal, usually at C_5, to anastomose with the anterior spinal artery. This branch is a source of collateral circulation.

After going through C_1, it travels in a groove around its posterior arch before entering the skull through the foramen magnum. In the suboccipital triangle, where it is covered only by soft tissues, it forms a loop akin to that of the carotid siphon and anastomoses freely with the occipital branch of the external carotid artery.

Clinical Correlation

1 The origin of the vertebral artery from the subclavian is a common site for the formation of atherosclerotic plaques which may stenose or occlude its ostium.

2 Congenital fibrous bands and muscles inserting into cervical ribs sometimes constrict the artery at this level. These obstructive effects are dependent, at least in part, on changes in the relation of the head and arm to the neck.

3 It is possible that kinking associated with elongation of the vessel may result in intermittent occlusion.

4 Osteoarthritis of the cervical vertebrae may lead to the production of osteophytes that protrude into the transverse foramina and impinge on the vertebral artery. Changes in the relationship of one vertebra to another as in flexion and extension, lateral bending, or rotation of the head may cause minimal to complete obstruction of flow through the vertebral artery and may result in signs and symptoms of brainstem ischemia, especially in individuals with associated disease of the carotid arterial system and those with atresia or disease affecting the other vertebral artery.

5 Rotatory movement of the head upon the neck occurs for the most part at the C_1 to C_2 level (the atlas upon the axis). There the vertebral artery winds around the atlas and is subject to a shearing force when the head is rotated. In normal persons, if flow through one vertebral artery is impaired temporarily by such movement, that through the other is increased, so that flow to the basilar artery and its branches remains constant. When one vertebral artery is congenitally absent or occluded by disease, such rotatory movement can produce episodic brainstem ischemia.

6 Acute injuries of the cervical spine producing transient dislocation of one cervical vertebra upon another (so-called "whiplash" or hyperextension injuries) can traumatize the vertebral arteries within their canals. The vasospasm that follows may lead to prolonged neurologic deficit. A similar mechanism may result from injudicious manipulation of the neck (as in chiropractic), extreme extension of the neck during intubation of the trachea or dental extraction and vigorous cervical traction.

7 Atlantoaxial dislocation, either acute or chronic, may also compromise blood flow through the vertebral artery.

8 In the Klippel-Feil syndrome (partial or total congenital fusion of the cervical vertebrae) and in basilar impression of the skull onto the atlas (C_1), bony compression of the arteries may produce signs of brainstem and/or cervical cord ischemia.

Intracranial Course of the Vertebral Arteries
Entering the skull through the foramen magnum, the two vertebral arteries pierce the dura mater and ascend along the ventrolateral aspects of the medulla oblongata, to which they give off numerous unnamed perforating arteries. At the junction between the pons and the medulla, the vertebrals join to form the unique anastomosis which initiates the basilar artery (Fig. 2-8A and B). Just after piercing the dura, each vertebral artery gives off its highly important anterior spinal ramus, which turns acutely downward on the lower medulla and angles toward the midline, where at the level of C_2 to C_3 it joins the anterior spinal ramus of the opposite side, and the two become a single artery which travels downward in the medial fissure of the cord to the conus medullaris (see Chap. 4).

Clinical Correlation
1 Although occlusion of the anterior spinal ramus in the medulla is rare, obstruction occurs occasionally at other levels, producing infarction of the cord with loss of function in the areas it supplies. The clinical result is paraplegia or tetraplegia with loss of sphincter control and a defect in pain and temperature perception, due to spinothalamic involvement. The function of the posterior columns is preserved, as is evidenced by normal perception of touch, vibra-

tion, and joint position. Before the days of specific treatment for syphilis, this disease was the most common cause of occlusion of the anterior spinal artery.

2 Compression of the anterior spinal artery by tumors of the cervical region may result in spastic tetraparesis, with wasting of the small muscles of the hands. The clinical picture bears a superficial resemblance to amyotrophic lateral sclerosis or syringomyelia.

3 Some believe that the symptoms associated with midline herniation of a cervical nucleus pulposus are due to compression of the artery by the disk. A more probable explanation is the interference with blood supplied to the cervical cord by medullary branches of the vertebral arteries.

Posterior Inferior Cerebellar Arteries

The posterior inferior cerebellar arteries (PICA) originate from the vertebral arteries about 1 cm below their junction to form the basilar artery. They are the largest and most variable branches of the vertebral arteries. Each PICA travels down and around the lateral surface of the medulla to the level of the foramen magnum before looping back up to supply portions of the cerebellum.

These arteries supply a wedge-shaped area of the medulla extending vertically from just

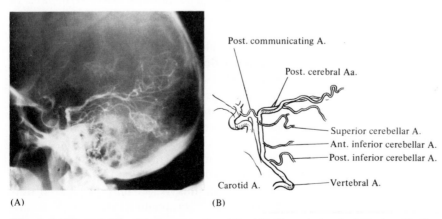

(A)

(B)

Post. communicating A.

Post. cerebral Aa.

Superior cerebellar A.
Ant. inferior cerebellar A.
Post. inferior cerebellar A.

Carotid A.

Vertebral A.

Figure 2-8(A) and (B) Arteriogram of vertebral-basilar arteries in lateral projection.

above the level of the cuneate and gracile nuclei to the upper limit of the medulla. On the surface, the area extends in an anteroposterior direction from just behind the inferior olivary nucleus to the inferior cerebellar peduncle. Centrally, the apex of the wedge approaches the floor of the fourth ventricle. The arteries also supply part of the surface of the cerebellar hemispheres and perhaps part of the dentate nuclei.

Clinical Correlation

1 Infarction (lateral medullary, or Wallenberg's syndrome) occurs more frequently in the distribution of this artery than in that of any other cerebellar artery. Such lesions are usually manifest by the sudden onset of vertigo, nystagmus, dysphagia, ataxia, nausea, and vomiting. Consciousness is not disturbed. There is a tendency to fall toward the involved side because of the cerebellar involvement, and spinothalamic function on the contralateral side of the body below the face is lost. Involvement of the descending root of the fifth cranial nerve causes homolateral loss of pain and temperature perception on the face. Homolateral Horner's syndrome may be seen.

2 When there is herniation of the tonsils of the cerebellum, the tonsillar branches of this artery may be displaced downward below the foramen magnum and may be visualized on a vertebral angiogram.

Basilar Artery

This artery is formed at the junction of the medulla with the pons and runs along the ventral aspect of the pons. It ends where the pons joins the midbrain, forming the two posterior cerebral arteries. As mentioned before, the posterior cerebrals are derived embryologically from the carotid system. Consequently, some anatomists consider the rostral termination of the basilar to be its mesencephalic branches which supply the tectum. However, because blood flow through the posterior cerebral arteries comes from the vertebral-basilar system in about 90 percent of individuals, we have chosen to consider the posterior cerebral arteries as the termination of the vertebral-basilar arterial system. In some persons the blood supply to the posterior cerebral arteries may come from both systems.

Branches

The branches of the vertebral-basilar system have been classified by Foix into *paramedian, short circumferential,* and *long circumferential arteries.* This same classification was applied to the branches of the internal carotid artery, previously described. Although their size and the areas they supply vary widely from individual to individual, these arteries have reasonable anatomic predictability (Fig. 2-9).

Internal Auditory Artery Particularly significant is the arterial supply of the inner ear, the semicircular canal, the saccule, the utricle, and the cochlea. In more than 80 percent of persons coming to autopsy, the auditory artery stems from the anterior inferior cerebellar artery. In most of the remainder, it originates directly from the basilar artery as the internal auditory artery.

Branches The auditory artery terminates in two branches, the cochlear and the vestibular. Each has a very tenuous anastomosis with the carotid circulation.

Clinical Correlation Just as the ophthalmic artery often affords the clue to disease of the carotid system, the internal auditory artery sometimes provides the first evidence of disease in the vertebral-basilar system. Because the auditory artery is in effect an end artery and because the semicircular canals are so exquisitely sensitive, reduction of blood pressure and/or flow through this vessel may produce disturbances of equilibrium to cause nausea, vomiting, and vertigo. Similar interruption of the

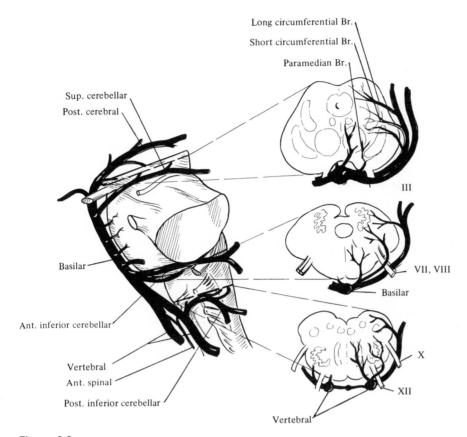

Long circumferential Br.
Short circumferential Br.
Paramedian Br.
Sup. cerebellar
Post. cerebral
III
VII, VIII
Basilar
Basilar
Ant. inferior cerebellar
X
Vertebral
Ant. spinal
XII
Post. inferior cerebellar
Vertebral

Figure 2-9

cochlear supply causes sudden loss of hearing. If both occur together, the syndrome produced can mimic Ménière's syndrome.

Anterior Inferior Cerebellar Artery This artery supplies the lateral portions of the tegmentum, the middle section of the brainstem, the inferior portion of the middle cerebellar peduncle, the inferior cerebellar peduncle, the flocculus, and the adjacent cerebellar hemisphere.

Clinical Correlation Occlusion of this artery is extremely unusual. When it does occur, the resulting infarction causes cerebellar dysfunction, facial palsy, deafness, and impairment of sensibility to light touch, pain, and temperature of the face on the side of the lesion; on the side

opposite the lesion there is incomplete loss of pain and temperature sensibility over the torso and extremities.

Superior Cerebellar Artery This vessel supplies the dorsolateral portion of the upper part of the brainstem, the superior cerebellar peduncle, the nuclei beneath the fourth ventricle, part of the dentate nucleus, part of the cortex of the superior part of the cerebellar hemisphere, and a variable part of the midbrain and pons.

The three arteries that supply the cerebellum—the posterior and anterior inferior cerebellars and the superior cerebellar—anastomose freely on the surface of the hemispheres.

Clinical Correlation Occlusion causes signs

of ipsilateral cerebellar dysfunction, abnormal movements of the upper and lower limbs on the same side, together with contralateral loss of appreciation of pain and temperature over the entire body.

Posterior Cerebral Arteries In the majority of people, the two posterior cerebral arteries are the terminal branches of the basilar artery, but in 5 to 30 percent one may originate from the internal carotid. They arise in the apex of the posterior fossa, pass above the oculomotor nerves, and move posteriorly in a curvilinear manner laterally around the midbrain, passing close to the sharp free edge of the tentorium cerebelli. Soon after their origin they anastomose with the posterior communicating arteries to complete the circle of Willis. They reach positions on the inferior and medial aspects of the temporal lobes of the cerebral hemispheres. Each then runs along the medial aspect of the temporal and occipital lobes to terminate at the occipital pole (Fig. 2-10A and B).

Branches Tiny *circumferential branches* supply the cerebral peduncle, the medial geniculate body, and the colliculi.

Thalamogeniculate arteries supply the pulvinar and other structures of the posterior thalamus and the lateral geniculate body.

The *posterior choroidal arteries* arise near the origin of the posterior cerebral arteries and enter the transverse fissure to terminate in the choroid plexus of the third ventricle. They supply portions of the thalamus and the splenium, and anastomose with terminal branches of the anterior choroidal artery.

The *anterior* and *posterior temporal,* the *parietooccipital,* and the *calcarine arteries*—supply the inferior surface of the temporal and occipital lobes of the brain. Their terminal branches anastomose with those of the anterior and middle cerebral arteries to form part of the leptomeningeal anastomotic circulation of the cerebral hemispheres.

Clinical Correlation

1 Because the oculomotor nerve runs between the superior cerebellar and the posterior cerebral arteries, an aneurysm on either of these arteries may produce paralysis of this nerve.

2 When increased intracranial pressure leads to herniation of the temporal lobe through the

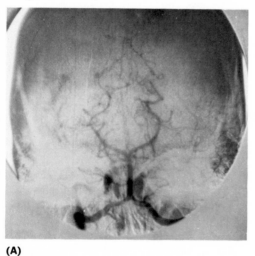

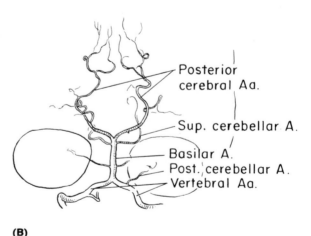

(A)   **(B)**

Figure 2-10(A) and (B) Arteriogram of the posterior fossa, showing normal arteries (Antero-posterior view).

incisura, compression of the posterior cerebral artery against the sharp edge of the tentorium may cause infarction of the occipital lobe with contralateral homonymous hemianopia. This mechanical compression and displacement can be seen in appropriate cerebral angiograms.

3 Ischemia or infarction of both occipital lobes leads to cortical blindness, in which pupillary responses to light are preserved but vision is lost bilaterally. The patient is sometimes unaware that he cannot see and will deny blindness. He may confabulate, describe imagined scenes, and walk unconcernedly into objects (Anton's syndrome). It is said that the ability to dream and to describe with the mind's eye is lost as well. A similar clinical picture may occur as a transient phenomenon complicating vertebral angiography.

4 Occlusion of the posterior cerebral artery on the dominant side may cause infarction of the homolateral visual cortex and the splenium of the corpus callosum. The resulting clinical deficit may be contralateral homonymous hemianopia. Splenial infarction causes dysconnection of the right occipital lobe from the speech area with resulting dyslexia without dysgraphia.

5 Occlusion of the thalamogeniculate branch of the posterior cerebral artery may result in the thalamic syndrome, in which pain and temperature perception are lost because of infarction in the portion of the thalamus which receives these impulses. This loss of pain sensation may be accompanied by a peculiar discomfort which has been called *anesthesia dolorosa.*

Brainstem Lesions

Because all the long tracts in the body, both ascending and descending, must pass through the brainstem, and because so many of the cranial nerve nuclei lie within it, vascular disease affecting this conglomeration of structures causes a variety of signs and symptoms. Chief among them are dysarthria, dysphagia, motor and sensory deficit, and disturbance of consciousness. The following phenomena are of such diagnostic importance that they must be enumerated specifically.

1 "Drop" attacks. These are sudden attacks in which loss of power in the lower extremities causes the patient to fall to the ground, fully conscious. The attacks subside as abruptly as they begin. No premonitory symptoms occur, but many patients believe that their attacks are precipitated by changes in the position of the head—particularly extension. It is tempting to think that these attacks represent ischemia of the cervicomedullary junction, related perhaps to temporary obstruction of flow through the vertebral arteries, caused by changing the position of the head upon the neck.

2 Attacks of vertigo, nausea, and vomiting. Often interpreted as atypical Ménière's syndrome, these may well be due to episodic ischemia of the structures of the inner ear or the brainstem. When they are accompanied by tinnitus and deafness, they are sometimes interpreted as evidence of otologic abnormality rather than of vertebral-basilar insufficiency.

3 "Blackout." Intermittent ischemia of the occipital lobes produces temporary loss of vision or complete blindness in both eyes known as "blackout."

4 Ocular abnormalities. Intermittent ischemia involving the medial longitudinal fasciculus or the abducens, para-abducens, and oculomotor nuclei can result in a variety of ophthalmologic abnormalities, the most frequent of which is diplopia. Lesions of the medial longitudinal fasciculus cause internuclear ophthalmoplegia, manifest by loss of conjugate movements of the eyes in one or another direction.

5 Crossed or alternate paralysis. Infarction or ischemic episodes occurring at various levels of the brainstem characteristically result in ipsilateral lower motor neuron cranial nerve paralysis with contralateral hemiparesis.

6 Myoclonus. Myoclonus involving the eyes, tongue, palate, larynx, and even the diaphragm can be caused by insufficiency or infarction of the central tegmental tract, the inferior olive, or

the contralateral dentate nucleus (the triangle of Guillain and Foix).

ANASTOMOTIC CHANNELS OF THE HEAD AND NECK

Extracranial Anastomoses

These collaterals exist between (1) the internal and external carotid arteries in the orbit, (2) the external carotid and the vertebral arteries, (3) branches of the subclavian and vertebral arteries, and (4) external carotid and subclavian arteries.

Clinical Correlation

1 When these collateral channels are adequate they help to decrease the neurologic deficit produced by extracranial arterial lesions.

2 Increased pulsations within these anastomoses may cause symptoms such as throbbing headache, audible bruits, and "queer" unpleasant or throbbing sensations over the head, neck, and chest.

3 Their pulsations, thrills, and audible bruits may give the physician clues to disease of the carotid or vertebral-basilar circulation.

Intracranial Anastomoses

Circle of Willis At the base of the brain is a network of blood vessels which is called the *circle of Willis*. This polygon is formed by the paired anterior cerebral, internal carotid, posterior cerebral, and posterior communicating arteries together with the unpaired anterior communicating artery. Variations are numerous, and a "normal" configuration is found in only about 50 percent of individuals. In the majority, however, the variations are related not to the number of the constituents but to the relative sizes of the component arteries (Fig. 2-11).

Clinical Correlation

1 The polygon provides an avenue for collateral circulation between the vascular channels of the two sides of the brain and between the

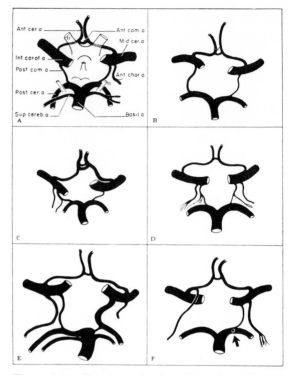

Figure 2-11 Diagrams showing different patterns of the circle of Willis. The posterior communicating arteries vary in origins, diameters, and branches. Sometimes a branch from the posterior communicating artery (C and D) parallels the anterior choroidal artery, giving off rami usually ascribed to the anterior choroidal artery. E: The left posterior cerebral artery is a major branch of the internal carotid artery. F: The right posterior communicating artery is absent; the right anterior choroidal artery branches from the right anterior cerebral artery. The arrow indicates a small aneurysm. *(Adapted from Lois A. Gillilan, J. Comp. Neurol., 112:59, 1959, Fig. 1.)*

carotid and vertebral-basilar circulations. These flow in either direction, depending on patency of the channels and their pressure gradients.

2 Its efficiency is one factor which determines the degree of neurologic deficit occurring after stenosis or occlusion of one or more of the arteries in the neck. Anomalies of the circle are associated with a higher incidence of cerebral infarction.

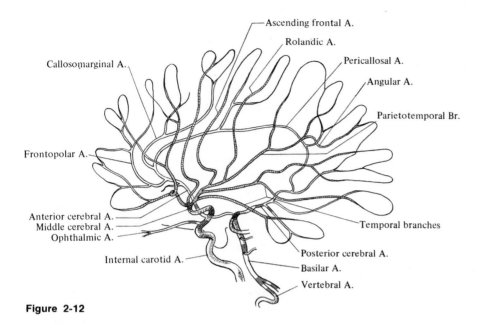

Ascending frontal A.

Rolandic A.

Callosomarginal A.

Pericallosal A.

Angular A.

Parietotemporal Br.

Frontopolar A.

Anterior cerebral A.
Middle cerebral A.
Ophthalmic A.

Temporal branches

Internal carotid A.

Posterior cerebral A.

Basilar A.

Vertebral A.

Figure 2-12

Leptomeningeal Anastomoses The anterior, middle, and posterior cerebral arteries branch and rebranch over the surface of the brain, forming a diffuse leptomeningeal network of arteries. These interconnect with one another, so that blood may course from what is normally anterior to middle to posterior cerebral territory (Fig. 2-12). At times anastomoses from the anterior and middle meningeal arteries are also prominent, providing a potential source of external carotid and collateral supply to the leptomeningeal network. In contrast to this rich interconnection are the perforating branches which spring from it. These are countless in number and supply the gray and white matter of the hemispheres. They have few if any anastomoses with their neighbors until they divide into their capillary terminations. The capillaries, on the other hand, do interconnect with those adjacent to them, but the resulting net is not effective as a source of collateral supply if one of the perforators is occluded.

SUGGESTED READINGS
General

Courville, C. B.: Vascular patterns of the encephalic gray matter in man, *Bull. Los Angeles Neurol. Soc.*, **23**:30, 1958.

Foley, J. M., Kinney, T. D., and Alexander, L.: The vascular supply of the hypothalamus in man, *J. Neuropathol. Exptl. Neurol.*, **1**:265, 1942.

Gillilan, L. A.: Observations on the anatomy of the cerebral blood vessels which may influence cerebral circulation, with clinical interpretations, *Arch. Neurol. Psychiat.*, **72**:116, 1954.

————: General principles of the arterial blood vessel patterns to the brain, *Trans. Am. Neurol. Assoc.*, **82**:65, 1957.

Kaplan, H. A.: "Embryology and anatomy of the blood vessels of the brain," in Pathogenesis and Treatment of Cerebrovascular Disease, edited by W. S. Fields, Charles C Thomas, Publisher, Springfield, Ill., 1961, pp. 5-35.

————, and Ford, D. H.: The Brain Vascular System, Elsevier Publishing Company, Amsterdam, 1966.

Klosovskii, B. N.: Blood Circulation in the Brain, Israel Program for Scientific Translations, Jerusalem, 1963.

Krayenbühl, H., and Yasargil, M. G.: Die vaskulären Erkrankungen im Gebiet der Arteria Vertebraillis und Arteria Basialis: Eine anatomische und pathologische, klinische und neuroradiologische Studie, Georg Thieme Verlag, KG, Stuttgart, 1957.

Lazorthes, G., Amaral-Gomes, F., Bastide, G., Compan, L., Espagno, J., Gaubert, J., Routhes, J., and Roulleau, J.: Vascularisation et circulation cérébrales, Masson et Cie, Paris, 1961.

Merritt, H. H., and Aring, C. D.: The differential diagnosis of cerebral vascular lesions, *Res. Pub. Assoc. Nerv. Ment. Dis.*, **18**:682, 1937.

Stephens, R. B., and Stilwell, D. L.: Arteries and Veins of the Human Brain, Charles C Thomas, Publisher, Springfield, Ill., 1969.

Van den Bergh, R.: Centrifugal elements in the vascular pattern of the deep intracerebral blood supply, *Angiology*, **20**:88, 1969.

Wolff, H. G.: The cerebral blood vessels—Anatomical principles, *Res. Pub. Assoc. Nerv. Ment. Dis.*, **18**:29, 1937.

Aortic Arch

Bosniak, M. A.: An analysis of some anatomic-roentgenologic aspects of the brachiocephalic vessels, *Am. J. Roentgenol.*, **91**:1222, 1964.

Daseler, E. H., and Anson, B. J.: Surgical anatomy of the subclavian artery and its branches, *Surg. Gynecol. Obstet.*, **108**:149, 1959.

Liechty, J. D., Shields, T. W., and Anson, B. J.: Variations pertaining to the aortic arches and their branches: With comments on surgically important types, *Quart. Bull. Northwestern Univ. Med. School*, **31**:136, 1957.

Carotid System in the Neck

Boldrey, E., Maass, L., and Miller, E. R.: The role of atlantoid compression in the etiology of internal carotid thrombosis, *J. Neurosurg.*, **13**:127, 1956.

Lehrer, H. Z.: Relative calibre of the cervical internal carotid artery. Normal variation with the circle of Willis, *Brain*, **91**:339, 1968.

Morris, G.: Delayed perforation of the internal ca-

rotid artery by an ingested foreign body, *Brit. J. Surg.*, **56**:711, 1969.

Roscher, A. A., Steele, B. C., and Woodard, J. S.: Carotid artery rupture after irradiation of larynx, *Arch. Otolaryngol.*, **83**:472, 1966.

Carotid System in the Head

Gillilan, L. A.: The arterial and venous blood supplies to the forebrain (including the internal capsule) of primates, *Neurology*, **18**:653, 1968.

Manigand, G.: Syndromes Artériels Encéphaliques, Expansion Scientifique, Paris, 1968.

Parkinson, D.: Collateral circulation of cavernous carotid artery: Anatomy, *Can. J. Surg.*, **7**:251, 1964.

Wallace S., Goldberg, H. I., Leeds, N. E., and Mishkin, M. M.: The cavernous branches of the internal carotid artery, *Am. J. Roentgenol.*, **101**:34, 1967.

Ophthalmic Artery

Bergland, R., and Ray, B. S.: The arterial supply of the human optic chiasm, *J. Neurosurg.*, **31**:327, 1969.

Brucher, J.: Origin of the ophthalmic artery from the middle meningeal artery, *Radiology*, **93**:51, 1969.

Kuru, Y.: Meningeal branches of the ophthalmic artery, *Acta radiol. (diagn.)*, **6**:241, 1967.

de Raad, R.: An angiographic study of the course of the ophthalmic artery in normal and pathological conditions, *Brit. J. Radiol.*, **37**:826, 1964.

Anterior Choroidal Artery

Abbie, A. A.: The clinical significance of the anterior choroidal artery, *Brain*, **56**:233, 1933.

Carpenter, M. B., Noback, C. R., and Moss, M. L.: The anterior choroidal artery: Its origins, course, distribution, and variations, *Arch. Neurol. Psychiat.*, **71**:714, 1954.

Herman, L. H., Fernando, O. U., and Gurdjian, E. S.: The anterior choroidal artery: An anatomical study of its area of distribution, *Anat. Rec.*, **154**:95, 1966.

Otomo, E.: The anterior choroidal artery, *Arch. Neurol.*, **13**:656, 1965.

Anterior Cerebral Artery

Ahmed, D. S., and Ahmed, R. H.: The recurrent

branch of the anterior cerebral artery, *Anat. Rec.,* **157**:699, 1967.

Baptista, A. G.: Studies on the arteries of the brain: II. The anterior cerebral artery: Some anatomic features and their clinical implications, *Neurology,* **13**:825, 1963.

Critchley, M.: The anterior cerebral artery and its syndromes, *Brain,* **53**:120, 1930.

Lazorthes, G., Gaubert, J., and Poulhes, J.: La distribution centrale et corticale de l'artère cérébrale antérieure; étude anatomique et incidences neurochirurgicales, *Neuro-Chirurgie,* **2**:237, 1956.

MacCarty, C. S., and Cooper, I. S.: Neurologic and metabolic effects of bilateral ligation of anterior cerebral arteries in man, *Proc. Staff Meetings Mayo Clinic,* **26**:185, 1951.

Morris, A. A., and Peck, C. M.: Roentgenographic study of the variations in the normal anterior cerebral artery; 100 cases studied in lateral plane, *Am. J. Roentgenol.,* **74**:818, 1955.

Ring, B. A., and Waddington, M. M.: Roentgenographic anatomy of the pericallosal arteries, *Am. J. Roentgenol.,* **104**:109, 1968.

Sohn, D., and Levine, S.: Frontal lobe infarcts caused by brain herniation. Compression of anterior cerebral artery branches, *Arch. Pathol.,* **84**:509, 1967.

Webster, J. E., Gurdjian, E. S., Lindner, D. W., and Hardy, W. G.: Proximal occlusion of the anterior cerebral artery, *Arch. Neurol.,* **2**:19, 1960.

Middle Cerebral Artery

Jain, K. K.: Some observations on the anatomy of the middle cerebral artery, *Can. J. Surg.,* **7**:134, 1964.

Ring, B. A., and Waddington, M.: Ascending frontal branch of middle cerebral artery, *Acta radiol. (diagn.),* **6**:209, 1967.

Sindermann, F., Dichgans, J., and Bergleiter, R.: Occlusion of the middle cerebral artery and its branches: Angiographic and clinical correlates, *Brain,* **92**:607, 1969.

Vertebral-Basilar Arterial System

Vertebral Artery

Jackson, R.: The Cervical Syndrome, 3d ed., Charles C Thomas, Publisher, Springfield, Ill., 1971.

Morris, L.: The anterior meningeal branch of the vertebral artery and other meningeal vessels arising from the internal carotid and vertebral arteries *(Proc. Soc. Brit. Neurol. Surg.) J. Neurol. Neurosurg. Psychiat.,* **32**:633, 1969.

Posterior Inferior Cerebellar Artery

Gillilan, L. A.: The arterial and venous blood supplies to the cerebellum of primates, *J. Neuropathol. Exptl. Neurol.,* **28**:295, 1969.

Greitz, T., and Sjogren, S. E.: The posterior inferior cerebellar artery, *Acta radiol. (diagn.),* **1**:284, 1963.

Takahashi, M., Wilson, G., and Hanafee, W.: The anterior inferior cerebellar artery: Its radiographic anatomy and significance in the diagnosis of extra-axial tumors of the posterior fossa, *Radiology,* **90**:-281, 1968.

Basilar Artery

Schechter, M. M., and Zingesser, L. H.: The radiology of basilar thrombosis, *Radiology,* **85**:23, 1965.

Wackenheim, A., and Braun, J. P.: Angiography of the Mesencephalon; Normal and Pathological Findings, Springer-Verlag, New York, 1970.

Branches

Adams, R. D.: Occlusion of the anterior inferior cerebellar artery, *Arch. Neurol. Psychiat.,* **49**:765, 1943.

Atkinson, W. J.: The anterior inferior cerebellar artery; its variations, pontine distribution, and significance in the surgery of cerebello-pontine angle tumours, *J. Neurol. Neurosurg. Psychiat.,* **12**:137, 1949.

Bebin, J.: The cerebellopontile angle, the blood supply of the brain stem and the reticular formation. Anatomical and functional correlations relevant to surgery of acoustic tumors, *Henry Ford Hosp. Med. J.,* **16**:61, 1968.

Luhan, J. A., and Pollack, S. L.: Occlusion of the superior cerebellar artery, *Neurology,* **3**:77, 1953.

Mani, R. L., and Newton, T. H.: The superior cerebellar artery: Arteriographic changes in the diagnosis of posterior fossa lesions, *Radiology,* **92**:1281, 1969.

Mazzoni, A., and Hansen, C. C.: Surgical anatomy of the arteries of the internal auditory canal, *Arch. Otolaryngol.,* **91**:128, 1970.

Plets, C.: Vascularisation topographique du thalamus humain, *Acta neurol. psychiat. belg.*, **66**:752, 1966.

Segarra, J.: Cerebral vascular disease and behavior: I. The syndrome of mesencephalic artery (basilar artery bifurcation), *Arch. Neurol.*, **22**:408, 1970.

Smith, C. G., and Richardson, W. F. G.: The course and distribution of the arteries supplying the visual (striate) cortex, *Am. J. Ophthalmol.*, **61**:1391, 1966.

Williams, D. J.: The origin of the posterior cerebral artery, *Brain*, **59**:175, 1936.

Brainstem Lesions

Gillilan, L. A.: The correlation of the blood supply to the human brain stem with clinical brain stem lesions, *J. Neuropathol. Exptl. Neurol.*, **23**:78, 1964.

Hassler, O.: Arterial pattern of human brain stem. Normal appearance and deformation in expanding supratentorial conditions, *Neurology*, **17**:368, 1967.

Schneider, R. C., and Crosby, E. C.: Vascular insufficiency of brain stem and spinal cord in spinal cord trauma, *Neurology*, **9**:643, 1959.

Anastomotic Channels of the Head and Neck

Berry, R. G.: Discussion of "collateral circulation of the brain," *Neurology*, **11**(4)(part 2):20, 1961.

Fields, W. S., Bruetman, M. E., and Weibel, J.: Collateral circulation of the brain, *Monographs Surg. Sci.*, **2**(3):183, 1965.

Extracranial Anastomoses

Gillilan, L. A.: The collateral circulation of the human orbit, *Arch. Ophthalmol.*, **65**:684, 1961.

Pakula, H., and Szapiro, J.: Anatomical studies of the collateral blood supply to the brain and upper extremity, *J. Neurosurg.*, **32**:171, 1970.

Schechter, M. M.: The occipital-vertebral anastomosis, *J. Neurosurg.*, **21**:758, 1964.

Toole, J. F.: Interarterial shunts in the cerebral circulation, *Circulation*, **33**:474, 1966.

Wolff, E.: The Anatomy of the Eye and Orbit; Including the Central Connections, Development, and Comparative Anatomy of the Visual Apparatus, 6th ed., revised by R. J. Last, W. B. Saunders Company, Philadelphia, 1968.

Intracranial Anastomoses

Gillilan, L. A.: Significant superficial anastomoses in the arterial blood supply to the human brain, *J. Comp. Neurol.*, **112**:55, 1959.

Weibel, J., and Fields, W. S.: Atlas of Arteriography in Occlusive Cerebrovascular Disease, W. B. Saunders Company, Philadelphia, 1969.

Circle of Willis

Alpers, B. J., and Berry, R. G.: Circle of Willis in cerebral vascular disorders: The anatomical structure, *Arch. Neurol.*, **8**:398, 1963.

——, ——, and Paddison, R. M.: Anatomical studies of the circle of Willis in normal brain, *Arch. Neurol. Psychiat.*, **81**:409, 1959.

Battacharji, S. K., Hutchinson, E. C., and McCall, A. J.: The circle of Willis—The incidence of developmental abnormalities in normal and infarcted brains, *Brain*, **90**:747, 1967.

Fisher, C. M.: The circle of Willis: Anatomical variations, *Vascular Diseases*, **2**:99, 1965.

Pallie, W., and Samarasinghe, D. D.: A study in the quantification of the circle of Willis, *Brain*, **85**:569, 1962.

Riggs, H. E., and Rupp, C.: Variation in form of circle of Willis. The relation of the variations to collateral circulation: Anatomic analysis, *Arch. Neurol.*, **8**:8, 1963.

Symonds, C.: The circle of Willis (Harveian oration), *Brit. Med. J.*, **1**:119, 1955.

Leptomeningeal Anastomoses

Vander Eeken, H. M.: The Anastomoses between Leptomeningeal Arteries of the Brain, Charles C Thomas, Publisher, Springfield, Ill., 1959.

Weidner, W., Hanafee, W., and Markham, C. H.: Intracranial collateral circulation via leptomeningeal and rete mirabile anastomoses, *Neurology*, **15**:39, 1965.

Chapter 3

Applied Anatomy of the Venous System

No part of the body is so full of veins as the brain.

William Harvey

Blood is drained from the cerebrum by superficial (external) and deep (internal) veins. The former group collects blood from the cortex and the adjacent white matter, while the latter drains the central structures. Both systems drain principally into the dural sinuses, which in turn empty into the internal jugular veins. Each internal jugular vein lies within the carotid sheath adjacent to the carotid artery and the vagus nerve; joining the subclavian veins in the superior mediastinum, they form the right and left brachiocephalic (innominate) veins. The brachiocephalics unite to form the superior vena cava, which empties into the right atrium (Fig. 3-1).

An accessory route, which usually removes smaller quantities of blood, is provided by the anastomoses connecting the dural sinuses, the diploic veins, and the emissary veins of the skull. The emissary veins, emerging through foramina in the outer table of the skull, anastomose with tributaries of the external jugular veins, which collect blood from the face, scalp, and cervical region. The external jugular veins descend through the neck and empty into the subclavian veins.

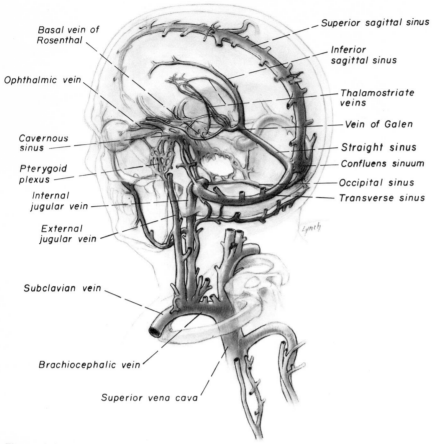

Basal vein of
Rosenthal

Ophthalmic vein

Cavernous
sinus

Pterygoid
plexus

Internal
jugular vein

External
jugular vein

Subclavian vein

Brachiocephalic vein

Superior vena cava

Superior sagittal sinus

Inferior
sagittal sinus

Thalamostriate
veins

Vein of Galen

Straight sinus

Confluens sinuum

Occipital sinus

Transverse sinus

Figure 3-1

SUPERFICIAL VENOUS SYSTEM

The superficial veins draining the cortex and the underlying white matter are divided into superior, middle (Sylvian), and inferior cerebral groups. They lie on the surface of the hemispheres and receive blood from pial branches ramifying over the convolutions of each side. Attached to the underside of this network are the emerging veins that traverse the Virchow-Robin spaces, bringing blood up from the depths of the brain.

Superior Group (Fig. 3–2)

The dorsal, dorsolateral, and medial aspects of each hemisphere above the corpus callosum are drained by 10 to 20 veins, through which blood flows upward into the superior sagittal sinus. Many of these veins join together to form four or five large trunks which are encased in cuffs of arachnoid membrane for about 0.2 to 3.0 cm as they traverse the subdural space before emptying into large venous lacunae adjacent to the superior sagittal sinus.

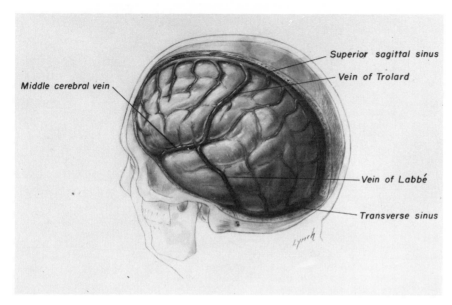

Middle cerebral vein

Superior sagittal sinus

Vein of Trolard

Vein of Labbé

Transverse sinus

Figure 3-2 Superficial drainage of the convexity of the cerebral hemisphere.

The frontal veins are somewhat smaller than those of the parietal region, and they join the superior sagittal sinus almost at right angles. However, those of the parietal region are angled posteriorly, so that they join the superior sagittal sinus at an acute angle which points toward the occiput. The frontal veins are the frontopolar and the inferior, middle, and superior frontal veins. In many instances these veins have a subdural course of as much as 3 cm (Fig. 3-3A and B).

Clinical Correlation

1 The venous lacunae sometimes lie in shallow excavations on the inner table of the skull, which appear in x-rays as radiolucencies near the midline.

2 The arachnoidal granulations (Pacchionian bodies) that develop within the venous lacunae of adults may possibly help to regulate cerebrospinal fluid pressure.

3 In occasional cases the foramina made by the emissary veins are large enough to mimic metastatic tumor in the skull x-ray.

4 Infections sometimes spread into the cranial cavity by way of the emissary veins.

5 Inflammation or thrombosis of the superficial veins may cause seizures and neurologic deficit, the nature of which depends upon the site and extent of the occlusion.

6 Subdural hematoma may be caused by rupture of one or more of the veins traversing the subdural space from the hemispheres to the dural sinuses.

7 The vein of Trolard is a rough guide for the identification of the central (Rolandic) fissure.

Middle Group

The insula and overlying operculum are drained by a collecting network of veins which anastomose with the distal tributaries of the superior and inferior groups of veins. The middle cerebral veins run through the Sylvian fissure to the base of the brain, where they empty into the cavernous, sphenoparietal, and middle meningeal sinuses. On the lateral surface of the hemisphere the vein of Trolard links them with the superior sagittal sinus above, and the lesser

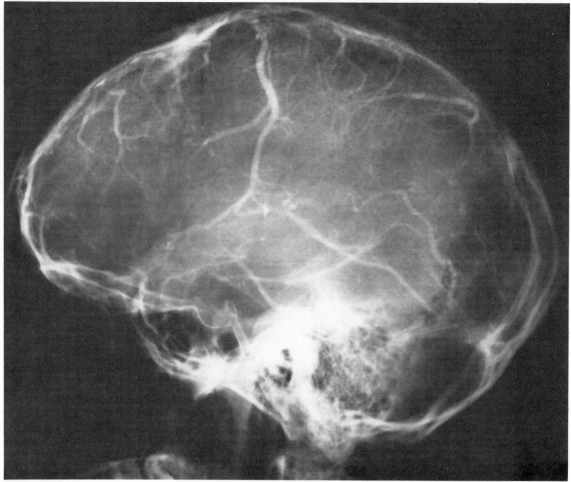

(A)

Figure 3-3(A) and (B) Venous phase of arteriogram in lateral projection showing superficial drainage.

anastomotic vein of Labbé connects them with the transverse sinus below. On the undersurface of the brain the middle cerebral veins interconnect with the basal cerebral vein (vein of Rosenthal).

Clinical Correlation Occlusion of veins in this group may cause focal motor seizures and central facial weakness. If the lesion lies in the dominant hemisphere aphasia may also occur.

Inferior Group

The inferior group of veins, including the vein of Labbé, drains the majority of the lateral surface of the temporal and occipital lobes and their undersurfaces. Blood collected from these regions is carried mainly into the transverse sinus. However, the inferior surface of the temporal lobe also drains into the superior petrosal

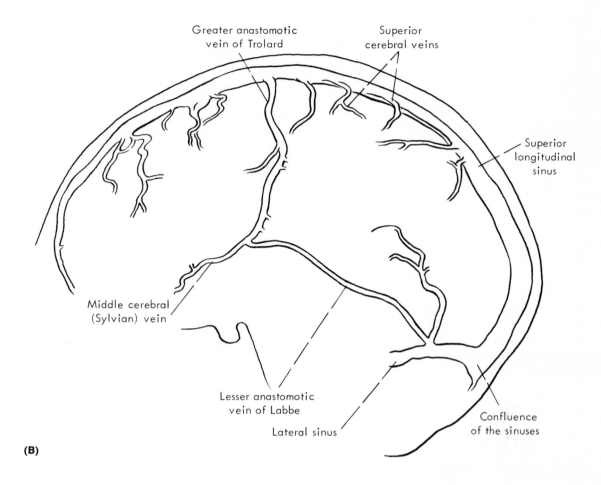

Greater anastomotic
vein of Trolard

Superior
cerebral veins

Superior
longitudinal
sinus

Middle cerebral
(Sylvian) vein

Lesser anastomotic
vein of Labbe

Lateral sinus

Confluence
of the sinuses

(B)

sinus and the basal cerebral vein of Rosenthal, while the inferior and medial surfaces of the occipital lobe empty into the great cerebral vein of Galen, as well as into the transverse sinus. Also present on the inferior surface of the temporal lobe is a series of one to six veins which have a long free course through the subdural space before they enter the transverse sinus, which also receives veins from the petrous portion of the temporal bone. These veins form a connecting link between the middle ear and the cranial cavity.

DEEP VENOUS SYSTEM

The deep system, which drains the paraventricular white matter, the basal ganglia, and other centrally placed structures, consists of the Galenic system and the paired basal veins of Rosenthal. This group collects blood from the territory perfused by the two carotid arteries and from a portion of the vertebral-basilar system.

Galenic System

The *septal vein* of each side becomes visible near the anterior tip of the lateral ventricle and runs posteriorly along the septum pellucidum to the foramen of Monro, where it joins the thalamostriate vein (Fig. 3-4A and B).

The *thalamostriate vein* becomes visible on the floor of the lateral ventricle in a groove between the caudate nucleus and the thalamus. It passes forward and receives blood from tributaries that drain the white matter near the lateral ventricles.

The *choroid vein* drains blood from the choroid plexus of the lateral ventricle.

The *internal cerebral vein* of each side arises from the confluence of the septal, thalamostriate, and choroid veins, which occurs at the foramen of Monro. The two internal cerebral veins run posteriorly in the roof of the third ventricle. They unite with each other to form the great vein of Galen just beneath the splenium of the corpus callosum and above the pineal gland.

The *great cerebral vein of Galen,* after curving upward around the splenium of the corpus callosum, empties into the straight sinus at an acute angle. It receives the two basal cerebral veins of Rosenthal, the posterior cerebral veins, the occipital veins, and the superior cerebellar veins, as well as small tributaries from the pineal gland and the tectum.

Clinical Correlation Displacement of these deeply situated veins may give the only angiographic clue to a centrally located tumor, because tumors in the central regions often do not displace the arteries on the surface of the brain.

1 The junction of the thalamostriate with the internal cerebral veins—"the venous angle"—is situated at the foramen of Monro and is visible in the venous phase on the lateral view of an angiogram. Tumors of the frontal lobe may distort this angle.

2 Lateral displacement of the internal cerebral veins, visible in anteroposterior angiograms, suggests a mass in the cerebral hemisphere.

3 The sweep of the thalamostriate veins, also visible in the anteroposterior study, is increased

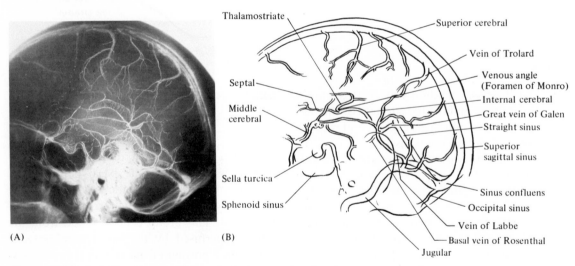

(A)   (B)

Figure 3-4(A) and (B) Venous phase of arteriogram showing deep venous system.

by dilatation of lateral ventricles as in hydrocephalus.

Basal Cerebral Veins (Veins of Rosenthal)

The basal vein of each side first becomes visible in the region of the anterior perforated substance. Each is formed by a union of the anterior cerebral vein, the inferior striate veins, and the deep middle cerebral vein. The basal vein passes posteriorly along the optic tract and around the cerebral peduncle, usually terminating in the great vein of Galen; occasionally, however, it ends in the internal cerebral vein or the straight sinus itself. The basal veins drain the medial pallidum, the preoptic region, the hypothalamus, the subthalamus, and areas of the upper part of the brainstem. They also receive the inferior choroidal veins from the temporal lobes.

Clinical Correlation In transtentorial herniation the downward displacement of the basal vein is sometimes visible on venograms. If this vein is pressed against the sharp edge of the tentorium cerebelli, the result may be edema and

hemorrhage in the upper part of the midbrain.

DURAL SINUSES

Superior Sagittal (Longitudinal) Sinus

This large venous sinus, triangular in cross section, lies in the line of attachment of the falx cerebri to the calvaria. It commences at the foramen caecum and crista galli and runs to the internal occipital protuberance, where it empties into the confluens sinuum (Fig. 3-5). Anterior to the coronal suture it carries only small quantities of blood, but posteriorly it enlarges rapidly and carries large volumes. Lateral to the sinus in the adjacent dura are many large venous lakes; arachnoid villi projecting into these lacunae may facilitate resorption of cerebrospinal fluid in adults.

The superior sagittal sinus receives the superior cerebral veins and veins from the diploë and dura mater, as well as those interconnecting with the veins of the scalp and with the pericranial and nasal veins.

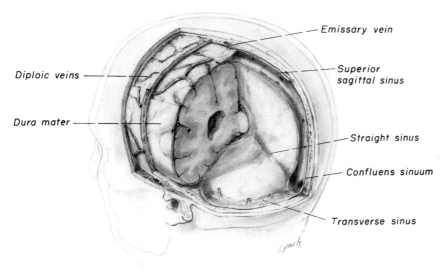

Figure 3-5

Clinical Correlation These are discussed in Chap. 21.

Inferior Sagittal (Longitudinal) Sinus

This relatively small sinus has a rounded lumen that increases in diameter throughout its course. Running in the posterior two-thirds of the free inferior margin of the falx cerebri, it receives veins from the corpus callosum and the cerebellum before it becomes continuous with the straight sinus.

Straight Sinus

The straight sinus, which has a triangular lumen, is formed by the union of the inferior sagittal sinus and the great vein of Galen. It runs backward in the junction between the falx cerebri and the falx cerebelli, and joins the confluens sinuum at the internal occipital protuberance.

Clinical Correlation
1 The straight sinus may sometimes be elevated by tumors of the posterior fossa.
2 Death may result from a hematoma in the posterior fossa following birth injuries that cause hemorrhage from the straight sinus.

Occipital Sinus

The occipital sinus, smallest of all intradural sinuses, is situated in the fixed margin of the falx cerebelli and runs upward from the foramen magnum to the confluens sinuum. Along the way it receives veins from the falx cerebelli and the medial aspect of the cerebellum. It also communicates with the vertebral venous plexus.
Clinical Correlation This sinus sometimes lies in a groove in the inner table of the occipital bone. This groove, when seen on x-ray films, may be confused with the excavation produced by a dermoid cyst.

Confluens Sinuum (Torcular Herophili)

The superior sagittal, the straight, and the occipital sinuses usually join together within the dura at the internal occipital protuberance to form the confluens sinuum, or torcular Herophili ("the winepress of Herophilus"). The majority of blood drained from the cerebrum, cerebellum, and upper part of the brainstem must therefore traverse this critical junction. In the confluens the superior sagittal sinus turns sharply to the right while the inferior sagittal and straight sinuses turn to the left, so that at times there is no mixing of blood within it.

Transverse (Lateral) and Sigmoid Sinuses

The transverse sinus begins at the confluens and runs within the fixed margin of the tentorium cerebelli to the base of the petrous pyramid, where it angles abruptly downward. Below this point it is called the *sigmoid sinus*. As it descends in its groove in the mastoid portion of the temporal bone, the sigmoid sinus lies in close proximity to the mastoid air cells of the middle ear. The sigmoid sinus leaves the skull at the jugular foramen, where it becomes known as the *internal jugular vein*. Emerging from the skull just medial to it are the glossopharyngeal, vagus, and spinal accessory nerves.

The transverse sinuses receive most of the inferior group of superficial cerebral veins and the superior and inferior petrosal sinuses, which in turn partially drain the cavernous sinus. The transverse sinuses communicate with scalp veins through emissary veins and with veins from the mastoid area.

Clinical Correlation
1 Mastoid infection may result in thrombosis of the transverse or sigmoid sinus, as discussed in Chap. 21.
2 Grooving of the inner table of the skull by the transverse sinuses is frequently visible on

plain films of the skull and is a fairly reliable guide to the size of the two sinuses.

3 The transverse sinuses usually differ in size, that on the right being the larger.

Sphenoparietal Sinus

This sinus runs along the lesser wing of the sphenoid bone to terminate in the cavernous sinus. Its tributaries are superficial veins from the middle and inferior groups of cerebral veins and a branch of the middle cerebral vein which usually interconnects it with the superior sagittal sinus.

Clinical Correlation Rupture of the sinus or of its tributary veins can cause a subdural hematoma in the middle fossa.

CAVERNOUS SINUSES

These paired plexuses of veins, situated on either side of the sella turcica, derive their name from the many interlacing filaments of fibrous tissue which divide the sinus into multiple cavities. They extend from the medial end of the sphenoid fissure to the apex of the petrous portion of the temporal bone. Passing through each but separated from the bloodstream by an endothelial wall are the internal carotid artery with its periarterial sympathetic plexus, the first two divisions of the trigeminal nerve, and the three nerves that control eye movement (Fig. 3-6).

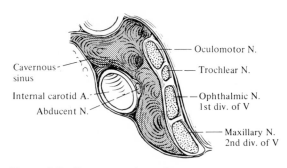

Cavernous sinus

Internal carotid A.

Abducent N.

Oculomotor N.

Trochlear N.

Ophthalmic N. 1st div. of V

Maxillary N. 2nd div. of V

Figure 3-6 Cavernous sinus diagram.

Tributaries of the cavernous sinus are the sphenoparietal sinus and the ophthalmic veins.

An extensive network of anastomosing veins provides multiple routes for the egress of blood from the cavernous sinuses. *Intracranial interconnections* within this network are as follows:

1 The superior petrosal sinus to the transverse sinus

2 The inferior petrosal sinus to the lowest portion of the sigmoid sinus

3 The middle group of superficial veins to the vein of Labbé and the transverse sinus

4 The middle group to the vein of Trolard and the superior sagittal sinus

5 The anterior and posterior intercavernous plexuses of veins which traverse the diaphragm of the sella and encircle the pituitary gland to form the circular sinus

6 The basal veins of Rosenthal to the straight sinus

The connections between *intracranial* and *extracranial vessels* are:

1 Cavernous sinus to superior ophthalmic vein, through the superior orbital fissure into the orbit and the facial veins

2 The inferior ophthalmic vein to the pterygoid plexus beneath the skull

3 Unnamed emissary veins connecting with the pterygoid plexus

Clinical Correlation

1 Because all the veins are valveless, blood may flow out of the skull or into it through these anastomoses. Thus infection from the eyes, nose, face, paranasal sinuses, pharynx, and teeth can be carried into the cavernous sinus and move rapidly from one vein to another if local pressure gradients are altered.

2 The intracavernous portion of the carotid artery may rupture, creating a caroticocavernous sinus fistula which may become symptomatic after a variable latent period. The symptoms and signs of such a fistula will depend in part on the patency and arrangement of the veins draining the sinus (see Chap. 25).

PETROSAL SINUSES

Superior Petrosal Sinus

This small, narrow sinus connecting the cavernous with the transverse sinus courses downward, backward, and laterally in the attachment of the tentorium cerebelli on the petrous portion of the temporal bone. It receives a few of the inferior occipital and cerebellar veins, and interconnects with veins in the middle ear.

Inferior Petrosal Sinus

Lying in the shallow groove at the junction of the petrous pyramid and the basioccipital bone, the inferior petrosal sinus connects the cavernous sinus with the superior bulb of the internal jugular vein. It receives veins from the inner ear, the pons, the medulla, and the undersurface of the cerebellum.

Clinical Correlation   When infection of the middle ear leads to thrombosis of this sinus, the result is Gradenigo's syndrome: unilateral otitis media with ipsilateral facial pain and abducens palsy.

VEINS OF THE CEREBELLUM AND BRAINSTEM

Cerebellar Veins

Near the midline on the superior surface of the cerebellum lie two to four *superior cerebellar veins* which drain blood from the parenchyma of the cerebellum into the great vein of Galen (Fig. 3-7).

The dentate nucleus and the inferior anterior surface of each cerebellar hemisphere are drained by anterior cerebellar veins which connect with the pontine venous plexus.

The *posterior cerebellar veins* drain the vermis and the posterior surface of the cerebellar hemisphere and empty into the straight or transverse sinuses.

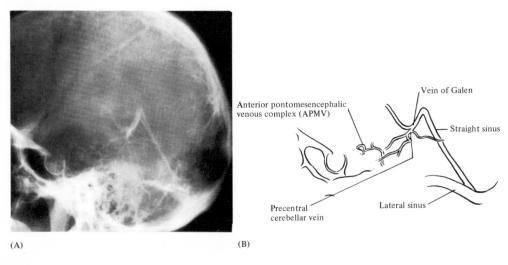

(A)   (B)

Figure 3-7

Clinical Correlation

1 During operations requiring exposure of the quadrigeminal plate, the superior cerebellar veins can be sacrificed without risk as long as the vein of Galen is not damaged.

2 Because of its proximity to the trigeminal nerve, the anterior cerebellar vein may be damaged during operations for tic douloureux.

Veins of the Brainstem

The central and lateral veins of the midbrain drain into the basal cerebral veins of Rosenthal.

The veins of the pons consist of a rich anastomotic network communicating with the petrosal veins on either side, with the basal veins of Rosenthal superiorly, and with the medullary veins inferiorly.

Veins of the medulla connect with cerebellar veins above, and with veins of the spinal cord and vertebral plexus below. They empty into the occipital sinus and, to a variable degree, into emissary veins.

Clinical Correlation

1 The rich anastomoses of the brainstem plexus, like those of the cavernous plexus, allow instantaneous readjustment of flow when some veins are obstructed.

2 Traction on the pons during removal of tumors in the cerebellopontine angle may result in fatal hemorrhage if pontile bridging veins are torn.

3 Because dural sinuses and veins of the brainstem connect with the vertebral (Batson's) plexus, they can serve as a means for the access of metastases to the cerebellum as well as to the skull and dural sinuses.

Basilar Plexus

The basilar plexus is a network of sinusoidal veins lying in the dura which covers the clivus. It communicates with the anterior vertebral venous plexus and with the inferior petrosal sinuses.

SECONDARY VENOUS DRAINAGE OF THE BRAIN

Emissary veins are channels connecting the intracranial venous sinuses to the tributaries of the external jugular vein or to the vertebral venous plexus.

The major emissary veins, together with their connections, are:

1 Ophthalmic (inferior ophthalmic vein and pterygoid plexus)
2 Ethmoidal (superior sagittal sinus and nasal veins)
3 Parietal (superior sagittal sinus and bone marrow of the skull and veins of the scalp)
4 Occipital (confluens sinuum and perivertebral plexus)
5 Mastoid (transverse sinus and occipital plexus)
6 Condyloid (sigmoid sinus and perivertebral plexus)
7 Hypoglossal (sigmoid sinus and vertebral veins)
8 Pharyngeal (cavernous and petrosal sinuses and pterygoid plexus)

At time almost a fourth of the blood flowing in the external jugular veins may be derived from the brain, but the usual proportion is substantially less. The exact quantities depend on the capacity of the channels just listed and on fluctuations in pressure relationships between the external and the internal jugular systems.

Clinical Correlation

1 Emissary veins are like a double-edged sword. In instances of intracranial sinus thrombosis venous outflow may be maintained by these channels as they flow into the perivertebral plexus. Since the vertebral venous plexus and the veins of the head and neck contain no valves, sudden increases of intrathoracic or intraabdominal and pelvic pressure (as in Valsalva maneuver) can reverse the direction of flow in the plexus and in the emissary veins, carrying septic or metastatic emboli into the venous systems of the spine and brain.

2 When the vertebral venous plexus is adequate (in young individuals or those who are not sedentary), removal of the external and internal jugular veins on one or both sides causes only minor and transient signs of intracranial hypertension.

3 In occasional patients, failure of jugular compression to cause a rise in spinal fluid pressure may be explained by a particularly rich vertebral venous plexus which drains off such large quantities of blood that spinal fluid pressure fails to rise when the jugular veins are compressed.

SUGGESTED READINGS

General

Kaplan, H. A.: The transcerebral venous system: An anatomical study, *Arch. Neurol.,* **1**:148, 1959.

Padget, D. H.: The cranial venous system in man in reference to development, adult configuration, and relation to the arteries, *Am. J. Anat.,* **98**:307, 1956.

Schlesinger, B.: The venous drainage of the brain with special reference to the Galenic system, *Brain,* **62**:274, 1939.

Woodhall, B.: Anatomy of the cranial blood sinuses with particular reference to the lateral, *Laryngoscope,* **49**:966, 1939.

———: Variations of the cranial venous sinuses in the region of the torcular Herophili, *Arch. Surg.,* **33**:297, 1936.

Superficial Venous System

Di Chiro, G.: Angiographic patterns of cerebral convexity veins and superficial dural sinuses, *Am. J. Roentgenol.,* **87**:308, 1962.

Wolf, B. S., Huang, Y. P., and Newman, C. M.: The superficial Sylvian venous drainage system, *Am. J. Roentgenol,* **89**:398, 1963.

Deep Venous System

Banna, M., and Young, J. R.: Normal anatomical variation and asymmetry of the Galenic venous system, *Brit. J. Radiol.,* **43**:126, 1970.

Hassler, O.: Deep cerebral venous system in man: A microangiographic study on its areas of drainage and its anastomoses with the superficial cerebral veins, *Neurology,* **16**:505, 1966.

Johanson, C.: Central veins and deep dural sinuses of brain; Anatomical and angiographic study, *Acta radiol. suppl.,* **107**:1, 1954.

Dural Sinuses

Superior Sagittal (Longitudinal) Sinus

Lerner, M. A.: The angiographic evaluation of the calvarial impressions and channels, and the clinical significance of the parasagittal sinusoidal cerebral veins, *Clin. Radiol.,* **20**:157, 1969.

Occipital Sinus

Das, A. C., and Hasan, M.: The occipital sinus, *J. Neurosurg.,* **33**:307, 1970.

Veins of the Cerebellum and Brainstem

Cerebellar Veins

Epstein, H. M., Linde, H. W., Crampton, A. R., Ciric, I. S., and Eckenhoff, J. E.: The vertebral venous plexus as a major cerebral venous outflow tract, *Anesthesiology,* **32**:332, 1970.

Gillilan, L. A.: The arterial and venous blood supplies to the cerebellum of primates, *J. Neuropathol. Exptl. Neurol.,* **28**:295, 1969.

Huang, Y. P., Wolf, B. S., Antin, S. P., and Okudera, T.: The veins of the posterior fossa—Anterior or petrosal draining group, *Am. J. Roentgenol.,* **104**:36, 1968.

Basilar Plexus

Vuia, O., and Alexianu, M.: Insuffisance veineuse du cerveau ramollissement et hémorragie cérébrale d'origine veineuse, *J. Neurol. Sci.,* **7**:495, 1968.

Clinical Significance

Bailey, P.: Peculiarities of the intracranial venous system and their clinical significance, *Arch. Neurol. Psychiat.,* **32**:1105, 1934.

Perese, D. M.: Superficial veins of the brain from a surgical point of view, *J. Neurosurg.,* **17**:402, 1960.

Perryman, C. R., Conlon, P. C., and Brust, R. W.: The value of cerebral vein study in carotid angiography, *Radiol. Clin. N. Am.,* **1**:145, 1963.

Chapter 4

Anatomy and Physiology of the Spinal Cord Vessels

The entire cervical and the upper thoracic segments of the spinal cord are supplied by branches of the vertebral arteries and by deep cervical, costocervical, and ascending cervical branches of the subclavian arteries. The remainder of the thoracic, lumbar, and sacral sections of the cord are nourished by branches of the thoracic and lumbar aortae and the iliac arteries (Fig. 4-1). Three types of arteries participate in the supply of the spinal cord and nerve roots.

1 Segmental arteries. Paired segmental arteries arise from vertebral arteries, the aorta, and the iliac arteries to perfuse paravertebral muscles, vertebrae, meninges, and nerve roots. Branches of these arteries travel with their respective segmental nerves through the vertebral foramina where they divide into anterior and posterior radicular arteries (Fig 4-2).

2 Radicular arteries. Radicular arteries arise from each of the segmental arteries and proceed through the vertebral foramina to supply the anterior and posterior nerve roots and sensory ganglia at their respective levels. They contribute little blood to the spinal cord.

3 Medullary arteries. Unpaired medullary arteries arise from some of the segmental arteries and travel without branching to the anterior median spinal artery or the posterior pial arteriolar plexus. Contrary to popular belief, medullary arteries do not arise at every segment and do not supply nerve roots.

In the cervical region three or four anterior medullary arteries arise from the vertebral arteries and the ascending and deep cervical arteries of each side. The upper few thoracic segments of the spinal cord are served by medullary branches of the deep cervical and/or superior intercostal arteries. The rest of the thoracic part of the cord is supplied by a few medullary arteries which arise from segmental branches of the thoracic aorta. This region has the most marginal blood supply of the entire cord and is most vulnerable to occlusion of a medullary artery.

The largest, and sometimes the only, lumbar medullary artery is called the *great anterior med-*

ullary artery (of Adamkiewicz). It is found usually at L_1 or L_2 but occasionally as high as T_{12} or as low as L_4. After joining the anterior median spinal artery, this artery furnishes all the blood supply of the anterior two-thirds of the entire lumbar and sacral segments of the cord, and sometimes the lower thoracic segments as well.

ANTERIOR MEDIAN SPINAL ARTERY

Two *anterior spinal rami* which arise as the first intracranial branches of the vertebral arteries descend on the anterior surface of the spinal cord to the level of the second or third cervical segment of the cord, where they unite to form a single anterior median spinal artery. Occasionally one of the anterior spinal rami is small or absent, and in rare cases the two run parallel as far as the lower cervical region or even to the sacral cord without joining together.

Throughout its length the anterior median spinal artery varies in caliber, being largest in its cervical and lumbar enlargements, probably because of the increased bulk of the cord which it must supply.

As it descends in the median fissure, the anterior median spinal artery receives contributions from the *anterior medullary arteries* sporadically at different levels. Although the average number is 7 to 10, there may be as few as 5 or as many as 17 (Fig. 4-3).

It is unique because, in total length, it is the longest artery in the body and because it is supplied by so many anastomoses.

Branches of the Anterior Median Spinal Artery

The anterior median spinal artery nourishes the anterior two-thirds of the spinal cord through *sulcal (paramedian) arteries* and branches to the ventrolateral portion of the *pial arteriolar plexus*. The sulcal arteries penetrate the median fissure until they reach the neural tissue, whereupon they turn alternately right and left into the

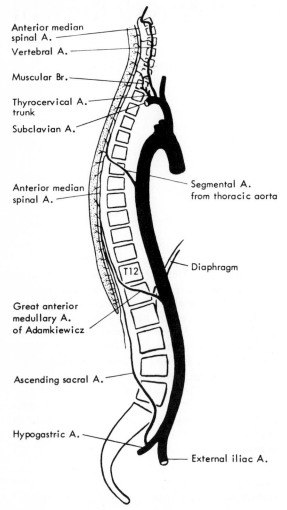

Figure 4-1 Diagram of the major sources of blood supply to the spinal cord. Anterior spinal rami are not shown.

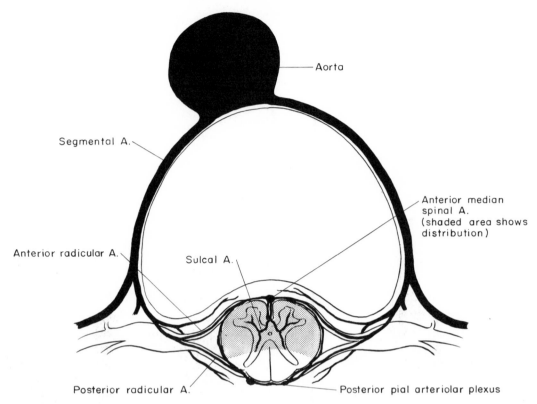

Figure 4-2

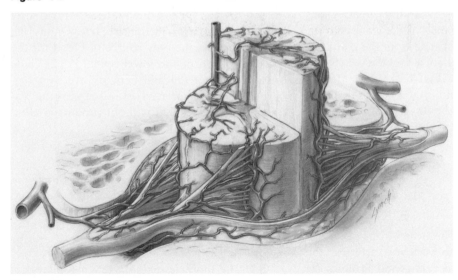

Figure 4-3

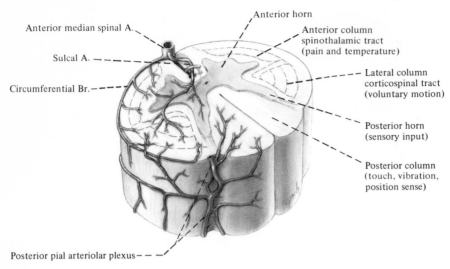

Anterior horn

Anterior median spinal A.

Sulcal A.

Circumferential Br.

Anterior column
spinothalamic tract
(pain and temperature)

Lateral column
corticospinal tract
(voluntary motion)

Posterior horn
(sensory input)

Posterior column
(touch, vibration,
position sense)

Posterior pial arteriolar plexus

Figure 4-4

parenchyma to supply the gray and white matter. Throughout the length of the cord their total number ranges from 250 to 300. Although there is little, if any, communication between the arteries of the two halves of the spinal cord, numerous capillary or precapillary anastomoses exist among those of the same side. This network is especially rich in the gray matter around cell bodies, where capillary density and blood flow are greater than in the white matter.

Penetrating branches arise from the pial arteriolar plexus and end in a capillary network with the sulcal arteries (Fig. 4-4). These arteries nourish the lateral and ventral spinothalamic tracts, the corticospinal pathways, and the anterior and lateral horns of the gray matter, all of which are contained in the anterior two-thirds of the spinal cord.

Posterior Spinal Rami and Pial Arteriolar Plexus

Arising as very small branches from the intracranial portion of the vertebral arteries, the paired posterior spinal rami wind around the lateral aspect of the cervicomedullary region to assume a position just lateral to the entrance of the posterior nerve roots on either side. They end at the second or third cervical segment of the cord by joining the lateral and ventral aspects of the pial arteriolar plexus. Throughout the length of the cord a variable number of posterior medullary branches from the segmental arteries of the cervical and thoracic regions terminate in this plexus. Below the thoracic level the great posterior medullary artery joins the network and is the only source of blood for the posterior third of the lower spinal cord. These anastomoses of the pial network are so extensive that any one or even several of the ramifications can be occluded without producing clinical deficit.

Clinical Correlation

1 The large number of arteries feeding into the spinal arterial system renders the spinal cord quite resistant to ischemic damage except in the zones of terminal supply (watershed areas), as in the midthoracic section of the cord, where the supply is least.

2 In the thoracic region a few medullary arteries carry the bulk of arterial blood to the cord. The lumbosacral portion of the cord is supplied by a single artery, obstruction of which may result in dysfunction of the anterior two-thirds of the lumbosacral cord.

3 Potential for collateral supply within the spinal cord exists at two levels: in the pial arteriolar plexus and at the capillary level. This collateral circulation is sufficient to prevent neural damage only in the region of the plexus which supplies the posterior third of the cord.

4 In contrast to the cerebral arteries, the intraspinal arteries are usually spared atherosclerosis of degree sufficient to produce symptoms.

5 Saccular aneurysms, so frequent in the cerebral arteries, are rare in the spinal arteries.

APPLIED VENOUS ANATOMY

Whereas the vessels on the anterior aspect of the cord are chiefly arterial, those on the posterior aspect are primarily venous. This venous system is plexiform, but within it six main channels can be distinguished—a posterior, two posterolateral, two anterolateral, and the anterior spinal veins. Most of the central veins draining the interior of the spinal cord empty into the anterior spinal vein, which runs throughout the length of the cord in the vicinity of the anterior median fissure.

The six longitudinal venous channels empty into the radicular veins accompanying the ventral and dorsal nerve roots. These spinal radicular veins, lying within the subarachnoid space, pierce the dura to join the epidural venous plexus, which in turn communicates with the internal vertebral venous plexus. The latter communicates with the inferior vena cava and the azygos system of veins through the perivertebral plexus.

In the cervical region the longitudinal cord veins and the internal vertebral plexus join the intracranial veins to form a continuous valveless system which may drain blood from the posterior fossa into the spinal canal, or in reverse direction from cord to posterior fossa.

PHYSIOLOGY OF THE SPINAL CORD CIRCULATION

Because the spinal cord is an extension of the brain, it is not surprising that, in general, the physiology of the spinal cord circulation is similar to that of cerebral circulation. The vessels autoregulate in response to changes in systemic arterial blood pressure; they dilate when the level of P_{CO_2} is increased and constrict when it is reduced.

The spinal cord perfusion is more closely related to changes in systemic blood pressure, however. It has been shown that a low peripheral vascular resistance leading to aortic hypotension diverts aortic outflow *away* from the spinal cord vessels and that when peripheral vascular resistance is high in the lower extremities, aortic outflow is diverted *toward* the spinal circulation, increasing pressure and possibly increasing perfusion itself.

Clinical Correlation

1 If the patient has hypertension and increased peripheral vascular resistance, the column of contrast medium remains static in the aorta during aortography and is diverted into the spinal cord circulation. If peripheral resistance is decreased, rapid forward flow occurs, and the aorta is virtually emptied at the end of one cardiac cycle.

2 The requirement for spinal cord blood flow increases with the activity of the neurons involved.

3 In some instances, at least, blood flow to the cord is redistributed between the other portions of the aortic circulation in response to changes in vasomotor tone initiated by reflexes. A specific and important reflex in animals and possibly in man is the diving reflex. Liquid applied to the face or snout area triggers a reflex over the afferent limb (the trigeminal nerve). Response through the efferent limb (the vagus nerve) and the splanchnic circulation induces bradycardia and a peripheral vasoconstriction with redistribution of blood to the brain and spinal cord.

The spinal cord is encased within a bony structure similar to that which protects the brain, so that any change in volume can take place only at the expense of the cerebrospinal fluid, the blood, or the spinal tissue itself. Furthermore, compression of the thoracic spinal cord may lead to a vasopressor response with slowing of the pulse rate owing to stimulation of the sympathetic nuclei from T_{12} to L_1.

In cats the blood flow is slower through the spinal cord than through the brain and has a value of 1.63 ml per Gm per min in the gray matter and 0.14 ml per Gm per min in the white matter.

It is believed that the average arterial pressure in the spinal cord is substantially lower than that in the aorta.

SUGGESTED READINGS

Types of Arteries Supplying the Cord and Nerve Roots

Lazorthes, G., Gouaze, A., Zadeh, J. O., Santini, J. J., Lazorthes, Y., and Burdin, P.: Arterial vascularization of the spinal cord. Recent studies of the anastomotic substitution pathways, *J. Neurosurg.,* **35**:253, 1971.

Doppman, J., and Di Chiro, G.: The arteria radicularis magna: Radiographic anatomy in the adult, *Brit. J. Radiol.,* **41**:40, 1968.

Corbin, J. L.: Anatomie et Pathologie Artériolles de la Moelle, Masson et Cie, Paris, 1961.

Gillilan, L. A.: "Arterial and venous anatomy of the spinal cord," in Cerebral Vascular Diseases, Transactions of the Seventh Princeton Conference, edited by J. Moossy and R. Janeway, Grune & Stratton, Inc., New York, 1971, pp. 3-9.

Hassler, O.: Blood supply to the human spinal cord: A microangiographic study, *Arch. Neurol.,* **15**:302, 1966.

Herren, R. Y., and Alexander, L.: Sulcal and intrinsic blood vessels of human spinal cord, *Arch. Neurol. Psychiat.,* **41**:678, 1939.

Romanes, G. J.: The arterial blood supply of the human spinal cord, *Paraplegia,* **2**:199, 1965.

Suh, T. H., and Alexander, L.: Vascular system of human spinal cord, *Arch. Neurol. Psychiat.,* **41**:659, 1939.

Turnbull, I. M., Brieg, A., and Hassler, O.: Blood supply of cervical spinal cord of man: A microangiographic cadaver study, *J. Neurosurg.,* **24**:951, 1966.

Willis, T. A.: Nutrient arteries of the vertebral bodies, *J. Bone Joint Surg.,* **31**-A:538, 1949.

Applied Venous Anatomy

Batson, O. V.: "The vertebral system of veins as a means for cancer dissemination," in Progress in Clinical Cancer, vol. 3, edited by I. M. Ariel, Grune & Stratton, Inc., New York, 1967, pp. 1-18.

———: The vertebral vein system, *Am. J. Roentgenol.,* **78**:195, 1957.

Di Chiro, G., and Doppman, J. L.: Endocranial drainage of spinal cord veins, *Radiology,* **95**:555, 1970.

Gillilan, L. A.: Veins of the spinal cord. Anatomic details; Suggested clinical applications, *Neurology,* **20**:860, 1970.

Vogelsang, H.: Intraosseous Spinal Venography, The Williams & Wilkins Company, Baltimore, 1970.

Physiology of the Spinal Cord Circulation

Di Chiro, G., and Fried, L. C.: Blood flow currents in spinal cord arteries, *Neurology,* **21**:1088, 1971.

Margolis, G.: "Circulatory dynamics of the spinal cord," in Cerebral Vascular Diseases, Transactions of the Seventh Princeton Conference, edited by J. Moossy and R. Janeway, Grune & Stratton, Inc., New York, 1971, pp. 10-17.

Palleske, H., and Herrman, H.-D.: Experimental investigations on the regulation of the blood flow of the spinal cord. I. Comparative study of the cerebral and spinal cord blood flow with heat clearance probes in pigs, *Acta neurochir.,* **19**:73, 1968.

———, Kivelitz, R., and Loew, F.: Experimental investigation on the control of spinal cord circulation. IV. The effect of spinal or cerebral compression on the blood flow of the spinal cord, *Acta neurochir.,* **22**:29, 1970.

Clinical Physiology of the Cerebral Circulation

One marked characteristic of literature dealing with the cerebral circulation is, we think, the contradictory nature of the results which have been obtained by different investigators.

C. S. Roy and C. S. Sherrington

Blood flow through the brain is kept relatively constant despite the phenomenal increases in cardiac output and arterial blood pressure which occur during exercise and the tendency for blood to pool in the legs while one is standing.

Whether one is awake or asleep, happy or angry, bending over, recumbent or erect, on the moon or submerged beneath the ocean, the adult brain requires 500 to 600 ml of oxygen and 75 to 100 mg of glucose each minute to support normal function. To supply these never-ending demands, about 1,000 ml (one-fifth of cardiac output) of oxygenated, glucose-laden blood circulates through the brain each minute, thus providing the source for the 30 watts of energy* the brain needs to function properly. In children, the cerebral circulation (about 400 ml

$$* \quad \frac{144 \text{ Gm glucose}}{24 \text{ hr}} \times \frac{4.3 \text{ Cal}}{\text{Gm glucose}} = \frac{619.2 \text{ Cal}}{24 \text{ hr}}$$

$$\frac{619.2}{24 \text{ hr}} \times \frac{4.185 \text{ joules}}{\text{Cal}} = \frac{2591350 \text{ joules}}{24 \text{ hr}}$$

$$= 107970 \text{ joules/hr}$$
$$= 30 \text{ joules/sec}$$

1 watt = 1 joule/sec, so the brain must use about 30 watts.

of blood per min) requires more than a third of the cardiac output.

In 24 hr, about 380† gal of blood circulates through the brain, which burns about 144 Gm of glucose as fuel and consumes 72 liters of oxygen in the process, or about two-thirds of the glucose and one-half of the oxygen required for an adult at rest. If the blood supply to the brain is interrupted for only 30 sec, neuronal metabolism suffers; in 2 min it ceases; and after 5 min cellular death begins.

EFFECTS OF SYSTEMIC FACTORS

The beating of the heart provides the propelling force for the circulation of blood, and the tone of the small peripheral arteries controls the arterial pressure. If either fails, the brain does also. Because all the vascular beds are irrigated by the same pump, each is to a certain extent in competition with the others for the available blood. When local requirements for blood are increased (for example, by exercise of the arms or legs), there must be an increase in cardiac output, an adjustment in vasomotor tone, and redistribution of flow if brain perfusion is to remain constant. However, the circulatory system has its own hierarchy. The brain, the heart, and the kidneys receive adequate perfusion even when other organs and skeletal muscles have become ischemic.

Cardiac Output

Each cardiac systole thrusts about 70 ml of blood from the left ventricle into the aorta, which in turn forces blood through the vascular system. At rest, the cardiac output is 70 ml times 70 contractions per min, or about 5,000 ml. Of this total, 1,000 ml is destined for the brain. During exercise output may increase to 15,000 ml, yet the brain continues to receive 1,000 ml.

† 380 gal/day × 365.25 days/year × 70 years/lifetime = 9.73 million gal/lifetime.

Clinical Correlation Abnormalities which appear to be the result of defective cerebral circulation may actually be produced by abnormalities of heart rate or rhythm which have decreased the cardiac output to critical levels.

Arterial Pressure

Arterial pressure may rise to tremendous heights during exercise, anger, excitement, fright, or Valsalva's maneuver (increase of intrapulmonic pressure by forcible exhalation against closed glottis). During changes in body posture it may fall rapidly. Such fluctuations are transmitted through the carotid and vertebral arteries and the circle of Willis directly to the cerebral arteries. Mean arterial pressure is only slightly lower at the circle of Willis than at the aortic arch, but it is progressively reduced to about 50 mm Hg at the arterioles, to 5 to 10 mm Hg in the capillaries, and to negative pressures in the larger veins. When the head is higher than the body in normal individuals the penetrating arteries and arterioles of the brain adjust their caliber in response to changes in mean arterial pressure. Thus, capillary pressure and perfusion remain constant unless mean arterial pressure falls below about 70 mm Hg or rises above 160 mm Hg.

Clinical Correlation
1 When mean arterial pressure rises above 160 mm Hg, the constrictive capacity of the arterioles is overcome. The result is increased pressure in the capillary bed, transudation of fluid, and the diapedesis of red blood cells into the extracellular spaces. Intense vasospasm may lead to distal microinfarction—the syndrome of hypertensive encephalopathy (see Chap. 19).
2 When arteriolar pressure of a person with atherosclerosis or long-standing hypertension falls because of the diminished capacity of the cerebral arterioles to dilate, he may experience syncope at levels tolerated by normal persons.

3 Rapid change in arterial pressure may exceed the capacity of the cerebral arterioles to respond and result in temporary changes in cerebral perfusion.

4 Reductions not sufficient to impede pressure or flow through the brain as a whole may produce reductions in a local vascular bed distal to point of stenosis and result in focal neurologic deficit.

Pulmonary Mechanics

Cerebral blood flow is also subject to alterations caused by the mechanics of respiration. Valsalva's maneuver can decrease cardiac output to such a degree that cerebral blood flow is reduced to critical levels. In persons with normal cerebral perfusion, slight giddiness is the only symptom noticed. In infants, however, breath-holding may lead to loss of consciousness; and in adults with diseased vessels, poor cardiac output, or pulmonary disease, syncope may result from lifting a heavy load, vigorous coughing, or unusual straining during a bowel movement or micturition.

Blood Viscosity

Provided that other variables remain constant, blood flow is related to blood viscosity. Flow is increased in anemic conditions and decreased when the blood becomes more viscous as a result of dehydration, for example, or of increases in plasma proteins or cellular constituents.

Clinical Correlation

1 In erythrocytosis or polycythemia rubra vera, the rate and volume of cerebral blood flow may be decreased sufficiently to cause symptoms of cerebrovascular insufficiency.

2 In cases of giant cell myeloma, the level of abnormal proteins in the circulating plasma may be so high that flow is impaired and cerebral symptoms result.

3 In certain disease states, the cellular elements may form aggregates or clumps which impede blood flow through the brain.

THE ARTERIAL SYSTEM

Cervicocranial Arteries

Each internal carotid supplies approximately 300 to 400 ml to the ipsilateral orbit and the cerebral hemisphere each minute. Most of this is destined for the middle cerebral artery and its branches. In contrast, less than 200 ml flows through the vertebral arteries to supply the muscles of the cervical region, the brainstem, the upper part of the spinal cord, the cerebellum, the occipital lobes, portions of the temporal lobes, and the inner ear.

Normally, the two internal carotids are about equal in caliber, and neither supplies blood to the territory of the other. The two vertebral arteries, however, are frequently asymmetric, and the one that carries the greater amount of blood supplies areas usually irrigated by the other. Because blood flowing through the carotid system does not normally mix with the vertebral-basilar blood, one may speak of the two cerebral circulations.

Blood flows faster in the carotid circulation than in the vertebral-basilar system—the transit time from common carotid to jugular vein being about 7 sec as compared to about 8 or 9 sec from the proximal vertebral to its venous collecting system. Yet, in each capillary bed a unit of blood spends only about 2 sec, and within this brief time metabolic exchange must take place. Another difference, not fully defined as yet, may be the vascular reactivity of the two systems to pharmacological agents and to changes in the blood gases.

Along the course of the carotid artery, there is little decrease in pressure from its origin to its intracranial branches. There should be no difference between arterial pressure in the carotid and the vertebral circulations because normally the circle of Willis equilibrates pressures.

Clinical Correlation

1 If anastomotic connections in the circle of Willis are inefficient because of congenital variations or atherosclerosis, pressure in each system may fluctuate independently of that in the other.

2 Stenosis of an artery alters pressure, velocity of flow, and volume of flow through that vessel. While the results of stenosis depend to a large extent upon the availability of alternate channels by which blood can bypass an obstruction, it must be recognized that the effects of a single donut-shaped or diaphragm-like constriction are different from those of long segments of narrowing and those of multiple stenoses within the course of a single artery. These effects will be considered in detail in Chaps. 10 and 13.

Microcirculation of the Brain

The terminal branches of the anterior, middle, and posterior cerebral arteries interconnect with one another through leptomeningeal anastomoses in such a way that blood may shunt through them as well as around the base of the brain via the circle of Willis.

From these large surface conducting arteries an interconnecting series of small distributing arteries ramifies over the surface of the brain, sending off arteries and arterioles that penetrate the brain to varying depths before dividing into terminal capillary networks for nutrition of the gray and white matter (Fig. 5-1). The capillary density is much greater in the gray matter (cortex and deep nuclei, comprising about 60 percent of brain weight) than in the white matter. The gray matter also receives three to five times as much blood as the white matter—undoubtedly because the cell bodies of the neurons contained in the gray matter need more blood to maintain cell metabolism than their axons and dendrites which constitute the bulk of the white

matter. In the cortex, layers 3, 4, and 5 (which contain the densest cell populations and have the highest metabolic rate) have the richest capillary networks.

Because the anastomotic intercapillary network within the substance of the brain is ineffective, occlusion of an arteriole is almost always accompanied by death of the tissues that it supplies. Although action of the arterioles normally maintains constant pressure and flow through the capillary network, there are many diseases that can alter this situation.

The anatomic configuration of the microcirculation varies in different regions of brain parenchyma (Fig. 5-2). In the archipallium the ar-

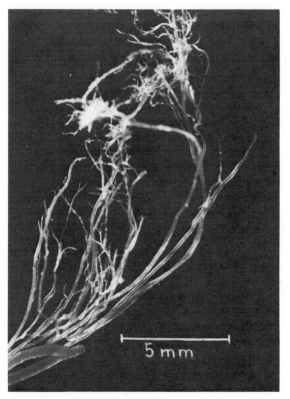

Figure 5-1 Corrosion preparation of the lenticulostriate group of arteries in a human brain showing penetrating arteries and arterioles.

teriolar network is sparse and poorly differentiated. Within the neopallium the inter-relation among arterioles, capillaries, and neurons is much more complicated and the vascularization is much richer. It is suspected that periodic constriction and dilatation occur in the closely approximated arteriole and venule

(A)

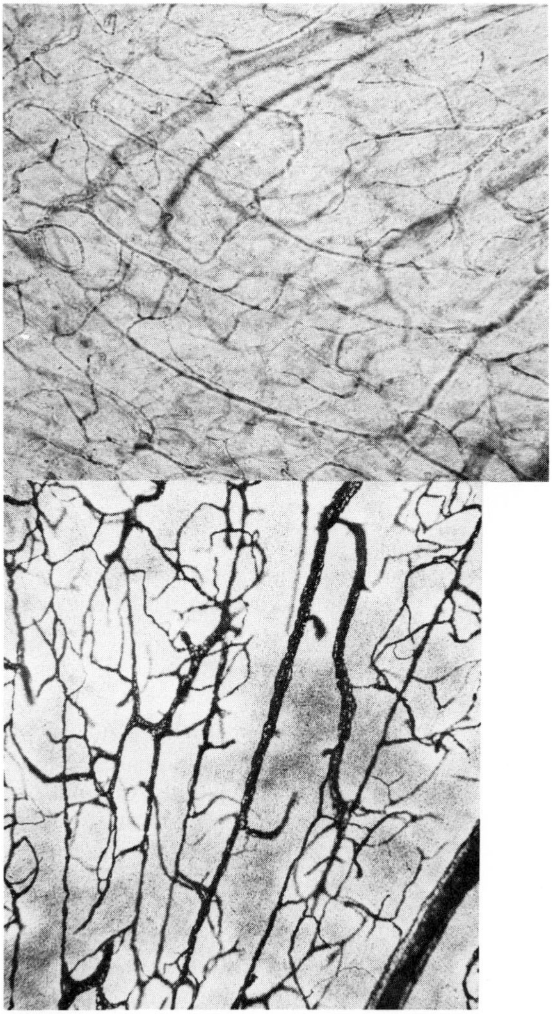

(B)

Figure 5-2 Photographs of the microcirculatory system in the cerebral cortex (A) and subcortex (B). (Metallic impregnation method.)

which, through their capillary network, serve a microcolumn of brain cells. In the aggregate, this change in caliber results in periodic increases and decreases in the flow of blood through various portions of the brain parenchyma—vasomotion.

This close approximation of the arteriole and venule may serve an important physiological function by permitting venous levels of CO_2, lactic acid, and histamine and the temperature of the venous effluent to be transmitted to the arteriole, providing it with the feedback necessary to allow it to regulate arteriolar inflow into the capillary beds.

Laminar Flow Blood flow is laminar in all arteries and veins, with blood flowing more slowly at the edge close to the walls of the vascular tube than at the center of the stream. In the major arteries the plasma and cellular constituents remain well mixed; but in the smaller vessels, such as arterioles and capillaries, the cellular elements are carried in the fast-flowing center and clear plasma can be seen next to the vessel walls. Streaming is pronounced, and in capillary branches which take off from the parent vessel at an appropirate angle, skimming results in lower ratios of red blood cells to plasma.

The red blood cells are normally carried through the arterioles and venules as a solid, closely packed column. At the capillary level the red blood cells are larger than the lumen and, consequently, assume an oblong shape.

Clinical Correlation

1 Irregularities on the lumen of arteries or arterioles disturb the laminar flow, and the resulting turbulence may lead to further changes within the vessel wall.

2 In some hematologic disorders, red blood cells may form into aggregates which interfere with their ability to travel through the capillary system. Sickle-cell anemia is one such disorder.

Autoregulation An arteriole is an endothelium-lined muscular tube which constricts against distending pressure in order to maintain constant capillary pressure and flow despite fluctuations in blood pressure (Bayliss effect). Since systemic pressure is continually changing, the caliber of the arteriole is constantly being readjusted. Furthermore, the arteriole responds to changes in metabolism of the cells it serves, adding a second governor to the regulation of arteriolar flow. Most investigators believe the control mechanism is the result of diffuse change in tone along the length of the arteriole, but some attribute it to Rouget cells (pericytes), which are located in the metarterioles and which act as precapillary sphincters.

Effects of Brain Metabolism Metabolism of the tissues served by the arteriole has a profound effect on blood flow within the vessel. Neuronal activity, for example, causes carbon dioxide, heat, and metabolites to accumulate in the local tissues. These products find their way to the venous capillaries and are eventually carried off; but first they cause arteriolar dilatation and increase of blood flow.

Clinical Correlation This phenomenon is dramatically demonstrated in focal convulsions.

When groups of neurons become active—e.g., when the lateral geniculate bodies or the visual cortex receive impulses from the retina, or when the motor cortex is stimulated to move an extremity—local P_{O_2} and glucose are decreased and P_{CO_2} and other metabolites accumulate, causing an increase of blood flow through that area of the brain.

Because the brain does not store glucose in any quantity and cannot shift to an effective anaerobic cycle, if blood flow is cut off even for 10 sec, neuron activity is impaired, lactic acid is produced, and soon the tissue ceases to function. Neurons and supporting glia remain alive but functionless for as long as 30 min before cellular death occurs. If blood flow is impaired but not completely cut off, neurons may be functionless but viable for 6 to 8 hr—rarely up to 48 hr.

When metabolism in brain tissue increases, blood flow also increases in order to satisfy tissue requirements for oxygen and glucose and to carry away heat, CO_2, and metabolites such as lactic acid, histamine, and water.

Arterioles dilate in response to an increase in hydrogen ions, including lactic acid. This effect occurs whether blood flowing through surrounding extracellular fluid is altered or not. As a consequence, one can imagine that blood flow through the millions of arterioles which serve the billions of cellular groups is constantly in a state of flux. When a finger moves or an iris changes in diameter, flow through the cellular elements controlling the involved muscles must alter. During convulsions, this response to lactic acid and hydrogen ions is carried to dangerous extremes because acid metabolites overwhelm the arterioles, producing maximal dilatation and hyperemia of the brain. The normal autoregulatory response of arterioles to changes in arterial pressure is overcome so that tissue perfusion fluctuates directly with changes in arterial pressure. Cortical hyperemia is so pronounced that oxygenated venous blood can be seen flowing from the site.

Clinical Correlation

1 When arterial or tissue P_{CO_2} or lactic acid is increased, cerebral blood flow increases, even if arterial pressure remains constant. Any increase in arterial pressure will be transmitted directly into the arteriolar-capillary network to create a dangerous increase in perfusion pressure. If arterial pressure falls, perfusion does also.

2 The possibility that restoration of flow during the interval between loss of neuron activity and tissue death might restore function is the basis for therapy of the evolving cerebral infarction. The clinical state of the patient during this time depends upon the area of the brain involved. For example, a large area in the nondominant hemisphere may become ischemic without causing any detectable abnormality; but if blood supply to a *small* area of mesencephalic gray matter in the upper brainstem is interrupted, coma ensues within 15 sec. Throughout our lives we hold a most tenuous link with consciousness.

Effects of Carbon Dioxide and Oxygen Although the tone of the cerebral arterioles is not modified by neural reflex, it is exquisitely responsive to variations in carbon dioxide tension in the arterial blood (Pa_{CO_2}). This tension is maintained normally at a pressure of about 40 torr. In the range of 20 to 55 torr each unit of change alters cerebral blood flow by about 1 ml per 100 Gm per min. When a person exhales excessive quantities of carbon dioxide, his Pa_{CO_2} may fall as low as 15 to 20 torr; cerebral vasoconstriction results and may reduce blood flow by 75 percent. The results of this reactive constriction can be seen in the electroencephalogram as diffuse slowing of brain rhythms. In the anxious individual who overbreathes at rest (hyperventilation syndrome) severe respiratory alkalosis can develop, leading to loss of consciousness and, in some cases, convulsions. Labored breathing following exercise does not produce cerebral vasoconstriction because muscle contraction results in the accumulation of lactate and carbon dioxide in the blood.

When a person inhales carbon dioxide mixed with air or when pulmonary disease prevents exhalation of the carbon dioxide normally produced by body metabolism, cerebral vasodilatation results and may increase blood flow by as much as 50 percent. In these situations, respiratory acidosis overcomes the intrinsic autoregulatory capacity of the cerebral vessels, causing intense vasodilatation and sometimes transudation of fluid. This leads to cerebral edema and increased intracranial pressure. Clinically this condition is seen in patients whose respiratory mechanics are impaired by obesity (Pickwickian syndrome), musculoskeletal diseases, and pulmonary diseases such as emphysema and alveolar capillary block.

Generally speaking, the effects of too much or too little oxygen are the opposite of those described for carbon dioxide. Arterial P_{O_2} is normally about 75 to 80 torr, while jugular venous P_{O_2} is about 34 torr. Oxygen tension in tissue is somewhat less than that in the capillaries because oxygen must diffuse from the blood through the capillary wall into the tissue surrounding it.

Although hypoxia results in some vasodilatation, this is seldom adequate to maintain constant oxygenation. Vasodilatation is maximal at an arterial P_{O_2} of about 25 torr. Consciousness is lost when the arterial P_{O_2} falls to 18 torr.

When supplementary oxygen is given to patients with deficient pulmonary gas exchange, the effect may be to depress respiration, thus causing a decrease in the exchange of oxygen and carbon dioxide. The resultant accumulation of carbon dioxide in the bloodstream may lead to carbon dioxide narcosis. The administration of oxygen to people with *normal* pulmonary exchange causes a slight increase in the volume of oxygen dissolved in the plasma. If oxygen pressure is increased as much as 3 atm, a much larger volume of O_2 is carried to the brain; but hyperoxia is toxic to the neurones and interferes with function.

Effects of Pharmacologic Agents Because of autoregulation, cerebral arterioles respond only indirectly to agents affecting systemic arterial blood pressure. Most drugs do not act directly upon the cerebral arteries but alter systemic arterial pressure by acting on vascular beds in other parts of the body. Some agents have a weak effect on the cerebral bed, but their effect on the systemic arterial pressure is so strong that it overshadows the cerebral effects. Only a few medications have been shown to have a clinically significant effect on the cerebral arteries and arterioles, and there is growing suspicion that some of these affect carotid and vertebral-basilar beds differently. Hypercapnia, hypoxia, and drugs such as papaverine and acetazolamide are all cerebral vasodilators of varying effectiveness. Many drugs marketed as cerebral vasodilators (e.g., nicotinic acid, pentylenetetrazol, and papaverine) have an extremely weak activity or have such profound effects on systemic vascular beds that their action in the vessels of the central nervous system is overshadowed. The net result may be that brain blood flow may be impaired rather than enhanced by their use. Both nicotinic acid and alcohol, for example, have at most a weak action on brain arteries but cause profound systemic vasodilatation. The result may be local or generalized reductions in cerebral perfusion pressure and flow. Aminophylline and propanolol (beta-adrenergic blocker) have a cerebral vasoconstrictor effect. Investigation of the effects of pharmacologic agents on the different cerebrovascular beds is in its infancy, and work on the alpha- and beta-adrenergic properties of cerebral vessels is badly needed.

It must be remembered also that the effect of pharmacologic agents upon diseased cerebral vessels may be quite different from the effects of these agents on normal arteries. In generalized cerebral atherosclerosis the arteries may be transformed from their normal supple, responsive state into rigid pipes which serve merely as conduits for the passage of blood. Such vessels may no longer be capable of responding to any agent, even carbon dioxide or oxygen. Hypertension and hypotension are also without effect on the vasomotor tone of sclerotic vessels. In such cases, abnormal elevations of blood pressure may be transmitted to the arterioles and capillaries, causing them to rupture, while even moderate hypotension may lead to profound ischemia and sometimes infarction.

Hydrostatic Effects Because gravity affects the columns of arterial and venous blood which interconnect the heart and brain, the hydrostatic force necessary to maintain a constant capillary perfusion pressure within the brain depends upon the position of the head in relation to the heart. When the head and the heart are on the same level, the arterial pressures within the circle of Willis and the middle cerebral artery, and presumably in the vertebral-basilar system, are all about equal to systemic arterial blood pressure. In the upright position, the hydrostatic effect of gravity ($+1\ g_z$) reduces pressure in the cerebral arteries by about 20 percent; but in a person doing a head stand, hydrostatic effects are reversed ($-1\ g_z$) and pressure in the arteries of the brain is increased (Fig. 5-3).

Cerebrospinal fluid pressure is similarly affected by gravity and acts to counterbalance variations in brain circulation that would otherwise be produced by postural changes. In the erect position, cerebrospinal fluid pressure is subatmospheric at the vertex of the cranial cavity and is nil at the cisterna magna. At the lumbar subarachnoid level the pressure is equal to that of a column of cerebrospinal fluid rising to the cisterna magna. The pressure of the spinal fluid on spinal arteries and veins is minimized to a degree by the subatmospheric pressure in the cranial cavity which tends to suspend the weight of the spinal fluid column. This protective mechanism does not operate when there is a defect in the cranial vault. In the horizontal position, spinal fluid pressure is the same at all levels of the cerebrospinal fluid system, and standing on one's head ($-1\ g_z$) reverses the pressure gradients.

During acceleration when aviators are exposed to high forces of $+3$ to $+6\ g_z$ the ability of the cerebral and peripheral vascular beds to accommodate the change in pressure is overcome, and the result is cerebrovascular insufficiency. Similar reactions are sometimes produced by the hydrostatic effect of standing upright in patients with abnormal cerebral or peripheral circulatory reflexes. If the systemic

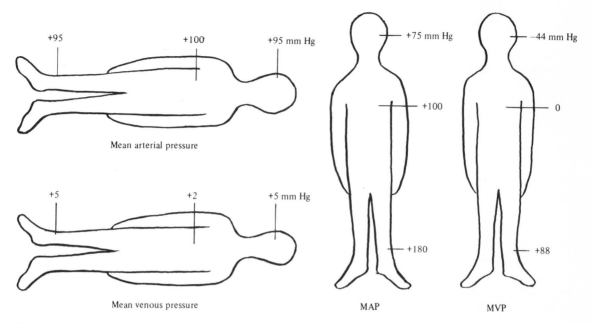

Figure 5-3

reflexes are impaired, blood may pool in the legs when the person stands motionless. In such cases pressure and flow to the head and eyes is reduced, even though cardiac output may be normal or high.

The first evidence of cerebrovascular insufficiency is fading of peripheral vision (called "gray-out" and interpreted by patients as blurred vision, "swimmy" vision, a veil, or haze), during which only macular or central vision remains. If perfusion pressure falls further, central vision is lost as well, and "blackout" results. At this stage of cephalic hypotension, the subject is blind but conscious with hearing intact, and the electroencephalogram shows normal brain rhythms. With further hypotension, cerebral circulatory stasis leads to hypoxia and loss of consciousness after about 10 sec of euphoria during which sounds become distant and muffled. Simultaneously, the electroencephalogram shows a slowing of brain rhythms.

Loss of vision precedes impairment of consciousness because intraocular pressure against the retinal arterioles and veins is 16 to 20 mm Hg. This means that pressure in the central artery of the retina is always less than that in the other cerebral arteries even though all are supplied by the internal carotid artery. Mean arterial pressure is normally about 60 to 70 mm Hg in the ophthalmic artery and about 80 to 90 mm Hg in the cerebral arteries. If intraocular pressure is normal, peripheral vision fades when the mean arterial pressure falls quickly to about 40 mm Hg, and at 20 mm Hg central vision disappears. In glaucomatous eyes, because of the elevated ocular pressure, even less reduction in the arterial pressure is required to produce loss of vision.

Effects of Neural Reflexes   Autonomic nerve fibers surround the carotid and vertebral arteries and their intracranial branches and form a dense plexus. Fibers follow the penetrating arteries into the substance of the brain and can be found in arterioles 20 μ in diameter. Their function is not known, although some authorities believe that they serve a vasoregulatory function.

It has already been pointed out that the ability of cerebral arteries and arterioles to regulate themselves is probably an intrinsic one, governed by the response of the muscularis to changes in arterial pressure and in the content of oxygen and carbon dioxide. This regulatory ability maintains a constant flow of blood through the brain and permits redistribution of blood within the brain in response to local metabolic requirements. There is some evidence to suggest that vasoregulatory neural fibers assist with this regional redistribution, and some investigators hypothesize that they play a major role in overall regulation. Parasympathetic dilator fibers pass from the facial nerve to the plexus surrounding the internal carotid artery via the greater superficial petrosal nerve.

The stellate, middle, and upper cervical sympathetic plexuses evidently contribute only a weak constrictor effect. Blocking the cervical sympathetics in normal people has no effect on brain blood flow; yet the diffuse vasospasm which may occur in some clinical states—e.g., embolism—may conceivably be mediated by overreaction of the sympathetic plexus to a foreign body in the arterial system.

The carotid sinus is uniquely innervated with mechanoreceptors whose function is to maintain blood pressure within a narrow range in the carotid and cerebral arteries. These pressoreceptors send impulses to medullary vasoregulatory centers via the glossopharyngeal nerve. In these centers they mediate two and possibly three reflex responses: (1) slowing of the heart action via the vagus; (2) systemic vasodilatation mediated through the thoracolumbar sympathetic nerves and leading to a fall in systemic blood pressure; and (3) possibly a primary cerebral vasoconstrictory reflex via sympathetic nerves

of the carotid system. External massage or compression over the normal sinus can elicit at least the first two of these reflex responses.

If the glossopharyngeal nerve is severed, the resultant effect on the regulatory tonus of the carotid sinus leads to an immediate, though transient, rise in systemic blood pressure. A steady state returns when the tonus of the sinus on the opposite side asserts itself.

Further investigations are needed to elucidate the effect, if any, of neural regulation of cerebral vasomotor tone.

Effect of Intracranial Pressure

The brain is encased within a bony cavity. Its specific gravity is somewhat greater than that of the cerebrospinal fluid which envelops it. In the erect position it hangs suspended from the veins that connect it to the dura, delicately poised upon the arteries and the bony structures below.

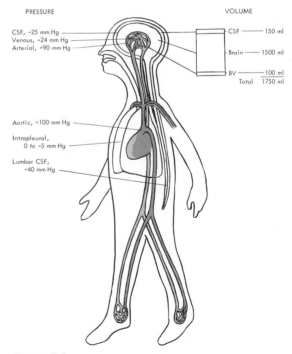

Figure 5-4

With each systole a pulse of blood courses through the cerebral arteries, transmitting an impulse to the brain and possibly increasing its volume somewhat. Under normal conditions, the brain itself probably distends little, if at all, because venous blood leaves the parenchyma as arterial blood enters. The amount of blood within the intracranial arteries and veins at any one time is normally between 50 and 100 ml. If for any reason the volume of blood in the brain changes, there must be a concomitant readjustment in the volume of the cerebrospinal fluid; otherwise, pressure within the skull will be altered because the brain is not compressible (Munro-Kellie doctrine) (Fig. 5-4).

Clinical Correlation Because skin overlying bony defects in the skull is seen to pulsate as the volume of blood in the cranium increases with each systole it is thought that the brain also pulsates.

Effect of Cerebrovascular Resistance

Cerebrovascular resistance (CVR) which depends chiefly on the resistivity of the cerebral arteriolar-capillary network and the resistance of the blood itself to flow through this tubular system can be calculated by the following equation:

$$CVR = \frac{perfusion\ pressure*}{cerebral\ blood\ flow}$$

Fluctuations in intracranial pressure affect the vascular bed and contribute to cerebrovascular resistance. In man, CVR approximates 1.6 mm Hg, which is the pressure required to force 1 ml of blood through 100 Gm of brain tissue in 1 min.

Clinical Correlation

1 If intracranial pressure is elevated, the brain is compressed, and resistance to flow is increased.

* Mean arterial pressure minus mean venous pressure.

2 Elevation of cerebrospinal fluid pressure increases cerebrovascular resistance and can result in decreased cerebral blood flow.

3 Tumors that prevent free communication along the subarachnoid pathways raise the cerebrospinal fluid pressure and alter the relationships of brain mass, cerebral blood, and cerebrospinal fluid volumes.

4 Intracranial tumors may cause edema of the brain by compressing cerebral veins. If they grow to sufficient size, the capacity for intracranial compensation is surpassed, and intracranial pressure rises. This increase in pressure may be so great that it compresses venous outflow and causes transudation of fluid, further swelling of cerebral tissue, and a cycle of accelerating increase in intracranial pressure.

5 Hydrocephalus can compress the brain from within, transmitting pressure to the capillaries and reducing blood flow.

6 In cerebral infarction and intracranial tumors, compression of the brain may cause loss of the autoregulatory capacity with vasomotor paralysis.

7 During occlusion, distal segments of an artery dilate to their maximum capacity. When obstruction is removed, reactive hyperemia floods the previously ischemic tissue with arterial blood. If the ability of the tissue to extract oxygen from this blood is exceeded, the venous outflow may contain oxygenated (red) blood—so-called luxury perfusion.

THE VENOUS SYSTEM

Cerebral venous pressure varies enormously, depending upon the position of the head in relation to the rest of the body. Understanding the effects of change in body position requires a detailed knowledge of the venous anatomy. Four points are essential for our purposes here:

1 The cortical veins are collapsible and are surrounded by cerebrospinal fluid.

2 The dural sinuses are rigid and noncollapsible, and their intraluminal pressure is not dependent upon changes in cerebrospinal fluid pressure.

3 The jugular veins are compressible and are exposed to external pressures.

4 The point at which change in body position does *not* cause alteration in venous pressure (the hydrostatic indifference point) is in the superior vena cava.

Because they are distensible, the cortical veins act as a capacitance system which can expand or reduce its blood pool. Because the rigid dural sinuses do not have this capacity, the response of the brain blood pool to changes in intracranial pressure and to compression of the jugular vein is dependent on changes in the quantity of blood in the cortical veins. Impairment of venous outflow distends cortical veins, expanding the brain blood pool by 10 to 15 percent; this mechanism is responsible for the increase in cerebrospinal fluid pressure that follows compression of the jugular veins.

Recumbent Position

When a person lies flat, his head is level with the superior vena cava and the right atrium, and the venous pressure gradients decrease progressively from the cortical veins (+3 mm Hg) through the dural sinuses and to the jugular veins and the right atrium (0 to −3 mm Hg). This gradient is not static but varies with phases of cardiac and respiratory cycles. During systole, atrial pressure rises and is transmitted into the brachiocephalic venous system, slowing cerebral venous return. During diastole, flow accelerates.

Respiration causes more complex changes in venous pressures because cerebrospinal fluid and cortical venous pressures are dependent upon pressures in the cerebrospinal fluid column and in the vertebral veins. During quiet inspiration the diaphragm descends, the viscera are compressed, and the outflow of venous blood from the vertebral veins is reduced; at the same time, however, outflow of blood from the cranial cavity is increased. Pressure in the rigid dural sinuses is reduced during inspiration, possibly creating negative pressures which draw blood from the capacitance (cortical) veins of the brain. During expiration jugular venous flow decreases and outflow from the vertebral veins increases.

Two results of this "see-saw" effect are (1) a tendency for cerebrospinal fluid to be pumped back and forth between the cranial and the spinal cavities and (2) diversion of venous blood up and down through the rich system of veins in the spinal canal and cranial cavities. The capacity of the cortical veins is two to three times that of the arterial system, so that they may expand and collapse with ease during the various phases of the respiratory cycle. Furthermore, even though the veins lack muscle fibers, it is suspected that they may have a valvelike action which produces a one-way system from brain to dural sinuses.

The arrival of an arterial pulse within the cranial cavity temporarily increases intracranial pressure and tends to squeeze blood from the cortical veins into the dural sinuses. Consequently, intracranial venous pulsations are synchronous with pulsations of the retinal veins within the hydraulic system of the eye.

The dural sinuses and the cortical veins also have a neural network, but its function is unknown. There is no information concerning the existence of pressure sensors in the cerebral venous system. Some authorities, however, suspect that the glomus jugulare might have such a function.

Upright Position

When one stands up, pressure in the jugular veins, the dural sinuses, and the cortical veins becomes negative, but the pressure gradient in the system remains unchanged. At the same time, pressure in the cerebrospinal fluid becomes negative at the vertex. If the intraluminal pressure created by venous blood were not greater than that of the cerebrospinal fluid, the cortical veins would collapse and blood would cease to flow.

Head-Down Position

When one is standing on one's head, cerebral venous pressure becomes so high that the delicate cortical veins would probably rupture if it were not for the fact that the cerebrospinal fluid pressure at the vertex becomes equally high, so that the transmural venous pressure is balanced. The mechanism responsible for the return of blood from the dependent cranial cavity into the jugular veins and right atrium is more complex; and, in fact, the return of blood from the head to the heart when the body is upside down appears physiologically impossible. The fact that it occurs leads one to conclude that more research is needed on the subject. The pooling of blood in the venous system is manifested by engorgement of the extracranial portions of this system: a feeling of fullness develops, the eyes bulge, and the face turns dusky red. During inspiration, blood is sucked into the chest cavity; but because the jugular veins have no valves, this is a relatively inefficient system.

Clinical Correlation

1 Because pressure within the jugular veins low in the neck is subatmospheric during diastole, venous blood from the skull is drawn into these veins. If they are severed, blood oozes from them during systole; but during diastole, the negative pressure may cause air to be sucked into them, creating an air embolism in the right atrium and ventricle.

2 If the jugular veins are ligated, the resultant increase in venous pressure is transmitted back into the capillaries of the brain, sometimes causing transudations of fluid, cerebral edema, and increased intracranial pressure. This effect rarely occurs when only one jugular vein is ligated and seldom causes clinical abnormalities even when both are occluded.

3 During high $+g_z$ acceleration, pressure in the jugular veins is greatly reduced. The suction

effect thus created may draw blood from the arterioles and capillary beds into the venous circulation.

MEASUREMENT OF CEREBRAL BLOOD FLOW

Anatomic and pathological changes in the large arteries and veins (dilatations, obstructions, and unusual configurations or anomalies) can be visualized by arteriography, and the transit time of opaque material through the system can be determined. However, angiography gives only indirect information about the microcirculation where metabolic exchange actually takes place. It is estimated, for example, that only 10 percent of the total arterial and venous circulation is visualized (Fig. 5-5). For this reason, measurements of total and regional cerebral blood flow have been enormously valuable in providing physiologic information about the cerebral circulation in healthy persons. Their application to the investigation of disease states has been only experimental, and they are not currently used in the care of patients.

Cerebral blood flow can be determined by the following equation:

$$CBF = \frac{MABP - CVP}{CVR}$$

where CBF = cerebral blood flow
MABP = mean arterial blood pressure (the diastolic plus half the pulse pressure)
CVP = cerebral venous pressure
CVR = cerebral vascular resistance

The basic principle underlying all studies for regional and total cerebral blood flow through the intact skull is that the quantity of a substance taken up by the brain in a unit of time is equal to the product of the blood flow through the organ and the difference between the arterial and the venous concentration of that sub-

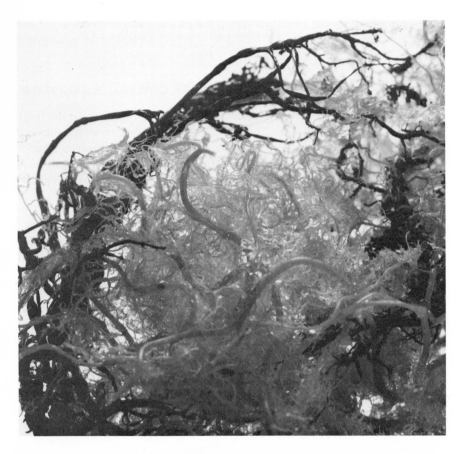

Figure 5-5 Only the larger arteries and veins within this tangled skein are visible with angiography.

stance. This principle can be expressed in the following equation:

$$t = \frac{Q_t}{C_a - C_v}$$

where t = flow in time
          Q_t = quantity of substance taken up in time
          C_a = concentration of substance in arterial blood
          C_v = concentration of substance in venous blood

Unlike most organs of the body that excrete identifiable metabolites, most of the brain secretes thought and action, which cannot be used as an end point for measuring cerebral blood flow or metabolism. Since the brain does absorb gases such as nitrous oxide and krypton, arteriovenous differences can be measured by the radioactivity of tagged isotopes, and this measurement can be used as an index of cerebral blood flow. Flow is expressed in terms of milliliters per 100 Gm of tissue per min, and total flow measurements are based on the supposition that the

Table 5-1 Physiologic and Pathologic States Involving Alterations in Cerebrovascular Resistance and Blood Flow

	Mean arterial blood pressure, mm Hg	Cerebral blood flow, cc/100 Gm/min	Cerebral O_2 consumption, cc/100 Gm/min	Cerebrovascular resistance, mm Hg/cc/100 Gm/min
Normal	85	54	3.3	1.6
Hyperventilation	98	34	3.7	2.9
CO_2 (5–7%)	93	93	3.3	1.1
O_2 (85–100%)	98	45	3.2	2.2
O_2 (10%)	78	73	3.2	1.1
Increased intracranial pressure	118	34	2.8	3.5
Primary polycythemia	108	25	3.0	4.3
Anemia	78	79	3.3	1.0
Cerebral arteriosclerosis	121	41	2.8	3.0
Cerebral hemangioma	75	164	3.3	0.5
Essential hypertension	159	54	3.4	3.0

Reproduced by permission of S. S. Kety, Circulation and metabolism of the human brain in health and disease, *Am. J. Med.*, **8**:205, 1950, p. 207.

average adult brain weighs 1,500 Gm. The measurements for total cerebral blood flow in a variety of conditions are given in Table 5-1.

Measurements of regional cerebral blood flow have demonstrated that flow through gray matter is about 80 ml per 100 Gm per min; flow through white matter is about 25 ml per 100 Gm per min. There is evidence to suggest that flow through the frontal lobes is greater during mental activity than during rest and that flow through the parietooccipital region is increased during the performance of mental arithmetic (a function normally residing in the parietal region). Surprisingly enough, total cerebral flow increases during sleep. During coma induced by most general anesthetics cerebral blood flow is decreased. For example, nitrous oxide 70 percent decreases cerebral blood flow to about 40 ml per 100 Gm of tissue per min and cyclopropane 5 percent to 26 ml per 100 Gm of tissue per min. Halothane and diethyl ether reduce cerebral blood flow the least, and thiopental has the most shocking effect of reduction to about 27 ml per 100 Gm of tissue per min.

Clinical Correlation

1 If regional cerebral blood flow (rCBF) in the frontal temporal region is reduced by more than 25 percent during clamping of the internal carotid at the time of operation, some degree of hemiparesis results.

2 Measurements of cerebral blood flow give a better indication of the microcirculation of the brain than measurements of flow through the proximal arteries. Measurements of rCBF, however, usually show significant increase following reconstruction of the carotid arteries.

SUGGESTED READINGS

General

Kety, S. S.: "The cerebral circulation," in Handbook of Physiology, vol. 3, Neurophysiology, American Physiology Society, Washington, D.C., 1960, p. 1751.

Luyendijk, W. (ed.): "Cerebral circulation," in Progress in Brain Research, vol. 30, Elsevier Publishing Company, New York, 1968.

Meyer, J. S., and Schade, J. P. (eds.): "Cerebral blood flow," in Progress in Brain Research, vol. 35, Elsevier Publishing Company, Amsterdam, 1972.

Naumenko, A. I., and Benua, N. N.: The Physiological Mechanisms of Cerebral Blood Circulation, Charles C Thomas, Publisher, Springfield, Ill., 1970.

Schmidt, C. F.: The Cerebral Circulation in Health and Disease, Charles C Thomas, Publisher, Springfield, Ill., 1950.

Sokoloff, L.: Aspects of cerebral circulatory physiology of relevance to cerebrovascular disease, *Neurology,* **11**(4)(part 2):34, 1961.

Wells, C. E.: The cerebral circulation: The clinical significance of current concepts, *Arch. Neurol.,* **3**:319, 1960.

Effects of Systemic Factors

Cardiac Output

Shapiro, W., and Chawla, N. P.: Observations on the regulation of cerebral blood flow in complete heart block, *Circulation,* **40**:863, 1969.

Arterial Pressure

Adams, J. H., Brierley, J. B., Connor, R. C. R., and Treip, C. S.: The effects of systemic hypertension upon human brain. Clinical and neuropathological observations in 11 cases, *Brain,* **89**:235, 1966.

Agnoli, A., Fieschi, G., Bozzao, L., Battistini, N., and Prencipe, M.: Autoregulation of cerebral blood flow. Studies during drug-induced hypertension in normal subjects and in patients with cerebral vascular diseases, *Circulation,* **38**:800, 1968.

Bevan, A. T., Honour, A. J., and Stott, F. H.: Direct arterial pressure recording in unrestricted man, *Clin. Sci.,* **36**:329, 1969.

Carlyle, A., and Grayson, J.: Blood pressure and the regulation of brain blood flow, *J. Physiol. London,* **127**:15P, 1955.

Gross, M.: Diurnal blood pressure variations in cerebrovascular disease, *Ann. Internal Med.,* **72**:823, 1970.

Himwich, W. A., and Spurgeon, H. A.: Pulse pressure contours in cerebral arteries, *Acta neurol. scand.,* **44**:43, 1968.

Pulmonary Mechanics

Comroe, J. H.: Physiology of Respiration; An Introductory Text, Year Book Medical Publishers, Inc., Chicago, 1965.

————, Forster, R. E., DuBois, A. B., Briscoe, W. A., and Carlsen, E.: The Lung: Clinical Physiology and Pulmonary Function Tests, Year Book Medical Publishers, Inc., Chicago, 1962.

Fazekas, J. F., McHenry, L. C., Jr., Alman, R. W., and Sullivan, J. F.: Cerebral hemodynamics during brief hyperventilation, *Arch. Neurol.,* **4**:132, 1961.

Klein, L. J., Saltzman, H. A., Heyman, A., and Sieker, H. O.: Syncope induced by Valsalva maneuver: A study of the effects of arterial blood gas tensions, glucose concentration, and blood pressure, *Am. J. Med.,* **37**:263, 1964.

Meyer, J. S., Gotoh, F., Takagi, Y., and Kakimi, R.: Cerebral hemodynamics, blood gases, and electrolytes during breath-holding and the Valsalva maneuver, *Circulation,* **33**–**34**(suppl. 2):35, 1966.

Walsh, R. E., Michaelson, E. D., Harkleroad, L. E., Zighelboim, A., and Sackner, M. A.: Upper airway obstruction in obese patients with sleep disturbance and somnolence, *Ann. Internal Med.,* **76**:185, 1972.

Arterial System

Adolph, R. J., Fukusumi, H., and Fowler, N. O.: Origin of cerebrospinal fluid pulsations, *Am. J. Physiol.,* **212**:840, 1967.

Cervicocranial Arteries

Fieschi, C., Garello, L., and Salan, A.: Comparative angiographic and radioisotopic study of the vertebro-basilar circulation, *Acta radiol. (diagn.),* **2**:41, 1964.

Hardesty, W. H., Roberts, B., Toole, J. F., and Royster, H. P.: Studies of carotid-artery blood flow in man, *New Engl. J. Med.,* **263**:944, 1960.

————, Whitacre, W. B., Toole, J. F., Randall, P., and Royster, H. P.: Studies on vertebral artery blood flow in man, *Surg. Gynecol. Obstet.,* **116**:662, 1963.

Kuhn, R.: The speed of cerebral circulation, *New Engl. J. Med.,* **267**:689, 1962.

McDonald, D. A., and Potter, J. M.: The distribution of blood to the brain, *J. Physiol.,* **114**:356, 1951.

Potter, J. M.: Redistribution of blood to the brain due to localized cerebral arterial spasm: The possible importance of the small peripheral anastomotic cerebral arteries, *Brain,* **82**:367, 1959.

Microcirculation of the Brain

Kennady, J. C., and Taplin, G. V.: Shunting in cerebral microcirculation, *Am. Surgeon,* **33**:763, 1967.

Rosenblum, W. I.: Cerebral microcirculation: A review emphasizing the interrelationship of local blood flow and neuronal function, *Angiology,* **16**:485, 1965.

Rowbotham, G. F., and Little, E.: A new concept of the circulation and the circulations of the brain: The discovery of surface arteriovenous shunts, *Brit. J. Surg.,* **52**:539, 1965.

Autoregulation

Altura, B. M.: Evaluation of neurohumoral substances in local regulation of blood flow, *Am. J. Physiol.,* **212**:1447, 1967.

Fujishima, M., Busto, R., Scheinberg, P., and Reinmuth, O. M.: Metabolic mechanisms in autoregulation of cerebral blood flow, *Neurology,* **20**:374, 1970.

Fulton, J. F.: Observations upon the vascularity of the human occipital lobe during visual activity, *Brain,* **51**:310, 1928.

Harper, A. M.: Autoregulation of cerebral blood flow: Influence of the arterial blood pressure on the blood flow through the cerebral cortex, *J. Neurol. Neurosurg. Psychiat.,* **29**:398, 1966.

———: Regulation of cerebral circulation, *Sci. Basis Med. Ann. Rev.,* 1969, pp. 60–81.

Jennett, W. B.: Experimental studies on the cerebral circulation: Clinical aspects, *Proc. Roy. Soc. Med.,* **61**:606, 1968.

Landau, W. M., Freygang, W. H., Rowland, L. P., Sokoloff, L., and Kety, S. S.: The local circulation of the living brain; values in the unanesthetized and anesthetized cat, *Trans. Am. Neurol. Assoc.,* **80**:125, 1955.

Lassen, N. A.: Autoregulation of cerebral blood flow, *Circulation Res.,* **15**(suppl. 1):201, 1964.

Meyer, J. S., and Marx, P.: Cerebral autoregulation and "dysautoregulation" and their relation to cerebral vascular symptoms, *Current Concepts Cerebrovascular Dis.—Stroke,* **6**:1, 1971.

Pálvölgyi, R.: Regional cerebral blood flow in patients with intracranial tumors, *J. Neurosurg.,* **31**:149, 1969.

Risberg, J., and Ingvar, D. H.: Regional changes in cerebral blood volume during mental activity, *Exptl. Brain Res.,* **5**:72, 1968.

Symon, L.: Experimental features and therapeutic implications of "intracerebral steal," *J. Neurol. Neurosurg. Psychiat.,* **32**:631, 1969.

Effects of Brain Metabolism

Posner, J. B., and Plum, F.: Independence of blood and cerebrospinal fluid lactate, *Arch. Neurol.,* **16**:492, 1967.

———, ———, and Zee, D.: Ventriculocisternal pH and cerebral blood flow, *Arch. Neurol.,* **20**:664, 1969.

Effects of Carbon Dioxide and Oxygen

Dunkin, R. S., and Bondurant, S.: The determinants of cerebrospinal fluid P_{O_2}: The effects of oxygen and carbon dioxide breathing in patients with chronic lung disease, *Ann. Internal Med.,* **64**:71, 1966.

Gotoh, F., Meyer, J. S., and Takagi, Y.: Cerebral effects of hyperventilation in man, *Arch. Neurol.,* **12**:410, 1965.

Lambertsen, C. J.: Medical implications of high oxygen pressures, *Trans. Stud. Coll. Physicians Philadelphia,* **33**:1, 1965.

Raichle, M. E., Posner, J. B., and Plum, F.: Cerebral blood flow during and after hyperventilation, *Arch. Neurol.,* **23**:394, 1970.

Schade, J. P., and McMenemey, W. H. (eds.): Selective Vulnerability of the Brain in Hypoxaemia, Blackwell Scientific Publications, Ltd., Oxford, 1963.

Woodbury, D. M., and Karler, R.: The role of carbon dioxide in the nervous system, *Anesthesiology,* **21**:686, 1960.

Effects of Pharmacological Agents

Barrett, R. E., Fraser, R. A. R., and Stein, B. M.: A fluorescence histochemical survey of monoaminergic innervation of cerebral blood vessels in primate and humans, *Trans. Am. Neurol. Assoc.,* **96**:39, 1971.

Karlsberg, P., Elliott, H. W., and Adams, J. E.: Effect of various pharmacologic agents on cerebral arteries, *Neurology,* **13**:772, 1963.

Sokoloff, L.: The action of drugs on cerebral circulation, *Pharmacol. Rev.,* **11**:1, 1959.

————, and Kety, S. S.: Regulation of cerebral circulation, *Physiol. Rev.,* **40**(suppl. 4):38, 1960.

To-day's Drugs: Cerebral vasodilators, *Brit. Med. J.,* 2:702, 1971.

Hydrostatic Effects

Patterson, J. L., Jr., and Warren, J. V.: Mechanisms of adjustment in the cerebral circulation upon assumption of the upright position, *J. Clin. Invest.,* **31**:653, 1952.

Physiology in the Space Environment, vol. I, circulation report of a study conducted by the Space Science Board of the National Academy of Sciences National Research Council 1966-67, National Academy of Sciences, Publication 1485 A, Washington, D.C., 1968.

Shenkin, H. A., Scheuerman, W. G., Spitz, E. B., and Groff, R. A.: Effect of change of position upon cerebral circulation of man, *J. Appl. Physiol.,* **2**:317, 1949.

Tindall, G. F., Craddock, A., and Greenfield, J. C., Jr.: Effects of the sitting position on blood flow in the internal carotid artery of man during general anesthesia, *J. Neurosurg.,* **26**:383, 1967.

Toole, J. F.: Effects of change of head, limb and body position on cephalic circulation, *New Engl. J. Med.,* **279**:307, 1968.

Effects of Neural Reflexes

Ask-Upmark, E.: The carotid sinus and the cerebral circulation: Anatomical, experimental, and clinical investigation, including some observations on rete mirabile caroticum, *Acta psychiat. neurol. scand., suppl.,* **6**:1, 1935.

Carrato-Ibanez, A., and Abadia-Fenoll, F.: Morphology and origin of the perivascular fibers into the brain substance, *Angiology,* **17**:771, 1966.

Fang, H. C.: Cerebral arterial innervations in man, *Arch. Neurol.,* **4**:651, 1961.

Heymans, C., and Neil, E.: Reflexogenic Areas of the Cardiovascular System, Little, Brown and Company, Boston, 1958.

Krog, J.: Autonomic nervous control of the cerebral blood flow in man, *J. Oslo City Hosp.,* **14**:25, 1964.

Linden, L.: The effect of stellate ganglion block on cerebral circulation in cerebrovascular accidents, *Acta med. scand.* 151 (suppl. 301) 1955.

Morgan-Hughes, J. A.: Cough seizures in patients with cerebral lesions, *Brit. Med. J.,* 2:494, 1966.

Rosenblum, W. I.: Cerebral arteriolar spasm inhibited by β-adrenergic blocking agents, *Arch. Neurol.,* **21**:296, 1969.

————: Neurogenic control of cerebral circulation, *Stroke,* **2**(5):429, 1971.

Effect of Intracranial Pressure

Brice, J. G., Dowsett, D. J., and Lowe, R. D.: The effect of constriction on carotid blood flow and pressure gradient, *Lancet,* **1**:84, 1964.

Fox, J. L.: Development of recent thoughts on intracranial pressure and the blood-brain barrier, *J. Neurosurg.,* **21**:909, 1964.

Greitz, T.: Effect of brain distention on cerebral circulation, *Lancet,* **1**:863, 1969.

Kety, S. S., Shenkin, H. A., and Schmidt, C. F.: Effects of increased intracranial pressure on cerebral circulatory functions in man, *J. Clin. Invest.,* **27**:493, 1948.

The Venous System

de Vlieger, M., Meijer, J. G., Krull, G. H., and de Clerck, D. E. P.: Influence of the venous system on movements in range of intracranial structures, *Neurology,* **19**:1051, 1969.

Eckenhoff, J. E.: The physiologic significance of the vertebral venous plexus, *Surg. Gynecol. Obstet.,* **131**:72, 1970.

Epstein, H. M., Linde, H. W., Crampton, A. R., Ciric, I. S., and Eckenhoff, J. E.: The vertebral venous plexus as a major cerebral venous outflow tract, *Anesthesiology,* **32**:332, 1970.

Hedges, T. R., and Weinstein, J. D.: Cerebrovascular responses to increased intracranial pressure, *J. Neurosurg.,* **21**:292, 1964.

Osterholm, J. L.: Reaction of the cerebral venous sinus system to acute intracranial hypertension, *J. Neurosurg.,* **32**:654, 1970.

Rapela, C. E., Machowicz, P., and Green, H. D.: Cerebral venous blood flow, *Federation Proc.,* **20**: 100, 1961.

Shenkin, H. N.: Air embolism from exposure of posterior cranial fossa in prone position, *J.A.M.A.,* **210**:726, 1969.

Measurement of Cerebral Blood Flow

"Cerebral blood flow; clinical and experimental results," in International Symposium on the Clinical Applications of Isotope Clearance Measurement of Cerebral Blood Flow, Mainz, 1969, edited by M. Brock, C. Fieschi, D. H. Ingvar, N. A. Lassen, and K. Schürmann, Springer-Verlag, Berlin, 1969.

Jensen, K. B., Høedt-Rasmussen, K., Sveinsdottir, E., and Lassen, N. A.: Regional cerebral blood flow determined by inhalation of xenon[133]. Summary of a methodological study, *Acta neurol. scand.*, **41**(suppl. 13)(part 1):309, 1965.

Lassen, N. A.: Cerebral blood flow and oxygen consumption in man, *Physiol. Rev.*, **39**:183, 1959.

McHenry, L. C., Jr.: Cerebral blood flow, *New Engl. J. Med.*, **274**:82, 1966.

Sapirstein, L. A.: Measurement of the cephalic and cerebral blood flow fractions of the cardiac output in man, *J. Clin. Invest.*, **41**(part 2):1429, 1962.

Skinhøj, E., Lassen, N. A., and Høedt-Rasmussen, K.: Cerebellar blood flow in man, *Arch. Neurol.*, **10**:464, 1964.

Chapter 6

Interview and Neurovascular Examination

Gentlemen, more mistakes are made, many more, by not looking than by not knowing.

Sir William Jenner

With all our varied instruments, useful as they are, nothing can replace the watchful eye, the alert ear, the tactful finger and the logical mind.

W. Keen

Interviewing patients with cerebrovascular disease is a subtle art, the goal of which is to extract an accurate history as rapidly as possible. Experienced clinicians assert that the patient's history gives the essential clues to diagnosis in 80 to 90 percent of cases, and one should allot at least half the time available at the initial examination to interviewing the patient and his family.

Defective memory and dysphasia caused by disease may make the task difficult, but the physician must never forget that an incomplete history is usually his own shortcoming, not the patient's; he has been trained in the art and the patient has not. The physician must ask his questions in terms that his patient can understand, must speak *to* him and not *about* him, and must always exhibit a warm and sympa-

72

thetic manner even under the most trying circumstances. Many a well-trained, thorough, and competent physician has made an incorrect diagnosis because he was so anxious to proceed with the neurologic examination that his impatient and condescending attitude caused his patient to give a perfunctory recitation.

INTERVIEW

The interview with the patient should be directed toward obtaining answers to the following questions:

1 What is the cause of the problem (etiology)?
2 What area of the brain is involved (location)?

The patient should be asked to begin his history with his first episode of illness, or with the time when he last felt completely well, rather than with the more recent episodes. This simple reorientation will often cause patients to recount important symptoms that they had thought to be inconsequential. Key points in the history are:

1 What was the patient doing when the difficulty began? Tradition says that ischemia or infarction usually occurs in repose, whereas hemorrhage begins during activity.
2 Was the onset instantaneous (apoplectic) as in hemorrhage or embolus, or stepwise and perhaps preceded by short-lived but similar episodes such as the transient ischemic attacks that often give warning of infarction?
3 How severe did the attack become before improvement began? Steady progression of symptoms suggests hemorrhage, whereas rapid recovery often follows an embolus.
4 Were there residual deficits?
5 How many attacks has the patient had? If they have been numerous, he should be asked to describe in detail the first, the most recent, and

the worst. At times it is helpful to diagram the events described by the patient.

After the patient has recounted his story, he should be questioned specifically about any of the following items that he has not already covered: (1) intellectual changes; (2) loss of consciousness; (3) difficulties with speech, reading, or writing; (4) paralysis or sensory disturbances involving any part of the body; (5) visual symptoms; (6) impairment of hearing or loss of balance; (7) headache; (8) trauma to the head; (9) systemic diseases such as diabetes, hypertension, cardiac disease, dysrhythmias, and anemia; and (10) medications that he may have been taking. Because information about these factors is so vital, they will be considered individually here, even though their relationship to specific diseases is discussed more fully in other chapters.

Intellectual Changes

The detail with which the patient describes his symptoms often affords information about his insight, judgment, and recent and remote recall. However, some patients do not realize they are losing portions of their memory and intellect and will deny impairment of mental function even in the presence of the most obvious defects. For this reason, one must always interview other members of the family to corroborate information about the patient's mental status, his memory, and his mood.

Loss of Consciousness

Loss of consciousness may occur without prodrome or after some seconds of light-headedness (giddiness or "swimmy-headedness"). Because unconsciousness is sometimes followed by amnesia for events surrounding the episode, patients may not be able to remember precipitants. It is essential, therefore, to have someone who observed the attack describe in detail the events surrounding it. Important points to be noted are:

1 The rapidity of onset. Was it without warning, as with most grand mal convulsions and with temporary cardiac arrest, or was it initiated by a feeling of light-headedness such as usually occurs in syncope, cardiac arrhythmia, and hypoglycemia?

2 The appearance of the patient during the attack. Pallor and sweating are typical of syncope and hypoglycemia; cyanosis suggests a convulsion. Patients with cardiac arrhythmias are often pale, while those with temporary asystole are suffused and cyanotic (Stokes-Adams attacks).

3 The rate and rhythm of the patient's heartbeat. If any of the bystanders has the presence of mind to take the patient's pulse during such an episode, this might provide the only clue to the diagnosis of an intermittent cardiac dysrhythmia.

4 Incontinence of feces or urine and any movements of the limbs or body. The presence of any of these findings suggests convulsion, since most patients who faint are limp and retain sphincter control. However, there are exceptions to this rule: certain patients with epileptic disorders are akinetic during the attack, and some patients suffering with syncope caused by one of a variety of disorders may have convulsive movements.

Difficulties with Speech, Reading, or Writing

Temporary alterations in comprehension of the spoken or written word may be ignored by the patient. Hence the physician must quiz the family carefully about lapses in conversation which could suggest temporary dysphasia or paraphasia, and the patient must be asked to read and to write.

Paralysis or Sensory Disturbances

The patient often uses the terms *numbness* and *paralysis* interchangeably, because many lay-

men do not realize that paralysis can occur without loss of sensation. The physician must do his best to differentiate between them. It is particularly important to distinguish hysterical paralysis from neurologic deficit. Abnormal neurologic signs may be present to confirm the latter diagnosis, but transient ischemia, for example, produces temporary numbness or paralysis without leaving residual abnormalities. In such cases, one must depend on the history given by the patient and his family. The following points are helpful in the differentiation of hysterical paralysis from paralysis that has a neurologic basis:

1 The onset. Cerebral ischemia, due to any cause, happens more frequently when the patient is at rest, whereas hysterical paralysis is likely to have a more dramatic onset in a public setting during a time of emotional stress.

2 The duration. Transient ischemic attacks seldom last longer than 24 hr; quite often the patient thinks his arm or leg has simply "gone to sleep" because of the position in which the extremity has been maintained. The hysterical episode usually lasts days or weeks.

3 The patient's attitude. The hysterical patient often has seeming lack of concern; but this is of little diagnostic value, since patients with transient ischemia are usually surprisingly calm even when an extremity is paralyzed.

4 Loss of sensation. Hysterical changes usually consist of total lack of feeling in the area involved, but the patient with neural deficit usually has some preservation of sensation even though it may be diminished. The pattern of sensory loss in hysteria does not usually follow anatomic distribution.

5 Personality. Hysterical attacks occur only in persons with immature personalities. If the patient has a personality disorder, some evidence of this fact can usually be obtained from the family. An attack occurring for the first time in a previously stable patient in the middle or upper age group is rarely hysterical in nature.

Another condition that may be difficult to distinguish from transient cerebral ischemia of any cause is a *focal motor seizure*. Because ischemic episodes do not usually cause cerebral irritability, convulsions are unusual manifestations. They do occur, however, and paralysis due to cerebral ischemia can be initiated by a focal seizure and is difficult to differentiate from temporary paralysis related to exhaustion of the cerebral cortex. The distinction cannot always be made on clinical grounds alone.

Visual Symptoms

The eyes may not be the mirror of the soul, but they do reflect cerebral vascular disease to a certain degree. Ophthalmologic symptoms are commonly associated with disorders of the carotid artery and of the vertebral-basilar system. For this reason, it is particularly important to inquire about visual phenomena.

Carotid Artery Syndrome Visual field defect caused by carotid artery disease may be the result of ischemia of the visual pathways or retina. Those of the brain are unusual and almost always affect the optic radiations resulting in homonymous hemianopic defect in the opposite visual field. The defect caused by retinal ischemia is either (1) a concentric constriction of the field in the homolateral eye caused by hypotension in the ophthalmic artery as in syncope or (2) an altitudinal defect described as a shade or veil being drawn across the upper or lower half of the visual field. These are caused by emboli which obstruct the upper or lower trunks of the central retinal arteriole (Fig. 6–1).

1 Amaurosis fugax. Episodes of monocular blindness lasting from seconds to minutes, especially when recurrent, are extremely suggestive of retinal ischemia due to insufficiency of the homolateral ophthalmic or carotid artery. Blindness due to cerebral vascular disease is most often sudden in onset, and the moment when it occurs is noted by the patient, who usually describes the attack as blurring of vision, "blackout," or "misty vision." Sometimes a yellowish or greenish hue is noted as peripheral vision is lost. Occasionally vision is lost and regained in an altitudinal fashion, the common complaint being that of a "veil" or "shade" descending or ascending in front of one eye. The loss may involve the whole visual field or only a segment (Fig. 6–2).

Because they do not cover one eye during an attack, most patients are unable to say whether just one eye or one-half of both visual fields was involved. Some patients are so upset by the abnormality that they believe both eyes to be blind when vision has become blurred or a scotoma has appeared in only one segment of the visual field. An intelligent and cooperative patient can be taught to test his own visual fields during possible subsequent attacks.

The common denominator of all these is retinal ischemia or infarction, which is usually secondary to obstruction of flow on the arterial side of the retinal circulation. Obstruction of the carotid or of the ophthalmic artery by thrombosis, embolus, or spasm may lower the pressure abruptly. At times phlebothrombosis may develop as a result of the lowering of venous pressure by arterial disease or phlebosclerosis. This results in prolonged impairment of vision because of retinal edema and hemorrhages.

2 Hemianopia. Whereas amaurosis fugax strongly suggests carotid artery disease, intermittent homonymous hemianopia is an unusual symptom of the carotid syndrome.

Vertebral-basilar Syndrome Disease in the vertebral-basilar system is associated with a wider variety of visual symptoms, including (1) diplopia, (2) visual field abnormalities, (3) visual hallucinations and illusions, and (4) oscillopsia.

1 Diplopia. Transient horizontal or vertical diplopia is a frequent symptom of vertebral-basilar insufficiency. Some patients describe double vision as "blurring of vision," even though

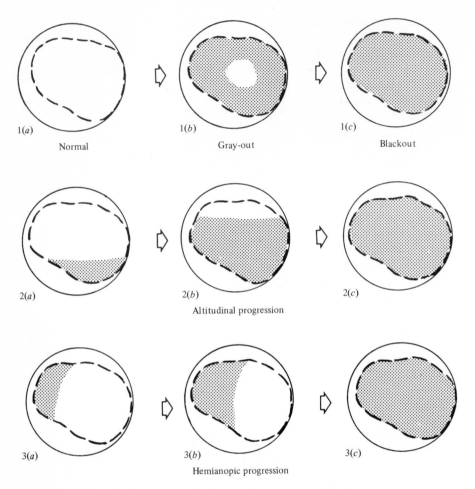

Figure 6-1 Modes of progression of visual defects in patients suffering with amaurosis fugax. *(Modified from C. C. Ewing, 1968.)*

Figure 6-2 Progression of an embolus from the ophthalmic artery through the central arteriole of the retina into branch arteries. Reading from top to bottom: Column (*a*). Altitudinal defect of visual field descending like a curtain and resolving in patchy scotomata. Column (*b*). Retinal ischemia rising upward. Column (*c*). Progression of an embolus into upper and lower retinal vessels. *(Modified from C. C. Ewing, 1968.)*

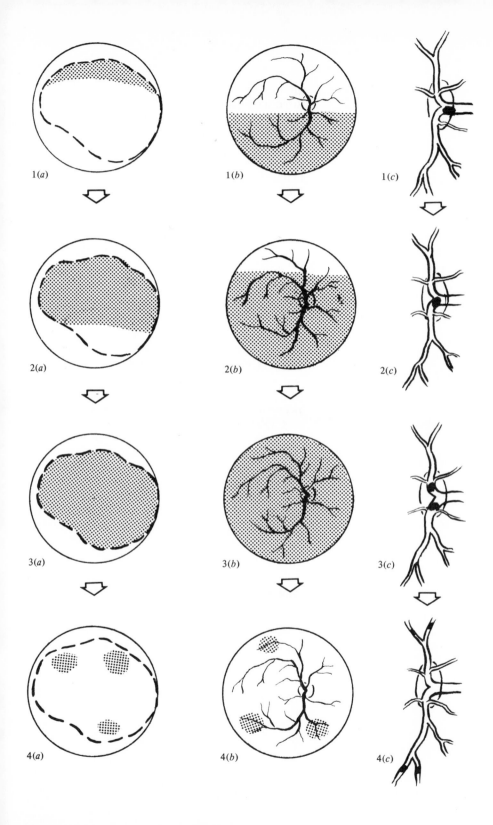

their vision is clear if one eye is kept closed. The attacks seldom last longer than 3 to 5 min and may be recurrent. Other conditions to be considered in the differential diagnosis of intermittent diplopia are palsies of cranial nerves III, IV, and VI, and disorders of the extraocular muscles themselves. These usually cause longer-lasting diplopia which only rarely is intermittent in nature.

2 Visual field abnormalities. These may take the form of homonymous defects or blindness.

a Homonymous defects. Such defects may result from interruption of function in the optic tract, the lateral geniculate body, the optic radiation, or the occipital lobe, all of which are supplied, at least in part, by branches of the basilar artery.

Sudden loss or impairment of vision which involves portions of both eyes suggests a homonymous field defect. Some patients first note the loss as a shadow or curtain obstructing vision; others say that parts of objects suddenly disappear or that words or letters seem to be missing from a page of print. Because central vision is usually preserved, quadrantanopia or hemianopia may be undetected by the patient until it leads to an unusual number of mishaps, such as stumbling into objects on the blind side or automobile accidents occasioned by the inability to see other cars from the "corner of the eye" on that side.

b Transient blindness or blurring of vision. Sometimes described as "blackout" or "the blind staggers," this condition has many causes, including hypotension, anemia, and occlusive disease of the vertebral-basilar arterial system. More often than not, such transient episodes presage serious sequelae. Rarely, cortical blindness occurs when homonymous hemianopia is followed at a later time by a defect in the other half of the field of vision.

Loss of vision in the presence of normal fundi and unimpaired pupillary reaction to light is the characteristic of cortical blindness. The condition can be distinguished from hysterical blindness by the absence of blinking reflex to visual threat, of optokinetic nystagmus, and of EEG changes in the occipital rhythms in response to

photic stimulation. The patient is often confused and disoriented, and he may deny blindness completely (Anton's syndrome).

Some patients with attacks of vertebral-basilar artery insufficiency have loss of their peripheral visual fields with preservation of macular vision. This constriction may be temporary, as in ischemia, or permanent, as in infarction of the occipital lobe. Acquired inability to read and failure to recognize objects, familiar surroundings, or the faces of people (visual agnosias) are due to an abnormality in the parieto-occipital association areas.

3 Visual hallucinations and illusions. These phenomena may arise from dysfunction in the parietal, temporal, or occipital lobes. Field defects due to occipital lobe dysfunction do not usually cause positive images, but they may cause *unformed* scotomata or photopsia. Formed, and at times very lifelike, visual images are associated most often with dysfunction of the parietal and temporal lobes, such as may occur in the vertebral-basilar syndrome.

4 Oscillopsia. An illusion of either horizontal or vertical movement occurs when a patient with nystagmus sees the images in his visual field as they move across his retina. The most common cause of either horizontal or vertical nystagmus is medication, barbiturates and hydantoinates being the major offenders. In the absence of drug intoxication, vertical nystagmus is an almost infallible sign of brainstem lesion which is perhaps vascular in nature.

Impairment of Hearing or Loss of Balance (Deafness, Vertigo, or Ataxia)

The auditory and vestibular apparatus encased in the petrous portion of the temporal bone is supplied by the vertebral-basilar arterial system. Episodes of vertigo, with or without accompanying loss of hearing, may be due to vascular disease in the brainstem or in the vestibular apparatus itself. Some attacks of ischemia are precipitated by changing the position of the head on the neck (as in looking up at a tall building), or by rotating the head to one side while backing an automobile or shaving. Sudden movement of the body or of the head may precipitate violent vertigo, oscillopsia, nausea, and vomiting. At times it is difficult to distinguish between vertigo (usually associated with a feeling of spinning) and the unsteady feeling that precedes syncope. Many patients with vertigo keep their eyes tightly closed and are unable to say whether objects seem to be moving or not, but they hear and are acutely aware of their environment. In syncope the eyes are not necessarily closed, but vision dims and sounds grow more distant as consciousness fades.

Some patients with vascular lesions have intermittent loss of hearing suggestive of Ménière's disease, and others complain of noises in the head which are not tinnitus but bruits. The patient should always be asked for a description of sounds he may have in his head, and should be questioned specifically about whether they are synchronous with the heartbeat. Occasionally the patient will insist that he has an intracranial sound synchronous with his hearbeat, even though the physician cannot hear it.

Headache

The vast majority of headaches result from abnormalities in pain-sensitive structures external to the skull, such as the arteries, nerves, periosteum, ligaments, muscles, paranasal sinuses, and teeth. Intracranial headaches originate in the meninges, the arteries, the dural sinuses, and the sensory portions of cranial nerves. Ache from the carotid arterial system is referred to the homolateral orbit or frontotemporal area, while that from the vertebral arteries is referred to the homolateral shoulder, neck, or suboccipital region, depending on the portion of the system involved. Pain secondary to disease of the basilar artery is referred to the midline of the occiput where it is felt as headache. Such headaches, commonly associated with migraine, at times will occur with rupture of an aneurysm or occlusion of an artery.

Although many cerebral vascular diseases are not accompanied by headache, this symptom may be a key to a precise diagnosis, particularly when the headache is unilateral, pounding or throbbing in nature, and preceded by an aura, as in migraine. If the headache invariably occurs on the same side of the head, it may suggest arteriovenous malformation. Contrary to common belief, aneurysm rarely causes headache until it ruptures, unless it happens to press on a cranial nerve.

Subdural hematoma almost always causes recurring dull headaches, which usually increase in severity as the hematoma enlarges. The headaches are made worse by Valsalva's maneuver, by bending over, or by jolting the head. Because most cerebral hematomata are located initially within the brain parenchyma, they do not at first stretch or put pressure upon pain-sensitive structures, and consequently headache occurs only after the hematoma has grown large enough to distort these structures. If hemorrhage dissects through to the surface or ruptures into the ventricular space, it immediately produces excruciating headache, usually with devastating neurologic deficit.

Cranial arteritis causes unremitting pain in the head which is not throbbing but is a gnawing discomfort. Cranial arteritis begins after middle age and is often accompanied by low-grade fever, malaise, and weight loss.

Although atherosclerosis of cerebral vessels may perhaps dull the senses, it does not cause headache. Occasionally acute obstruction of the internal carotid artery may cause unilateral headache which resembles that of migraine or even cranial arteritis. This pain is thought to be due to compensatory dilatation of the external carotid arteries.

Trauma to the Head

In older patients, especially those with underlying diseases such as diabetes or hypertension, and in patients who are receiving anticoagulant medication, even minor trauma may cause a subdural hematoma to accumulate.

At times trauma may tear the intima of cervical or intracranial segments of the carotid arteries, causing dissection and obstruction of the lumen of the artery.

Systemic Diseases

Particularly important are anemia, polycythemia, hypertension, coronary artery disease with or without previous myocardial infarctions, pulmonary diseases, and diabetes mellitus, all of which can impair oxygenation or perfusion of the brain.

Medications

Medications that the patient has been taking, especially phenothiazine derivatives and hypotensive drugs, may cause or aggravate his problem by inducing postural hypotension and transient attacks. Steroids, when administered for a prolonged period, sometimes have secondary effects on the cerebral circulation, and anticoagulants can initiate intracranial bleeding. An important, though unusual, complication of use of amine-oxidase inhibitor psychotropic medications is hypertensive crisis after eating cheese or drinking Chianti wine. This combination can cause cerebral vascular episodes. Alcohol, hypoglycemic drugs, progestational contraceptives, Dilantin, and barbiturates are other examples of medications that may affect the central nervous system and produce symptoms which simulate cerebral vascular disease.

Synthesis

The physician must weigh the evidence elicited from the patient and his family, allowing for possible distortion resulting from confabulation and memory loss, or from suppression of facts because of underlying neurosis and fear. Elicitation of a history is dynamic and often cannot be confined to one interview. Like an artist, the skillful physician often paints his picture by sketching in the background on the first interview and adding details and color on subsequent occasions.

NEUROVASCULAR EXAMINATION

The physical and neurologic examination of a patient with cerebral vascular disease must include special observations for the following: (1) abnormal pulsations in an artery or arterial branch supplying the head; (2) cranial or cervical bruit; (3) a hypersensitive carotid sinus reflex; (4) unequal blood pressures in the arms; (5) postural hypotension or diminished cardiac output during Valsalva's maneuver; (6) abnormal ophthalmic artery pressures; and (7) certain retinal abnormalities. The assessment of these special points makes up what we call the *neurovascular examination*. These observations are made as a part of the customary physical and neurologic examinations but are considered separately in this chapter in order to emphasize them.

Palpation

Technique The following arteries in the neck and head must be palpated in sequence bilaterally and simultaneously: the superficial temporal, facial, supra- and infraorbital arteries, and occipital branches of the external carotid arteries, followed by the common carotids at the bifurcation behind the angle of the jaw and low in the neck, the subclavian arteries above and below the clavicle, and the radial and ulnar arteries. The abdominal aorta, the iliac and femoral arteries, and the pedal pulses should be palpated next. Comparison of one pulse with another may reveal an increase, a decrease, or even absence of pulsations in one or more arteries. It is particularly important to palpate the two radial arteries simultaneously to determine

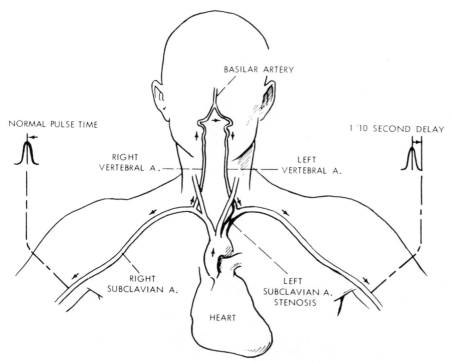

Figure 6-3 Mechanism by which pulse delay in the radial artery occurs in subclavian steal syndrome. Arterial blood on the side of occlusion or stenosis must traverse a circuitous route through the vertebral arteries and the arrival time of the pulse at the wrist is consequently delayed and damped.

the possibility of delay in the arrival time of pulse on one side, which when found is almost diagnostic of subclavian steal syndrome (Fig. 6-3). See Chap. 12.

The internal carotid artery can be palpated inside the mouth with the tip of a gloved finger placed on the tonsillar fossa. This maneuver is helpful in detecting disease of the internal carotid, but it is rather cumbersome to perform.

Occasionally, palpation of the other arteries will uncover unsuspected disease, such as an abdominal or popliteal aneurysm, which is unrelated to the main problem at hand.

Evaluation of Results

1 Diminution or absence of pulsations in one of the superficial temporal or occipital arteries suggests disease of that vessel or of the ex-

ternal or common carotid artery. If the artery is tender, cranial arteritis should be considered (Fig. 6-4); if it is not, atherosclerotic occlusion is the probable cause.

2 Increased pulsation of the superficial temporal or facial artery sometimes indicates stenosis or occlusion of the homolateral internal carotid artery, with the development of collateral flow through the external system.

3 Inability to palpate the common carotid, combined with the finding of good pulsations in the superficial temporal and occipital arteries, suggests a tortuous common carotid artery lying behind the trachea.

4 Absence of pulsations in one carotid in the pharynx is diagnostic of carotid occlusion; failure to find pulsations in both carotids is often due to poor technique.

5 If pulses in the subclavian artery are di-

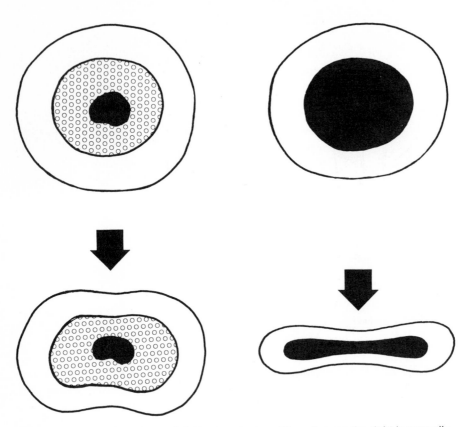

Figure 6-4 Palpation of superficial temporal artery. The artery on the right is normally compressible. The one on the left depicts a thickened artery with decreased compressibility.

minished or absent, the proximal portion of the vessel is diseased.

6 In the absence of anemia or aortic stenosis, a thrill felt over any artery usually indicates disease at the site of the thrill.

7 Pulse delay in one radial artery is almost diagnostic of disease of the subclavian artery proximal to the origin of the vertebral artery on that side.

8 Absence of a radial, ulnar, or pedal pulse occurs in occlusive disease of the large vessels and should suggest the possibility of generalized atherosclerosis or embolism.

9 Absence of aortic, femoral, and pedal pulses is due to occlusion of the aorta by coarctation, embolus, or atherosclerosis.

10 Reappearance of previously absent pulses suggests spasm, recanalization of arteries, or temporary diversion of blood flow.

Auscultation

Where to Listen After listening to the heart and lungs in the usual manner over the thorax and precordium, one should attempt to detect murmurs caused by disease of the aortocranial arteries. One should listen along the course of the vertebral and carotid arteries, auscultating for murmurs, particularly at the subclavian-vertebral junction, over the mastoids, along the common carotid artery, and at the carotid bifurcation just beneath the angle of the jaw (Fig. 6-5). Because of its extreme importance, the carotid bifurcation must be auscultated with particular care with the patient's head first in the neutral position and then turned to one side and then the other. Bruits that are not heard with the head in the neutral position may become evident when it is turned. The explanation may lie in the kinking or compressing of the artery by turning the head, but it is just as likely that the sternocleidomastoid muscle, moving across the artery as the head is turned, alters the audibility of bruits. At times the lateral mass of the first cervical vertebra (the atlas) can compress the artery from behind when the head is turned and produce turbulent flow.

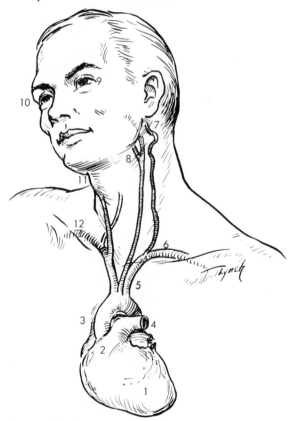

Figure 6-5 Sites for aortocranial auscultation. *(By permission of American Heart Association.)*

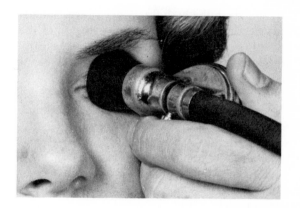

Figure 6-6 Technique for auscultating the orbit. The patient is asked to close both eyes, and the bell is then placed over one eye. The patient is asked to open his eyes and to fix on a distant object.

Next the *orbits* must be auscultated by placing the bell of the stethoscope gently but firmly on the closed eyelid. The patient is then instructed to open his eyes and fix his gaze on a distant object, thus relaxing the orbicularis oculi muscle and eliminating adventitious sounds produced by muscle and eyeball movements. The patient is asked to stop breathing momentarily so that breath sounds which are often heard over the cranial cavity cease and soft bruits become distinct (Fig. 6-6). The presence of such bruits, audible only in the orbit, is thought to be related to the conical construction of the orbit, the apex of which is situated near the central regions of the skull close to the internal carotid artery and its branches. This megaphone-shaped receptacle is thought to conduct sound from the depths of the head to the surface. Whatever the reason, cephalic murmurs are often audible over the orbits.

The *mastoid* is another region to which murmurs are transmitted, perhaps because the dense petrous portion of the temporal bone conducts sound well. It will be recalled that the carotid artery passes through this bone and that the vertebral and basilar arteries lie close to it.

The *skull* has a characteristic resonating frequency of about 300 cps, so that it tends to filter out sounds in the high-frequency range. Sounds may be audible in one or another region of the calvarium, but the parietal region is usually chosen for auscultation because it is free of overlying muscle.

How to Listen Intracranial and cervical murmurs vary in their sound frequencies, so that some murmurs can be heard with the bell and not with the diaphragm. In rare cases, they are audible with neither and yet can be heard easily when one ear is placed against the patient's head or neck.

Inexperienced examiners sometimes create murmurs by compressing an artery. This is particularly easy to do when auscultating the carotid arteries. Although some neurologists advocate compression of one carotid to obliterate soft murmurs or to increase flow through the opposite one and "bring out" bruits, this technique can be dangerous and should be used only with extreme caution, if at all. Compression of both jugular veins low in the neck will usually obliterate venous hums and increase bruits caused by caroticocavernous fistulae.

The importance of turning the head to different positions during auscultation has already been mentioned. The patient should also be examined lying down and sitting up with his arms placed in various positions. Since the subclavian artery runs behind the clavicle and can be compressed between the clavicle and the first rib when the arm is extended, the intensity of subclavian murmurs varies with the position of the arm.

Sometimes murmurs are made audible by having the patient exercise, thus increasing his cardiac output and velocity of flow. Other methods that have been suggested but not fully explored are hyperventilation to create cerebral vasoconstriction, and the inhalation of carbon dioxide or amyl nitrite to enhance the audibility of murmurs by altering blood flow to the head.

What Murmurs Signify Even though loud murmurs are sometimes audible in patients with no symptoms and others with severe vascular disease have no bruit, listening for murmurs is the best bedside method for detection of atherosclerosis. The site of maximum intensity usually overlies the lesion but does not necessarily give a clue to its cause or severity because volume, pitch, and transmission characteristics are not reliable indices of the degree of constriction in the vascular lumen. The common denominator of all bruits is turbulent flow, which may be the result of one or several of the following: abnormal blood viscosity, change in velocity of flow, irregularities in the lumen or in the intimal wall of the artery, and the relation of focal constriction to poststenotic dilatation of the artery.

Whether this turbulence produces vortices in the bloodstream or flitter movements of the wall, the end result is a systolic murmur of variable intensity which may be prolonged into diastole.

As mentioned before, not all bruits are diagnostic of disease of the vessel; in many cases they may be induced artificially by using excessive pressure on the artery with the stethoscope. They can be the result also of increased velocity of flow due to anemia. Murmurs audible in the head, orbits, or neck may result from changes in blood flow occurring with anemia, exertion, hyperthyroidism, anxiety, fever, or pregnancy. In interpreting the significance of bruits, therefore, one must consider the age of the patient, the presence of systemic disease, and the presence or absence of symptoms of cerebrovascular disease (Fig. 6-7).

Arterial disease is by far the most common cause of cervical murmurs heard in adults. Consequently, a bruit over the carotid or vertebral arteries of a patient with symptoms suggestive of aortocranial disease should cause one to suspect extracranial lesions which might be removed surgically.

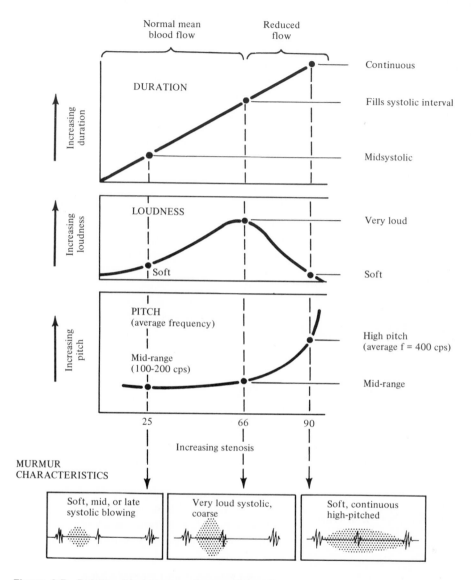

Figure 6-7 Relationship between characteristics of arterial murmurs and the degree of stenosis in patients with normal cardiac output and blood viscosity. The exact timing of a murmur in relation to heart sounds depends on the distance of the lesion from the heart. The greater the distance, the later the murmur will occur. *(Modified from a diagram by Merrill P. Spencer.)*

On the other hand, absence of bruits should not lull one into a false sense of security. People with severe stenosis or obstruction of one, two, or even three of these major vessels may have no murmurs in the chest, neck, head, or orbits. When there is no flow, there is no murmur.

Cephalic Murmurs Soft systolic bruits can be heard over the cranium in almost 50 percent of normal infants and children because their circulation is rapid and the volume of flow through sharply angulated cerebral vessels is proportionately great (about 40 percent of cardiac output). Some neurologists believe they can distinguish between physiologic souffles and pathologic murmurs caused by increased intracranial pressure—the physiologic souffle being short and soft and the pathologic bruit, rasping, higher pitched, and more prolonged. In adults, cephalic bruits must be considered pathologic until proved otherwise since they are found in less than 1 percent of "normal" adults. These murmurs suggest arteriovenous malformations or, rarely, a highly vascular neoplasm, intracranial hematoma, or Paget's disease of the skull.

Any intracranial murmur extending into diastole is abnormal, but venous murmurs in the neck (such as venous hums) are normal and can be distinguished from arterial murmurs by their disappearance during gentle compression of the jugular veins on the side of the sound. Furthermore, venous hums, in contrast to pathologic bruits, usually cease or diminish in intensity when the patient lies down, whereas pathologic bruits do not.

Cervical Murmurs These may be heard in all age groups as a physiologic sound. The physiologic murmur is situated low in the neck, usually on the right side, and is a soft, early systolic sound. In adults, the most common cause of murmurs over the carotid and vertebral arteries is atherosclerosis with roughening of the intima

and stenosis of the lumen. Consequently, the finding of a neck bruit in a patient with signs suggestive of aortocranial disease is strongly suggestive of a lesion in one of the extracranial vessels.

In patients with atherosclerotic cerebrovascular disease, bruits are heard more frequently over the region of the carotid bifurcation. They may be localized here or may be transmitted cranially through the internal carotid, to be heard in the region of the mastoid and, at times, in the temporal area as well. A short, early systolic bruit heard over the common carotid in the base of the neck is less commonly associated with disease of the carotid itself than with disease of the aortic valve; on the other hand, a bruit primary at the carotid bifurcation is most often secondary to stenosis or occlusion of the carotid in this location. The bruit may be caused by external, internal, or common carotid disease. If heard over the orbit as well, it is probably an internal carotid sound.

Because obstruction of one carotid or vertebral artery is accompanied by increased flow through the opposite one, murmurs are sometimes heard over the less involved carotid bifurcation or the vertebral artery contralateral to the obstruction. In other patients with no bruit in the neck, a souffle can be heard over the orbit because of the increased flow through the sinous carotid siphon opposite the occluded carotid.

Venous hum is common in children but unusual in adults. When heard, it should suggest intracranial arteriovenous malformation if no other systemic cause can be found.

Carotid Massage and Compression

When examining the patient in the office or at the bedside, it is tempting to massage the sinus to ascertain if the patient may be having episodes secondary to hypersensitivity, but we believe that the test should be performed only by the methods to be described in Chap. 8.

Blood Pressure

Blood pressures must be taken and compared in each arm with the patient lying and standing, as well as during and after Valsalva's maneuver. A difference exceeding 20 mm Hg in the systolic pressures between the two sides is strongly suggestive of subclavian artery disease. The blood pressure may fall precipitously when the arm with the obstruction is exercised, and if the blood pressure is measured simultaneously in both arms, a perceptible delay in arrival of the pulse wave will be noted on the affected side.

The patient must then stand up, and repeated measurements must be made for several minutes, because blood pressure may be normally sustained for a minute or two before it begins to fall to hypotensive levels. While standing, the patient should be asked to perform Valsalva's maneuver. The erect position may reduce arterial blood pressure and the straining decrease cardiac output, thus placing a maximum strain on cerebrovascular reserve which may precipitate symptoms of insufficiency. At this time the blood pressure may be measured using the cuff technique.

Blood pressures in the ophthalmic arteries must also be measured and correlated with brachial pressures. See Chap. 7.

Ophthalmoscopic Examination

Most physicians perform an ophthalmoscopic examination by the direct method, which gives a restricted view of the optic fundus.

A much better total picture is obtained by indirect ophthalmoscopy with the pupil dilated by midriatics. The more peripheral parts of the retina can be seen with this method.

Atherosclerosis of the retinal arterioles produces the following changes, detectable with the ophthalmoscope and classified by Scheie as:

Grade 0   Hypertensive patient without any evidence of sclerosis

Grade I   Increase or broadening of the light streak with minimal arteriovenous compression
Grade II   Changes more marked
Grade III   Arteriovenous compression more marked; light streak occupies most of the arteriole, which has a burnished-copper appearance
Grade IV   Changes of grade III, but in addition the vessel wall is opaque and has a silver-wire appearance

Although there has been some question as to whether these changes reflect alterations in vessels supplying the brain, we believe that they provide valuable clues to the degree of atherosclerosis in the intracranial arterioles. However, a misleading picture may be produced by plaques within the ophthalmic artery or the carotid siphon where they may protect retinal arterioles while advanced changes are taking place in other intracranial arterioles.

Atherosclerosis of any portion of the carotid artery proximal to the origin of the ophthalmic artery may be accompanied by reduction of pressure in the ophthalmic artery. When pressure is low enough, retinal ischemia produces attacks of loss of vision in that eye (amaurosis fugax), as well as hemorrhages and exudates secondary to endothelial hypoxia. If infarction of the optic nerve and retina occurs, the retina is pale, the disk is white, the arteries are difficult to see, and the veins are attenuated.

Perhaps because of slowing of the circulation through the retina, disease of the carotid artery may also lead to thrombosis of retinal veins. This is seen through the ophthalmoscope as loss of pulsation in and engorgement of the central retinal vein, accompanied by edema, hemorrhages, and exudates in the retina. Occlusion of one of the branches of the retinal vein produces a similar picture in one segment of the retina.

Refractile bodies, which vividly reflect the light of the ophthalmoscope, can occasionally be seen lodged in the arterioles. These are cholesterol spicules which have been cast off from atheromatous plaques situated in the aorta or carotid artery. They can sometimes be seen to migrate along the course of the artery; they are long and narrow, and lodge in but do not obstruct the artery. When digital pressure exceeding the diastolic pressure is gently applied to the globe, the bloodstream imparts a pulsatile appearance to cholesterol plaques, indicating their intraluminal origin.

In contrast, platelet emboli are creamy white and produce spasm of the arterioles, with segmentation of the distal blood column. This segmentation or "boxcar effect" is seen in the vein draining the region. Clinicians who have observed the fundus during an attack of amaurosis fugax state that they have seen slowing of the arteriolar flow and segmentation of the blood column, with rouleaux formation. This segmentation also occurs in patients about to faint and in aviators during blackout caused by the high force of gravity. Retinal microemboli of calcium following mitral valvulotomy are said to appear as chalky-white intravascular fragments in contrast to those seen after carotid endarterectomy, in which they are refractile.

When the ocular fundi show grade III or grade IV hypertensive retinopathy, hypertensive encephalopathy may be suspected. We classify hypertensive retinopathy on the basis of the Keith-Wagener scale. See the following table.

Grade I	Irregularity of the arteriolar blood column (spasm)
Grade II	Spasm with beading of the arterioles
Grade III	Hemorrhages and exudates in addition to spasm and beading
Grade IV	All the above findings plus papilledema

Subarachnoid hemorrhage at times causes ophthalmoscopic findings resembling those of hypertensive retinopathy, but the hemorrhages are large, crescent-shaped, and subhyaloid (preretinal), in contrast to the minute, flame-shaped retinal hemorrhages of hypertension. Subhyaloid hemorrhages may develop within hours after the onset of subarachnoid hemorrhage. They may obstruct vision and are indicative of an acute rise in intracranial pressure, usually, but not necessarily, due to subarachnoid bleeding. Their shape slowly alters with changes in the patient's position. Flame-shaped and globular hemorrhages are contained within the substance of the retina and do not affect vision or change their shape.

Examination of the conjunctivae for petechiae and for sludging should be done when indicated.

Neovascularization of the retina is sometimes seen in a patient with chronic carotid artery disease due to any cause.

Rubeosis oculi is a circumlimbal proliferation and dilatation of capillaries in the bulbar conjunctiva associated with extreme degrees of external and internal carotid artery obstruction. The red rim of vessels around the cornea resembles that sometimes seen in acute iritis.

In this chapter, no attempt has been made to describe the more unusual but nonetheless important findings that may be uncovered by interview or examination of the patient. Signs and symptoms associated with specific disease entities will be considered in the appropriate chapters, which follow.

SUGGESTED READINGS

General

Aring, C. D.: Differential diagnosis of cerebrovascular stroke, *Arch. Internal Med.*, **113**:195, 1964.

Shapiro, H. M., Ng, L., Mishkin, M., and Reivich, M.: Direct thermometry, ophthalmodynamometry, auscultation and palpation in extracranial cerebrovascular disease: An evaluation of rapid diagnostic methods, *Stroke,* **1**:205, 1970.

Toole, J. F.: Diagnosis and Management of Stroke, American Heart Association, New York, 1968.

Interview

Toole, J. F.: "Some aspects of the neurologic interview," in Special Techniques for Neurologic Diagnosis (Contemporary Neurology Series, 3), edited by J. F. Toole, F. A. Davis Company, Philadelphia, 1969, pp. 1–9.

Visual Symptoms

Bender, M. B.: "Disorders in visual perception," in Problems of Dynamic Neurology, edited by L. Halpern, The Department of Nervous Diseases of the Rothschild Hadassah University Hospital and The Hebrew University Hadassah Medical School, Jerusalem, Israel, 1963, pp. 319–375.

Dailey, E. J., Holloway, J. A., Murto, R. E., and Schlezinger, N. S.: Evaluation of ocular signs and symptoms in cerebral aneurysms, *Arch. Ophthalmol.*, **71**:463, 1964.

Dark, A. J., and Rizk, S. N.: Progressive focal sclerosis of retinal arteries: A sequel to impaction of cholesterol emboli, *Brit. Med. J.*, **1**:270, 1967.

Eadie, M. J., Sutherland, J. M., and Tyrer, J. H.: Recurrent monocular blindness of uncertain cause, *Lancet*, **1**:319, 1968.

Ewing, C. C.: Recurrent monocular blindness, *Lancet*, **1**:1035, 1968.

Fisher, C. M.: Some neuro-ophthalmological observations, *J. Neurol. Neurosurg. Psychiat.*, **30**:383, 1967.

Hoyt, W. F.: Transient bilateral blurring of vision: Considerations of an episodic ischemic symptom of vertebral-basilar insufficiency, *Arch. Ophthalmol.*, **70**:746, 1963.

Karjalainen, K.: Occlusion of the central retinal artery and retinal branch arterioles. A clinical, tonographic and fluorescin angiographic study of 175 patients, *Acta ophthalmol. suppl.*, **109**:1, 1971.

Kearns, T. P., and Hollenhorst, R. W.: Venous-stasis retinopathy of occlusive disease of the carotid artery, *Proc. Staff Meetings Mayo Clinic*, **38**:304, 1963.

Minor, R. H., Kearns, T. P., Millikan, C. H., Siekert, R. G., and Sayre, G. P.: Ocular manifestations of occlusive disease of the vertebral-basilar arterial system, *Arch. Ophthalmol.*, **62**:84, 1959.

Rose, F. C.: Transient blindness, *Brit. Med. J.*, **3**:763, 1969.

Symonds, C., and Mackenzie, L.: Bilateral loss of vision from cerebral infarction, *Brain*, **80**:415, 1957.

Impairment of Hearing and Loss of Balance (Deafness, Vertigo, or Ataxia)

Bergan, J. J., Levy, J. S., Trippel, O. H., and Jurayj, M.: Vascular implications of vertigo, *Arch. Otolaryngol.*, **85**:292, 1967.

Edwards, C. H.: Ischaemia of the brain, *Proc. Roy, Soc. Med.*, **55**:177, 1962.

Fisher, C. M.: Vertigo in cerebrovascular disease, *Arch. Otolaryngol.*, **85**:529, 1967.

Sheehy, J. L.: The dizzy patient: Eliciting his history, *Arch. Otolaryngol.*, **86**:18, 1967.

Drugs

Spillane, J. P.: Drug-induced neurological disorders, *Proc. Roy. Soc. Med.*, **57**:135, 1964.

Neurovascular Examination

Palpation

Fisher, C. M.: Facial pulses in internal carotid artery occlusion, *Neurology*, **20**:476, 1970.

Garrison, G. E., Floyd, W. L., and Orgain, E. S.: Exercise in the physical examination of peripheral arterial disease, *Ann. Internal Med.*, **66**:587, 1967.

Auscultation, General

Allen, N.: The significance of vascular murmurs in the head and neck, *Geriatrics*, **20**:525, 1965.

————, and Mustian, V.: Origin and significance of vascular murmurs of the head and neck, *Medicine*, **41**:227, 1962.

Howells, D. P. M.: Arterial auscultation in a relative atheroma-free population, *Lancet*, **2**:242, 1971.

Janeway, R.: The art of listening, *Current Concepts Cerebrovascular Dis.—Stroke*, **6**:17, 1971.

————, and Toole, J. F.: "Diagnostic techniques in cerebrovascular disease," in Medical Basis for Comprehensive Community Stroke Programs, edited by N. O. Borhani and J. S. Meyer, in collaboration with the Special Task Force of the Joint Council's Subcommittee on Cerebrovascular Disease (National Heart Institute and National Institute of Neurological Diseases and Blindness), National Institutes of Health, June 1, 1968.

McDowell, F., and Ejrup, B.: Arterial bruits in cerebrovascular disease. A follow-up study, *Neurology*, **16**:1127, 1966.

Myers, J. D., Murdaugh, H. V., McIntosh, H. D., and Blaisdell, R. K.: Observations on continuous murmurs over partially obstructed arteries; Explanation for continuous murmur found in aortic arch syndrome, *Arch. Internal Med.*, **97**:726, 1956.

Silverstein, A.: Auscultation, palpation and compression of the neck and head, *J. Mt. Sinai Hosp.*, **33**:265, 1966.

Toole, J. F., and Janeway, R.: "Diagnostic techniques," chap. 10 in Handbook of Clinical Neurology, vol. II, edited by P. J. Vinken and G. W. Bruyn, North-Holland Publishing Company, Amsterdam, 1972.

Ziegler, D. K., Zileli, T., and Dick, A.: Correlation of bruits over the carotid artery with angiographically demonstrated lesions, *Neurology,* **20**:374, 1970.

Auscultation, in Head

Dalsgaard-Nielsen, T.: Studies on intracranial vascular sounds, *Acta psychiat. neurol.*, **14**:69, 1939.

Fisher, C. M.: Augmentation bruit of the vertebral artery, *J. Neurol. Neurosurg. Psychiat.*, **29**:343, 1966.

Gareeboo, H.: Severe anemia as a cause of cranial bruit, *Brit. Med. J.*, **1**:294, 1968.

Hardison, J. E.: Cervical venous hum. A clue to the diagnosis of intracranial arteriovenous malformations, *New Engl. J. Med.*, **278**:587, 1968.

Mackenzie, I.: The intracranial bruit, *Brain,* **78**:350, 1955.

Merendino, K. A., and Hessel, E. A., II: The "murmur on top of the head" in acquired mitral insufficiency. Pathological clinical significance, *J.A.M.A.*, **199**:892, 1967.

Wadia, N. H., and Monckton, G.: Intracranial bruits in health and disease, *Brain,* **80**:492, 1957.

Auscultation, in Neck

Crevasse, L.: Carotid artery murmurs: Clinical and pathophysiologic correlation, *Neurology,* **11**(4)(part 2):100, 1961.

Crevasse, L. E., and Logue, R. B.: Carotid artery murmurs; continuous murmurs over carotid bulb—new sign of carotid artery insufficiency, *J.A.M.A.,* **167**:2177, 1958.

Fowler, N. O., and Marshall, W. J.: The supraclavicular arterial bruit, *Am. Heart J.,* **69**:410, 1965.

Hammond, J. H., and Eisinger, R. P.: Carotid bruits in 1,000 normal subjects, *Arch. Internal Med.,* **109**:563, 1962.

Jones, F. L., Jr.: Frequency, characteristics and importance of the cervical venous hum in adults, *New Engl. J. Med.,* **267**:658, 1962.

Kartchner, M. M., and McRae, L. P.: Auscultation for carotid bruits in cerebrovascular insufficiency, *J.A.M.A.,* **210**:494, 1969.

Nelson, W. P., and Hall, R. J.: The innocent supraclavicular arterial bruit—Utility of shoulder maneuvers in its recognition, *New Engl. J. Med.,* **278**:778, 1968.

Siekert, R. G., and Millikan, C. H.: Changing carotid bruit in transient cerebral ischemic attacks, *Arch. Neurol.,* **14**:302, 1966.

Carotid Massage and Compression

Toole, J. F.: Bruits, ophthalmodynamometry, carotid compression tests and other diagnostic procedures, *Res. Pub. Assoc. Nerv. Ment. Dis.,* **41**:267, 1961.

Blood Pressure

Bannister, R., Ardill, L., and Fentem, P.: Defective autonomic control of blood vessels in idiopathic orthostatic hypotension, *Brain,* **90**:725, 1967.

Ophthalmoscopic Examination

AtLee, W. E., Jr.: Talc and cornstarch emboli in eyes of drug abusers, *J.A.M.A.,* **219**:49, 1972.

Baghdassarian, S. A., Crawford, J. B., and Rathbun, J. E., Jr.: Calcific emboli of the retinal and ciliary arteries, *Am. J. Ophthalmol.,* **69**:372, 1970.

Breslin, D. J., Gifford, R. W., Jr., Fairbairn, J. P., II, and Kearns, T. P.: Prognostic importance of ophthalmoscopic findings in essential hypertension, *J.A.M.A.,* **195**:335, 1966.

Cogan, D. G., Kuwabara, T., and Moser, H.: Fat emboli in the retina following angiography, *Arch. Ophthalmol.,* **71**:308, 1964.

David, N. J., Klintworth, G. K., Friedberg, S. J., and Dillon, M.: Fatal atheromatous cerebral embolism associated with bright plaques in the retinal arterioles: Report of a case, *Neurology,* **13**:708, 1963.

Fisher, C. M.: Observations of the fundus oculi in transient monocular blindness, *Neurology,* **9**:333, 1959.

Frayser, R., Houston, C. S., Bryan, A. C., Rennie, I. D., and Gray, G.: Retinal hemorrhage at high altitude, *New Engl. J. Med.,* **282**:1183, 1970.

Godtfredsen, E.: Choked disc or hypertensive retinopathy IV? *Acta ophthalmol.,* **42**:387, 1964.

Hoefnagels, K. L. J.: Rubeosis of the iris associated with occlusion of the carotid artery, *Ophthalmologica,* **148**:196, 1964.

Hollenhorst, R. W.: Significance of bright plaques in the retinal arterioles, *J.A.M.A.,* **178**:23, 1961.

———: Vascular status of patients who have cholesterol emboli in the retina, *Am. J. Ophthalmol.,* **61**:1159, 1966.

Ide, C. H., Almond, C. H., Hart, W. M., Simmons, E. M., and Wilson, R. J.: Hematogenous dissemination of microemboli. Eye findings in a patient with Starr-Edwards aortic prosthesis, *Arch. Ophthalmol.,* **85**:614, 1971.

Keith, N. M., Wagener, H. P., and Barker, N. W.: Some different types of essential hypertension: Their course and prognosis, *Am. J. Med. Sci.,* **197**:332, 1939.

McBrien, D. J., Bradley, R. D., and Ashton, N.: The nature of retinal emboli in stenosis of the internal carotid artery, *Lancet,* **1**:697, 1963.

Russell, R. W. R.: The source of retinal emboli, *Lancet,* **2**:789, 1968.

Scheie, H. G.: Evaluation of ophthalmoscopic changes of hypertension and arteriolar sclerosis, *Arch. Ophthalmol.,* **49**:117, 1953.

Van Buchem, F. S. P., v.d. Heuvel-Aghina, J. W. M. T., and v.d. Heuvel, J. E. A.: Hypertension and changes of the fundus oculi, *Acta med. scand.,* **176**:539, 1964.

Walsh, F. B., and Hoyt, W. F.: Clinical Neuro-ophthalmology, 3d ed., The Williams & Wilkins Company, Baltimore, 1969.

Walsh, T. J., Garden, J. W., and Gallagher, B.: Obliteration of retinal venous pulsations: During elevation of cerebrospinal-fluid pressure, *Am. J. Ophthalmol.,* **67**:954, 1969.

Additional Reference

Moore, R. Y., and Baumann, R. J.: Intracranial bruits in children, *Develop. Med. Child Neurol.,* **11**:650, 1969.

Chapter 7

Ophthalmodynamometry

Technical expressions are a danger for every system of philosophy, whether Indian or European. For they may become formulae which hinder the natural development of thought in the same way as ruts in a road hinder traffic.

Albert Schweitzer

Ophthalmodynamometry (ODM), the measurement of pressure in the ophthalmic artery, was popularized in the early 1920s by Bailliart. The ophthalmodynamometer (Fig. 7-1), which he invented, is a spring-loaded gauge calibrated in grams, the footplate of which is designed to be applied to the sclera of the eye (Fig. 7-2). Pressure is exerted on the instrument while the central arteriole of the retina is observed with an ophthalmoscope. Normally this vessel has no visible pulse. But when diastolic pressure is exceeded, arterial pulsations appear; and when systolic pressure is reached, they cease.

Since about 90 percent of carotid obstructions occur below the origin of the ophthalmic artery, the test often provides the clue that leads to the diagnosis of aortocranial occlusive disease.

Some physicians who have tried to learn the technique have abandoned the effort because they lacked skill in using the ophthalmoscope or in manipulating the ophthalmodynamometer. Others have been discouraged by the misleading results obtained in occasional cases. Despite these limitations, we recommend ODM to any physician who must manage patients with cere-

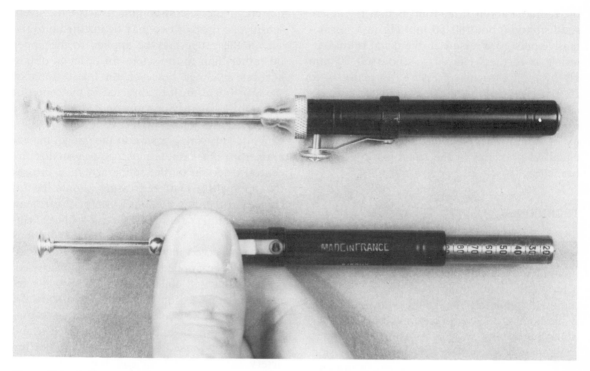

Figure 7-1 Balliart ophthalmodynamometers. A pressure of 85 Gm has been applied to the lower instrument, and the sliding scale locked by pressure on the thumbpiece. *(With permission of F. A. Wood and J. F. Toole, J.A.M.A., 165:1266, 1957.)*

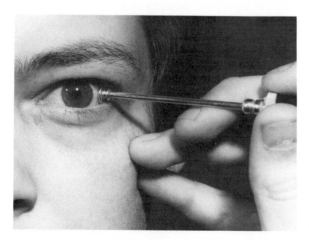

Figure 7-2 Footplate is placed against the lateral sclera while gaze is fixed at a distance. *(Permission of F. A. Wood and J. F. Toole, J.A.M.A., 165:1266, 1957.)*

brovascular diseases. The test is harmless and painless, requires only minutes to perform, and often provides information of great value in assessing the patient's problem and evaluating its course.

GENERAL PRINCIPLES

Because the internal carotid ascends from its origin in the neck to the circle of Willis without any major branches other than the ophthalmic artery, pressure in the ophthalmic artery reflects pressure in the carotid itself. Normally the pressure in the proximal portion of the ophthalmic artery is almost equal to that in the carotid siphon, while pressure in the central arteriole of the retina is about three-fourths that in the carotid siphon (about 80/50 mm Hg in a normotensive person). Pressure in the distal retinal arteriole is further reduced to about 60/30 mm Hg by the intraocular pressure (normally 16 to 20 mm Hg). Ophthalmic pressure does not necessarily reflect the pressure in the other branches of the carotid system because the circle of Willis, unless it is diseased or anomalous, equalizes pressures in the distal carotid and its branches.

TECHNIQUES

Although an occasional physician prefers to have an assistant manipulate the ophthalmodynamometer while he observes the central retinal arteriole, it is not difficult to master the technique of applying the gauge with one hand while holding the ophthalmoscope in the other. Some physicians, instead of using an ophthalmoscope, ask the patient to report loss of vision, which occurs at the instant the gauge pressure exceeds the systolic pressure in the ophthalmic artery. While this indirect method is less accurate than direct observation of the retinal arteriole, it is useful for those who are not adept with an ophthalmoscope.

Whenever possible, the test should be performed with the patient sitting because the effects of hydrostatic pressure cause ophthalmic pressures to be lower in the upright than in the recumbent position. In some cases inequalities of pressure between the two eyes can be observed only with the patient upright.

Direct Method

The footplate of the gauge is applied to the sclera of the eye while the patient fixes his gaze on a distant object. If light is subdued, the pupils will usually dilate adequately; if they do not, a short-acting mydriatic agent can be employed. Topical anesthesia is not usually re-

quired; if the scleral conjunctiva is excessively sensitive, a drop or two may be instilled into the sac, or the gauge may be applied to the upper lid rather than to the sclera. In order to obtain accurate readings, however, the line of force of the instrument must be directed to the center of the globe and the gauge must not slip behind or above the eye.

While applying pressure to the gauge, the examiner uses his ophthalmoscope to visualize the central arteriole of the retina where it crosses the optic disk. Gauge pressure should be increased at the rate of about 5 Gm per heartbeat. Some examiners apply pressure in a linear fashion; others use a stepwise system. Pulsations will be observed in the retinal veins before 10 Gm has been applied. As pressure is increased, retinal veins will collapse at the disk while remaining engorged on the retina; and soon the central retinal arteriole will be observed to pulsate. If pressure is applied too rapidly, the end point will be passed between pulsations of the artery. At the first brief collapse of the blood column in the arteriole, the gauge reading is recorded as the diastolic pressure. Pressure is then increased until the arteriole becomes bloodless at the disk throughout the cardiac cycle. The systolic pressure reading is noted, and pressure is immediately released.

Since carotid obstruction often reduces the systolic pressure more than the diastolic, both measurements must be made in all cases. The test is repeated on the other eye, and pressures on the two sides are recorded and compared.

Indirect Method

The patient is instructed to cover one eye and look off into the distance while the gauge is applied to the other eye. He is asked to report the instant at which his vision begins to "fade out." With some preliminary instruction, most reasonably intelligent and objective patients can pinpoint with a fair degree of accuracy the instant at which peripheral vision fades while central vision remains. At this moment retinal diastolic arterial pressure has been equaled or exceeded, and the gauge is read. Pressure is again increased until the patient reports that vision has faded completely. Pressure is immediately released, and the gauge reading at this point is recorded as the systolic pressure. As with the direct method, pressures in the two eyes are measured and compared.

The reader will find it instructive to press the outer canthus of his eye with a finger while looking off into the distance with the other eye closed. As the slightest pressure is applied, a negative image is projected from the retina near the inner canthus. When pressure is increased, vision quickly begins to fade concentrically from the periphery, until suddenly all vision is lost. The slightest decrease in pressure allows vision to return almost immediately. Many of us inadvertently do this several times daily when we rub our eyes so hard that we are momentarily blinded. Do not exert pressure sufficient to maintain blindness more than a moment or two as retinal damage could result.

INTERPRETATION OF RESULTS

Because pressures in the ophthalmic artery vary somewhat from minute to minute, as does systemic arterial pressure, one cannot compare pressures taken at different times, except in the most general way. Pressures in the two eyes are usually equal—the maximum variation being 15 percent in the systolic pressure and 10 percent in the diastolic pressure. Greater differences usually indicate obstruction somewhere between the aortic arch and the retinal artery on the side with the lower pressure.

Under normal conditions the intraocular pressures of the eyes are equal, and it is seldom necessary to measure ocular pressure when dynamometry is performed. If pressure in one eye is elevated by glaucoma or reduced by injury,

however, the dynamometer pressure necessary to exceed ophthalmic arterial pressure in that eye will be altered. To arrive at actual values for ophthalmic artery pressure, the ocular and dynamometer pressures must be added together. The relation between ocular pressure and ophthalmodynamometer pressure is not purely additive, however, since it is affected by individual variables such as the elasticity of the sclera and the length of time that pressure is applied by the dynamometer.

CLINICAL APPLICATIONS

Ophthalmodynamometry has three principal uses: (1) diagnosis of aortocranial occlusive disease; (2) evaluation of the results of ligation or reconstruction of the carotid artery in the neck; and (3) determination of arterial pressure within the cerebral circulation.

Diagnosis of Aortocranial Occlusive Disease
In about 75 percent of patients with occlusion or stenosis of more than 50 percent of the carotid artery, ophthalmic pressures on the diseased side are abnormally low. The exceptions occur principally in patients with old occlusions in whom collateral circulation may develop between the vertebral-basilar and the external carotid systems. In such cases arterial reconstruction is seldom feasible.

When disease is present in both carotids, pressures may be equally reduced on both sides. In such cases, comparison of ophthalmic pressures with brachial blood pressure will show the latter to be relatively high (Table 7–1). This situation is reversed when both subclavian arteries are stenosed and the carotid system is patent, as in bilateral subclavian steal. Normally, ophthalmic pressures (measured in grams) are a little more than half the brachial blood pressures (measured in millimeters of mercury). Nomograms have been constructed for accurate

Table 7-1   Relationship of Blood Vessel Obstruction and Blood Pressure

	Pressure	
Vessel obstructed	Brachial artery, mm Hg	Ophthalmic artery, Gm
One carotid artery	Equal	Low on involved side
Both carotid arteries	Equal	Bilaterally low compared with brachials
Brachiocephalic artery	Right low	Right low
Proximal subclavian artery (subclavian steal)	Unequal	Equal
Vertebral-basilar artery	Equal	Equal
Both subclavian arteries	Equally low	Equally high

comparison of the two, but they contribute little to the clinical evaluation of the patient.

Measurement of Ophthalmic Artery Pressure before and after Carotid Ligation for Intracranial Aneurysm   This valuable guide to the degree of pressure reduction has not been fully exploited by neurosurgeons. Measurements made periodically for months or years help to determine whether collateral circulation is being established.

Evaluation of Carotid Artery Reconstructive Surgery   Pre- and postoperative determinations of ophthalmic artery pressures give objective evidence of the success of arterial reconstruction and are essential for the assessment of continued patency of the artery (see Chap. 17).

Determination of Arterial Pressure within the Cerebral Circulation   Some cases have been reported in which intracranial blood pressure appeared to be higher than systemic arterial pressure (so-called "central hypertension"). One theory that has been offered to explain such regional hypertension is that a change in the caliber of intracranial arterioles produces reflected or standing arterial waves that may increase blood pressure locally. A more likely explanation is that an occasional patient with arterial hypertension as measured by ODM has "normal" brachial blood pressures because of stenosis of both subclavian arteries.

CONTRAINDICATIONS AND COMPLICATIONS

The only contraindication to this test is recent retinal detachment or ophthalmic surgery. Aside from rare and harmless subconjunctival hemorrhages, the only complications that have been reported were due to inept handling of the instrument. Corneal abrasions have occurred in a few cases, and there are one or two reports of permanent blindness following the test; this probably resulted from prolonged pressure of the instrument against the globe. As we have stated, the pressure must be released from the globe as soon as retinal systolic pressure is exceeded, so that the blood flow can be reestablished immediately.

IMPORTANT CONSIDERATIONS

1 The ophthalmodynamometer measures *pressure* and not *flow* in the ophthalmic artery. Low pressures can exist with high flow, and the reverse is also true.

2 Pressure on the globe by the ophthalmodynamometer causes a small quantity of aqueous humor to be squeezed from it. Consequently, at least 5 min must be allowed to elapse between measurements on the same eye, so that the volume of aqueous humor can reestablish itself.

3 If the heartbeat is unusually slow or irregular, as in cases of atrial fibrillation or frequent premature ventricular contractions with compensatory pauses, the vessel may become exsanguinated during asystole. In such cases it is impossible to measure accurately the diastolic and systolic end points.

4 We do not recommend compression of the carotid artery in conjunction with ophthalmodynamometry. Although this test does give information regarding patency of the carotid, it also stimulates the carotid sinus and may produce serious side effects, as described in Chap. 8.

5 In rare instances the ophthalmic artery arises from the middle meningeal branch of the external carotid rather than from the carotid artery itself. More commonly, a variable degree of anastomosis exists between the two. In such cases, the reduction in ophthalmic pressures resulting from disease of the carotid artery depends upon the degree of this anastomosis.

6 If occlusion of the carotid artery occurs gradually, as it usually does with atherosclerosis, the development of collateral circulation may prevent reduction of pressure in the ophthalmic artery despite extensive disease of the carotid.

7 Spontaneous arterial pulsations can be seen when intraocular pressure is high, and when arterial pulse pressure is wide or very low.

8 An unusually wide pulse pressure in the ophthalmic artery suggests systolic hypertension, aortic insufficiency, or low peripheral resistance. Rare causes are arteriovenous fistulae and occlusion of the opposite carotid.

9 Obstruction of the carotid just distal to the origin of the ophthalmic artery may cause an abnormal elevation of ophthalmic pressure on the side of the occlusion.

SUGGESTED READINGS

General Principles

Kjer, P., Eiken, M., and von Wowern, F.: Ophthalmodynamometry in apoplectic patients with hemispherical infarction or transitory hemispherical symptoms, *Acta ophthalmol.*, **48**:700, 1970.

Palena, P. V., Jaeger, E. A., Behrendt, T., and Duane, T. D.: Quantitative effect of increased intraocular pressure on blackout, *Arch. Ophthalmol.*, **83**:84, 1970.

Toole, J. F.: Ophthalmodynamometry, *Neurology*, **11**:97, 1961.

Weigelin, E., and Lobstein, A.: Ophthalmodynamometry, Hafner Publishing Company, Inc., New York, 1963.

Wood, F. A., and Toole, J. F.: Carotid artery occlusion and its diagnosis by ophthalmodynamometry, *J.A.M.A.*, **165**:1264, 1957.

Wunsh, S. E.: Ophthalmodynamometry, *New Engl. J. Med.*, **281**:446, 1969.

Techniques

Indirect Method

Toole, J. F.: Ophthalmodynamometry—A simplified method, *Arch. Internal Med.*, **112**:981, 1963.

Interpretation of Results

Borras, A., Martinez, A., and Mendez, M. S.: Carotid compression test and direct measurement of ophthalmic artery pressure in man, *Am. J. Ophthalmol.*, **67**:688, 1969.

Drake, W. E., Jr., McAuliffe, M., and Stone, D. W.: Ophthalmic artery profiles in cerebrovascular disease: An angiographic correlation, *Neurology*, **14**:386, 1964.

Ewing, C. C.: Ophthalmodynamometry in retinal infarction. The difficulty of differentiating internal carotid from central retinal artery occlusion, *Am. J. Ophthalmol.*, **58**:759, 1964.

Goldstein, J. E., Peczon, J. D., and Cogan, D. G.: Intraocular pressure and ophthalmodynamometry, *Arch. Ophthalmol.*, **74**:175, 1965.

Hedges, T. R., Weinstein, J. D., Kassell, N. F., and Langfitt, T. W.: Correlation of ophthalmodynamometry with ophthalmic artery pressure in the rhesus monkey, *Am. J. Ophthalmol.*, **60**:1098, 1965.

Smith, M. C., and Hoyt, W. F.: Chronic occlusive disease of the carotid arteries with nondiagnostic or misleading pressures on the retinal arteries, *Am. J. Surg.*, **102**:661, 1961.

Clinical Applications

Hollenhorst, R. W., Kublin, J. G., and Millikan, C. H.: Ophthalmodynamometry in the diagnosis of intracerebral orthostatic hypotension, *Proc. Staff Meetings Mayo Clinic*, **38**:532, 1963.

Liversedge, L. A., and Smith, V. H.: The place of ophthalmodynamometry in the investigation of cerebrovascular disease, *Brain*, **84**:274, 1961.

Russell, R. W., and Cranston, W. I.: Ophthalmodynamometry in carotid artery disease, *J. Neurol. Neurosurg. Psychiat.*, **24**:281, 1961.

Contraindications and Complications

Hollwich, F.: Question and answer: Damage to the eye after pressure on the eyeball: Could repeated pressure on the eyeball to stop attacks of paroxysmal tachycardia cause damage to the eye? *German Med. Monthly*, **10**:297, 1965.

Important Considerations

Calderon, R. G.: Postural ophthalmodynamometry in carotid artery occlusive disease, *J.A.M.A.*, **185**:826, 1963.

Szapiro, J., and Pakula, H.: Anatomical studies of collateral blood supply to brain and the retina, *J. Neurol. Neurosurg. Psychiat.*, **26**:414, 1963.

Zappia, R. J., Winkelman, J. Z., Roberson, G. H., Rosenbaum, H. E., and Gay, A. J.: Progressive intracranial arterial occlusion syndrome. Report of a case with unusually high ophthalmodynamometry (O.D.M.) values, *Arch. Ophthalmol.*, **86**:455, 1971.

Carotid Sinus Massage and Carotid Compression Test

Mammals are distinguished, not merely by suckling their young, but also by a dilatation on the dominant cerebral artery before it enters the skull.

W. E. Adams

Even though the physical examination and laboratory studies prove to be negative, the examination of a patient complaining of syncope is not complete until the effect of hyperventilation, of pressure on the carotid sinus, and of motionless standing have been determined.

Eugene Stead

Since time immemorial, compression of the carotid artery has been performed to render people senseless,* and its effects on the cerebral circulation have been debated almost as long

* The adjective *carotid* is derived from the Greek *karos* meaning "heavy sleep."

(Fig. 8-1). Although some physicians question the reliability of tests involving manipulation of the carotid and others fear disastrous consequences, we believe that massage of the carotid sinus and compression of the carotid artery, performed in the manner described in this chapter, are extremely valuable aids in the diagnosis and

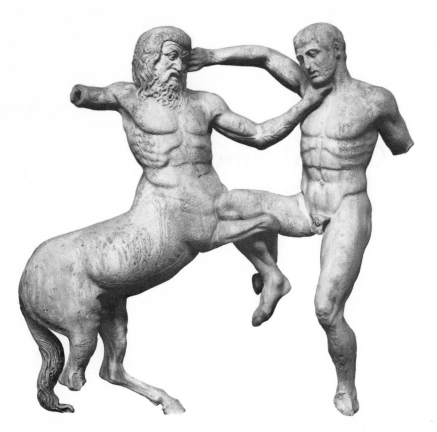

Figure 8-1 Carotid compression has been known since antiquity, as illustrated by the thirty-first sculpture on the south side of the Parthenon (Elgin marbles). Left carotid compression, producing adverse seizure to the right. *(Reproduced by permission of the British Museum.)*

evaluation of the obstructive forms of aortocranial disease. The tests should be done only after a complete physical and neurologic examination and certain preliminary studies have been made. Some physicians perform both tests in the office or at the bedside, but we are convinced that compression of the artery should never be done except in a laboratory where changes in the electroencephalogram, electrocardiogram, and blood pressure can be monitored. The information thus recorded can then be analyzed to show the correlation between

brain activity, heart function, and blood pressure.

PHYSIOLOGY OF THE CAROTID SINUS REFLEX

The key to understanding the effects of massage or compression lies in recalling that the carotid sinus is situated on the internal carotid artery just distal to the bifurcation of the common carotid. The sinus is richly supplied with sensory endings, primarily of the glossopharyngeal nerve. Immediately adjacent to it lies the carotid body, similarly supplied. The carotid body is sensitive to changes in blood gases and has pneumoregulatory effects.

The carotid sinus has two and possibly three normal regulatory effects which arise in receptors situated in the adventitia of the sinus and in immediately adjacent regions of the internal, common, and external carotid arteries. Impulses travel over afferent fibers of the glossopharyngeal nerve to nuclei in the brainstem reticular formation, where "centers" initiate efferent impulses, with the following effects:

1 The heart is slowed and cardiac output is decreased by vagal inhibitory reflexes transmitted down the vagus nerve to the sinoatrial node of the heart.

2 Vasodepressor impulses travel to the thoracolumbar regions of the spinal cord, thence via the spinal nerves to the paravertebral sympathetic chains. The resultant dilatation of the splanchnic and limb arterial beds causes a fall in arterial blood pressure.

3 It is possible that impulses from brainstem "centers," traveling a vaguely described efferent pathway such as that outlined in the preceding paragraph or following a direct intracranial route in parasympathetic fibers of the facial nerve, might cause constriction of the cerebral arteries and arterioles.

Clinical research initiated by Dr. Soma Weiss during the late 1920s and early 1930s led him to conclude that one or more of these normal reflexes might become hypersensitive, resulting in syncope or even convulsions in some patients. He believed that he could distinguish clearly the three effects just described: (1) the vagal inhibitory reflex with cardiac slowing or standstill, (2) the vasodepressor responses with a precipitous fall in blood pressure but no slowing of the heart, and (3) cerebral vasoconstriction. He also ascertained that one or more of these reflexes could lead to signs of cerebral vascular insufficiency.

He found the vagal inhibitory effect to be parasympathetic in nature and readily overcome by blockage and atropine. The vasodepressor effect, being sympathetic, is suppressed by vasoconstrictor agents such as epinephrine or ephedrine. The "direct cerebral effect" responds to neither type of drug.

No one has questioned the accuracy of his conclusions concerning the existence of the first and second forms of sinus hypersensitivity. There is a school of thought, however, which believes that Dr. Weiss, whose investigations were performed prior to the advent of cerebral arteriography and electroencephalography, produced his so-called cerebral response by occluding the carotid artery and reducing cerebral blood flow. Consequently, a clear distinction must be made between *massage of the sinus* and *compression of the artery* either at the sinus or below it, since the effects elicited may be quite different. The former initiates a reflex, while the latter simply reduces blood flow by manual obstruction of the vessel.

The reflexes described can be elicited in most persons, but only in a few can signs and symptoms of syncope, vertigo, dizziness and, occasionally, seizures be produced. In these people the carotid sinus is said to be "hypersensitive."

Because of its unusual construction, the region of the carotid bifurcation and the carotid sinus just distal to it are predisposed to the accumulation of atheromatous plaques. These plaques render the carotid sinus reflex hyperreactive by making the artery stiff and destroying its normal expansile characteristics. In many persons, they also obstruct the lumen of the vessel, so that those who have carotid sinus hypersensitivity may also have signs and symptoms of carotid artery insufficiency. Consequently, even gentle massage of the artery may temporarily obliterate the lumen of the vessel. The bifurcation is also a site of predilection for the angiopathy of Takayasu (Chap. 28), and symptoms secondary to hypersensitivity of the carotid sinus are common in patients with this disease.

Rarely irritation or neuralgias of the glossopharyngeal nerve may cause convulsions secondary to hypotension or bradycardia.

TECHNIQUES

Sinus Massage

Massage may safely be performed in the office or at the bedside, provided that lead II of the electrocardiograph and blood pressure are properly monitored. A syringe containing atropine, 1/50 grain, should be handy for emergency use, although the need for it is extremely rare.

The examiner places a finger of one hand on the superficial temporal artery and several fingers of the other hand on the carotid sinus, which is usually felt as a bulbous dilatation just beneath the angle of the jaw medial to the sternocleidomastoid muscle. The head should not be turned to either side, since this may impair flow through one of the carotid or vertebral arteries. The carotid is stroked very gently for 30 sec unless the heart slows unduly or arrhythmia develops, in which case the vessel is immediately released. The other side is then similarly massaged. If massage is tolerated on both sides without signs of vagal inhibition, the test should be repeated with the patient sitting up, in order to assess the possibility of a vasodepressor reflex. Under no circumstances should the vessel be compressed. The pulse in the superficial temporal artery must be monitored throughout the test to be certain that no compression of the carotid has occurred as a result of overenthusiastic massage. After each massage, a record should be made of any symptoms and signs that develop during the procedure.

Carotid Compression

Compression of the artery, which calls for a more formal test, must be preceded by a complete electrocardiogram to be certain that the patient has no myocardial damage or cardiac arrhythmia, and by a base-line electroencephalogram to eliminate the possibility of cerebral dysrhythmias.

There is a slight but very real hazard associated with carotid artery compression, and the test must not be employed unless serious consideration is being given to surgical reconstruction of the carotico-vertebral-basilar system. Even then the decision must be tempered by the realization that some patients are in too precarious a condition to tolerate it. Patients with angina pectoris or recent myocardial infarction should not be tested. The cardiac rate and rhythm and the brain waves should be normal. If the base-line electrocardiogram or electroencephalogram is abnormal, it is difficult to tell whether changes occurring during the test are spontaneous variations or are precipitated by the carotid manipulation.

Electroencephalographic leads are applied to the frontal and temporal regions of each hemisphere and, with the patient securely strapped to the tilt table in the supine position, the electrocardiograph lead II and blood pressure cuff are attached. An objective measure of the external carotid pulse can be made by attaching a photoresistive cell to the pinna of each ear.

The first procedure to be carried out is the sinus massage just described. If massage on either side produces vagal inhibition or vasodepression without reproducing the patient's symptoms, atropine or a vasopressor agent should be used to block the reflex response before proceeding further. An alternative method is to infiltrate the region of the carotid sinus with procaine to block the afferent limb of the reflex arc, but we do not recommend this procedure.

If massage elicits no reflex response or if one desires to determine the degree of obstructive aortocranial disease that may exist along with carotid sinus hypersensitivity, the common carotid may be compressed below the sinus. Each internal carotid artery normally perfuses its hemisphere with 300 to 400 ml of blood per min. Compression of the vessel compromises cerebral circulation, and if disease has obstructed flow through the opposite carotid artery, even temporary occlusion of the vessel will initiate signs of cerebral vascular insufficiency. If it is to occur at all, slowing of the EEG to theta and delta range begins after about 10 to 15 sec of compression and is followed in another 5 to 10 sec by fading of vision and symptoms of cerebral ischemia. At the instant the EEG changes are seen and before clinical evidence of ischemia occurs, the vessel is released and blood pressure is recorded (Fig. 8-2). The patient is asked what symptoms, if any, he experienced; usually he will report none. He is not to be given any clue as to what is expected, since sug-

gestible patients will report imagined symptoms.

If compression of the carotid on each side is tolerated without precipitating symptoms or signs, the table is tilted to an angle of 70°, with the patient's head up. He is asked to remain motionless and relaxed while the blood pressure is taken at intervals of 15 sec. If the pressure remains stable for 3 min, carotid compression is performed again in the same manner as before. Because of the vasodepressor reflex and added hydrostatic effects, compression which has been tolerated in the recumbent position may not be tolerated in the upright. If the test is tolerated in each carotid with the face front, compression is repeated again, with the head turned to one side and then to the other.

By this series of maneuvers it is possible to test the patient systematically for all three types of carotid sinus hypersensitivity—the vagal inhibitory, the vasodepressor, and the so-called cerebral type—and also to test his cerebrovascular reserve and the effect of body posture and

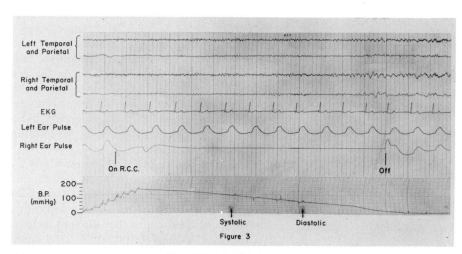

Figure 8-2 Right temporoparietal slowing of the brain rhythms produced by right carotid compression. Alteration in the cardiac rate or rhythm is proved by the EKG and the blood pressure record. The ear pulse monitor serves as an index to the adequacy of compression.

head position on cerebral blood flow and reserve. The three distinct effects that may result from these maneuvers are (1) a reflex effect, produced by massage of the carotid sinus; (2) a mechanical effect from compression of the artery; and (3) an anatomic effect secondary to change of body posture and head position.

The test should be terminated whenever a positive result is obtained at any stage of the procedure, unless the reflex effects are blocked pharmacologically or the response of the other side is to be tested. If, for example, massage of either carotid sinus produces cardiac standstill, one must not proceed to carotid compression without blocking the vagal effect by infiltrating the carotid sinus with procaine or, better, by giving the patient an intravenous injection of atropine, 1/150 to 1/100 grain. If, in another case, carotid massage produces no effect but compression of the right carotid in the recumbent position results in slowing of brain rhythms over the right hemisphere, one should perform no further compressive maneuvers on the right carotid. The left carotid, however, should be compressed for 30 sec, after allowing an interval of 1 to 2 min for the cerebral flow to recover; the test should then be discontinued. Finally, if both massage and compression are tolerated in the recumbent position, the patient should be tilted to 70° head up and the maneuvers repeated. Again the test must be stopped if a positive effect is obtained at any point.

Despite its seeming simplicity, the proper performance of the carotid compression test requires a knowledge of the fundamentals on which it is based and awareness of the following points:

1 The risks involved and the preparations necessary to handle the emergencies that could result. The physician must know the rudiments of interpreting the electroencephalogram and electrocardiogram and, when he performs the test, should situate himself in such a manner that he can supervise the personnel with whom he is working.

2 Variations in the location of the carotid sinus. In some patients it is high behind the angle of the mandible; in others, it lies at the level of the thyroid cartilage. One cannot always be certain whether the sinus or the common carotid artery is being tested.

3 The different effects of compressing the common carotid. In some patients this maneuver reverses flow from the external carotid artery, so that some flow toward the head continues through the internal carotid artery despite the compression. In other patients flow through the internal carotid artery is reversed and actually siphons blood from the brain to the external carotid system. It is preferable, therefore, to carry out carotid compression just below the carotid sinus, so that both the common and the external carotid system may be effectively occluded.

4 The necessity for frequent blood pressure readings. The blood pressure must be taken just before compression, midway through it, and immediately after the vessel is released. The vasodepressor response is usually abrupt in onset, the blood pressure falling almost immediately after compression begins and returning to baseline values within seconds after the carotid is released. In many instances a vasodepressor reflex is unrecognized because the examiner does not determine blood pressure during the test and because other neurologic events overshadow the hypotension. It should be emphasized that the *rate of fall,* not only the degree of hypotension, is the important factor in precipitating cerebrovascular insufficiency.

5 The significance of facial pallor. Many patients become noticeably pale just before electroencephalographic slowing begins. This pallor may result from constriction of the vessels in the external carotid system as they attempt to redistribute flow to the intracranial circulation. Whatever the cause, facial pallor is a good clinical sign of impending cerebral vascular insufficiency and should alert the examiner.

6 Hyperventilation due to stimulation of the

carotid body. Once it is recognized that hyperventilation is based on mechanical causes as well as on anxiety, the hyperpnea can be ignored.

7 The danger of massaging or compressing both carotid sinuses at the same time. This should never be done under any circumstances.

Testing the Oculocardiac Reflex

If the results of carotid massage and compression tests are normal, the explanation for episodes suggestive of cerebrovascular insufficiency may be found by testing the oculocardiac reflex. This is done by pressing the globe into the orbit hard enough to cause pain, thus initiating afferent impulses over the ophthalmic division of the trigeminal nerve. These impulses, traversing an ill-defined route to vagal nuclei in the brainstem, may produce cardiac slowing or asystole. This reflex response is said to occur in patients who have orthostatic hypotension due to vasovagal reflexes.

Testing the Diving Reflex

The trigeminal nerve is sensitive to water applied to the skin, particularly over the ophthalmic division. This causes vagal slowing of the heart, peripheral vasoconstriction with redistribution of blood flow to the brain, and increase in systemic arterial blood pressure, and in theory could cause increased cerebral blood flow in patients with cerebrovascular disease, although this has not yet been assessed.

INDICATIONS FOR CAROTID MASSAGE AND COMPRESSION

The tests should be reserved for patients suspected of having episodes of cerebrovascular insufficiency or carotid sinus hypersensitivity whose condition is such that the information provided might be of value in selecting appropriate therapy. If cerebrovascular insufficiency

is precipitated by the tests, angiography should be considered with a view toward the surgical correction of any extracranial vascular lesion that might be found.

Carotid compression is also used for evaluating the feasibility of ligating the carotid in patients with intracranial aneurysm. In these cases, the artery should be compressed for 10 min, if necessary, to rule out hypersensitivity of the carotid sinus and cerebrovascular insufficiency. In patients with either abnormality, the vessel must be occluded gradually with a clamp, possibly after denervating the sinus. Some of these patients, however, cannot tolerate occlusion by any method. If the test is not performed before angiography, it must be delayed until the tenderness resulting from hematoma and trauma to the artery has subsided.

INTERPRETATION OF RESULTS

The results obtained from the carotid massage and compression tests must be assessed in relation to the patient's history and his neurovascular examination.

Results of Carotid Sinus Massage

In many older patients hypersensitivity to carotid sinus massage is asymptomatic and bears no relation to the patient's problem. On the other hand, if the results obtained duplicate the patient's symptoms and particularly if the patient volunteers the remark that the symptoms reproduce his clinical attacks, one is usually safe in concluding that the patient's problem is related to a hypersensitive carotid sinus. The most frequent basis of hypersensitivity of the carotid sinus reflex is aortocranial atherosclerosis.

Orthostatic Hypotension

A rapid fall in blood pressure when the patient is tilted into the 70° upright position indicates spontaneous loss of vasomotor tone. This may be related to (1) medications which the patient is taking; (2) unsuspected endocrine abnormalities such as hypoadrenalism, hypopituitarism, or salt depletion; (3) peripheral neuropathies of any type, but most often diabetic in origin; or (4) orthostatic hypotension on a psychogenic basis—although it is surprisingly rare for this to occur during the performance of the test.

Results of Carotid Compression

Carotid compression is valuable in assessing cerebral vascular reserve and gives clues to the patency of the carotid arterial system. When one common carotid is compressed, there is a compensatory increase in flow—sometimes as much as 50 percent—through the other carotid and through each of the two vertebral arteries unless a sinus reflex response with hypotension or cardiac slowing occurs simultaneously. Normally this increase is accompanied by a redistribution of flow intracranially through the circle of Willis, so that the area usually supplied by the compromised artery is perfused by blood flowing through the opposite carotid and the vertebral-basilar system. In the presence of disease such as atherosclerosis of the aortocranial system, or when congenital anomalies lead to inadequate crossover through the circle of Willis (particularly through the anterior and posterior communicating arteries), compression of the carotid precipitates signs and symptoms of cerebral vascular insufficiency.

Results obtained from carotid compression are interpreted as follows:

1 If the patient tolerates compression of either carotid for 30 sec, his cerebral vascular reserve is probably adequate, although he may still have obstruction to an extra- or intracranial artery. We have seen many patients with occlusion of one or even both of the internal carotid arteries in the neck who tolerated compression of either artery without symptoms. The explanation probably lies in the presence of adequate collateral supply through the vertebral-basilar or external carotid circulations and in the fact

that arteries already occluded can be compromised no further.

2 If electroencephalographic changes result from pressure on one side but not on the other, one may conclude that the carotid on the positive side is essential for adequate brain perfusion (Fig. 8-3). The most frequent causes of this situation are *(a)* severe stenosis or occlusion of the artery on the negative side; *(b)* an anomaly in the circle of Willis, causing most of the cerebral flow to traverse the carotid artery on the positive side; and *(c)* occlusion of the proximal portion of the anterior cerebral artery, so that collateral flow is prevented.

3 If neither carotid sinus is hypersensitive but compression is not tolerated on either side, both internal carotid arteries are patent, but cerebral reserve is borderline and collateral flow from one carotid to the other (through the anterior communicating artery) or from the posterior to the anterior circulation (through the posterior communicating arteries) is not adequate. Another possible explanation is bilateral occlusion of the vertebral arteries or bilateral subclavian steal; in such cases both the anterior and the posterior circulations are totally dependent on the two internal carotid arteries.

4 If carotid compression produces EEG changes only when the head is turned to one side, one should suspect that flow through the vertebral arteries is compromised by the change of head position or that flow through the opposite carotid is impaired by kinking or looping.

5 If compression of either carotid artery causes loss of consciousness without a change in the electroencephalogram, the probable cause is either a psychophysiologic reaction or vascular insufficiency in the brainstem combined with disease of the vertebral-basilar artery.

6 Vertical nystagmus just prior to the onset of encephalographic changes suggests insufficiency of the basilar artery.

COMPLICATIONS

In rare cases, manipulation of atherosclerotic carotid arteries leads to permanent cardiac or neurologic damage. This may be caused by the

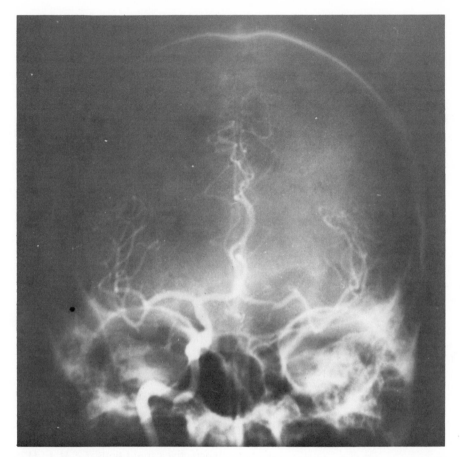

Figure 8-3 Injection of the right carotid artery during compression of the left carotid artery in a patient with an adequate anterior communicating artery resulting in filling of the left anterior and middle cerebral arteries.

abrupt decrease in cardiac output that results from hypersensitivity of the carotid sinus reflex, or by an acute decrease in cerebral blood flow secondary to carotid compression. Even more rarely, the vessel is damaged by compression, or cerebral emboli occur when atheromatous plaques are dislodged.

Another possibility is prolonged cardiac asystole or cardiac arrest with ventricular fibrillation following the initiation of a vagal reflex. Even though this complication has been reported very rarely in the world literature, a defibrillator should be available and the team should be proficient in cardiac-pulmonary resuscitation.

SUGGESTED READINGS

General

Engel, G. L.: On the existence of the cerebral type of carotid sinus syncope, *Neurology,* **9**:565, 1959.

Gastaut, H., Naquet, R., and Regis, H.: L'ictus larynge ou syncope tussive: Forme particulière du syndrome d'hyperréflexie sinucarotidienne, *Presse med.,* **67**:2229, 1959.

Gurdjian, E. S., Webster, J. E., Hardy, W. G., and

Lindner, D. W.: Nonexistence of the so-called cerebral form of carotid sinus syncope, *Neurology*, **8**:818, 1958.

Kong, Y., Heyman, A., Entman, M. L., and McIntosh, H. D.: Glossopharyngeal neuralgia associated with bradycardia, syncope, and seizures, *Circulation*, **30**:109, 1964.

Lown, B., and Levine, S. A.: The carotid sinus: Clinical value of its stimulation, *Circulation*, **23**:766, 1961.

Weiss, S., and Baker, J. P.: The carotid sinus reflex in health and disease: Its role in the causation of fainting and convulsions, *Medicine*, **12**:297, 1933.

Carotid Sinus Syndrome

Anderson, G. M.: The carotid sinus syndrome, *J. Louisiana Med. Soc.*, **116**:54, 1964.

Golding-Wood, P. H.: The laryngologist and vertigo: The carotid sinus and its syndromes, *Proc. Roy. Soc. Med.*, **55**:180, 1962.

Hutchinson, E. C., and Stock, J. P.: The carotid-sinus syndrome, *Lancet*, **2**:445, 1960.

Webster, J. E., Gurdjian, E. S., and Martin, F. A.: Mechanism of syncope due to unilateral compression of carotid bifurcation, *Arch. Neurol. Psychiat.*, **74**:556, 1955.

Techniques

Fuster, B., Ferreiro, C., Cleaves, F., and Coleman, W. G.: The carotid compression test. The questionable value of the ear lobe pulse as monitor of the blood flow to the brain through the compressed carotid, *Acta neurol. latinoam.*, **11**:391, 1965.

Silverstein, A., Doniger, D., and Bender, M. B.: Manual compression of the carotid vessels, carotid sinus hypersensitivity and carotid artery occlusions, *Ann. Internal Med.*, **52**:172, 1960.

Toole, J. F.: Stimulation of the carotid sinus in man: I. The cerebral response; II. The significance of head positioning, *Am. J. Med.*, **27**:952, 1959.

Sinus Massage

Thomas, J. E.: Hyperactive carotid sinus reflex and carotid sinus syncope, *Mayo Clinic Proc.*, **44**:127, 1969.

Voss, D. M., and Magnin, G. E.: Demand pacing and carotid sinus syncope, *Am. Heart J.*, **79**:544, 1970.

Indications for Carotid Massage and Compression

Meyer, J. S., Leiderman, H., and Denny-Brown, D.: Electroencephalographic study of insufficiency of the basilar and carotid arteries in man, *Neurology*, **6**:455, 1956.

Terzian, H.: The diagnostic value of carotid artery .compression in cerebral vascular insufficiency, *Electroencephalog. Clin. Neurophysiol.*, **7**:441, 1955.

Toole, J. F., and Bevilacqua, J. E.: The carotid compression test: Evaluation of the diagnostic reliability and prognostic significance, *Neurology*, **13**:601, 1963.

Complications

Askey, J. M.: Hemiplegia following carotid sinus stimulation, *Am. Heart J.*, **31**:131, 1946.

Greenwood, R. J., and Dupler, D. A.: Death following carotid sinus pressure, *J.A.M.A.*, **181**:605, 1962.

Hilal, H., and Massumi, R.: Fatal ventricular fibrillation after carotid-sinus stimulation, *New Engl. J. Med.*, **275**:157, 1966.

Marmor, J., and Sapirstein, M. R.: Bilateral thrombosis of anterior cerebral artery following stimulation of a hyperactive carotid sinus, *J.A.M.A.*, **117**:1089, 1941.

Meredith, H. C., Jr., and Beckwith, J. R.: Development of ventricular tachycardia following carotid sinus stimulation in paroxysmal supraventricular tachycardia, *Am. Heart J.*, **39**:604, 1950.

Zeman, F. D., and Siegal, S.: Monoplegia following carotid sinus pressure in the aged, *Am. J. Med. Sci.*, **213**:603, 1947.

Treatment

Greeley, H. P., Smedal, M. I., and Most, W.: The treatment of the carotid-sinus syndrome by irradiation, *New Engl. J. Med.*, **252**:91, 1955.

Herman, M., and Levy, E. S.: Carotid sinus syncope treated with roentgen therapy, *Arch. Internal Med.*, **109**:287, 1962.

Ray, B. S., and Stewart, H. J.: The treatment of hypersensitive carotid sinus by glossopharyngeal nerve section, *J. Neurosurg.*, **1**:338, 1944.

Webster, J. E., and Gurdjian, E. S.: Carotid artery compression as employed both in the past and in the present, *J. Neurosurg.*, **15**:372, 1958.

Interpretation of Results

Brodie, R. E., and Dow, R. S.: Studies in carotid compression and sinus sensitivity, *Neurology*, **18**:1047, 1968.

Gastaut, H., and Fischer-Williams, M.: Electroencephalographic study of syncope: Its differentiation from epilepsy, *Lancet*, **2**:1018, 1957.

Gurdjian, E. S., and Webster, J. E.: Digital carotid artery compression with occlusion of the anterior cerebral artery, *Neurology*, **7**:635, 1957.

Janeway, R.: "The carotid compression test: Arteriographic correlations and observations on carotid sinus sensitivity," in Cerebral Vascular Diseases, Transactions of the Sixth Princeton Conference, edited by R. G. Siekert and J. P. Whisnant, Grune & Stratton, Inc., New York, 1968, pp. 220-231.

Lewis, T.: Vasovagal syncope and the carotid sinus mechanism with comments on Gower's and Nothnagel's syndrome, *Brit. Med. J.*, **1**:873, 1932.

Meyer, J. S., Gotoh, F., and Favale, E.: Effects of carotid compression on cerebral metabolism and electroencephalogram, *Electroencephalog. Clin. Neurophysiol.*, **19**:362, 1965.

Schluger, J.: Treatment of angina pectoris by nonmanual autostimulation of the carotid sinus, *Am. Heart J.*, **82**:277, 1971.

Solomon, S.: Evaluation of carotid artery compression in cerebrovascular disease. An electroencephalographic-clinical correlation, *Arch. Neurol.*, **14**:165, 1966.

Aortocervical Atherosclerosis

... disease of old age, which might surprise a man, and yet not immediately kill him, and of which there might possibly be a removal, at least for a season, that there might some space be given him to recover a little strength, before he goes home and be no more seen.

John Smith

Atherosclerosis is a noninflammatory degenerative disease that can affect segments of almost any artery in the body. It is by far the commonest vascular disorder and is the underlying cause of death in most persons over 50. Because atheromata have been seen as incidental findings in the arteries of young adults, children, or even infants who have died of accidental causes, atherosclerosis is known to begin in early life. However, it usually does not become symptomatic until later because the crippling effects of the disease are not due to the sclerosis but are secondary to decrease in the amount of blood supplied to tissues.

A discussion of the causes and prevention of atherosclerosis is not within the scope of this book, but a few important facts should be recorded:

1 Judging from the fact that atherosclerosis of the arteries supplying the brain has been found in Egyptian mummies preserved from 4000 B.C., this disease has probably afflicted man ever since he indulged his gastronomic urges by eating the forbidden fruit.

2 Atherosclerosis is not necessarily a result of "civilized" human living. It occurs spontaneously in primitive tribes as well as in baboons, monkeys, and pigeons and can be induced in

rabbits and chickens maintained on appropriate diets.

3 Despite years of research, the etiology and pathogenesis of atheromatosis are still obscure. Among the many factors believed to influence its occurrence are heredity, the dietary fat content, endocrine changes, chronic psychic stress, the use of tobacco, and lack of exercise.

4 Some believe that the prevention of atherosclerosis lies in the hands of the food producers not the physicians.

5 Atherosclerosis is of greatest clinical importance when it occurs in the coronary arteries, the arch of the aorta and its aortocranial branches, the renal arterial tree, and the aorto-

iliac area. Persons with extensive atherosclerosis in any of these locations may remain asymptomatic until some superimposed event suddenly reduces blood flow to the distal areas below a critical level. Although atherosclerosis of the aortocranial arteries is the subject of this chapter, the clinician must consider it in relation to the more generalized disease.

PATHOGENESIS

Lipid and cholesterol deposits are laid down beneath the intima of the arteries supplying the brain, particularly at angulations, bifurcations, and areas of dilatation or tortuosity. It is

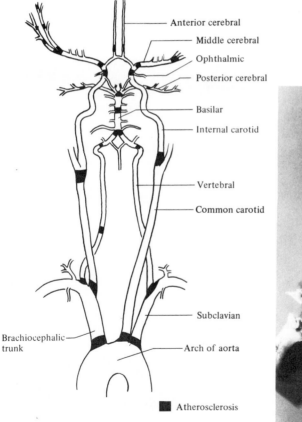

Anterior cerebral
Middle cerebral
Ophthalmic
Posterior cerebral
Basilar
Internal carotid
Vertebral
Common carotid
Subclavian
Brachiocephalic trunk
Arch of aorta

■ Atherosclerosis

(A)

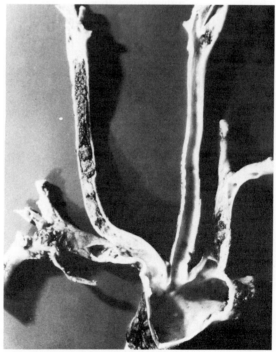

(B)

Figure 9-1 (A) Sites of predilection for atherosclerotic plaques in aortocranial arteries. (B) Segmental atherosclerosis and clot in branches of the aortic arch.

thought that these deposits create turbulence and eddy currents in the bloodstream, resulting in injury to the smooth endothelium, after which high-density chylomicrons and lipoproteins tend to collect in these roughened areas. Whatever the ultimate cause, severe involvement of such important sites as the origins of the aortocranial arteries from the arch of the aorta, the origin of the vertebral from the subclavian artery, the bifurcation of the common carotid, the carotid sinus, and angulations such as the carotid siphon may occur, and yet areas in between may remain free of disease (Fig. 9-1A and B).

In the vertebral and basilar arteries, however, the distribution of atherosclerotic plaques is more general. Some authorities believe that the lipid deposits in the vertebral arteries which occur in the segments between the transverse processes of the cervical vertebrae are possibly related to greater pulsation of these segments. In the region of the sixth cervical vertebra, where the vertebral artery *usually* enters the transverse foramen, atherosclerotic plaques often appear first at the point where the artery lies close to the transverse process and the posterior root ganglion. Perhaps these plaques are related to direct pressure of these structures against the arterial wall.

Under normal conditions blood moves through the aortic arch and great vessels in a laminar fashion, the velocity being greater at the center of the column than next to the endothelial wall. The brachiocephalic, left common carotid, and left subclavian arteries branch off from the aortic arch at angles that allow smooth progress of the blood column. If atherosclerosis causes the arch to become elongated and uncoiled, these angles are changed, so that laminar flow is distorted and the resulting eddy currents further damage the arteries and accelerate the atherosclerotic process.

The sites most frequently and severely involved within the skull are the carotid siphon,

the circle of Willis, and the proximal portions of the anterior, middle, and posterior cerebral arteries. The intracranial portion of the vertebrals and the basilar artery are often affected as well; other sites are the leptomeningeal arteries and the branches of the basilar artery.

PATHOLOGIC FINDINGS

The lesions of atherosclerosis begin in the intima of the large and medium-sized arteries, where they are first visible as fatty streaks. With the passage of time, the atheromata encroach on the arterial lumen and extend into the media.

An atherosclerotic artery may be normal in length and circumference or may be dilated, elongated, and tortuous. In the early stages its normally thin and translucent wall is infiltrated

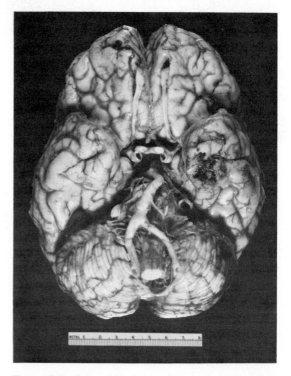

Figure 9-2 Base of the brain showing fusiform dilatation of the vertebral and basilar arteries secondary to atherosclerosis.

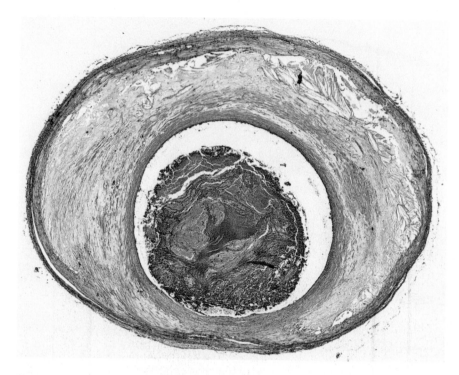

Figure 9-3 Carotid artery in late stage of atherosclerosis. Note narrowing of the lumen. (H & E stain.)

by patches of yellowish opacities. In advanced disease the artery is rigid and thick, and it may be dilated, especially in the carotid siphon and in basilar arteries where fusiform aneurysms may develop (Fig. 9-2).

The appearance on cross section depends on the site at which the cut is made. The lumen may be eccentric and narrowed, even slitlike, or it may be larger than normal. Beneath the intima, which may be ulcerated, friable, or covered with thrombus, are found atheromatous plaques containing grumous material (Fig. 9-3). Beneath the plaques there may be fresh or old hemorrhage resulting from rupture of the vasa vasorum.

Concomitant weakening of the arterial wall may lead to dilatation, aneurysm formation, or subintimal dissection; or ulceration of the endothelium may allow the contents of the plaque to

be discharged into the bloodstream as emboli (Fig. 9-4).

When an artery is occluded by thrombus or embolus, blood flow in the distal segment is arrested and clots are formed as far as the next branch, where flow is maintained by collateral channels. For example, when the internal carotid artery becomes occluded at its sinus, thrombus usually extends up to the caroticotympanic or ophthalmic artery, where collateral flow develops and prevents clotting; at times, however, it may continue past these branches into the ophthalmic, anterior, and middle cerebral branches of the carotid and result in optic atrophy and extensive hemispheric infarction.

Later on, fibroblastic proliferation causes the clot to adhere firmly to the wall of the vessel, with resultant organization of the clot and, in

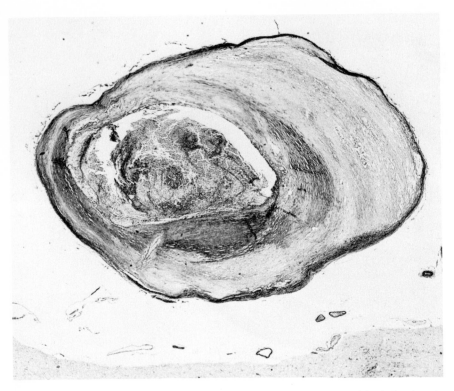

Figure 9-4 Basilar artery with prominent atherosclerosis, laceration of the intimal coat, and formation of a thrombus. Note narrowing of the lumen. (H & E stain.)

about 3 weeks, beginning fibrosis of the artery. Eventually the occluded artery is so reduced in diameter that it becomes a dense cord. If the process includes the intracranial branches of the internal carotid, the disorder which some classify as "cerebral thromboangiitis obliterans" occurs.

On microscopic examination, plaques containing foam cells swollen with fat are the characteristic feature. In addition cholesterol crystals which may initiate a foreign-body giant-cell reaction are found in the subintimal layers. In advanced cases the internal elastic membrane is ruptured and the medial coat of the artery also shows degenerative changes.

PATHOPHYSIOLOGY

It must be emphasized that *atheromatous plaques in themselves produce no symptoms and* *that no method is available at present to indicate the cases in which symptomatic atherosclerotic cerebral vascular disease will develop in the future.* Although hyperlipemia, or symptomatic coronary artery disease, and retinal or renal arteriopathies are all frequently associated with manifestations of aortocranial atherosclerosis, any of these conditions may exist without clinical signs of the others. Yet these processes are all interrelated, and impairment of function of one organ by the atherosclerotic process may cause malfunction in another. In the presence of underlying cerebral atherosclerosis, for example, cardiac decompensation secondary to coronary atherosclerosis may precipitate cerebral vascular insufficiency. In such cases correction of the heart failure ameliorates the neurologic dysfunction.

A plaque occluding the lumen of the vertebral or even the basilar artery will produce no signs of neurologic deficit in many patients but will have disastrous consequences in others. The clinical effect in an individual case depends on the availability of collateral blood supply for the area normally irrigated by the occluded vessel. This in turn depends on the construction of the intracranial vessels in that individual and the rapidity with which occlusion develops. If the posterior communicating arteries are widely patent, a short segment of the basilar artery may be occluded without producing dysfunction unless the penetrating arteries are affected. On the other hand, the person whose posterior communicating arteries are threadlike or absent will probably suffer a crippling or fatal infarction of the brainstem if a segment of the basilar artery is obstructed in any location. In summary, the two most important factors in determining the clinical effects of atherosclerotic cerebral vascular disease are the pattern of the aortocranial vessels laid down during embryogenesis and the distribution of the atheromatous plaques.

The vessels coming off the aortic arch to supply the brain, as well as those in the circle of Willis at the base of the brain, have varying patterns of configuration, which will be considered in Chap. 13. The development of collateral circulation following the occlusion of an artery depends not only on these configurations but also, to a certain degree, on the rapidity with which occlusion occurs. Postmortem injection studies and cerebral arteriograms have demonstrated that when the anastomoses within the circle of Willis and the leptomeningeal (surface conducting) vessels are present at all, they are patent at all times and are available for almost immediate use whenever the need arises. The widely held concept that an appreciable length of time is required for these vessels to dilate or for existing channels to compensate is probably incorrect. The ebb and flow of cerebral circulation is such that compensatory flow into an area with impaired circulation begins the instant pressure in one system is lowered and continues until equilibration of pressures is attained. This state-

ment, however, does not imply that compensatory dilatation of a vessel cannot be an important factor later on.

Sclerotic changes may take years to reduce the lumen of a vessel. During this period the section of the artery just distal to the point of constriction may slowly dilate, and arteries which act as potential sources of collateral flow may also have a compensatory increase in diameter. By this means collateral channels may develop into luxuriant anastomoses.

It has been shown that almost 90 percent of the cross-sectional area of the lumen of the extracranial segments of the carotid or vertebral must be blocked before its flow is significantly diminished. However, its perfusion pressure will be reduced, but unless the hemispheric branches contain other stenotic or occlusive lesions, perfusion in the distal arteries will be kept adequate by the intrinsic reserve and by dilatation of portions of the circle of Willis and of the leptomeningeal arteries. Unfortunately, atherosclerosis usually involves many arteries simultaneously, so that these anastomoses may also be involved by the process.

An additional factor to be considered is the difference between the critical closing and opening pressures of the sclerotic arteries. Whenever arterial pressure falls below a certain level, the artery collapses (critical closing pressure). Because of endothelial adhesiveness, the pressure necessary to reopen such a collapsed vessel is higher than that required to keep it open, and if pressures cannot be raised adequately, the artery remains collapsed and infarction of distal tissues may occur. This may be the basis for the "no reflow phenomenon" which occurs after arrest of brain circulation for longer than 5 to 7 min. In this situation flow cannot be reestablished through the brain vascular bed despite elevation of arterial pressure far above normotensive levels.

Other factors that enter into the clinical picture produced by aortocranial atherosclerosis are (1) pulmonary diseases which reduce oxygenation of the blood, (2) fluctuations in the systemic arterial blood pressure, (3) variations in the cardiac output, and (4) abnormalities in the viscosity of the blood and in its content of hemoglobin, oxygen, and glucose. Any of these, alone or in combination, may produce symptoms and signs of cerebral vascular insufficiency. Whether the insufficiency involves the entire brain or only portions of it depends on the interrelationships between the collateral flow available for maintaining cerebral circulation and the rapidity with which the change takes place. Whereas syncope may be produced by a *sudden* fall in systemic blood pressure or by anemia due to *acute* blood loss, slowly developing hypotension or anemia of the same degree can be tolerated without any symptoms. When superimposed on stenosis of one or more aortocranial vessels, however, even slowly developing hypotension or anemia may produce symptoms of insufficiency in the area of brain tissue normally perfused by the affected vessel or vessels. This effect is particularly apparent when sources of collateral supply are inadequate, either because of the congenital pattern of the cerebral vessels or because of acquired disease.

CLINICAL FEATURES

Even though the arteries of the cerebral circulation and their diseases will be discussed separately, it is a mistake to think of disease of the aortocranial arteries as solely extracranial or intracranial, or to consider abnormality of one carotid artery independent of that of the other or of disease of the vertebral-basilar system. These arteries function as a unit, contributing to one another, equilibrating from side to side, and from front to back. To emphasize this interdependence, some neurologists have used the term *caroticovertebral disease*. Because of the therapeutic implications, however, discussions of cerebral vascular disease usually classify the causes of symptoms referable to the cerebral tree as either extracranial or intracranial and as carotid or vertebral-basilar.

Per se, atherosclerosis of the aortic arch seldom produces symptoms. At times an elongated and tortuous artery may cause a visible pulsation behind the sternal notch or above the sternoclavicular joint. Such an artery occasionally becomes aneurysmal, and in such cases the enlargement may be great enough to cause the patient concern. At times dilatation of the brachiocephalic (innominate) artery can compress the left brachiocephalic vein, causing the left jugular vein to be distended; and rarely an artery may cause dysphagia by pressing on the esophagus.

EXAMINATION OF THE PATIENT

There may be visible pulsation of an artery which is normally quiet, and palpation may reveal a hyperpulsatile mass. This usually represents a kink in the artery but is occasionally a true aneurysm. In other patients the palpable portions of the carotid and subclavian arteries, though not tortuous, are rigid and incompressible, and a thrill may be felt.

If the ascending portion of the aortic arch is roughened by atheromatosis, auscultation may reveal systolic murmurs above the aortic area. These may be transmitted into the carotid artery at the base of the neck. Bruits which may be audible along the course of the subclavian, vertebral, and carotid arteries will be considered in detail in appropriate chapters.

Blood pressure readings in the arms may show characteristic systolic hypertension with widened pulse pressure.

LABORATORY EXAMINATIONS
X-Ray Findings

Posteroanterior views of the chest may show a prominent ascending and transverse aorta and widening of the superior mediastinal shadow. The aortic arch is uncoiled and the thoracic aorta may be tortuous. Calcification may be visible in the walls of the arteries, particularly in

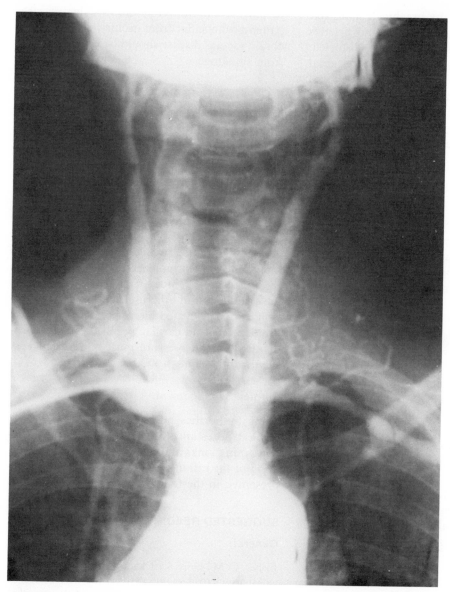

Figure 9-5   Aortic arch injection via the right subclavian artery, illustrating evidence of diffuse aortocervical atherosclerosis. Note the stenosis of the right vertebral and the right internal carotid arteries near their origins. The left subclavian artery is kinked and stenosed, and the left vertebral artery is not opacified. Perhaps it is occluded.

the ascending and transverse aorta. Cervical films may reveal calcification in the carotid bifurcations. These calcifications are said to give a very good indication of the presence of internal carotid stenosis or occlusion.

Arteriography

The lumen of the aortic arch is wide, and the artery is elongated so that it lies higher than normal in the thorax. The resultant changes in the angles of origin of the brachiocephalic, left common carotid, and left subclavian arteries may cause these vessels to be kinked, distorted, and perhaps stenotic. In the neck the vertebral and carotid arteries may appear tortuous and may contain visible kinks (Fig. 9-5). The angle formed by the external and internal carotid arteries is normally acute, but in atherosclerosis of these vessels it will often be widened.

TREATMENT

Medical Management

By the time aortocervical atherosclerosis has developed to such a degree that the patient has symptoms or signs caused by it, there are no measures which have been shown to reverse the process. However, its progression is believed by many to be slowed by proper management of general medical diseases such as hypertension, diabetes mellitus, and gout as well as by the measures outlined below.

Diet Because low-fat, low-carbohydrate diets may reduce serum lipids, atherosclerotic patients should restrict their intake of these foods. Such a regimen will decrease postprandial lactescence and may retard atherogenesis.

The obese patient should have his caloric intake restricted until his weight has reached the minimum recommended for his height and body build. In addition to decreasing the likelihood of further cerebral episodes, weight reduction will also make it easier for the patient with a neurologic deficit to become ambulatory once more.

Exercise Although there is no basis for believing that exercise prevents cerebral atherosclerosis, daily exercise is to be recommended as a good measure of health.

Avoidance of Nicotine In view of the strong evidence that nicotine increases the incidence of cardiovascular and cerebral vascular diseases, patients who suffer from occlusive forms of cerebral vascular disease should be urged to refrain from smoking.

Other Therapies Cholesterol-reducing agents have not proved popular for patients with levels of serum lipids refractory to dietary restriction. Atherosclerosis is less frequent in premenopausal women than in men of the same age; therefore, some suggest the use of estrogen therapy in postmenopausal women.

Control of Hypertension Sustained systolic and diastolic hypertension accelerates atherogenesis. Consequently, blood pressure should be maintained at normotensive levels as a preventive measure. Unfortunately, many patients have concomitant atherosclerosis and hypertension, so that elevated blood pressure is vital for brain, renal, and cardiac perfusion. In these individuals blood pressure must be reduced very slowly and to only a moderate degree.

Surgical Management

Some authorities advocate surgery to remove focal stenoses and to shorten elongated arteries containing kinks and loops. A detailed consideration of the rationale of surgical management is presented in the following chapters.

SUGGESTED READINGS

General

Fisher, C. M., Gore, L., Okabe, N., and White, P. D.: Atherosclerosis of the carotid and vertebral arteries—Extracranial and intracranial, *J. Neuropathol. Exptl. Neurol.*, **24**:455, 1965.

Leading article: Carotid or vertebral? *Lancet*, **1**:1005, 1965.

Martin, M. J., Whisnant, J. P., and Sayre, G. P.: Occlusive vascular disease in the extracranial cerebral circulation, *Arch. Neurol.*, **3**:530, 1960.

Task Force on Arteriosclerosis. Report by the National Heart and Lung Institute, National Institutes of Health, vols. I and II, Bethesda, Md., 1971-1972.

Pathogenesis

Caro, C. G., Fitz-Gerald, J. M., and Schroter, R. C.: Arterial wall shear and distribution of early atheroma in man, *Nature*, **223**:1159, 1969.

Constantinides, P.: Experimental Atherosclerosis, Elsevier Publishing Co., New York, 1965.

Cumings, J. N., Grundt, I. K., Holland, J. T., and Marshall, J.: Serum lipids and cerebrovascular disease, *Lancet*, **2**:194, 1967.

Fredrickson, D. S., Levy, R. I., and Lees, R. S.: Fat transport in lipoproteins—An integrated approach to mechanisms and disorders, *New Engl. J. Med.*, **276**:34-44, 94-103, 148-156, 215-225, 273-281, 1967.

Geer, J. C., and McGill, H. C., Jr.: "The evolution of the fatty streak," in Atherosclerotic Vascular Disease; A Hahnemann Symposium, edited by A. N. Brest and J. H. Moyer, Appleton-Century-Crofts, New York, 1967, pp. 8-22.

———, Panganamala, R. V., Newman, H. A. I., and Cornwell, D. G.: "Mural metabolism," in Atherosclerosis; Proceedings of the Second International Symposium, edited by R. J. Jones, Springer-Verlag, New York, 1970, pp. 6-12.

Greenhouse, A. H.: Blood lipids and strokes; Are they related? *J. Chronic Diseases*, **23**:823, 1971.

Gross, M., and Marshall, J.: Blood pressure lability in ischaemic cerebrovascular disease, *Clin. Sci.*, **38**:563, 1970.

Holman, R. L., and Moossy, J.: "The natural history of aortic, coronary and cerebral atherosclerosis," in Pathogenesis and Treatment of Cerebrovascular Disease, edited by W. S. Fields, Charles C Thomas, Publisher, Springfield, Ill., 1961, p. 39.

Lloyd, J. K., and Wolff, O. H.: A pediatric approach to the prevention of atherosclerosis, *J. Atheroscler. Res.*, **10**:135, 1969.

McGill, H. C., Jr., Geer, J. C., and Strong, J. P.: "Natural history of human atherosclerotic lesions," in Atherosclerosis and Its Origin, edited by M. Sandler and G. H. Bourne, Academic Press, New York, 1963, pp. 39-65.

Pickering, G. W.: Pathogenesis of myocardial and cerebral infarction: Nodular arteriosclerosis, *Brit. Med. J.*, **1**:517, 1964.

Prineas, J., and Marshall, J.: Hypertension and cerebral infarction, *Brit. Med. J.*, **1**:14, 1966.

Pathologic Findings

Adams, J. H., and Graham, D. L.: Twelve cases of fatal cerebral infarction due to arterial occlusion in the absence of atheromatous stenosis or embolism, *J. Neurol. Neurosurg. Psychiat.*, **30**:479, 1967.

Fisher, C. M., Gore, I., Okabe, N., and White, P. D.: Calcification of the carotid siphon, *Circulation*, **32**:538, 1965.

Giertsen, J. C.: Atherosclerosis in an autopsy series. 3. Interrelationship between atherosclerosis in the aorta, the coronary and the cerebral arteries, *Acta pathol. microbiol. scand.*, **63**:391, 1965.

Klassen, A. C., and Sung, J.-H.: Histological changes in cerebral arteries with increasing age, *J. Neuropathol. Exptl. Neurol.*, **27**:607, 1968.

Pickering, G.: Arterial occlusion especially of the coronary arteries and of the subclavian and carotid arteries, Lecture 1, *Bull. Johns Hopkins Hosp.*, **113**:105, 1963.

———: Other examples of arterial thrombosis, Lecture 2, *Bull. Johns Hopkins Hosp.*, **113**:124, 1963.

Schwartz, C. J., and Mitchell, J. R.: Atheroma of the carotid and vertebral arterial systems, *Brit. Med. J.*, **2**:1057, 1961.

Smith, E. B.: Intimal and medial lipids in human aortas, *Lancet*, **1**:799, 1960.

Gross Appearance

Adams, R. D., and vander Eecken, H. M.: Vascular disease of the brain, *Ann. Rev. Med.*, **4**:213, 1953.

Blackwood, W., Hallpike, J. F., Kocen, R. S., and Mair, W. G. P.: Atheromatous disease of the carotid arterial system and embolism from the heart in cerebral infarction: A morbid anatomical study, *Brain*, **92**:897, 1969.

Pathophysiology

Fazekas, J. F., Yuan, R. H., Callow, A. D., Paul, R. E., Jr., and Alman, R. W.: Studies of cerebral hemodynamics in aortocranial disease, *New Engl. J. Med.*, **266**:224, 1962.

Ingvar, D. H.: The pathophysiology of occlusive cerebrovascular disorders related to neuroradiological findings, EEG, and measurements of regional cerebral blood flow, *Acta neurol. scand.,* **43**(suppl. 31):-93, 1967.

Lowe, R. D.: Adaptation of the circle of Willis to occlusion of the carotid or vertebral artery: Its implication in caroticovertebral stenosis, *Lancet,* **1**:395, 1962.

Moossy, J.: Cerebral infarcts and the lesions of intracranial and extracranial atherosclerosis, *Arch. Neurol.,* **14**:124, 1966.

Texon, M., Imparato, A. M., and Helpern, M.: The role of vascular dynamics in the development of atherosclerosis, *J.A.M.A.,* **194**:1226, 1965.

Yates, P. O., and Hutchinson, E. C.: Cerebral infarction: The role of stenosis of the extracranial cerebral arteries, *Med. Res. Council Spec. Rept. Ser.,* **300**:1, 1961.

Clinical Features

Aarli, J. A.: Neurological manifestations in hyperlipidemia, *Neurology,* **18**:883, 1968.

Gurdjian, E. S., Darmody, W. R., and Thomas, L. M.: Recurrent strokes due to occlusive disease of extracranial vessels, *Arch. Neurol.,* **21**:447, 1969.

Hardesty, W. H.: Minimum brain deficiency with occlusion of carotid and vertebral arteries bilaterally, *J.A.M.A.,* **205**:527, 1968.

Nizzoli, V., and Nicola, G. C.: Completely asymptomatic multiple extracranial vascular obstruction, *Europ. neurol.,* **3**:105, 1970.

Poser, C. M., Zosa, A. M., and Hardin, C. A.: Psychiatric manifestations of cerebrovascular insufficiency, *Dis. Nervous System,* **25**:611, 1964.

Whisnant, J. P., Martin, M. J., and Sayre, G. P.: Atherosclerotic stenosis of cervical arteries; clinical significance, *Arch. Neurol.,* **5**:429, 1961.

Examination of the Patient

Cooper, D., Hill, L. T., Jr., and Edwards, B. A.: Detection of early arteriosclerosis by external pulse-recording, *J.A.M.A.,* **199**:449, 1967.

Puls, R. J., and Heizer, K. W.: Pulse-wave changes with aging, *J. Am. Geriat. Soc.,* **15**:153, 1967.

Laboratory Findings

Baüer, R., Sheehan, S., and Meyer, J. S.: Arteriographic study of cerebrovascular disease: II. Cerebral symptoms due to kinking, tortuosity and compression of carotid and vertebral arteries in neck, *Arch. Neurol.,* **4**:119, 1961.

Boström, K., and Hassler, O.: Radiological study of arterial calcification: I. Aortic arch and large cervical vessels, *Neurology,* **15**:941, 1965.

Faris, A. A., Poser, C. M., Wilmore, D. W., and Agnew, C. H.: Radiologic visualization of neck vessels in healthy men, *Neurology,* **13**:386, 1963.

Feild, J. R., Robertson, J. T., and DeSaussure, R. L., Jr.: Complications of cerebral angiography in 2,000 consecutive cases, *J. Neurosurg.,* **19**:775, 1962.

Gilroy, J.: The evolution of cerebral arteriography, *Am. J. Roentgenol.,* **92**:948, 1964.

Gurdjian, E. S., Hardy, W. G., Lindner, D. W., and Thomas, L. M.: Four vessel angiography: Experiences with three hundred consecutive cases, *Clin. Neurosurg.,* **10**:251, 1964.

Hodges, F. J., III: Developments in cerebral angiography: Current application and future utilization, *Radiol. Clin. N. Am.,* **2**:515, 1964.

Lavy, S., Stern, S., Herishianu, Y., and Carmon, A.: Electrocardiographic changes in ischemic stroke, *J. Neurol. Sci.,* **7**:409, 1968.

Muller, R., Greitz, T., Liliequist, B., and Hellstrom, L.: Aortocervical angiography in occlusive cerebrovascular disease, *Neurology,* **14**:136, 1964.

Shapiro, H. M., Ng, L., Mishkin, M., and Reivich, M.: Direct thermometry, ophthalmodynamometry, auscultation and palpation in extracranial cerebrovascular disease: An evaluation of rapid diagnostic methods, *Stroke,* **1**:205, 1970.

Weibel, J., and Fields, W. S.: Atlas of Arteriography in Occlusive Cerebrovascular Disease, W. B. Saunders Company, Philadelphia, 1969.

Treatment

Fredrickson, D. S., and Levy, R. I.: Treatment of essential hyperlipidaemia, *Lancet,* **1**:191, 1970.

Gillespie, J. A. (ed.): Extracranial Cerebrovascular Disease and Its Management, Appleton-Century-Crofts, New York, 1969.

Additional References

Edwards, E. A.: Dynamic consequences of arterial stenosis, *J. Cardiovascular Surg.*, **8**:386, 1967.

Fogelholm, R.: Occlusive lesions of the cervical arteries in patients with ischemic cerebrovascular disease. A clinical and angiographic study of 213 patients, *Acta neurol. scand.*, **46**:suppl. 42, 1970.

Kolakowska, T., Mowery, G. L., and Zwang, H. J.: Comparative value of brain scan, electroencephalography and arteriography in intracranial neoplasms and cerebrovascular lesions, *Clin. Electroencephalog.*, **2**:136, 1971.

Carotid Artery Syndrome

The question of localization is only an application of the common physiology of the nervous system, of the facts that should be familiar to every student, and can be relearned, if necessary, with ease by every practitioner.

W. R Gowers

That digital compression of one or both of the common carotid arteries may sometimes produce aphasia, weakness of the opposite side of the body, and loss of consciousness was known before the time of Hippocrates. After Sir Thomas Willis made the initial report on his famous circle in 1664, it was also recognized that the internal carotid artery may sometimes be occluded without producing any effect (Fig. 10-1). The extreme variability in symptoms and signs of carotid lesions has resulted in confusion which persists to this day. In this chapter we will attempt to clarify this situation somewhat.

ETIOLOGY

There are a variety of causes of internal carotid obstruction. The artery may be congenitally absent or atretic; these conditions are asymptomatic because of compensatory collateral circulation. Rarely tonsillitis or otitis media may involve the internal carotid artery in the tonsillar fossa or the tegmen tympani, leading to carotid thrombosis. Occasionally an embolus or nonseptic arteritis will occlude the artery. Other unusual causes include (1) external compression or invasion of the artery by tumor or cicatrix;

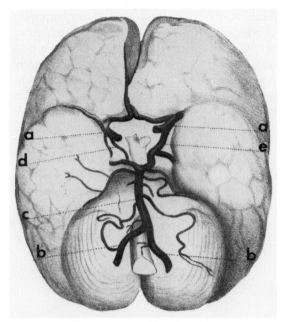

Figure 10-1 Illustration by Sir Astley Cooper in 1821 showing compensatory dilatation of the left posterior communicating artery in a patient who had had a previous left carotid ligation in the neck. *(Reprinted from Guy's Hospital Rept., 1:58, 1836.)*

(2) trauma with subintimal hematoma and dissection; (3) compression from behind by the lateral mass of the atlas; (4) fibromuscular dysplasia; and (5) inflammatory arteritis (Takayasu's disease, see Chap. 28). By far the most frequent cause of carotid obstruction is atherosclerosis, the only form to be discussed in this chapter.

INCIDENCE

The incidence of atherosclerotic occlusion of the carotid artery varies with the means of study employed and the population selected. In the Orient it is unusual, but in the United States it is a problem of epidemic proportions. Men are affected almost twice as often as women, and the peak age incidence is 50 to 70 years, although we have seen atherosclerotic carotid obstruction in men and women in their twenties.

In autopsies on the white population of the United States over 60 years of age *without symp-*

toms of cerebral ischemia or infarction during life, the incidence of atherosclerotic internal carotid occlusions is about 6 percent, while that of intimal roughening and stenosis is very much greater. In patients *with symptoms* of cerebrovascular disease, the incidence of "significant" carotid disease found at arteriography has been as high as 40 percent in some series. In Negroes carotid or vertebral obstruction by atherosclerosis in the neck is very unusual, but disease of the intracerebral arteries is more common.

PATHOGENESIS

The clinical effects of stenosis or occlusion of the carotid artery depend on many factors. The syndrome produced by sudden occlusion of the artery is quite different from that caused by slowly progressive stenosis culminating finally in occlusion.

Although the degree of stenosis produced by the atherosclerotic plaques remains constant in a given patient, the effective arterial lumen may vary because of external compression and kinking induced by turning the head. Fluctuations in systemic arterial blood pressure; alterations in blood sugar, carbon dioxide, oxygen, and lipids; and changes in blood composition with anemia or erythrocytosis produce a dynamic situation in which the only constant is the never-ceasing requirement of the brain for an adequate quantity of blood under sufficient pressure to provide it with oxygen and nutrient materials. To supply this, the compensatory mechanisms described in detail in Chap. 5 come into play.

Patients with the carotid artery syndrome often have recurring attacks of reversible neurologic deficit, commonly termed "transient ischemic attacks." In some cases these attacks are caused by local or systemic hypotension, which reduces perfusion pressure in the areas supplied by the carotid artery or its branches below the critical closing pressure of the leptomeningeal (surface conducting or pial) and perforating arteries. In most instances, however, microemboli in the form of cholesterol crystals, fibrin, or platelet aggregates cast off from the atherosclerotic plaques travel through the carotid tree until they finally lodge in one of the smaller arteries (Fig. 10-2). Obstruction of a small vessel produces neurologic deficit, the duration of which depends on the adequacy of collaterals or on further distal movement of the embolus. See Chap. 15 for details.

PATHOLOGIC FINDINGS

In about 90 percent of patients with internal carotid occlusion, the initial obstruction is found in the region of the sinus. Other locations, in order of frequency, are the intracavernous portion of the carotid siphon (less than 8 percent), the supracavernous segment, and rarely its petrous portion. Atheromatous stenosis or occlusion in other parts of the internal carotid is extremely rare, and even when severe disease is present at the sinus and in the siphon the area between is usually spared. Lesions may calcify, turning the artery into a rigid pipe. Because the vessel also lengthens when it becomes sclerotic, the two factors, lengthening and rigidity, may combine to produce a kink in the artery which may further impair flow.

If collateral circulation through the orbital

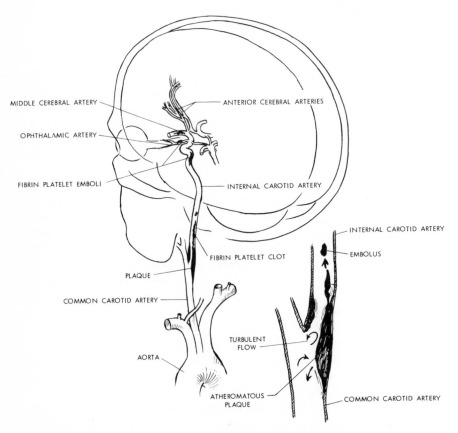

MIDDLE CEREBRAL ARTERY

ANTERIOR CEREBRAL ARTERIES

OPHTHALMIC ARTERY

FIBRIN PLATELET EMBOLI

INTERNAL CAROTID ARTERY

INTERNAL CAROTID ARTERY

EMBOLUS

FIBRIN PLATELET CLOT

PLAQUE

COMMON CAROTID ARTERY

TURBULENT FLOW

AORTA

ATHEROMATOUS PLAQUE

COMMON CAROTID ARTERY

Figure 10-2 Atheromatous plaques at the carotid artery bifurcation can be a source of cerebral microemboli.

and leptomeningeal arteries and the circle of Willis is adequate, occlusion of the internal carotid will cause no deficit (Fig. 10-3A and B). If it is not, occlusion causes infarction in the area supplied by the anterior or middle cerebral artery or in the area supplied by both.

In most patients with internal carotid occlusion, scattered areas of softening signify infarction in the area supplied by its middle cerebral branch. Such an infarction may involve, in addition to the cortex, the lenticulate nucleus and the head of the caudate nucleus, the genu, the anterior limb, and the anterior portion of the posterior limb of the internal capsule. Isolated lesions in the distribution of the anterior cerebral branch are less common and usually occur in association with involvement of the area supplied by the middle cerebral artery. Hemispheric swelling accompanies the larger infarctions and at times is of such degree that intracranial pressure rises and the midbrain is compressed by herniation of the uncus through the tentorial notch.

PATHOPHYSIOLOGY

The internal diameter of the carotid artery at postmortem examination averages 6 mm (normal range, 3 to 10 mm) at the carotid sinus and 3.3 mm in its intradural portion, where the normal range is 2 to 5 mm; in vivo the artery may be somewhat larger. It is believed that the cross-sectional area of the normal lumen must be reduced by 50 percent before distal pressure is affected. Flow is decreased only when the lumen is decreased by 90 percent. Theoretically, then, the lumen of the internal carotid artery must be reduced to less than 5 sq mm before the distal perfusion pressure is lowered. The length of the stenosis is another factor of some importance, but a series of stenoses along the course of an artery does not have an additive effect. When the lumen is reduced to less than 2 sq mm, mean pressure in the distal artery always falls, and

flow is reduced throughout the length of the artery until the point where the first major collateral vessel enters it. Distal to this point, flow is augmented by the collaterals even though pressure may remain low.

Under normal conditions pressure falls only slightly from the origin of the carotid artery to the ophthalmic and the cerebral arteries. However, the intraocular pressure exerted against the retinal arterioles reduces the pressure in the retinal arterioles and capillaries, so that retinal arterioles are often the first to be affected by reduction of pressure in the carotid system. Therefore, retinal ischemia with fading of vision or temporary blindness in the homolateral eye (amaurosis fugax) may precede hemispheric symptoms and signs.

CLINICAL FEATURES

Clinically, it is impossible to distinguish between the symptoms produced by carotid stenosis and occlusion with absolute certainty. The signs and symptoms produced by both depend on the following factors:

1 The segment involved—whether above or below the origin of the ophthalmic artery
2 The rapidity of development of the obstruction—whether gradual, as in progressive atheromatous deposits, or sudden, as by thrombus or embolus
3 The availability and adequacy of collateral circulation
4 The area of brain affected—whether in the distribution of the anterior cerebral artery or of the middle cerebral artery

More than 40 percent of patients with carotid artery disease have warning symptoms of transitory neurologic dysfunction (transient ischemic attacks) before a permanent deficit develops. About a third of the patients who have these transient attacks continue to have them for a variable length of time before they abate spon-

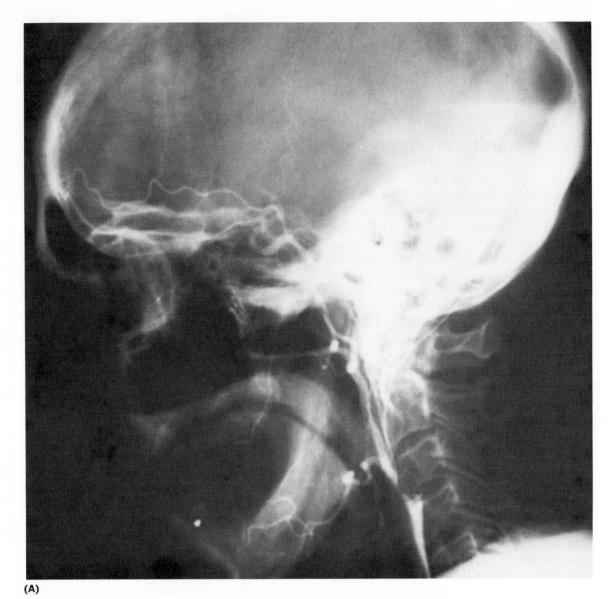

(A)

Figure 10-3(A) and (B)   Carotid arteriogram showing an apparent internal carotid artery occlusion with minimal collateral circulation. (B) Subtraction of film shown in (A).
The extracranial circulation is displayed vividly, and the internal carotid is shown to be
stenosed rather than occluded.

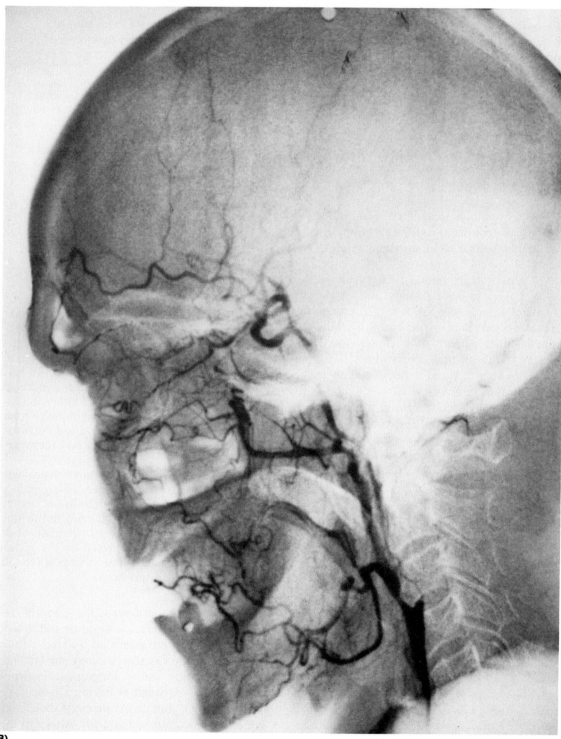

taneously; permanent damage eventually occurs in another third, while the remainder continue to have reversible attacks indefinitely.

A sudden onset of the type one usually associates with infarction occurs in more than 30 percent of the patients, but the majority have a steplike or gradually progressive onset, at times evolving over a period of weeks, so that one suspects a neoplasm. In some patients headaches on the homolateral side and occasionally pain over the carotid artery in the neck may precede the episode.

Visual symptoms sometimes herald the ictus; they usually consist of transient loss of vision in the homolateral eye, interpreted by some patients as "spots," "gray-out," or "steamy vision." Occasionally retinal infarction may develop, leading to optic atrophy; but usually the collateral arterial supply is so great that this does not occur. Some patients feel light-headed and at times actually lose consciousness for varying lengths of time. Premonitory focal motor seizures are reported to occur, usually in the early stages of infarction.

Most often infarction caused by carotid artery disease is heralded by paresthesias and numbness of the opposite side of the body, weakness, difficulty with comprehension and communication, and perhaps personality change.

The extreme variability of the clinical picture makes it impossible to formulate a description which is applicable to all instances of carotid artery syndrome (Table 10-1). The symptomatic cases may be divided roughly into three groups:

1 Those with recurring attacks of neurologic deficit which subside completely within minutes or hours. In this group, homolateral amaurosis fugax occurring in combination with paresis or sensory deficit on the contralateral side is pathognomonic of the carotid artery syndrome. In some patients with carotid disease the manifestations are those of vertebral-basilar syndrome,

Table 10-1   Approximate Frequency of Symptoms in Carotid Artery Syndrome

Symptom	Percent of cases
Hemiplegia or hemiparesis	80+
Aphasia	30–60
Headache	20–50
Mental disturbance	20
Hemianesthesia or hemihypesthesia	15
Unconsciousness	15
Monoplegia or monoparesis	10–15
Visual disturbances	10–30
Paresthesias of one extremity	10
Seizures	10–20
Homonymous field defect	5–12
Optic atrophy	5–10
Homolateral loss of vision with contralateral hemiparesis	15–20

and lesions are found diffusely distributed throughout the carotid and vertebral-basilar systems.

2 Those with an apoplectic onset characterized by hemiplegia without previous episodes of insufficiency. This type occurs in 35 to 40 percent of patients with carotid artery syndrome and is compatible with disease of either the carotid artery or its middle cerebral branch. Other conditions to be considered in the differential diagnosis are cerebral embolism and intracerebral hemorrhage.

3 Those with slowly progressive neurologic deficit compatible with a variety of expanding intracranial lesions, particularly brain tumor. From 15 to 25 percent of the cases fall in this group. About 2 to 3 percent of patients with symptoms and signs interpreted by the physicians as due to intracranial neoplasms are found to have internal carotid obstruction.

Of particular importance is the group of patients whose symptoms are so subtle and slowly progressive that no events of sudden nature would suggest a vascular etiology for intellectual deterioration and quadriparesis. Such patients may be classified as having a dementing illness which simulates Alzheimer's disease or *état lacunaire* (Chaps. 13 and 19). Although the data are difficult to assess, a body of literature suggests that depression, irritability, drowsiness, disorientation, confusion, and emotional lability, as well as dementia, may result from otherwise asymptomatic occlusion of one or both of the internal carotid arteries. Many authorities believe that these symptoms are but an exaggeration of premorbid personality traits.

It is tempting, but probably incorrect, to think that the intellectual deterioration which is considered to be a normal part of the aging process is in actual fact due to progressive changes in the carotid trees. Unless there is other clinical evidence of carotid artery insufficiency, it is unwise to postulate a causal relationship between dementia and unilateral or bilateral carotid artery disease.

EXAMINATION OF THE PATIENT

Findings depend on which type of syndrome the patient presents: (1) recurrent episodes of reversible neurologic deficit; (2) apoplectic or stepwise onset; (3) a slowly progressive neurologic deficit.

Recurrent Episodes of Reversible Neurologic Deficit (Transient Ischemic Attacks)

If the patient happens to be seen during an episode, he will present all the phenomena to be described in the next section. Otherwise, the findings in the neurologic examination are normal. The examiner may or may not hear a bruit over the region of the carotid bifurcation. It must be remembered that the presence of bruits depends on many factors which are constantly in a state of flux, and that repeated auscultation of the head and neck is necessary in order to rule out a bruit of changing intensity. Two other significant points to be kept in mind are (1) that a murmur localized over the carotid bifurcation suggests an abnormality in that region but does not mean that *extracranial* vascular disease is

the cause of the patient's neurologic problem; (2) that the intensity of the murmur correlates very poorly with the degree of stenosis. Still, bruit is the clinical sign most suggestive of extracranial vascular disease.

Although it is clear that no invariable rule regarding the significance of carotid murmurs can be given, a high-pitched systolic murmur heard in the region of the carotid bifurcation usually means stenosis in that location. Occlusion usually abolishes the murmur, but the diversion of blood into the external carotid may also cause a loud murmur. Furthermore, a holosystolic murmur prolonged into or through diastole indicates increased flow through a stenosis and strongly suggests occlusion of the opposite internal carotid artery. Similarly, a systolic bruit heard over one orbit is a strong indication of increased blood flow through the sclerotic carotid siphon on that side and suggests occlusion of the opposite carotid. At times the sudden disappearance of a murmur or a change in its character suggests that a stenosed artery has become occluded.

Aside from bruit, abnormally low pressure in the ophthalmic artery is the most reliable indication of carotid artery disease in patients with transient episodes. This measurement is described in detail in Chap. 7.

Palpation of the carotid artery in the neck occasionally reveals a thrill or diminished pulsations. Although the thrill is a clue to stenosis, the diminution of pulsations may mean nothing. Kinked or tortuous common carotid arteries may lie behind the trachea where they cannot be palpated. In these patients the superficial temporal arteries are usually found to be pulsating well, so that the examiner can be certain that the common and external carotid arteries are not occluded. In palpating the carotid artery, the examiner should remember that some patients have such a sensitive carotid sinus that even gentle massage or compression will cause bradycardia and hypotension.

Hyperpulsation of the superficial temporal artery suggests occlusion of the internal carotid with collateral circulation through the external carotid. Hypopulsation or absence of pulsations in the superficial temporal artery, which is rare, suggests atherosclerotic involvement of the external carotid artery or cranial arteritis.

The internal carotid artery in the pharynx may be palpated (using topical anesthesia, if necessary) by placing a gloved fingertip against the tonsillar fossa. If pulsation is absent in one carotid artery and present in the opposite artery, one can assume that the carotid is occluded in the neck. If, on the other hand, neither can be palpated, one usually discovers that the arteries are patent but the technique of palpation is faulty, although occasionally both carotids are found to be occluded.

Of interest is the finding that skin temperatures and pulse amplitude over the medial aspects of the forehead may be decreased on the side of internal carotid occlusion, presumably because of decreased flow through the ophthalmic artery.

In some patients with internal carotid stenosis, ophthalmoscopic examination will reveal bright cholesterol crystals in the retinal arterioles and, rarely, retinal venous thrombosis with hemorrhages and exudates. These findings are discussed further in Chap. 6.

If the cervical sympathetic plexus which travels on the carotid has been affected, an incomplete Horner's syndrome is apparent on the homolateral side.

Apoplectic or Stepwise Onset

The patient most often has the abrupt onset of dysphasia or of a deficit (motor, sensory, or both) affecting the contralateral arm, leg, or half of the face. The progressive deficit may or may not have been preceded by previous episodes of reversible neurologic deficit. If these episodes have occurred, the progressive one may begin

with the same clinical picture but does not end with rapid recovery.

Results of palpation and auscultation are similar to those described in the preceding section. Pressures in one or both of the ophthalmic arteries are usually reduced to levels which are diagnostic of carotid occlusion.

Slowly Progressive Neurologic Deficit

At times there is no sudden episode to suggest vascular abnormality. Instead, slowly progressive dementia, convulsions, and a progressive motor and/or sensory dysfunction of the face, arm, or leg suggest the possibility of an expanding intracranial lesion such as a subdural hematoma or neoplasm. However, these patients may have bilateral carotid stenosis or occlusion without clearly localized or lateralized signs. The ophthalmic pressures are equally reduced in both eyes, so that the results must be compared with the brachial blood pressures. If both ophthalmic pressures are quite low in relation to the brachial blood pressures, bilateral carotid disease should be suspected.

In patients with slowly progressive neurologic deficit, bruits such as those described earlier in this chapter are often heard. In occasional patients stenosis or occlusion in the regions of the carotid bifurcation and the carotid siphon may be combined with disease in the vertebral-basilar system, creating such a variety of hemodynamic effects that accurate interpretation of the meaning of the murmurs is impossible.

LABORATORY FINDINGS

Blood count, urinalysis, and spinal fluid examination usually produce normal findings except in the presence of massive infarction of the hemisphere with cerebral edema. In such cases the spinal fluid may be under increased pressure, and in the occasional patient with a hemorrhagic infarction, blood will be found in the spinal fluid.

X-ray Findings

X-rays of the neck may reveal calcification of the arteries in the region of the carotid bifurcation. Skull films are usually normal. If the pineal gland is calcified, it can be seen in midline, except in cases of massive infarction when cerebral edema causes a shift of the hemisphere to the opposite side. Calcification of the internal carotid arteries adjacent to the sella turcica does not give a clue to the site of carotid occlusion and probably should be disregarded.

Electroencephalogram

Recordings made during an attack of reversible neurologic deficit or during the progressive stage of cerebral infarction secondary to carotid occlusion may show slow waves over the involved hemisphere. The electrical activity tends to revert to normal with the passage of time.

Echoencephalogram

In patients with marked unilateral cerebral

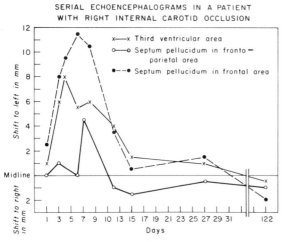

SERIAL ECHOENCEPHALOGRAMS IN A PATIENT WITH RIGHT INTERNAL CAROTID OCCLUSION

x—x Third ventricular area
o—o Septum pellucidum in fronto-parietal area
•—• Septum pellucidum in frontal area

Figure 10-4 Echoencephalogram. The position of the third ventricle has been plotted against time. As edema subsides, the structure returns to the midline position.

edema, the echoencephalogram shows displacement of midline structures away from the occluded side (Fig. 10-4).

Ultrasonography

In patients with occlusion of the internal carotid artery there is usually increased flow through the superficial temporal, facial, and angular branches of the external carotid which anastomose with terminal branches of the internal carotid. Blood flows retrograde through these arteries into the ophthalmic and then to the internal carotid. The direction of flow can be assessed by using a transcutaneous Doppler flowmeter and compressing the accessible external carotid branches. If flow through the ophthalmic decreases when one of them (for example, the superficial temporal artery) is compressed, then the internal carotid is occluded and the external carotid is the major source of collateral supply.

If there is stenosis only, pressure may be sufficiently lowered in the ophthalmic so that flow ceases in diastole, a finding easily diagnosed by Doppler ultrasonography.

Radioisotopic Brain Scan

This valuable screening procedure should be done on all patients suspected of having disease of the carotid artery as a help in differential diagnosis of an intracranial lesion such as a subdural hematoma or neoplasm. The size and stage of evolution of infarction determine whether an increased uptake will be visible in areas of necrosis or neovascularization. Small infarcts cannot be distinguished from background activity; but larger ones usually can be (Fig. 10-5A and B). This increased uptake may be visible for months. Although the size, shape, and distribution of radioactivity give some aid in the differentiation of infarction from neoplasm, serial scans are more helpful.

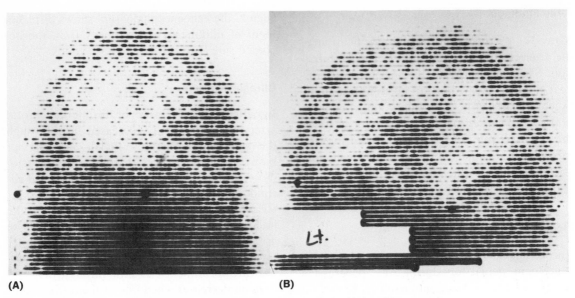

(A)   **(B)**

Figure 10-5 Abnormal concentration of 99m$_{Tc}$ in an area of cerebral infarction caused by left internal carotid artery occlusion. (A) Anteroposterior view. (B) Left lateral view.

Isotope Angiography

A bolus of radioisotope such as 99m$_{Tc}$ (technetium) is injected intravenously and its course through the cervical and cranial arteries is monitored with a gamma camera. In normal subjects the arrival and transit of the radioactivity through the two carotids in the neck and anterior and middle cerebral arteries intracranially should be simultaneous. In the case of carotid occlusion, radioactivity is absent in the neck and the middle cerebral shows later on the occluded side than on the patent side. In occlusion of major arteries in the cranium the middle cerebral artery does not become visible.

Carotid Compression Test

This test, described in Chap. 8, should be performed only on patients who are being evaluated for possible reconstructive surgery. *It should not be done* on patients with progressive neurologic deficit or evolving stroke, or on pa-

tients with old cerebral infarction unless the possibility of reconstructive surgery is being considered.

Forehead Skin Temperature Measurement

Skin temperature as an index of cutaneous and subcutaneous flow has been used in the assessment of peripheral vascular disease for many years. Its recent application to the evaluation of aortocranial vascular disease may prove to be a valuable new diagnostic method. The skin of the medial aspect of the supraorbital region is supplied by the terminal branches of the internal carotid artery, and it has been observed that in patients with occlusion or stenosis of the internal carotid artery there may be a local reduction of forehead skin temperature by 0.5 to 1°C. Several methods are currently being evaluated in an effort to provide a measurement of this reduction in temperature. These include skin thermometry, thermography, and thermo-

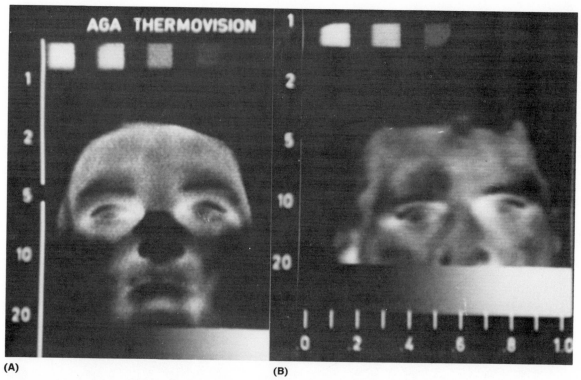

Figure 10-6 Thermograms. (A) Normal control. (B) Abnormal facial thermogram (cool area over right eye). *(Courtesy of Dr. T. D. Capistrant.)*

chromic paints (Fig. 10-6). It seems probable that with refinements of technique, methods for the rapid evaluation of local thermal changes about the forehead and perhaps even the occipital region in patients with vertebral-basilar artery disease may prove to be a valuable adjunct to the diagnosis of cerebral vascular syndromes.

Aortocranial Angiography

Although arteriography will usually reveal the exact location of obstructions in the aortocranial circulation, it should be carried out only under the following circumstances: (1) when the diagnosis is in doubt, (2) when surgical reconstruction is contemplated, or (3) occasionally when other arteries are being studied, as in aor-

tic arch reconstructions. Arteriography should never be undertaken by anyone who is not skilled in the management of patients with cerebrovascular disease, and it should not be done unless facilities for immediate reconstructive vascular surgery are available (see Chap. 17). In addition to visualization of the arch and the origins of the aortocranial arteries, selective injections (Fig. 10-7) of the cervical arteries are necessary for detailed evaluation.

DIFFERENTIAL DIAGNOSIS

Three major possibilities must be considered: (1) despite the presence of symptoms and signs suggestive of carotid artery syndrome, the patient has an unrelated intracranial lesion such as

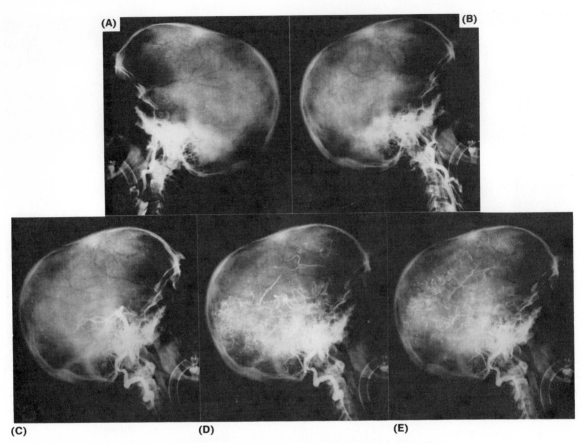

Figure 10-7 Arteriograms of aortocranial circulation in a patient with intellectual deterioration, showing occlusion of both internal carotid arteries just distal to their origins (A and B). In (C), (D), and (E) the vertebral-basilar system is seen to supply the majority of the cerebral circulation. *(Reprinted from J. F. Toole, Interarterial shunts in the cerebral circulation, Circulation, vol. 33, March 1966, by permission of the American Heart Association, Inc.)*

abscess, tumor, or subdural hematoma; (2) the offending lesion is located in one of the intracranial branches of the carotid artery, such as the middle cerebral artery; (3) the lesion in one carotid artery is accompanied by disease in other extracranial or intracranial arteries such as the opposite carotid or the vertebral-basilar system.

1 Laboratory tests, particularly the radioactive brain scan, are extremely helpful in eliminating the possibility of a brain tumor. The presence of a bruit at the region of the carotid

bifurcation gives strong support to a diagnosis of vascular disease. In some cases, however, carotid arteriography must be performed to rule out intracranial neoplasm. If the carotid artery is occluded in the neck, the intracranial arteries will not be visualized; in such cases an air-contrast study offers the only hope for establishing a definitive diagnosis.

2 The finding of a bruit in the neck at the region of the carotid bifurcation, together with reduced pressure in the ophthalmic artery, is almost diagnostic of obstruction in the extracranial portion of the artery. If the extracranial arteries are stenosed and not occluded, reduction in ophthalmic artery pressures may be equivocal and a bruit may be the only positive finding. Other possibilities, when ophthalmic artery pressures are not reduced, are that the carotid lesion is so old that collateral circulation has developed or that the lesion lies distal to the origin of the ophthalmic artery—perhaps in the middle cerebral itself. It is said that a hemisensory deficit is more commonly found in obstruction of the middle cerebral or a branch artery because the possibility of collateral circulation is not so great as it is in obstruction of the carotid artery in the neck.

3 The symptoms produced by obstruction of either carotid in the neck and by obstruction in the vertebral-basilar system depend in part on the interrelationship of the two carotid arteries through the circle of Willis; for this reason, localization of the lesion is often difficult. In many cases of atherosclerosis, stenosis of the carotid artery in the region of the carotid sinus occurs so slowly that there is ample time for collateral circulation to develop before complete obstruction of the carotid finally occurs. Such patients have no symptoms until the opposite carotid artery or the vertebral-basilar system also becomes involved. At this time there may be catastrophic bilateral cerebral damage or a cerebral episode in the *opposite* hemisphere. It may not be possible to determine clinically which artery provided the final insult, since both carotid arteries and one or more of the vertebral-basilar arteries may be obstructed.

MANAGEMENT

Recurrent Episodes of Reversible Neurologic Deficit

Patients with such episodes constitute the greatest diagnostic and therapeutic challenge. If a correct diagnosis can be made and proper management instituted before there is permanent damage to one or both of the cerebral hemispheres, a disastrous neurologic deficit can sometimes be avoided. Once the diagnosis of ex-

tracranial vascular disease has been made, the physician has a choice of one of three courses of action:

1 To use general supportive measures while allowing the neurovascular illness to take its course
2 To institute long-term anticoagulant therapy
3 To consider reconstructive surgery

Since the choice depends on individual circumstances, few general principles can be laid down. It is safe to say, however, that old, debilitated patients in whom the symptoms of carotid disease are only part of a general picture of deterioration should not be considered for either anticoagulants or surgery. On the other hand, individuals in good general condition should be given the benefit of a complete neurovascular study.

First, it must be ascertained that the patient's symptoms are not those of a generalized disease such as arteritis, anemia, or polycythemia. If the process is believed to be atheromatous and the possibility of surgery is to be considered, it is a good idea to perform a carotid artery compression test in order to ascertain the degree of cerebral vascular reserve in each carotid artery. Unless compression of one of the carotid arteries produces symptoms of insufficiency, one may reasonably assume that the symptoms are not the result of diminished carotid blood flow alone, but are due to some other superimposed triggering mechanisms, of which microembolism and episodic hypotension are two possibilities. If, on the other hand, symptoms develop when either artery is temporarily obstructed during the carotid compression test, one may consider the feasibility of arterial reconstruction to increase the patient's cerebral vascular reserve. With these circumstances, aortocranial arteriography is recommended.

Both carotids and the vertebral-basilar arte-

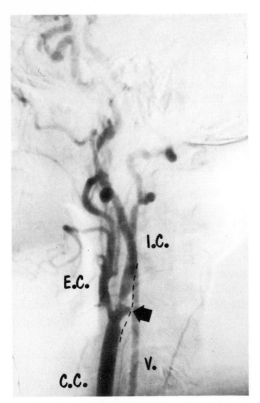
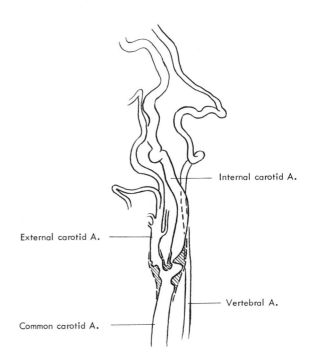

Figure 10-8 Ulcerated plaque at the internal carotid artery. *(Courtesy of Dr. F. Farrell, Department of Radiology, Bowman Gray School of Medicine.)*

ries should be visualized from their origins in the arch of the aorta to their intracranial branches. The angiographer must pay particular attention to the region of the carotid bifurcation and look for ulcerations which can serve as the source for emboli (Fig. 10-8). If there is any doubt whatsoever about the cause, the intracranial branches must be visualized in detail with contrast material injected by catheter placed in the ostia of the cervical arteries, or by direct arterial puncture.

Progressive Neurologic Deficit

Operation for patients with evolving cerebral infarction is not only useless but dangerous. Even though the artery may be successfully reopened, improvement does not result, and at times, the infarcted area may be converted from an anemic to a hemorrhagic one by the restoration of high pressure in the carotid artery. Such hemorrhages occasionally expand rapidly, producing a fatal increase in intracranial pressure.

Probably the best course of action in this group of patients is to administer anticoagulants in an attempt to forestall the propagation of the thrombus or embolization from it. Anticoagulants given during the stage of progressive neurologic deficit may prevent extension of the thrombotic process from the carotid artery into the intracranial branches. The decision to employ long-term anticoagulant therapy is dependent on many factors discussed in Chap. 16.

Static Neurologic Deficit

In patients with cerebral infarction due to long-standing carotid occlusion, both surgery and anticoagulants are useless. If, however, as sometimes occurs, such patients begin to experience symptoms of reversible neurologic deficit secondary to involvement of the other carotid artery or of the vertebral-basilar system, consideration should be given to the use of one of these therapeutic measures.

SUGGESTED READINGS

General

Daly, D., Svien, H. J., and Yoss, R. E.: Intermittent cerebral symptoms with meningiomas, *Arch. Neurol.,* **5**:287, 1961.

Gunning, A. J., Pickering, G. W., Robb-Smith, A. H. T., and Russell, R. R.: Mural thrombosis of the internal carotid artery and subsequent embolism, *Quart. J. Med.,* **33**:155, 1964.

Ottenberg, R.: Occlusion of internal carotid artery: Clinical diagnosis and therapy, *J. Mt. Sinai Hosp. N. Y.,* **22**:99, 1955.

In Childhood

Bickerstaff, E. R.: Aetiology of acute hemiplegia in childhood, *Brit. Med. J.,* **2**:82, 1964.

Dyken, M.: Angiographic study of the middle cerebral artery in chronic infantile hemiplegia, *J. Neurol. Neurosurg. Psychiat.,* **27**:326, 1964.

Pitner, S. E.: Carotid thrombosis due to intra-oral trauma: An unusual complication of a common childhood accident, *New Engl. J. Med.,* **274**:764, 1966.

Shillito, J.: Carotid arteritis: A cause of hemiplegia in childhood, *J. Neurosurg.,* **21**:540, 1964.

Wisoff, H. S., and Rothballer, A. B.: Cerebral arterial thrombosis in apparently healthy children, *Arch. Neurol.,* **4**:213, 1961.

Kinking and Tortuosity

Derrick, J. R., Kirksey, T. D., Estess, M., and Williams, D.: Kinking of the carotid arteries: Clinical considerations, *Am. Surgeon,* **32**:503, 1966.

Harrison, J. H., and Davalos, P. A.: Cerebral ischemia: Surgical procedure and cases due to tortuosity and buckling of cervical vessels, *Arch. Surg.,* **84**:85, 1962.

Najafi, H., Javid, H., Dye, W. S., Hunter, J. A., and Julian, O. C.: Kinked internal carotid artery: Clinical evaluation and surgical correction, *Arch. Surg.,* **89**:134, 1964.

Etiology

Andersen, P. E.: Fibromuscular hyperplasia of the carotid arteries, *Acta radiol. (diagn.),* **10**:90, 1970.

Bland, J. E., Perry, M. O., and Clark, K.: Spasm of the cervical internal carotid artery, *Ann. Surg.,* **166**:987, 1967.

Hunt, T. K., Blaisdell, F. W., and Okimoto, J.: Vascular injuries of the base of the neck, *Arch. Surg.,* **98**:586, 1969.

McDowell, F. H., Potes, J., and Groch, S.: The natural history of internal carotid and vertebral-basilar artery occlusion, *Neurology,* **11**(4)(part 2):153, 1961.

Mandel, M. M., and Strimel, W. H., Jr.: Bilateral carotid artery occlusion in a young adult. Clinicopathological report of a case associated with oral contraceptives, *J.A.M.A.,* **208**:145, 1969.

Mandelbaum, I., and Kalsbeck, J. E.: Extrinsic compression of internal carotid artery, *Ann. Surg.,* **171**:434, 1970.

Mastaglia, F. L., Savas, S., and Kakulas, B. A.: Intracranial thrombosis of the internal carotid artery after closed head injury, *J. Neurol. Neurosurg. Psychiat.,* **32**:383, 1969.

Matthew, N. T., Abraham, J., Taori, G. M., and Iyer, G. V.: Internal carotid artery occlusion in cavernous sinus thrombosis, *Arch. Neurol.,* **24**:11, 1971.

Polin, S. G.: Carotid artery fibromuscular hyperplasia: Three cases and review of the literature, *Am. Surgeon,* **35**:501, 1969.

Smith, K. R., Jr., Nelson, J. S., and Dooley, J. M., Jr.: Bilateral "hypoplasia" of the internal carotid arteries, *Neurology,* **18**:1149, 1969.

Pathogenesis

Landolt, A. M., and Millikan, C. H.: Pathogenesis of cerebral infarction secondary to mechanical carotid artery occlusion, *Stroke,* **1**:52, 1970.

Rundles, W. R., and Kimbell, F. D.: The kinked carotid syndrome, *Angiology*, **20**:177, 1969.

Pathologic Findings

Berry, R. G., and Alpers, B. J.: Occlusion of the carotid circulation. Pathologic considerations, *Neurology*, 7:223, 1957.

Castaigne, P., Lhermitte, F., Gautier, J.-C., Escourolle, R., and Derouesné, C.: Internal carotid artery occlusion. A study of 61 instances in 50 patients with post-mortem data, *Brain*, **93**:231, 1970.

Fieschi, C., and Bozzao, L.: Transient embolic occlusion of the middle cerebral and internal carotid arteries in cerebral apoplexy, *J. Neurol. Neurosurg. Psychiat.*, **32**:236, 1969.

Fisher, M.: Occlusion of the internal carotid artery, *Arch. Neurol. Psychiat.*, **65**:346, 1951.

Pathophysiology

Barnett, H. J. M., Wortzman, G., Gladstone, R. M., and Lougheed, W. W.: Diversion and reversal of cerebral blood flow. External carotid artery "steal," *Neurology*, **20**:1, 1970.

Davies, E. R., and Sutton, D.: Pseudo-occlusion of the internal carotid artery in raised intracranial pressure, *Clin. Radiol.*, **18**:245, 1967.

Desai, M.: The internal carotid artery and tumours of the neck, *Neurology (India)*, **16**:70, 1968.

Eklöf, B., and Schwartz, S. I.: Effects of critical stenosis of the carotid artery and compromised cephalic blood flow, *Arch. Surg.*, **99**:695, 1969.

Fogelholm, R., and Vuolio, M.: The collateral circulation via the ophthalmic artery in internal carotid artery thrombosis, *Acta neurol. scand.*, **45**:78, 1969.

Lhermitte, F., Gautier, J.-C., and Derouesné, C.: Anatomopathologie et physiopathologie des sténoses carotidiennes, *Rev. neurol.*, **115**:641, 1966.

Stern, W. E.: Circulatory adequacy attendant upon carotid artery occlusion, *Arch. Neurol.*, **21**:455, 1969.

Suzuki, J., Takaku, A., Hori, S., Ohara, I., and Kwak, R.: Spasm of the cervical portion of the carotid artery and its surgical treatment, *J. Neurosurg.*, **27**:94, 1967.

Clinical Features

Crompton, M. R.: Retinal emboli in stenosis of the internal carotid artery, *Lancet*, **1**:886, 1963.

Dunning, H. S.: Detection of occlusion of internal carotid artery by pharyngeal palpation, *J.A.M.A.*, **152**:321, 1953.

Ford, F. R.: The carotid pain syndrome: Report of two cases which suggest that, in some instances, migraine is responsible, *Bull. Johns Hopkins Hosp.*, **114**:266, 1964.

Hedges, T. R., Jr.: Ophthalmoscopic findings in internal carotid artery occlusion, *Am. J. Ophthalmol.*, **55**:1007, 1963.

Hollenhorst, R. W.: The ocular manifestations of internal carotid arterial thrombosis, *Med. Clin. N. Am.*, **44**:897, 1960.

Kellogg, D. R., and Smith, L. L.: Recurrent monocular blindness due to a redundant carotid artery, *Arch. Surg.*, **95**:908, 1967.

O'Doherty, D. S., and Green, J. B.: Diagnostic value of Horner's syndrome in thrombosis of the carotid artery, *Neurology*, **8**:842, 1958.

Olivarius, B. de F.: The external carotid artery sign, *Acta neurol. scand.*, **41**:539, 1965.

Roseman, D. M.: Carotidynia. A distinct syndrome, *Arch. Otolaryngol.*, **85**:81, 1967.

Sindermann, F., Bechinger, D., and Dichgans, J.: Occlusions of the internal carotid artery compared with those of the middle cerebral artery, *Brain*, **93**:199, 1970.

———, Dichgans, J., and Bergleiter, R.: Occlusion of the middle cerebral artery and its branches: Angiographic and clinical correlates, *Brain*, **92**:607, 1969.

Trotsenburg, L. V., and Vinken, P. J.: Fatal cerebral infarction simulating an acute expanding lesion, *J. Neurol. Neurosurg. Psychiat.*, **29**:241, 1966.

Examination of the Patient

Fisher, C. M.: Cranial bruit associated with occlusion of the internal carotid artery, *Neurology*, 7:299, 1957.

———: Facial pulses in internal carotid artery occlusion, *Neurology*, **20**:476, 1970.

Hørven, I. H., Nornes, H., and Tønjum, A.: Ophthalmological approaches to the diagnosis of carotid occlusive disease, *Acta neurol. scand.*, **47**:272, 1971.

Zeigler, D. K., Zileli, T., and Dick, A.: Correlation of bruits over the carotid artery with angiographically demonstrated lesions, *Neurology,* **20**:374, 1970.

Recurrent Episodes of Reversible Neurologic Deficit (Transient Ischemic Attacks)

Baker, R. N., Ramseyer, J. C., and Schwartz, W. S.: Prognosis in patients with transient cerebral ischemic attacks, *Neurology,* **18**:1157, 1968.

Slowly Progressive Neurologic Deficit

Clarke, E., and Harris, P.: Thrombosis of the internal carotid artery simulating an intracranial space-occupying lesion, *Lancet,* **1**:1085, 1958.

Raskind, R.: Frontal lobe abscess simulating "stroke" in two women, one pregnant, *Angiology,* **17**:264, 1966.

Laboratory Findings

Echoencephalogram

Brinker, R. A., Landiss, D. J., and Croley, T. F.: Detection of carotid artery bifurcation stenosis by Doppler ultrasound. Preliminary report, *J. Neurosurg.,* **29**:143, 1968.

Brisman, R., Grossman, B. L., and Correll, J. W.: Accuracy of transcutaneous Doppler ultrasonics in evaluating extracranial vascular disease, *J. Neurosurg.,* **32**:529, 1970.

Kristensen, J. K., Eiken, M., and von Wowern, F.: Ultrasonic diagnosis of carotid artery disease, *J. Neurosurg.,* **35**:40, 1971.

McKinney, W. M.: "Echoencephalography," in Special Techniques for Neurologic Diagnosis (Contemporary Neurology Series, 3), edited by J. F. Toole, F. A. Davis Co., Philadelphia, 1969, pp. 195–210.

Radioisotopic Brain Scan and Thermometry

Austin, J. H., and Sajid, M. H.: Direct thermometry in ophthalmic-internal carotid blood flow, *Arch. Neurol.,* **15**:376, 1966.

———, and ———: A simple method of direct thermography for the clinical estimation of ophthalmic-internal carotid artery blood flow, *Trans. Am. Neurol. Assoc.,* **90**:223, 1965.

Conrad, M. C., Toole, J. F., and Janeway, R.: Thermistor recording of forehead skin temperature as an index of carotid artery disease, *Circulation,* **39**:126, 1969.

Heinz, E. R., Goldberg, H. I., and Taveras, J. M.: Experiences with thermography in neurologic patients, *Ann. N. Y. Acad. Sci.,* **121**:177, 1964.

Price, T. R., and Heck, A. F.: Correlation of thermography and angiography in carotid arterial disease: Thermographic measurement as a screening technique, *Neurology,* **20**:398, 1970.

Aortocranial Angiography

Hugh, A. E., and Fox, J. A.: The precise localisation of atheroma and its association with stasis at the origin of the internal carotid—a radiographic investigation, *Brit. J. Radiol.,* **43**:377, 1970.

Ivan, L. P., and Marian, J. J.: Angiographic occlusive patterns of the internal carotid artery, *J. Neurosurg.,* **30**:233, 1969.

Lehrer, H. Z.: Cervical internal carotid artery caliber: Variation with arterial occlusions, *Acta neurol. scand.,* **45**:277, 1969.

Maddison, F. E., and Moore, W. S.: Ulcerated atheroma of the carotid artery: Arteriographic appearance, *Am. J. Roentgenol.,* **107**:530, 1969.

Najafi, H., Cagle, J. E., Javid, H., and Julian, C. C.: Bilateral carotid arteriography; its adequacy in cerebrovascular insufficiency evaluation, *Arch. Surg.,* **98**:53, 1969.

Wortzman, G., Barnett, H. J. M., and Lougheed, W. M.: Bilateral internal carotid occlusion: A clinical and radiological study, *Can. Med. Assoc. J.,* **99**:1186, 1968.

Differential Diagnosis

Lascelles, R. G., and Burrows, E. H.: Occlusion of the middle cerebral artery, *Brain,* **88**:85, 1965.

Lhermitte, F., Gautier, J.-C., Derouesné, C., and Guiraud, B.: Ischemic accidents in the middle cerebral artery territory. A study of the causes of 122 cases, *Arch. Neurol.,* **19**:248, 1968.

Clinical Course

Bradshaw, P., and Casey, E.: Outcome of medically treated stroke associated with stenosis or occlusion of the internal carotid artery, *Brit. Med. J.,* **1**:201, 1967.

Hardy, W. G., Lindner, D. W., Thomas, L. M., and Gurdjian, E. S.: Anticipated clinical course in carotid artery occlusion, *Arch. Neurol.,* **6**:138, 1962.

Javid, H., Ostermiller, W. E., Jr., Hengesh, J. W., Dye, W. S., Hunter, J. A., Najafi, H., and Julian, O. C.: Natural history of carotid bifurcation atheroma, *Surgery,* **67**:80, 1970.

Lougheed, W. M., Elgie, R. G., and Barnett, H. J. M.: The results of surgical management of extracranial internal carotid artery occlusion and stenosis, *Can. Med. Assoc. J.,* **95**:1279, 1966.

Marshall, J.: The management of occlusion and stenosis of the internal carotid artery, *Neurology,* **16**:1087, 1966.

———, and Meadows, S.: The natural history of amaurosis fugax, *Brain,* **91**:419, 1968.

Williams, M., and McGee, T. F.: Psychological study of carotid occlusion and endarterectomy, *Arch. Neurol.,* **10**:293, 1964.

Additional References

Brice, J. G., Dowsett, D. J., and Lowe, R. D.: The effect of constriction on carotid blood-flow and pressure gradient, *Lancet,* **1**:84, 1964.

Capistrant, T. D., and Gumnit, R. J.: Thermography and extracranial cerebrovascular disease. Preliminary report of a new provocative technique, *Arch. Neurol.,* **22**:499, 1970.

———, and ———: Thermography following a carotid transient ischemic episode, *J.A.M.A.,* **211**:656, 1970.

Clark, O. H., Moore, W. S., and Hall, A. D.: Radiographically occluded, anatomically patent carotid arteries, *Arch. Surg.,* **102**:604, 1971.

Gado, M., and Marshall, J.: Clinico-radiological study of collateral circulation after internal carotid and middle cerebral occlusion, *J. Neurol. Neurosurg. Psychiat.,* **34**:163, 1971.

Gomensoro, J. B., Maslenikov, V., Azambuja, N., Fields, W. S., and Lemak, N. S.: Joint study of extracranial arterial occlusion. VIII. Clinical-radiographic correlation of carotid bifurcation lesions in 177 patients with transient cerebral ischemic attacks, *J.A.M.A.,* **224**:985, 1973.

Gurdjian, E. S., Audet, B., Sibayan, R. W., and Thomas, L. M.: Spasm of the extracranial internal carotid artery resulting from blunt trauma demonstrated by angiography, *J. Neurosurg.,* **35**:742, 1971.

Hass, W. K., and Goldensohn, E. S.: Clinical and electroencephalographic considerations in the diagnosis of carotid artery occlusion. A review of 35 verified cases, *Neurology,* **9**:575, 1959.

Isaacs, J. P., Swanson, H. S., and Smith, R. A.: Transient childhood strokes from internal carotid stenosis. Successful surgical treatment, *J.A.M.A.,* **207**:1859, 1969.

Javid, H., Ostermiller, W. E., Hengesh, J. W., Dye, W. S., Hunter, J. A., Najafi, H., and Julian, O. C.: Carotid endarterectomy for asymptomatic patients, *Arch. Surg.,* **102**:389, 1971.

Lippman, H. H., Sundt, T. M., and Holman, C. B.: The poststenotic carotid slim sign: Spurious internal carotid hypoplasia, *Mayo Clinic Proc.,* **45**:762, 1970.

Marshall, J., and Wilkinson, I. M. S.: The prognosis of carotid transient ischaemic attacks in patients with normal angiograms, *Brain,* **94**:395, 1971.

Najafi, H., Javid, H., Dye, W. S., Hunter, J. A., Wideman, F. E., and Julian, O. C.: Emergency carotid thromboendarterectomy. Surgical indications and results, *Arch. Surg.,* **103**:610, 1971.

Sarkari, N. B., Holmes, J. M., and Bickerstaff, E. R.: Neurological manifestations associated with internal carotid loops and kinks in children, *J. Neurol. Neurosurg. Psychiat.,* **33**:194, 1970.

Wake, J. G., Larson, C. P., Jr., Hickey, R. F., Ehrenfeld, W. K., and Severinghaus, J. W.: Effects of carotid endarterectomy on carotid chemoreceptor and baroreceptor function in man, *New Engl. J. Med.,* **282**:823, 1970.

Vertebral-Basilar Artery Syndrome

Perfectly exact truth is but rarely to be seen.

Hippocrates

The medical literature of the late nineteenth century contains isolated reports of cases in which thrombosis of the basilar artery was found at autopsy. Not until 1946, when Kubik and Adams published their classic work on the effects of occlusion of the basilar artery, was the syndrome established and the diagnosis made during life. Description of vertebral-basilar insufficiency states is even more recent.

The delay in recognizing the syndromes associated with disease of the vertebral-basilar system can be explained to a certain extent by the inaccessibility of the cervical portion of the vertebral arteries. Clinicians and pathologists had attempted to make clinicopathologic correlations from the more readily available intracranial branches. The intracranial branches of the vertebral and basilar arteries were minutely studied, and a syndrome was described for each, prompting a cynic to remark that the neurologic equivalent of the Hall of Fame is a brainstem eponym.

The concept of cerebrovascular insufficiency—more specifically, carotid and vertebral-basilar insufficiency—has already brought about great simplification in neurologic terminology. We feel safe in predicting that the eponymic syndromes of brainstem vascular disease which have been the bane of medical students will soon pass into oblivion.

ETIOLOGY AND PATHOGENESIS

Trauma

Trauma to the vertebral arteries inflicted by hyperextension or sudden rotary movements of the neck can produce disastrous brainstem disease. The most common causes of such trauma seem to be hyperextension or "whiplash" injuries of the neck, overenthusiastic chiropractic manipulation in which the head is forcibly turned and snapped, and freak accidents which occasionally occur during such athletic activities as football and swimming. A rarer cause is extension of the head on the neck for dental extraction or for intubation during general anesthesia.

Puncture of the midcervical portion for arteriography occasionally results in neural deficit. This procedure has been known to cause subintimal dissection leading to acute occlusion of the vessel; it can also initiate vasospasm which may result in signs and symptoms of cerebrovascular insufficiency.

Atherosclerosis

An atherosclerotic plaque in the vertebral artery can serve as a nidus for the formation of a thrombus which may occlude the vessel acutely or be cast off as an embolus and ascend into the intracranial branches of the artery. Because the caliber of the vertebral artery is smaller than that of the basilar, any embolus which arises in the vertebral will probably navigate through and lodge in the rostral end of the basilar or in one of its branches.

Osteoarthritis

A factor that may be of importance in some instances of the vertebral-basilar syndrome is osteoarthritis of the cervical spine (Fig. 11-1).

OSTEOARTHRITIS AND ATHEROSCLEROSIS

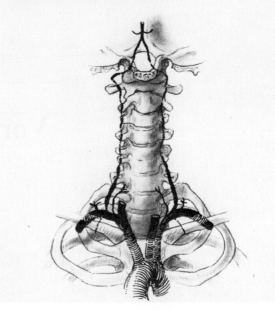

Figure 11-1 The vertebral arteries course through the cervical spine, where they can be impinged upon by osteoarthritic spurs. When associated with atherosclerotic plaques in the arteries, these spurs may cause vertebral-basilar artery insufficiency.

When osteoarthritic spurs protruding into the canal impinge upon one of the vertebral arteries or narrow the space in which it lies, movement of one vertebra in relation to another may stretch or pinch the artery. Under most circumstances when flow through one vertebral artery is diminished, flow through the other increases and compensates. When one vessel is hypoplastic, stenosed, or occluded in atherosclerosis, this compensation may not occur, and movements of the head can precipitate vascular insufficiency.

Bony Anomalies

Other possible etiologic factors are congenital anomalies of the cervical spine, such as the Klippel-Feil syndrome and basilar impression, either of which may be associated with anomalies of the vertebral arteries themselves. More important, however, are the osseous deformities which, by limiting normal movement of the vertebral arteries within the foramina, may lead to symptoms of vascular insufficiency when the head is moved in relation to the neck.

Cervical Rib and Fibrous Bands

When the arm is extended, a cervical rib can cause forward displacement of the vertebral artery, causing it to be distorted and, in some people, temporarily occluded near its origin. Fibrous bands extending from such a cervical rib, or even from a normal rib to the vertebra, occasionally press upon the artery and occlude it when the head, neck, and arm are in certain relationships to one another. Compression by slips of muscle from the insertion of the longus

colli and scalenus anticus at C_6 can also produce temporary arterial obstruction when the head is turned to one side.

Kinks and Loops

In some instances, congenital anomalies or atherosclerosis may cause the vertebral artery to be unusually long, so that kinks or knuckles develop in it when arm-neck relations are changed. These kinks may obstruct flow through the artery (Fig. 11-2).

PATHOPHYSIOLOGY

Normally, the vertebral artery is about half the diameter of the internal carotid. The two carotid arteries are usually equal in caliber, while one vertebral artery is frequently much smaller

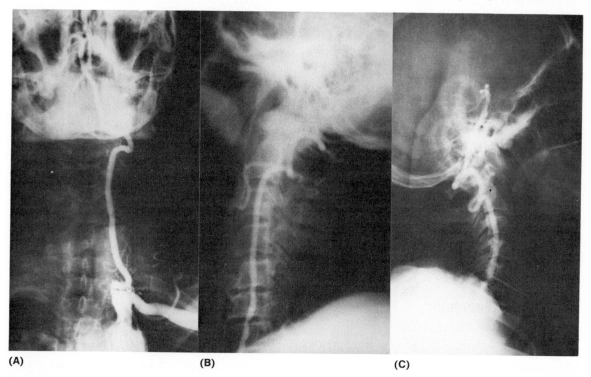

(A)   (B)   (C)

Figure 11-2 Vertebral arteriograms showing (A) kinking, (B) external compression by osteoarthritic spurs, and (C) looping.

than the other and in some cases is obviously incapable of carrying a significant quantity of blood to the brain. In most patients with such a pattern the opposite vertebral is unusually large, so that the total quantity of blood flowing through the basilar artery is not altered.

In other cases, two vertebral arteries of normal size do not join in the usual fashion. In these instances one vertebral artery continues as the basilar and the other as the posterior inferior cerebellar artery. Under some circumstances such anomalies can play an important role in the production of varying clinical manifestations of the vertebral-basilar syndromes.

Unlike the internal carotid, which has no branches or anastomoses between its origin in the common carotid and its intracranial portion, the vertebral artery gives off numerous branches as it ascends through the neck. It has a rich series of anastomoses with the thyrocervical trunk, the vertebral artery of the opposite side, and the occipital branch of the external carotid. Any of these anastomoses may bypass segmental occlusions.

When normal individuals face front, pressures within the two vertebral arteries are equal and their bloodstreams remain separate throughout the length of the basilar artery, the left vertebral supplying the left side of the cerebellum and brainstem, and the right vertebral supplying the right side. If pressure relations are altered by head turning or by pathologic situations such as the subclavian steal syndrome (discussed in Chap. 12), blood from one vertebral may fill the entire lumen of the basilar artery and nourish all structures supplied by it.

PATHOLOGIC FINDINGS

Arterial Lesions

Atheromatous plaques are usually deposited at the point where the vertebral artery branches off from the subclavian, and along the course of the first part of the artery before it enters the foramen of the transverse process of the cervical vertebra. Somewhat less commonly the atheromatous process also affects the second part of the artery, which ascends through the vertebral canal; the regions between the transverse processes are particularly susceptible. It is surprising that atheromatous deposits are more common in the second, straight portion of the artery than in the third portion, which bends around the transverse process of the atlas. The fourth portion, above the foramen magnum and below the junction of the two vertebral arteries, is usually involved only to a moderate degree.

The basilar artery, although it has no bends, is often affected by atherosclerotic plaques near its origin, its termination, and at junctions with its branches. It has been theorized that the confluence of currents from the two vertebral arteries may set up eddies within the stream of blood flowing through the basilar artery and that these eddies traumatize the vessel and lead to the formation of atheromas.

Lesions in the Brain

At autopsy, the brain of a patient with vertebral-basilar disease may show infarcts scattered in the occipital lobes, the undersurfaces of the temporal lobes, the thalamus, the entire brainstem, the cerebellum, and the upper part of the spinal cord. Whether infarctions are single or multiple depends on the interplay of atherosclerotic lesions in the collateral vessels, the leptomeningeal arteries, and the posterior communicating artery that connects the carotid with the vertebral-basilar system (Fig. 11-3).

CLINICAL FEATURES

Blood carried in the vertebral-basilar system nourishes 10 of the 12 cranial nerves, all the ascending and descending tracts, the end organs for hearing and balance, and parts of the cerebral hemispheres. Hence disease within this sys-

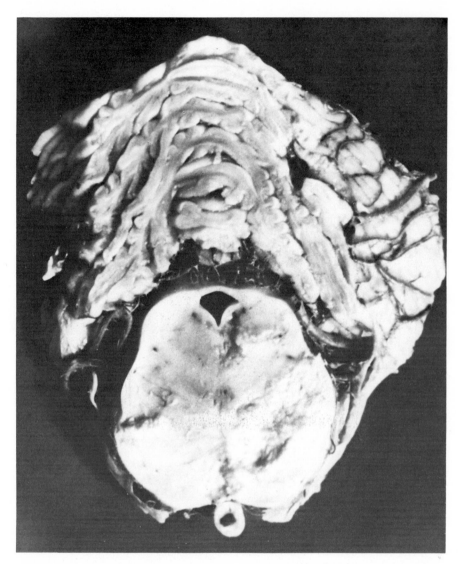

Figure 11-3 Basilar artery stenosis and pontile softening secondary to atherosclerosis.

tem can lead to a myriad of symptoms and signs (Table 11-1). The constellation of symptoms occurring in an individual case, however, usually clusters around one region of the brain. One patient, for example, may have episodes of blindness with no vertigo, whereas another may have severe vertigo and loss of hearing without any evidence whatsoever of involvement of the occipital lobes of the brain. In the first case the symptoms are secondary to ischemia within the distribution of both posterior cerebral arteries; in the second, to ischemia in the cochlea and semicircular canals or their neural counterparts in the brainstem.

Table 11-1   Some Symptoms and Signs Produced by Vertebral-Basilar Disease

Location of disease	Symptoms and signs
Upper spinal cord and lower brainstem (anterior spinal artery)	Weakness or paralysis of legs or all four extremities (drop attacks) with preservation of consciousness Weakness and vertigo precipitated by head rotation or extension Ataxia Dysarthria and dysphagia Unilateral or bilateral hypalgesia
Cerebellum (posterior and anterior inferior cerebellar, and superior cerebellar arteries)	Ataxia Dysmetria Dyssynergia
Labyrinth and cochlea (internal auditory artery)	Vertigo, nausea, and vomiting Tinnitus Sudden deafness
Pons and midbrain (basilar artery)	Occipital headache Light-headedness and/or syncope Stupor or coma Diplopia Ocular palsies Unilateral or bilateral hypalgesia or weakness Peduncular hallucinosis Paroxysmal hypertension
Thalamus	Anesthesia dolorosa Tremor
Subthalamus	Ballism
Cerebral hemispheres, occipital lobes, and temporoparietal areas (posterior cerebral artery)	Homonymous or quadrantanopic visual field loss Blindness, cortical type Temporal lobe seizures Amnestic syndrome (bilateral hemispheric involvement) Dyslexia without agraphia (dominant hemisphere) Visual agnosia

It is estimated that about 70 percent of patients who eventually suffer infarction in the distribution of the vertebral-basilar arterial system have one or many episodes of reversible neurologic deficit (transient ischemic attacks) before infarction occurs. These attacks, similar in etiology to those associated with the carotid artery syndrome, may be precipitated by one or more of the following factors: (1) changes in systemic blood pressure, usually hypotension but occasionally hypertension; (2) changes in blood viscosity; (3) anemia or erythrocytosis; (4) hypoglycemia; (5) movements of the head upon the neck; (6) trauma to the arteries; and (7) cardiac arrhythmias.

Episodic vertigo and diplopia, often accompanied by nystagmus and at times by nausea and vomiting, are characteristic of vertebral-basilar insufficiency. Such vertigo may wrongly be attributed to Ménière's or pseudo-Ménière's syndrome. The correct diagnosis can sometimes be made by differential caloric tests and by testing for positional nystagmus. It is not known whether vascular insufficiency causing attacks of vertigo affects the semicircular canals or the vestibular nuclei in the brainstem.

Hemiparesis and hemiplegia with cranial nerve palsies are common, the clinical picture depending on the level of involvement of the brainstem. Cranial nerve involvement of the lower motor neuron type on one side occurring simultaneously with hemiparesis on the other is pathognomonic of brainstem abnormality.

Also strongly suggestive of vertebral-basilar insufficiency is the "drop attack," in which the patient suddenly loses body tone and falls to the ground. In this characteristic syndrome, the weakness usually subsides more slowly than it begins, and the patient apparently retains consciousness during the attack. He frequently attributes the fall to stumbling and looks for an obstruction in his path. Such attacks are thought to be due to episodic ischemia of the lower brainstem or upper cervical cord with involvement of either the corticospinal tract or the reticular formation.

A throbbing headache in the occipital region, sometimes radiating down the neck along the course of the vertebral artery, may be the first symptom of impending vertebral-basilar insufficiency. Although the genesis of such headaches is uncertain, they are possibly related to hyperpulsation following sudden obstruction to flow within the vertebral artery. The increased pulsa-

tions may be within the vertebral artery itself or within the anastomotic channels, particularly the occipital artery, which may bypass an obstructing lesion. Another possible cause is ischemia of the cervical muscles.

Occasionally a patient suspected of having a vertebral-basilar syndrome deteriorates rapidly. The clinical picture is of intracranial hypertension due to the development of an obstructive hydrocephalus resulting from a swollen, necrotic cerebellum which compresses the aqueduct of Sylvius and the exit foramina of the fourth ventricle.

EXAMINATION OF THE PATIENT

Pulsations of the arteries, ophthalmoscopic examination, and ophthalmodynamometry give scant clues to vertebral-basilar disease—and unless the patient is seen during an attack or during the evolution of infarction no neurologic deficit will be found. The patient's temperature is normal, but his blood pressure may be elevated.

Clues which suggest the presence of vertebral-basilar disease are (1) a bruit over the subclavian or vertebral-basilar artery; (2) unequal blood pressures in the two arms, which might occur with the subclavian steal syndrome; and (3) bruises on the knees, which may give mute evidence of previous "drop attacks." Even these clues may be absent in some patients with severe vertebral-basilar disease who have recurrent attacks of insufficiency. Rarely, brachial blood pressures may be equal and low even though ophthalmic artery and femoral pressures are high; this combination of findings is strongly suggestive of bilateral subclavian artery disease, which may involve the vertebral-basilar system as well.

In patients seen during an attack or during the evolution of infarction, one of the following groups of abnormalities may be found: (1) homonymous hemianopia, with or without macular sparing (secondary to ischemia or infarction of the occipital lobes of the brain); (2) visual or auditory hallucinations related to a disturbance in the temporal lobe; (3) disturbances of consciousness with akinetic mutism or coma; (4) hemiparesis or quadriparesis accompanied by cranial nerve deficit, dysmetria, ataxia, dyssynergia, dysarthria, and dysphagia (secondary to brainstem involvement); (5) positional nystagmus; (6) internuclear ophthalmoplegia; and (7) various sensory deficits.

LABORATORY FINDINGS

No abnormalities are found in blood count, urinalysis, spinal fluid examination, skull x-rays, echoencephalograms, or radioisotopic brain scan. Even in patients with infarction of the brainstem, edema is seldom if ever sufficient to cause laboratory evidence suggestive of a shift of brain structures.

Electroencephalography

Most patients have normal electroencephalograms; the abnormality seen most frequently is electrical slowing over both the temporal lobes. Compression of one carotid artery while the patient's head is turned to the opposite side may produce electrical slowing over the cerebral hemispheres, particularly in the temporal regions. If the carotid compression test is positive only when the head is turned, one may suspect that the vertebral artery is compressed by the head-turning maneuver.

Aortocranial Angiography

Angiography to reveal the location of suspected vascular obstructions should be carried out only when the patient is being considered for surgical reconstruction of the extracranial portion of the artery, as considered in Chap. 17, or to eliminate other etiologic possibilities.

DIFFERENTIAL DIAGNOSIS

The following signs are helpful in the diagnosis of vertebral-basilar artery disease:

1 Bruits at the subclavian-vertebral junction and along the course of the vertebral artery to the mastoid
2 Unequal blood pressures in the two arms (subclavian steal syndrome)
3 Arm blood pressures reduced in relation to ophthalmic artery pressures (bilateral subclavian steal)

Because of the large number of structures supplied by the vertebral-basilar system, disease of these arteries can mimic multiple sclerosis; a tumor within the cerebellopontile angle (such as an acoustic neuroma or a basilar artery aneurysm); cerebellar tumor, usually metastatic; drug intoxication, especially by barbiturates or tranquilizers; postural hypotension, with or without symptoms of vascular disease involving the brainstem; carotid sinus hypersensitivity; hypoglycemic attacks; Ménière's or pseudo-Ménière's syndrome; neurotic complaints related to hyperventilation or hysteria; migraine involving the vertebral-basilar system; and fluid or electrolyte imbalance.

Points in favor of a vascular etiology are recurrent episodic attacks which closely resemble one another, a murmur along the course of the vertebral arteries, and inequality of brachial blood pressures. Even when these findings are all present, however, the underlying vascular disease may not be the cause of the patient's symptoms.

A diligent search for the factors that precipitate or trigger the attacks of reversible neurologic deficit often uncovers the cause of the problem. Attacks caused by changes in the position of the head upon the neck strongly suggest osteoarthritis with insufficiency of the vertebral-basilar system. If head-neck movement has no effect, but sudden change from the recumbent to the erect posture does, one must consider postural hypotension or anemia.

Demyelinating diseases such as multiple sclerosis characteristically begin in younger patients and cause attacks of longer duration which usually leave a lasting neurologic deficit. The spinal fluid in cases of multiple sclerosis sometimes shows an abnormal colloidal-gold curve and an elevated gamma-globulin level.

Tumors of the cerebellopontile angle usually have a more gradual onset and cause lasting neurologic deficit, which is particularly evident on caloric and audiometric tests. Cerebellar tumors, at least in their early stages, generally cause symptoms and signs of a localized lesion: ataxia, dyssynergia, and dysmetria without vertigo or involvement of the long tracts. It may be very difficult to distinguish Ménière's syndrome, in which there may be sudden and recurring episodes of tinnitus, deafness, and vertigo from vertebral-basilar arterial insufficiency. Differential caloric tests may provide helpful information.

A differential diagnosis between vertebral-basilar insufficiency due to atherosclerosis and that due to aneurysm of the basilar artery often cannot be made on the basis of the history and physical examination alone.

MANAGEMENT

The most important aspect of the management of the patient with symptomatic vertebral-basilar disease due to atherosclerosis is to determine and correct, if possible, the mechanisms which trigger the attacks; correction of the underlying disease is seldom feasible. Patients suffering postural hypotension should be warned against rapid changes of head or body position. Those with polycythemia, anemia, or hypoglycemia should be given appropriate medical treatment. Patients with symptomatic cervical spondylosis are sometimes relieved by wearing a neck brace.

When no mechanisms triggering the intermittent attacks can be found and corrected, the patient may be a candidate for long-term anticoagulant therapy or for remedial surgery. As a rule, surgery is feasible only when arteriography shows kinks, external compression by osteophytes or fascial bands, or isolated atherosclerotic plaques situated in the proximal subclavian artery or in the vertebral artery before it enters the transverse process of the cervical vertebra. Patients with diffuse atherosclerosis extending throughout the vertebral artery and into the basilar system, and those with plaques in inaccessible locations may be selected for anticoagulant therapy. The medical and surgical management of patients with atherosclerosis is discussed in Chaps. 16 and 17. Anticoagulants are more valuable than surgery, however.

SUGGESTED READINGS

General

Biemond, A.: Thrombosis of the basilar artery and the vascularization of the brain stem, *Brain,* **74**:300, 1951.

Denny-Brown, D.: Basilar artery syndromes, *Bull. New Engl. Med. Center,* **15**:53, 1953.

De Villiers, J. C.: A brachiocephalic vascular syndrome associated with cervical rib, *Brit. Med. J.,* **2**:140, 1966.

Fields, W. S., Ratinov, G., Weibel, J., and Campos, R. J.: Survival following basilar artery occlusion, *Arch. Neurol.,* **15**:463, 1966.

Hiller, F.: The vascular syndromes of the basilar and vertebral arteries and their branches, *J. Nervous Mental Disease,* **116**:988, 1952.

Kubik, C. S., and Adams, R. D.: Occlusion of the basilar artery—clinical and pathological study, *Brain,* **69**:73, 1946.

Loeb, C., and Meyer, J. S.: Strokes Due to Vertebrobasilar Disease: Infarction, Vascular Insufficiency and Hemorrhage of the Brain Stem and Cerebellum, Charles C Thomas, Publisher, Springfield, Ill., 1965.

Etiology and Pathogenesis

Alajouanine, T., Castaigne, P., Cambier, J., and Lia-
nantonikis, E.: Le rôle des positions abnormales et
prolongées de la tête et du cou dons le détermin-
isme des certains accidents vasculaires du tronc cé-
rébral, *Bull. soc. med. hôp. (Paris)*, **74**:21, 1958.

Arseni, C., Popescu, C., and Ghitescu, M.: Brain
stem ischaemia as the presenting feature in a case
of cerebellar tumor, *J. Neurol. Sci.*, **8**:507, 1969.

Ford, F. R.: Syncope, vertigo and disturbances of
vision resulting from intermittent obstruction of
vertebral arteries due to defect in odontoid process
and excessive mobility of second cervical vertebra,
Bull. Johns Hopkins Hosp., **91**:168, 1952.

———, and Clark, D.: Thrombosis of basilar artery
with softenings in cerebellum and brain stem due
to manipulation of neck: A report of 2 cases with
one post-mortem examination: Reasons are given
to prove that damage to vertebral arteries is responsible, *Bull. Johns Hopkins Hosp.*, **98**:37, 1956.

Fowler, M.: Two cases of basilar artery occlusion in
childhood, *Arch. Disease Childhood*, **37**:78, 1962.

Green, D., and Joynt, R. J.: Vascular accidents to the
brain stem associated with neck manipulation,
J.A.M.A., **170**:522, 1959.

Harder, H. I., and Brown, A. F.: Embolization of
basilar artery by myocardial fragment; report of a
case, *Arch. Internal Med.*, **95**:587, 1955.

Hardin, C. A.: Vertebral artery insufficiency produced by cervical osteoarthritic spurs, *Arch. Surg.*,
90:629, 1965.

———, and Poser, C. M.: Rotational obstruction of
the vertebral artery due to redundancy and extra-
luminal cervical fascial bands, *Ann. Surg.*, **158**:133,
1963.

———, Williamson, W. P., and Steegman, A. T.:
Vertebral artery insufficiency produced by cervical
osteoarthritic spurs, *Neurology*, **10**:855, 1960.

Janeway, R., Toole, J. F., Leinbach, L. B., and
Miller, H. S.: Vertebral artery obstruction with
basilar impression: An intermittent phenomenon
related to head turning, *Arch. Neurol.*, **15**:211,
1966.

McDowell, F. H., Potes, J., and Groch, S.: The natural history of internal carotid and vertebral-basilar
artery occlusion, *Neurology*, **11**(4)(part 2):153,
1961.

Powers, S. R., Jr., Drislane, T. M., and Nevins, S.:
Intermittent vertebral artery compression: A new
syndrome, *Surgery*, **49**:257, 1961.

Schwarz, G. A., Geiger, J. K., and Spano, A. V.:
Posterior inferior cerebellar artery syndrome of
Wallenberg after chiropractic manipulation, *Arch.
Internal Med.*, **97**:352, 1956.

Tissington Tatlow, W. F., and Bammer, H. G.: Syndrome of vertebral artery compression, *Neurology*,
7:331, 1957.

Toole, J. F., and Tucker, S. H.: Influence of head
position upon cerebral circulation. Studies on
blood flow in cadavers, *Arch. Neurol.*, **2**:616, 1960.

Yates, P. O.: Birth trauma to the vertebral arteries,
Arch. Disease Childhood, **34**:436, 1959.

Trauma

Carpenter, S.: Injury of neck as cause of vertebral
artery thrombosis, *J. Neurosurg.*, **18**:849, 1961.

Nick, J., Contamin, F., Nicolle, M. H., Lauriers, A.
des, and Ziegler, G.: Incidents et accidents neu-
rologiques dus aux manipulations cervicales (à
propos de trois observations), *Bull. soc. med. hôp.
(Paris)*, **118**:435, 1967.

Sights, W. P., Jr.: Incarceration of the basilar artery
in a fracture of the clivus, *J. Neurosurg.*, **28**:588,
1968.

Simeone, F. A., and Goldberg, H. I.: Thrombosis of
the vertebral artery from hyperextension injury to
the neck, *J. Neurosurg.*, **29**:540, 1968.

Osteoarthritis

Holt, S., and Yates, P. O.: Cervical spondylosis and
nerve root lesions. Incidence at routine necropsy,
J. Bone Joint Surg., **48B**:407, 1966.

Bony Anomalies

Bell, H. S.: Basilar artery insufficiency due to atlanto-
occipital instability, *Am. Surgeon*, **35**:695, 1969.

Bernini, F. P., Elefante, R., Smaltino, F., and Tedes-
chi, G.: Angiographic study on the vertebral artery
in cases of deformities of the occipitocervical joint,
Am. J. Roentgenol., **107**:526, 1969.

Cervical Rib and Fibrous Bands

Husni, E. A., and Storer, J.: The syndrome of mechanical occlusion of the vertebral artery; further
observations, *Angiology*, **18**:106, 1967.

Symonds, C. P.: Cervical rib: Thrombosis of subclavian artery. Contralateral hemiplegia of sudden onset, probably embolic, *Proc. Roy. Soc. Med.,* **20**:1244, 1927, and in Studies in Neurology, Oxford University Press, New York, 1970, pp. 78-79.

Kinks and Loops

Zimmerman, H. B., and Farrell, W. J.: Cervical vertebral erosion caused by vertebral artery tortuosity, *Am. J. Roentgenol.,* **108**:767, 1970.

Pathophysiology

Fisher, C. M., and Karnes, W. E.: Local embolism, *J. Neuropathol. Exptl. Neurol.,* **24**:174, 1965.

Pathologic Findings

Fisher, C. M., Karnes, W. E., and Kubik, C. S.: Lateral medullary infarction—The pattern of vascular occlusion, *J. Neuropathol. Exptl. Neurol.,* **20**:323, 1961.

Gillilan, L. A.: The correlation of the blood supply to the human brain stem with clinical brain stem lesions, *J. Neuropathol. Exptl. Neurol.,* **23**:78, 1964.

Clinical Features

Bradshaw, P., and McQuaid, P.: The syndrome of vertebro-basilar insufficiency, *Quart. J. Med.,* **32**:279, 1963.

Eadie, M. J., and Tyrer, J. H.: Giddiness in vertebro-basilar arterial insufficiency, *Med. J. Australia,* **2**:251, 1968.

Fields, W. S., and Weibel, J.: "Effects of vascular disorders on the vestibular system," in Neurological Aspects of Auditory and Vestibular Disorders, compiled and edited by W. S. Fields and B. R. Alford, Charles C Thomas, Publisher, Springfield, Ill., 1964, p. 305.

Fisher, C. M.: Occlusion of the vertebral arteries causing transient basilar symptoms, *Arch. Neurol.,* **22**:13, 1970.

————: Vertigo in cerebrovascular disease, *Arch. Otolaryngol.,* **85**:529, 1967.

————, and Caplan, L. R.: Basilar artery branch occlusion: A cause of pontine infarction, *Neurology,* **21**:900, 1971.

Herrschaft, H.: Die Zirkulationsstorungen der Arteria vertebralis, *Arch. Psychiat. Nervenkr.,* **218**:22, 1970.

Jaffe, B. F.: Sudden deafness. An otologic emergency, *Arch. Otolaryngol.,* **86**:55, 1967.

Kemper, T. L., and Romanul, F. C. A.: State resembling akinetic mutism in basilar artery occlusion, *Neurology,* **17**:74, 1967.

Kubala, M. J., and Millikan, C. H.: Diagnosis, pathogenesis and treatment of "drop attacks," *Arch. Neurol.,* **11**:107, 1964.

Millikan, C. H., and Siekert, R. G.: Studies in cerebrovascular disease: I. The syndrome of intermittent insufficiency of the basilar arterial system, *Proc. Staff Meetings Mayo Clinic,* **30**:61, 1955.

————, ————, and Whisnant, J. P.: The syndrome of occlusion of the labyrinthine division of the internal auditory artery, *Trans. Am. Neurol. Assoc.,* **84**:11, 1959.

Montgomery, B. M.: The basilar artery hypertensive syndrome, *Arch. Internal Med.,* **108**:559, 1961.

Schneider, R. C., and Crosby, E. C.: Vascular insufficiency of brain stem and spinal cord in spinal trauma, *Neurology,* **9**:643, 1959.

————, and Schemm, G. W.: Vertebral artery insufficiency in acute and chronic spinal trauma with special reference to the syndrome of acute central cervical spinal cord injury, *J. Neurosurg.,* **18**:348, 1961.

Segarra, J. M.: Cerebral vascular disease and behavior. I. The syndrome of the mesencephalic artery (basilar artery bifurcation), *Arch. Neurol.,* **22**:408, 1970.

Williams, D., and Wilson, T. G.: The diagnosis of the major and minor syndromes of basilar insufficiency, *Brain,* **85**:741, 1962.

Neurootologic Features

Aschan, G.: "Nystagmography and caloric testing," in Neurological Aspects of Auditory and Vestibular Disorders, compiled and edited by W. S. Fields and B. R. Alford, Charles C Thomas, Publisher, Springfield, Ill., 1964, p. 216.

Cawthorne, T.: "Otological aspects in the differential diagnosis of vertigo," in Neurological Aspects of Auditory and Vestibular Disorders, compiled and edited by W. S. Fields and B. R. Alford, Charles C Thomas, Publisher, Springfield, Ill., 1964, p. 271.

Neuroophthalmologic Features

Hoyt, W. F.: Transient bilateral blurring of vision: Consideration of an episodic ischemic symptom of vertebral-basilar insufficiency, *Arch. Ophthalmol.*, **70**:746, 1963.

Masucci, E. F.: Bilateral ophthalmoplegia in basilar-vertebral artery disease, *Brain*, **88**:97, 1965.

Minor, R. H., Kearns, T. P., Millikan, C. H., Siekert, R. G., and Sayre, C. P.: Ocular manifestations of occlusive disease of vertebral-basilar arterial system, *Arch. Ophthalmol.*, **62**:84, 1959.

Redlich, F. C., and Dorsey, J. F.: Denial of blindness by patients with cerebral disease, *Arch. Neurol. Psychiat.*, **53**:407, 1945.

Westby, R. K., and Dietrichson, P.: Insufficiency of the vertebral-basilar arterial system; with special reference to ocular symptoms and signs, *Acta ophthalmol.*, **41**:416, 1963.

Examination of the Patient

Chase, T. N., Moretti, L., and Prensky, A. L.: Clinical and electroencephalographic manifestations of vascular lesions of the pons, *Neurology*, **18**:357, 1968.

Soffin, G., Feldman, M., and Bender, M. B.: Alterations of sensory levels in vascular lesions of lateral medulla, *Arch. Neurol.*, **18**:178, 1968.

Laboratory Findings

Electroencephalography

Kooi, K. A., and Sharbrough, F. W.: Electrophysiological findings in cortical blindness. Report of a case, *Electroencephalog. Clin. Neurophysiol.*, **20**:260, 1966.

Otomo, E.: Beta wave activity in the electroencephalogram in cases of coma due to acute brain-stem lesions, *J. Neurol. Neurosurg. Psychiat.*, **29**:383, 1966.

Phillips, B. M.: Temporal-lobe changes associated with the syndromes of basilar-vertebral insufficiency: An electroencephalographic study, *Brit. Med. J.*, **2**:1104, 1964.

Tucker, J. S.: The electroencephalogram in brain stem vascular disease: Some observations relating electroencephalographic findings to various combinations of infarction and vascular insufficiency, *Electroencephalog. Clin. Neurophysiol.*, **10**:405, 1958.

Weintraub, M. I., and Smith, B. H.: Vertigo: Epileptic manifestation of vertebral-basilar artery insufficiency, *N. Y. State J. Med.*, **69**(part 1):1141, 1969.

Aortocranial Angiography

Currier, R. D., Schneider, R. C., and Preston, R. E.: Angiographic findings in Wallenberg's lateral medullary syndrome, *J. Neurosurg.*, **19**:1058, 1962.

Meyer, J. S., Sheehan, S., and Bauer, R. B.: An arteriographic study of cerebrovascular disease in man: I. Stenosis and occlusion of the vertebral-basilar system, *Arch. Neurol.*, **2**:27, 1960.

Robinson, F., Porro, R. S., and Scatliff, J. H.: Angiographic recognition of occipital lobe infarction, *Neurology*, **16**:1016, 1966.

Schechter, M. M., and Zingesser, L. H.: The radiology of basilar thrombosis, *Radiology*, **85**:23, 1965.

Tatsumi, T., and Shenkin, H. A.: Occlusion of the vertebral artery, *J. Neurol. Neurosurg. Psychiat.*, **28**:235, 1965.

Weibel, J., and Fields, W. S.: Angiography of the posterior cervicocranial circulation, *Am. J. Roentgenol.*, **98**:660, 1966.

Differential Diagnosis

Streeto, J. M.: Acute hypercalcemia simulating basilar-artery insufficiency, *New Engl. J. Med.*, **280**:427, 1969.

Management

Gortvai, P.: Insufficiency of vertebral artery treated by decompression of its cervical part, *Brit. Med. J.*, **2**:233, 1964.

Additional References

Castaigne, P., Lhermitte, F., Gautier, J.-C., Escourolle, R., Derouesné, C. der Agopian, P., and Popa, C.: Arterial occlusions in the vertebro-basilar system; a study of forty-four patients with post-mortem data, *Brain*, **96**:133, 1973.

Nordgren, R. E., Markesbery, W. R., Fukuda, K., and Reeves, A. G.: Seven cases of cerebromedullospinal disconnection: The "locked-in" syndrome, *Neurology*, **21**:1140, 1971.

Ouvier, R. A., and Hopkins, I. J.: Occlusive disease of the vertebro-basilar arterial system in childhood, *Develop. Med. Child Neurol.*, **12**:186, 1970.

Chapter 12

Subclavian Steal Syndrome

Feel the pulse with two hands and ten fingers.

Sir William Osler

Under physiologic conditions, arterial pressure is lower in the intracranial arteries than in the aortic arch or its branches. As long as this normal pressure gradient is maintained, arterial blood ascends through the carotid and vertebral arteries to supply the intracranial contents. However, obstructions situated in strategic locations may invert these gradients and cause blood to flow in the reverse direction from the head toward the heart and upper extremities (Fig. 12-1). This unique pathophysiologic situation, in which blood is diverted from the brain and used to supply the upper extremities, has been named the *subclavian steal.*

PATHOLOGY

Atherosclerosis, usually involving the portion of the subclavian artery proximal to the origin of the left vertebral, is by far the most common form of obstructive lesion found in patients with reversed flow. Congenital lesions include coarctation of the aorta and atresia of the proximal subclavian artery. Inflammatory angiopathy produced by such conditions as Takayasu's disease can also cause reversed flow. The Blalock-Taussig operation (anastomosis of the proximal subclavian to the pulmonary artery) for the tetrad of Fallot will also produce reversed flow un-

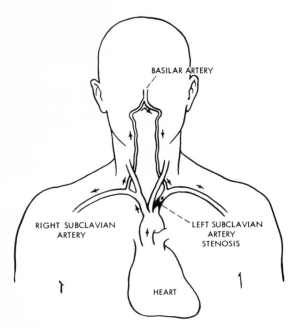

Figure 12-1 Hemodynamic pattern in subclavian steal syndrome.

less the left vertebral artery is also ligated. A few patients have had symptoms of cerebral vascular insufficiency following this or other surgical procedures on the aortic arch or great vessels—e.g., correction of dysphagia lusoria, in which the right subclavian artery arises from the thoracic aorta and courses behind the esophagus. In isolated instances, subintimal dissection of the proximal subclavian artery following trauma has resulted in the subclavian steal syndrome.

PATHOPHYSIOLOGY

Obstructions in different locations produce different forms of "steals" (Figs. 12-2 to 12-4). In all of them the volume and direction of abnormal flow depend on (1) the anatomy of the aortocranial arteries, which may be normal or anomalous; (2) the location of obstructions; and (3) the balance between demands of the limb and cerebral vascular beds for blood.

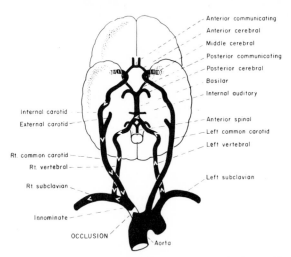

Figure 12-2 Brachiocephalic artery occlusion with reversal of carotid and vertebral artery flow.

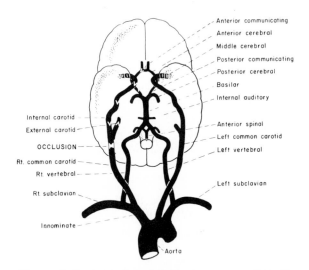

Figure 12-3 Occlusion of right common carotid with reversal of flow through the internal carotid artery.

The anatomy and location of lesions remain the same, but the needs of the interconnected vascular beds are constantly changing. This causes the volume of reversed flow to fluctuate. For example, cutaneous vasodilatation and muscular exercise cause vasodilatation of limb vascular beds and augment the siphoning effect.

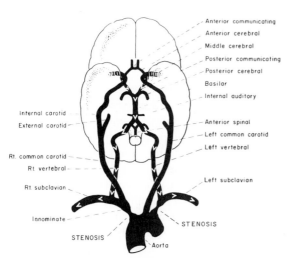

Internal carotid
External carotid

Rt. common carotid
Rt. vertebral
Rt. subclavian

Innominate
STENOSIS
Aorta

Anterior communicating
Anterior cerebral
Middle cerebral
Posterior communicating
Posterior cerebral
Basilar
Internal auditory

Anterior spinal
Left common carotid
Left vertebral

Left subclavian

STENOSIS

Figure 12-4 Stenosis of brachiocephalic and left sub-clavian arteries siphoning blood from the carotid circulation through both vertebral arteries. Brachial blood pressures may be equal.

Symptoms of vascular insufficiency in the brain or the upper extremity will occur only if the metabolic needs of these tissues exceed the amount of blood available to them. In patients with collateral channels adequate to provide this nutrient requirement, extensive volumes of blood may be siphoned without producing cerebral vascular insufficiency. In other patients small volumes may exceed reserve and produce symptoms.

CLINICAL FEATURES

The symptoms that may be produced are of three different types:

1 Arm symptoms. Some patients complain of claudication, numbness, and tingling when the involved limb is exercised. Permanent weakness, wasting of the muscles, and vasomotor phenomena in the involved extremity are rare.
2 Symptoms of vertebral-basilar insufficiency. Although syncope, dizziness, vertigo, unsteadiness, and occipital headache are the most frequent complaints, any of the other

symptoms of vertebral-basilar insufficiency (Chap. 11) may be seen.
3 Symptoms of carotid artery insufficiency. Symptoms due to carotid artery insufficiency are rare but may occur in patients with stenosis of the brachiocephalic (innominate) artery or of both proximal subclavian arteries.

EXAMINATION OF THE PATIENT

Because neural dysfunction is episodic, interictal examination fails to reveal any abnormality of the central nervous system. If abnormal neurologic signs are present between attacks, it is likely that another disease is also present.

General physical examination reveals the radial pulse on the affected side to be diminished. In addition, the arrival time of the pulse on the involved side is usually palpably delayed—a sign that is almost pathognomonic of subclavian steal. Auscultation over the subclavian or vertebral artery frequently reveals a systolic bruit, usually on the ipsilateral side but occasionally on the contralateral side, caused by the altered hemodynamics. Systolic blood pressure readings in the two arms show a difference of at least 20 mm Hg, but diastolic pressures may remain equal. The disparity of blood pressure between the two may be accentuated if measured with the patient standing erect and after exercise of the two arms. On occasion a significant blood pressure difference may be discovered only if pressures are recorded frequently over a 24-hr period, suggesting that the disparity in arm pressures may fluctuate and that reversal may be intermittent.

In some patients, exercising the involved arm also induces claudication, causes the ipsilateral radial pulse to disappear, and accentuates the supraclavicular bruit, all signs of increased demand for blood by the exercising muscles. In occasional patients, this test will precipitate vertigo, syncope, and headache, suggesting that some structures normally supplied by the vertebral-basilar system have been deprived of blood.

DIFFERENTIAL DIAGNOSIS

In all patients suffering with vertebral-basilar insufficiency, especially if they have symptoms of arm claudication or if symptoms of neurologic deficit are precipitated by arm exercise, one should always suspect the subclavian steal syndrome. These historical features, together with a pulse delay, a subclavian-vertebral bruit, and a difference of at least 20 mm Hg in the blood pressures of the two arms, form the tetrad of this syndrome. The only other abnormalities which will also produce blood pressure inequality and pulse delay are (1) coarctation in the aorta located proximal to the subclavian origin and (2) aneurysm of the proximal portion of the subclavian artery or aortic arch.

More often than not, patients with symptomatic subclavian steal syndrome have concomitant atheromatous involvement of the carotid or vertebral artery, or both. In such instances, it may be difficult to decide which lesion is causing the patient's symptoms.

LABORATORY FINDINGS

Digital Plethysmography

This procedure may be used to record abnormal pulse contour and to confirm delay in pulse arrival time on the involved side. As has already been stated, such a delay is almost pathognomonic of the steal syndrome.

Bilateral Simultaneous Sphygmomanometry

Inequality of the two brachial blood pressures can be demonstrated by taking pressures simultaneously in the two arms. In equivocal instances the pressure difference can be made greater if the arms are exercised; pressure in the

involved arm will be decreased while that in the normal arm will be maintained.

Arteriography

The diagnosis of the subclavian steal syndrome is a clinical one, and arteriography is justified only when surgery is contemplated. In this case the abnormal flow patterns should be displayed and the exact site and extent of the obstructive lesion must be demonstrated for the surgeon (Fig. 12-5A and B). To accomplish this, serial exposures or cineradiography following injection of contrast material into the aortic arch confirms the reversal of blood flow and pinpoints the offending lesion. This technique also reveals the extracranial course of the carotid and vertebral arteries, which often show atherosclerotic changes. In some cases of the subclavian steal syndrome the reversal of flow is intermittent and can be demonstrated only by having the patient exercise his arm during the arteriography. Because an obstructive lesion may also be located in the intracranial vessels, separate injection of the vessels in the neck is often needed.

At times retrograde vertebral artery flow will be demonstrated during arteriography of the vertebral arteries when none is present on subsequent occasions. It is believed that this artifact is the result of sudden fall in systemic blood pressure occurring during the injection of contrast material. This sudden hypotension changes pressure relationships and may cause a temporary reversal of blood flow.

COURSE AND PROGNOSIS

Because this syndrome was recognized so recently, its natural history and prognosis are not known. It has been established, however, that symptoms do not occur in all individuals with reversed direction of flow. In some of the symptomatic cases the development of collateral cir-

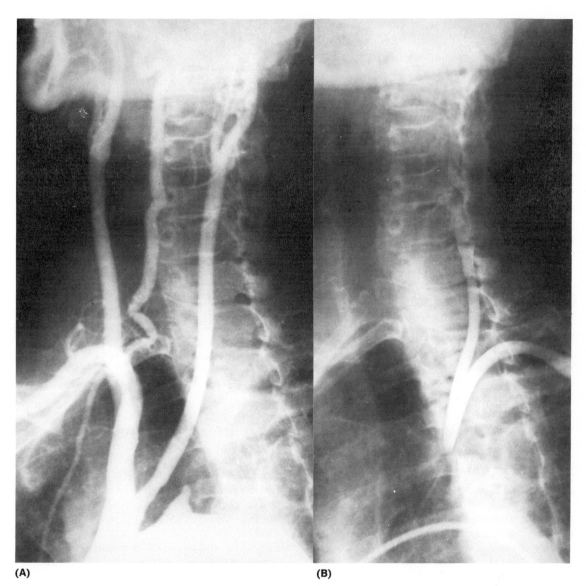

(A)   **(B)**

Figure 12-5 (A)   Aortogram (retrograde femoral approach) depicting anomalous origin of left common carotid artery from brachiocephalic trunk; occlusion of left subclavian artery (2 cm from its origin); right vertebral artery shows kinking. (B) Later phase shows left vertebral artery filling in retrograde fashion. *(Courtesy of Dr. F. Farrell, Department of Radiology, Bowman Gray School of Medicine.)*

culation eventually leads to a spontaneous re-mission.

MANAGEMENT

Asymptomatic patients need no treatment. In those with arm claudication or symptoms of cerebral vascular insufficiency, surgical correction offers the only hope of relief unless spontaneous remission occurs.

The best technique for restoring normal blood flow is endarterectomy with patch grafting. Some surgeons, however, prefer to bypass the obstruction by grafting the subclavian artery to the aorta or the carotid. The advantage of caroticosubclavian anastomosis is that it can be performed through the supraclavicular approach without performing a thoracotomy. In patients who are poor surgical candidates, the vertebral artery or the third part of the ipsilateral subclavian artery can be ligated through a cervical exposure.

Surgical results are gratifying; postoperatively, the radial pulses and blood pressures are usually equal and the patient is relieved of his symptoms of vertebral-basilar insufficiency.

SUGGESTED READINGS

General

Agee, O. F.: Two unusual cases of subclavian steal syndrome: Bilateral steal and steal secondary to tumor thrombus, *Am. J. Roentgenol.,* **97**:447, 1966.

Berger, R. L., Sidd, J. J., and Ramaswamy, K.: Retrograde vertebral-artery flow produced by correction of subclavian-steal syndrome, *New Engl. J. Med.,* **277**:64, 1967.

Editorial: A new vascular syndrome—"The subclavian steal," *New Engl. J. Med.,* **265**:912, 1961.

Miller, J. D. R., Grebneff, A., and Ross, C.: Postsurgical reversed vertebral flow, *Vascular Diseases,* **3**:221, 1966.

Patel, A. N.: Birth of the subclavian steal syndrome, *Neurology (India),* **16**:14, 1968.

———, and Toole, J. F.: Subclavian steal syndrome—Reversal of cephalic blood flow, *Medicine,* **44**:289, 1965.

Poker, N., Finby, N., and Steinberg, I.: The subclavian arteries: Roentgen study in health and disease, *Am. J. Roentgenol.,* **80**:193, 1958.

Reivich, M., Holling, H. E., Roberts, B., and Toole, J. F.: Reversal of blood flow through the vertebral artery and its effect on cerebral circulation, *New Engl. J. Med.,* **265**:878, 1961.

Sokol, S., Narkiewicz, M., and Billewicz, O.: Subclavian steal syndrome after Blalock-Taussig anastomoses, *J. Cardiovascular Surg.,* **10**:350, 1969.

Pathophysiology

Dardik, H., Gensler, S., Stern, W. Z., and Glotzer, P.: Subclavian steal syndrome secondary to embolism: First reported case, *Ann. Surg.,* **164**:171, 1966.

Editorial: Problem—To define theft, *New Engl. J. Med.,* **277**:103, 1967.

Lord, R. S. A., Adar, R., and Stein, R. L.: Contribution of the circle of Willis to the subclavian steal syndrome, *Circulation,* **40**:871, 1969.

Clinical Features

Barnett, H. J. M., Wortzman, G., Gladstone, R. M., and Lougheed, W. M.: Diversion and reversal of cerebral blood flow. External carotid artery "steal," *Neurology,* **20**:1, 1970.

Behrman, S.: Episodic retinal ischemia caused by reduced cerebral vascular resistance ("brain steal"), *Brit. J. Ophthalmol.,* **51**:269, 1967.

Editorial: Vascular thievery, *J.A.M.A.,* **209**:1899, 1969.

Heidrich, H., and Bayer, O.: Symptomatology of the subclavian steal syndrome, *Angiology,* **20**:406, 1969.

Mozes, M., Bank, H., and Wortreich, B.: Subclavian-steal syndrome and motor accidents, *Lancet,* **2**:533, 1967.

Piccone, V. A., Jr., Karvounis, P., and LeVeen, H. H.: The subclavian steal syndrome, *Angiology,* **21**:240, 1970.

Pratesi, F., Capellini, M., Macchini, M., Nuti, A., Deidda, C., and Caramelli, L.: The innominate steal, *Vascular Diseases,* **5**:214, 1968.

Differential Diagnosis

Yahr, W. Z., Furman, S., and Robinson, G.: Innominate artery steal syndrome, *N. Y. State J. Med.*, **67**(part 1):1328, 1967.

Laborabory Findings

Conrad, M., Toole, J. F., and Janeway, R.: Hemodynamics of the upper extremities in subclavian steal syndrome, *Circulation*, **32**:346, 1965.
Grossman, B. L., Brisman, R., and Wood, E. H.: Ultrasound and the subclavian steal syndrome, *Radiology*, **94**:1, 1970.

Bilateral Simultaneous Sphygmomanometry

King, G. E.: Taking the blood pressure, *J.A.M.A.*, **209**:1902, 1969.
Toole, J. F., and Tulloch, E. F.: Bilateral simultaneous sphygmomanometry: A new diagnostic test for subclavian steal syndrome, *Circulation*, **33**:952, 1966.

Radiology

Curry, J. L., and Howland, W. J.: Subclavian steal syndrome: Pitfalls in its diagnosis, *Am. J. Roentgenol.*, **91**:1254, 1964.
Gonzalez, L., Weintraub, R. A., Wiot, J. F., and Lewis, C.: Retrograde vertebral artery blood flow: A normal phenomenon, *Radiology*, **82**:211, 1964.
Klinkhammer, A. C.: Aberrant right subclavian artery: Clinical and roentgenologic aspects, *Am. J. Roentgenol.*, **97**:438, 1966.
Newton, T. H., and Wylie, E. J.: Collateral circulation associated with occlusion of the proximal subclavian and innominate arteries, *Am. J. Roentgenol.*, **91**:394, 1964.
Shockman, A. T.: Retrograde vertebral artery flow as an artifact of technique, *Am. J. Roentgenol.*, **91**:1258, 1964.

Course and Prognosis

Dumanian, A. V., Frahm, C. J., Pascale, L. R., Teplinsky, L. L., and Santschi, D. R.: The surgical treatment of the subclavian steal syndrome, *J. Thoracic Cardiovascular Surg.*, **50**:22, 1965.
Fields, W. S., and Lemak, N. A.: Joint study of extracranial arterial occlusion. VII. Subclavian steal—a review of 168 cases, *J.A.M.A.*, **222**:1139, 1972.
Finkelstein, N. M., Byer, A., and Rush, B. F., Jr.: Subclavian-subclavian bypass for the subclavian steal syndrome, *Surgery*, **71**:142, 1972.
Mandelbaum, I., Nahrwold, D. L., and Dzenitis, A. J.: Spontaneous resolution of traumatic subclavian steal syndrome, *Ann. Surg.*, **165**:314, 1967.
North, R. R., Fields, W. S., DeBakey, M. E., and Crawford, E. S.: Brachial-basilar insufficiency syndrome, *Neurology*, **12**:810, 1962.
Resnicoff, S. A., DeWeese, J. A., and Rob, C. G.: Surgical treatment of the subclavian steal syndrome, *Circulation*, suppl. 41 and 42, part 2, p. 147, 1970.

Cerebral Atherosclerosis

Arteriosclerotic dementia: a diagnosis made when your elders disagree with what you say.

Anonymous

And all the conduits of my blood froze up, yet hath my night of life some memory, my wasting lamps some fading glimmer left.

William Shakespeare
The Comedy of Errors (Act V, Scene 1)

For purposes of classification, the intracranial branches of the carotid and vertebral arteries have customarily been considered separately from their extracranial arterial trunks. This artificial division has no sound basis in anatomy or physiology, because the aortocranial system functions almost as a unit, from thoracic origin to intracranial capillary bed. Because of long usage, a tremendous literature has accumulated about "cerebral" atherosclerosis, and it is often regarded as if it were a separate entity. Nothing could be further from the truth (Fig. 13-1)!

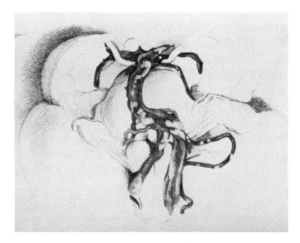

Figure 13-1 Richard Bright's illustration of atherosclerosis in the vertebral-basilar system.

PATHOPHYSIOLOGY

The circle of Willis and the arteries on the surface of the brain form a network which distributes and regulates the flow of blood into the brain parenchyma. Systemic arterial blood pressure is transmitted into these arteries, and pressure differences equilibrate within the surface network. With increasing atherosclerosis, the capacity of the cerebral circulation to distribute blood is reduced, both in degree and in rapidity of response, rendering the brain more and more vulnerable to sudden reduction in systemic arterial blood pressure. In addition, the margin of safety for focal areas is further diminished by a decrease in flow through individual sclerotic arteries. However, so great is the built-in reserve that local flow may be reduced by a third before signs of neurologic deficit begin to develop.

It is important to realize that regional cerebral blood flow may differ remarkably because of (1) individual variations in vascular configuration, which are determined during embryogenesis, and (2) the vagaries of atherosclerosis, which may destroy different segments of this anastomotic system. Both these factors affect the potential for collateral circulation to any given region of the brain and may produce regional deficiencies in blood flow while total cerebral blood flow may be normal. Superimposed upon these local deficiencies, systemic stresses (such as reduction in systemic blood pressure, alterations in blood and plasma viscosity, anemia, hypoxia, and hypoglycemia) can act as triggering mechanisms which result in neurologic deficit in the areas of brain most compromised by atherosclerosis.

PATHOLOGIC FINDINGS

Gross Examination

At autopsy the arteries of patients who have atherosclerosis may show advanced changes without any visible alterations in the brain (Fig. 13-2). In other brains with atherosclerotic arteries there is a reduction in brain weight, the interhemispheric and interlobar fissures are broad, the convolutions are small, and the sulci are widened, particularly in the frontal and temporal lobes; the circumference of the brainstem is smaller than normal, and the bulk of the cerebellum is reduced (Fig. 13-3).

It has been impossible to determine a direct cause-and-effect relation between atherosclerosis and brain atrophy, but on the other hand, the cervical portions of the brain arteries have not been examined in a large enough series to allow for valid correlations to be made. When such an atrophic brain is sectioned, the cortical ribbon is seen to be narrowed and the bulk of the white matter beneath is decreased. The ventricles are symmetrically dilated. The cut ends of the sclerotic penetrating arteries may protrude above the cut surface, and old infarctions of varying ages may be seen irregularly scattered throughout the substance of the brain. Even in retrospect one finds that many such small infarctions do not cause recognizable symptoms or signs during life.

Multiple, tiny irregular cavities visible in the internal capsule, putamen, thalamus, pons, and

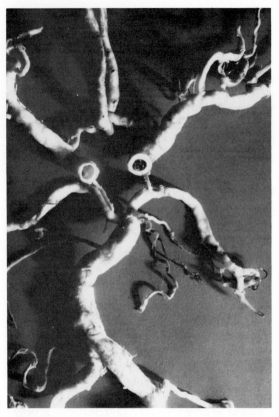

Figure 13-2 Arteries of the base of the brain showing severe atherosclerosis with thickening, tortuosity, and elongation of the vessels. Note the fusiform dilatation of the basilar artery.

posterior cerebral arteries, where the smaller branches of one artery form anastomoses with those of another. Local arterial pressures in these watershed areas are normally the lowest of any in the system, so that any generalized reduction first reaches critical levels in these terminal branches (Fig. 13-4A and B).

The more deeply situated infarctions of the cerebrum are most commonly found in the region of the internal capsule in the distribution of the penetrating branches of the middle cerebral artery (the lenticulostriate arteries).

Cerebral infarctions change their appearance with age. Although the most recent are not visible, they are palpable as circumscribed areas of softening within the substance of the brain. Later on, the infarcted tissue becomes necrotic and the structure of the infarcted brain may collapse, so that a cavity is formed. If infarction has involved the cortex or the subjacent white matter, a depression is visible on the surface of the brain.

Infarctions due to atherosclerosis are usually pale, signifying a lack of blood supply. They may become hemorrhagic under certain circumstances: (1) if the underlying mechanism is an embolus; (2) in some instances when anticoagulants have been used; or (3) when, following an infarction secondary to hypotension, the blood pressure is elevated and the necrotic area is again flooded with blood.

Microscopic Examination

In the aged brain the cortical neurons may be shrunken and the supporting glia may show degeneration in the perivascular feet of the astrocytes. The brain capillaries are somewhat thickened and have an excess number of loops. In advanced degeneration the cerebral parenchyma contains pale zones that retain the ghost-like shadows of degenerated neurons. The astrocytes are pyknotic and thickened.

In   infarcted   areas   the   microscopic

sometimes cerebellum constitute a condition called *état lacunaire* (lacunar state). These are the remains of very small infarctions and contain disintegrated brain parenchyma or fluid-filled vacuoles surrounding arteries that may contain small thrombi. Another condition which is identified by the presence of pinhole-sized dilatations situated in the centrum semiovale is called *état criblé*. These cavities are markedly dilated perivascular spaces of Virchow-Robin and may have no clinicopathologic significance.

Superficial infarctions have a predilection for the terminal areas of the anterior, middle, and

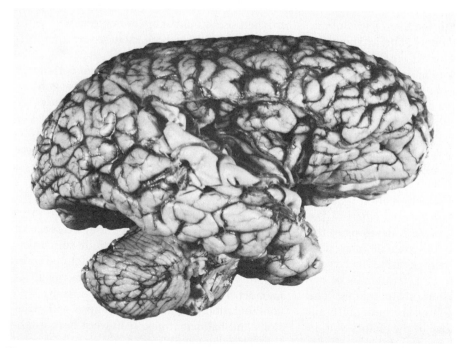

Figure 13-3 Atrophic brain with concomitant atherosclerosis.

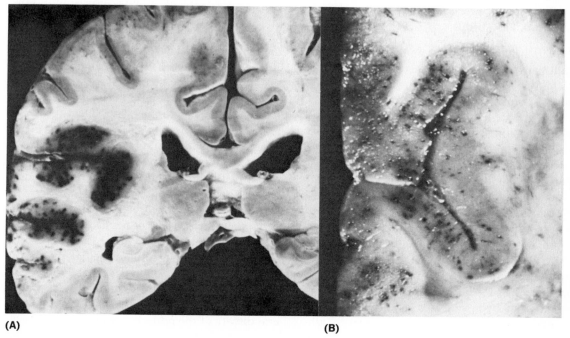

(A)

(B)

Figure 13-4(A) and (B) Hemorrhagic infarction in the distribution of the middle cerebral artery.

appearance changes with the age of infarction. The first microscopically detectable changes are sludging and aggregation of red blood cells within the arterioles, capillaries, and venules of the affected area. Later on, further degeneration is visible, the walls of the capillaries become ectatic, and some diapedesis of red blood cells takes place. The astrocytes and neurons become swollen, and local edema sometimes develops.

As the healing process occurs, the infarcted area gradually becomes knit by the process of neovascularization and scar formation (gliosis). The new-vessel formation does not benefit the patient, except perhaps when it develops in the marginal zones around the area of infarction. This type of formation may occasionally be seen as a cloud or blush on the arteriograms of patients who have had cerebral infarctions. The gliosis causes contraction of surrounding brain substance and may be one of the factors that, in later years, trigger epileptiform discharges from the zones surrounding the infarction.

CLINICAL FEATURES

It is unfortunate that the numerous symptoms and signs of neural dysfunction described as "senility" have been attributed to "cerebral" atherosclerosis. Some patients who are considered senile are actually depressed or intoxicated by medication; others are suffering from subdural hematomata, from malignancies that produce disorders of the sensorium, from nutritional, metabolic, or endocrine insufficiency, or even from unrecognized cardiac or pulmonary decompensation—all treatable illnesses. Another possibility is hydrocephalic dementia (normal pressure hydrocephalus) in which obstruction to the free flow and resorption of cerebrospinal fluid causes hydrocephalus which in turn results in dementia. Removal of the obstruction or bypassing it with a shunt restores mental function. A diagnosis of "cerebral" atherosclerosis should not be entertained until these disorders have been excluded by appropriate studies.

At least five syndromes have been considered by some authorities to be the result of atherosclerotic changes in the aortocranial vessels. Although these are discussed separately, it must be recognized that there may be considerable overlapping among them and that about some there is much controversy.

Dementia

Mental changes occurring without evidence of focal neurologic deficit may include subtle personality deterioration ("second childhood"), irritability with mood swings, impairment of memory for recent events with garrulity and confabulation, and at times psychosis with delusions and hallucinations. It has not been established how many of these so-called classic symptoms of "cerebral" atherosclerosis are actually due to aortocranial atherosclerosis and how many are due to an involutional process in the glia, the ground substance, or in the neurons themselves (Alzheimer's disease).

One form of dementia, an isolated loss of the ability to form new memories, is due to lesions in both the hippocampal and fornical systems. Patients with such lesions have intact recall for remote events, normal speech, and in many cases a remarkable ability to hide their deficit in recent memory. The pathologic cause is to be found in the hippocampal gyrus of both sides.

The situation is quite different, however, in patients with focal neurologic deficits such as hemiparesis, dysphasia, or hemianopia. Aphasia is usually accompanied by some loss of comprehension and slowing of intellectual processes. Patients with infarction in the frontal lobe, particularly if it involves the dominant hemisphere, may have subtle personality change. With bilateral disease of the posterior cerebral artery or of the vertebral-basilar system, infarction may occur in the inferomedial portions of both temporal lobes, the fornix, the mammillary bodies, and the hippocampal formations of both sides. Patients with such conditions may have profound defects in recent memory, with retrograde amnesia and loss of the ability to learn new skills (Korsakoff's psychosis).

Binswanger's Disease

Some neurologists deny that this condition exists as a specific entity; others identify it as atherosclerosis which involves the penetrating arteries of the temporal and occipital lobes of the two hemispheres. Infarction of these regions causes the symptoms and signs of Binswanger's disease: progressive mental deterioration, cortical blindness, seizures, and a variable amount of corticospinal and extrapyramidal dysfunction.

Parkinsonism

Most authorities believe that atherosclerosis per se cannot cause parkinsonism. In those patients whose syndrome resembles parkinsonism, they find associated pyramidal dysfunction, dementia, and/or pseudobulbar signs in addition to the extrapyramidal disorder. In those patients with diffuse disease, *état lacunaire* is often found in the brain at postmortem examination.

Others make a diagnosis of atherosclerotic parkinsonism when the acute onset of signs of extrapyramidal disorder affords clearly localized evidence of vascular disease, probably atherosclerosis. In these instances the characteristic tremor of parkinsonism begins suddenly, and the most logical explanation seems to be that atherosclerosis has caused infarction of a critical area of the brain.

Pseudobulbar Palsy

Even though the clinical signs associated with this condition are superficially suggestive of primary medullary (bulbar) dysfunction, the abnormality is secondary to bilateral lesions in the corticobulbar tracts which result in supranuclear paralysis of lower cranial nerves characterized by dysarthria, dysphagia, and an immobile facies. The most common location of lesions is in the internal capsules. Since one side is usually involved before the other, most patients have a history of previous hemiparesis, followed by more recent paralysis on the opposite side and superimposed pseudobulbar signs.

The patient has difficulty in speaking and protruding his tongue because of spasticity. Movements of the larynx are disturbed, and respiration may be impaired. The jaw jerk is abnormally brisk, as are the circumoral myotactic reflexes. The bilateral corticospinal tract lesions cause the gait to be slow, clumsy, unsteady, and shuffling *(marche-à-petit-pas)*; tendon reflexes are abnormally brisk, and Hoffmann's and Babinski's signs may be present on both sides. Diffuse cerebral involvement may cause personality changes, with inappropriate and uncontrolled laughter or crying as an overreaction to minor emotional stimuli.

Cranial Nerve Palsies

Pressures of the rigid atherosclerotic arteries may occasionally cause one of the cranial nerves at the base of the brain to lose its function. Binasal hemianopia is ascribed to dilated and calcified internal carotid arteries which compress the lateral margins of the optic nerves and chiasm (Fig. 13-5). A dilated, tortuous basilar artery pressing against cranial nerves sometimes causes a cerebellopontile angle syndrome, tic douloureux of the trigeminal nerve, bilateral sixth or seventh nerve palsies, or hemifacial spasm. Elongation of the terminal portion of the basilar artery may invaginate the third ventricle and is thought to result at times in internal hydrocephalus, causing dementia (Fig. 13-6A and B).

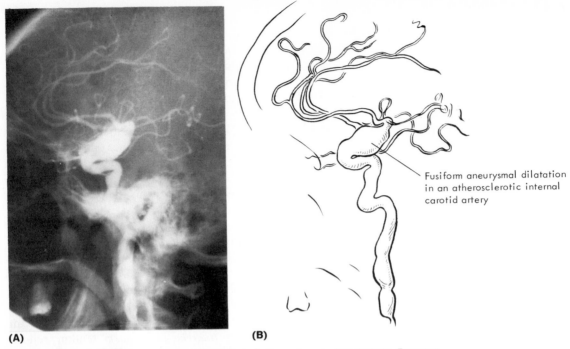

(A)

(B)

Fusiform aneurysmal dilatation
in an atherosclerotic internal
carotid artery

Figure 13-5(A) and (B) *(Courtesy of Dr. F. Farrell, Department of Radiology, Bowman
Gray School of Medicine.)*

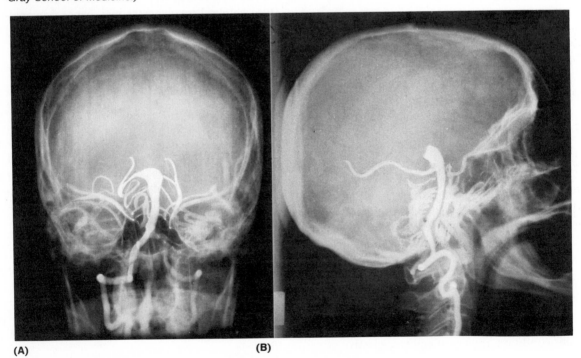

(A)

(B)

Figure 13-6(A) and (B) Elongation and tortuosity of the basilar artery secondary to
atherosclerosis. *(Courtesy of Dr. Jacques E. Botton.)*

DIFFERENTIAL DIAGNOSIS

The diagnosis of neurologic deficit caused by atherosclerosis is made by exclusion. Senescence per se, even when combined with the finding of atherosclerosis in other parts of the body, is not sufficient grounds for ascribing neurologic change in an aged patient to atherosclerosis. Whenever one is tempted to make a diagnosis of senile dementia or "chronic brain syndrome" secondary to atherosclerosis, one should first eliminate the following possibilities, among others, for each of which specific therapy is available:

1 Drug intoxication (by tranquilizers, sedatives such as barbiturates or bromides, hypotensive drugs, or agents employed in the treatment of parkinsonism)
2 Subdural hematoma
3 Intracranial neoplasm
4 Nutritional deficiency (avitaminosis B_1 or B_{12})
5 Profound anemia of any cause
6 Hypothyroidism, hypopituitarism, or hypoadrenalism
7 Cardiopulmonary disease with hypoxia or hypercapnia
8 Renal disease with uremia
9 Occult carcinoma with secondary encephalopathy
10 Endogenous depression
11 Neurosyphilis
12 Chronic congestive heart failure
13 Hepatic encephalopathy
14 Occult hydrocephalus
15 Hypoglycemia

After a complete history, physical, and neurologic examination with particular attention to the clues which suggest aortocervical vascular disease, the following minimal group of screening tests must be performed:

1 Skull and chest x-ray
2 Blood count, urinalysis, and serologic tests for syphilis

3 Determinations of the blood content of urea nitrogen, protein-bound iodine, sodium, potassium, carbon dioxide, and liver function tests
4 Determination for blood level of barbiturates and bromides
5 Radioisotopic study of arterial flow and brain scan
6 Spinal fluid examination
7 Electroencephalograms
8 Tests for free gastric acid
9 Schilling's test or serum vitamin B_{12} levels if the patient is achlorhydric
10 Echoencephalogram if the pineal gland is not calcified
11 In some instances, radioisotope iodinated serum albumin (RISA) cisternography, arteriography, or pneumoencephalography

Even when the history, physical examination, and neurologic findings are normal and laboratory studies are negative, one must still consider the possibility of depression, drug intoxication, or both.

LABORATORY FINDINGS

Blood Cholesterol and Triglycerides

Except in people under age 55, no clear correlation has been demonstrated between levels of blood cholesterol or triglycerides and the incidence of cerebral atherosclerosis.

Lumbar Puncture

The patient with cerebral atherosclerosis will have normal spinal fluid pressure and contents. If the brain is atrophic, the volume of spinal fluid may be increased; this abnormality, however, will not be evident unless total-drainage pneumoencephalography is performed.

X-Ray Findings

Skull films may reveal calcification in the carotid siphon and occasionally in the basilar artery. Calcifications in the circle of Willis and its branches are almost never visible.

Arteriography

Arteriographic findings in the extracranial portions of the carotid and vertebral arteries were considered in the preceding chapters. Intracranially, the vessels may be dilated, tortuous, and elongated. Indentations in the column of contrast material, giving it a serrated appearance, suggest the presence of atheromatous plaques protruding into the lumen of the artery. These indentations, most often visible in the carotid siphon, are occasionally seen in the middle, anterior, and posterior cerebral arteries. Elongation and tortuosity may give a sinuous appearance to the branches of these three arteries.

In the early phases of the arteriogram, occlusion of one or more arteries causes nonfilling of the area normally supplied by that vessel. In later phases, the contrast material may proceed into the area in a reverse direction through collateral channels (Fig. 13-7A and B). At this time, a faint cloud or stain of opaque material may suggest the presence of neovascularization.

Delay in transit time of the contrast material, indicating prolonged circulation time, does not necessarily occur.

Pneumoencephalography

This procedure must be used sparingly and with caution in patients suffering with dementia or atherosclerosis because it may aggravate the condition. Every effort should be made to fill the parasaggital cortical area with air, thereby excluding "normal pressure" hydrocephalus.

In cerebral atrophy symmetric dilatation of the ventricles will be seen, perhaps more in the frontal and temporal horns than in the occipital. The third ventricle, the aqueduct of Sylvius, and the fourth ventricle are usually dilated. The most striking finding is the puddling of air in the sulci over the frontal, insular, Rolandic, and temporal areas. At times air in the sulci may render the convolutions of the brain apparent. In patients with hydrocephalic dementia the ventricles are large but there is no outline of the convexity of the brain because air is trapped below the tentorium cerebelli by adhesions in the region of the incisura.

Radioisotopic Brain Scan

Unless there has been recent infarction, the brain scan is normal in patients with "cerebral" atherosclerosis.

Electroencephalography

Some authorities believe that "cerebral" atherosclerosis causes slowing of the normal brain rhythms into the theta range. In patients who have had recent cerebral infarctions close to the surface of the brain, there may be focal high-

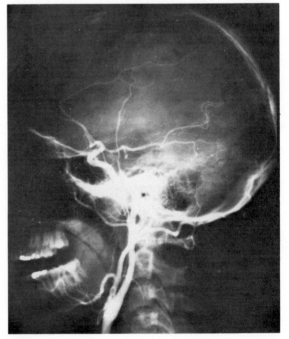

(A)

Figure 13-7(A) and (B) Arteriogram showing middle cerebral arterial occlusion. (A) Nonfilling of the middle cerebral artery. (B) Later phase showing reversed filling through collateral channels.

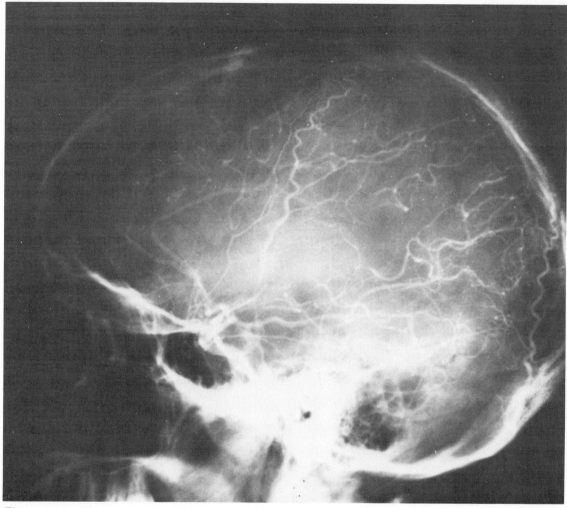

(B)

voltage delta rhythm overlying the area. Small or deeply situated infarctions, however, seldom produce discernible disturbance in the electro-encephalogram unless they occur in the reticular formation of the brainstem; small infarctions involving this area may cause diffuse disturbance of brain-wave activity.

Patients with old, long-healed infarctions may have episodic sharp-wave activity emanating from the zone surrounding the gliotic area. These sharp waves may be evidence of an irritative focus. It is estimated that 10 to 25 percent of patients who have healed cerebral infarctions eventually suffer with focal or generalized convulsions which originate in the zone surrounding the old infarction. Even in patients who have no seizures following infarction, disturbance of the EEG rhythms is usually seen.

MANAGEMENT

If all the procedures outlined in the section on differential diagnosis fail to reveal a cause for the patient's mental deterioration, one may occasionally be justified in attributing the symptoms to atherosclerosis. In such cases the physician and the patient's family must watch the gradual decline of a once fertile intellect without succumbing to the temptation to try meddlesome therapy. Tranquilizers or psychic energizers may aggravate rather than forestall the deterioration and therefore must be reserved for the occasional agitated or depressed patient. Barbiturates often excite these patients. So-called cerebral vasodilators such as nikethamide (Coramine) and pentylenetetrazol (Metrazol) are ineffective. Alcohol in small quantities may improve the patient's appetite, render him euphoric, and keep him tractable.

By far the most important aspect of therapy is support to the patient's family as they adjust to the situation. It is usually the family, not the patient, who suffers most from this distressing condition.

SUGGESTED READINGS

General

Adler, E., Adler, C., Magora, A., Shanan, J., and Tal, E.: Stroke in Israel 1957–1961: Epidemiological, Clinical, Rehabilitation and Psycho-Social Aspects, Polypress, Ltd., Jerusalem, 1969.

Baker, A. B., Flora, G. C., Resch, J. A., and Loewenson, R.: The geographic pathology of atherosclerosis: A review of the literature with some personal observations on cerebral atherosclerosis, *J. Chronic Diseases,* **20**:685, 1967.

———, Resch, J. A., and Loewenson, R. B.: Hypertension and cerebral atherosclerosis, *Circulation,* **39**:701, 1969.

Constantinides, P.: Pathogenesis of cerebral artery thrombosis in man, *Arch. Pathol.,* **83**:422, 1967.

Heyden, S., Heyman, A., and Camplong, L.: Mortality patterns among parents of patients with atherosclerotic cerebrovascular disease, *J. Chronic Diseases,* **22**:105, 1969.

Kannel, W. B.: Current status of the epidemiology of brain infarction associated with occlusive arterial disease, *Stroke,* **2**:295, 1971.

———, Wolf, P. A., Verter, J., and McNamara, P. M.: Epidemiologic assessment of the role of blood pressure in stroke. The Framingham study, *J.A.M.A.,* **214**:301, 1970.

Kurtzke, J. F.: Epidemiology of Cerebrovascular Disease, Springer-Verlag, New York, 1969.

Malmros, H.: Dietary prevention of atherosclerosis, *Lancet,* **1**:94, 1970.

Mints, A. Ya., and Sachuk, N. N.: Studies of cerebral atherosclerosis in old and very old individuals, *Federal Proc. Trans. Suppl.,* **24**(6)(part 2):T967, 1965.

Moossy, J.: "Cerebral atherosclerosis: Intracranial and extracranial lesions," in Pathology of the Nervous System, vol. 2, edited by J. Minckler, McGraw-Hill Book Company, New York, 1971, pp. 1423–1432.

———: Cerebral infarction and intracranial arterial thrombosis, *Arch. Neurol.,* **14**:119, 1966.

Paffenbarger, R. S., Jr., and Williams, J. L.: Chronic disease in former college students. V. Early precursors of fatal stroke, *Am. J. Pub. Health,* **57**:1290, 1967.

———, and Wing, A. L.: Characteristics in youth predisposing to fatal stroke in later years, *Lancet,* **1**:753, 1967.

———, Laughlin, M. E., Gima, A. S., and Black, R. A.: Work activity of longshoremen as related to death from coronary heart disease and stroke, *New Engl. J. Med.,* **282**:1109, 1970.

Page, I. H.: Atherosclerosis: A personal overview, *Circulation,* **38**:1164, 1968.

Solberg, L. A., McGarry, P. A., Moossy, J., Tejada, C., Loken, A. C., Robertson, W. B., and Donoso, S.: Distribution of cerebral atherosclerosis by geographic location, race, and sex, *Lab. Invest.,* **18**:601, 1968.

Stallones, R. A.: Epidemiology of cerebrovascular disease. A review, *J. Chronic Diseases,* **18**:859, 1965.

Strong, J. P., and McGill, H. C., Jr.: The pediatric aspects of atherosclerosis, *J. Atheroscler. Res.,* **9**:251, 1969.

Wallace, D. C.: The natural history of cerebral vascular disease, *Am. Heart J.*, **75**:285, 1968.

Pathophysiology

Di Chiro, G., and Libow, L. S.: Carotid siphon calcification and cerebral blood flow in the healthy aged male, *Radiology*, **99**:103, 1971.

Gilroy, J., and Meyer, J. S.: Pituitary insufficiency with cerebrovascular symptoms: A new clinical syndrome, *New Engl. J. Med.*, **269**:1115, 1963.

Hassler, O.: Vascular changes in senile brains: A micro-angiographic study, *Acta neuropathol. (Berlin)*, **5**:40, 1965.

Hedlund, S., Köhler, V., Nylin, G., Olsson, R., Regnström, O., Rothström, E., and Aström, K. E.: Cerebral blood circulation in dementia, *Acta psychiat. scand.*, **40**:77, 1964.

Shenkin, H. A., Novak, P., Goluboff, B., Soffe, A. M., and Bortin, L.: The effects of aging, arteriosclerosis, and hypertension upon the cerebral circulation, *J. Clin. Invest.*, **32**:459, 1953.

Pathologic Findings

Adams, R. D.: "Pathology of cerebral vascular diseases. B. Cranial cerebral lesions," in Cerebral Vascular Diseases, Transactions of the Second Princeton Conference, edited by C. H. Millikan, Grune & Stratton, Inc., New York, 1958, pp. 23–39.

Baker, A. B.: Structure of the small cerebral arteries and their changes with age, *Am. J. Pathol.*, **13**:453, 1937.

Blackwood, W., Hallpike, J. F., Kocen, R. S., and Mair, W. G. P.: Atheromatous disease of the carotid arterial system and embolism from the heart in cerebral infarction: A morbid anatomical study, *Brain*, **92**:897, 1969.

Fisher, C. M.: The arterial lesions underlying lacunes, *Acta neuropathol. (Berlin)*, **12**:1, 1969.

———, Gore, I., Okabe, N., and White, P. D.: Atherosclerosis of the carotid and vertebral arteries— Extracranial and intracranial, *J. Neuropathol. Exptl. Neurol.*, **24**:455, 1965.

Flora, G. C., Baker, A. B., Loewenson, R. B., and Klassen, A. C.: A comparative study of cerebral atherosclerosis in males and females, *Circulation*, **38**:859, 1968.

Grunnet, M.: Changes in cerebral arteries with aging, *Arch. Pathol.*, **88**:314, 1969.

Moossy, J.: Cerebral infarcts and the lesions of intracranial and extracranial atherosclerosis, *Arch. Neurol.*, **14**:124, 1966.

Routsonis, K. G.: Histopathological changes in the intracranial portion of the optic nerves in cerebral atherosclerosis, *Acta neuropathol. (Berlin)*, **16**:77, 1970.

Clinical Features

Alman, R. W., and Fazekas, J. F.: Disparity between low cerebral blood flow and clinical signs of cerebral ischemia, *Neurology*, **7**:555, 1957.

Ang, R. T., and Utterback, R. A.: Seizures with onset after forty years of age; role of cerebrovascular disease. *South. Med. J.*, **59**:1404, 1966.

Aring, C. D.: Supranuclear (pseudobulbar) palsy, *Arch. Internal Med.*, **115**:198, 1965.

Evans, J. H.: Transient loss of memory, an organic mental syndrome, *Brain*, **89**:539, 1966.

Faris, A. A.: Limbic system infarction. A report of two cases, *Neurology*, **19**:91, 1969.

Fisher, C. M., and Curry, H. B.: Pure motor hemiplegia of vascular origin, *Arch. Neurol.*, **13**:30, 1965.

———, and Adams, R. D.: Transient global amnesia, *Acta neurol. scand.*, **40**(suppl. 9):7, 1964.

Lhermitte, F., Gautier, J.-C., and Derouesné, C.: Nature of occlusions of the middle cerebral artery, *Neurology*, **20**:82, 1970.

Ring, B. A.: Angiographic recognition of occlusions of isolated branches of the middle cerebral artery, *Am. J. Roentgenol.*, **89**:391, 1963.

———: The Neglected Cause of Stroke. Occlusion of the Smaller Intracranial Arteries and Their Diagnosis by Cerebral Angiography, Warren H. Green, Inc., St. Louis, 1969.

Sindermann, F., Dichgans, J., and Bergleiter, R.: Occlusion of the middle cerebral and its branches: Angiographic and clinical correlates, *Brain*, **92**:607, 1969.

Waddington, M. M., and Ring, B. A.: Syndromes of occlusions of middle cerebral artery branches. Angiographic and clinical correlation, *Brain*, **91**:685, 1968.

Wood, M. W., and Murphey, F.: Obstructive hydro-

cephalus due to infarction of a cerebellar hemisphere, *J. Neurosurg.,* **30**:260, 1969.

Dementia

Allen, E. B.: Psychiatric aspects of cerebral arteriosclerosis, *New Engl. J. Med.,* **245**:677, 1951.

Banshchikov, V. M., and Stoliarov, G. V.: Arteriosclerotic psychoses: A review of the foreign literature from 1940-1956, *J. Nervous Mental Disease,*
128:160, 1959.

Benton, A. L. (ed.): Behavioral Changes in Cerebrovascular Disease, Harper & Row, Publishers, New
York, 1970.

de Boucaud, P., Vital, C., and de Boucaud, D.: Dé-
mence thalamique d'origine vasculaire, *Rev. neurol.,* **119**:461, 1968.

Boudin, G., Brion, S., Pépin, B., and Barbizet, J.:
Syndrome de Korsakoff d'étiologie artériopath-
ique, par lésion bilatérale, asymetrique du système
limbique, *Rev. neurol.,* **119**:341, 1968.

Breig, A., Ekbom, K., Greitz, T., and Kugelberg, E.:
Hydrocephalus due to elongated basilar artery: A
new clinicoradiological syndrome, *Lancet,* **1**:874,
1967.

Ekbom, K., Greitz, T., and Kugelberg, E.: Hydrocephalus due to ectasia of the basilar artery, *J.
Neurol. Sci.,* **8**:465, 1969.

Karp, H. R.: Dementia in cerebrovascular disease
and other systemic illnesses, *Current Concepts Cerebrovascular Dis.—Stroke,* **7**:11, 1972.

Rothschild, D.: Neuropathologic changes in arteriosclerotic psychoses and their psychiatric significance, *Arch. Neurol. Psychiat.,* **48**:417, 1942.

Torvik, A., Endresen, G. K. M., Abrahamsen, A. F.,
and Godal, H. C.: Progressive dementia caused by
an unusual type of generalized small vessel thrombosis, *Acta neurol. scand.,* **47**:137, 1971.

Victor, M.: The amnesic syndrome and its anatomical basis, *Can. Med. J.,* **100**:1115, 1969.

———, Adams, R. D., and Cole, M.: The acquired
(non-Wilsonian) type of chronic hepatocerebral
degeneration, *Medicine,* **44**:345, 1965.

———, Angevine, J. B., Jr., Mancall, E. L., and
Fisher, C. M.: Memory loss with lesions of hippocampal formation: Report of a case with some remarks on the anatomical basis of memory, *Arch.
Neurol.,* **5**:244, 1961.

Binswanger's Disease

Olszewski, J.: Subcortical arteriosclerotic encephalopathy: Review of the literature on the so-called
Binswanger's disease and presentation of two
cases, *World Neurol.,* **3**:359, 1962.

Van Bogaert, L., and Martin, J.-J.: Analyse critique
de la pathologie de l'angiomatose cerebroméningée
diffuse noncalcifiante et de l'encéphalopathie de
Binswanger, *J. Neurol. Sci.,* **14**:301, 1971.

Parkinsonism

Eadie, M. J., and Sutherland, J. M.: Arteriosclerosis
in Parkinsonism, *J. Neurol. Neurosurg. Psychiat.,*
27:237, 1964.

Cranial Nerve Palsies

Gardner, W. J., and Sava, G. A.: Hemifacial spasm
—A reversible pathophysiologic state, *J. Neurosurg.,* **19**:240, 1962.

Sunderland, S.: Neurovascular relations and anomalies at the base of the brain, *J. Neurol. Neurosurg.
Psychiat.,* **11**:243, 1948.

Taptas, J. N.: Les dilatations et allongements de l'artère carotide interne: États fonctionnels et orga-
niques, *Rev. neurol.,* **80**:338, 1948.

Differential Diagnosis

Adams, R. D., Fisher, C. M., Hakim, S., Ojemann, R.
G., and Sweet, W. H.: Symptomatic occult hydrocephalus with "normal" cerebrospinal-fluid pressure: A treatable syndrome, *New Engl. J. Med.,*
273:117, 1965.

Aita, J. A.: Neurologic Manifestations of General
Diseases, Charles C Thomas, Publisher, Springfield, Ill., 1964.

Hill, M. E., Lougheed, W. M., and Barnett, H. J. M.:
A treatable form of dementia due to normal-pres-
sure, communicating hydrocephalus, *Can. Med.
Assoc. J.,* **97**:1309, 1967.

Müller, C., and Ciompi, L. (eds.): Senile Dementia,
Clinical and Therapeutic Aspects, The Williams &
Wilkins Company, Baltimore, 1968.

Ojemann, R. G., Fisher, C. M., Adams, R. D., Sweet,
W. H., and New, P. F. J.: Further experience with
the syndrome of "normal" pressure hydrocephalus,
J. Neurosurg., **31**:279, 1969.

Laboratory Findings

Arteriography

Kapp, J., Cook, W., and Paulson, G.: Chronic brain syndrome: Arteriographic study in elderly patients, *Geriatrics,* **21**:174, 1966.

Silverstein, A.: Arteriography of stroke: II. Factors relating to the normal angiogram, *Arch. Neurol.,* **13**:441, 1965.

Siqueira, E. B.: Cerebral angiography in the elderly patient, *Geriatrics,* **20**:835, 1965.

Wilson, McC.: Angiography in cerebrovascular occlusive disease, *Am. J. Med. Sci.,* **250**:554, 1965.

Encephalography

Alker, G. J., Glasauer, F. E., and Leslie, E. V.: Long-term experience with isotope cisternography, *J.A.M.A.,* **219**:1005, 1972.

Dyken, M. L., and Nelson, G.: Cerebral circulatory and metabolic studies related to pneumoencephalography, *Acta neurol. scand.,* **44**:148, 1968.

Silverman, D.: Serial electroencephalography in brain tumors and cerebrovascular accidents, *Arch. Neurol.,* **2**:122, 1960.

Management

Chynoweth, R., and Foley, J.: Pre-senile dementia responding to steroid therapy, *Brit. J. Psychiat.,* **115**:703, 1969.

Heyden, S., and Gerber, C. J.: Atherosclerotic cerebrovascular disease—Its nature and management, *Am. J. Med.,* **46**:763, 1969.

Brain Infarction

Disease is from of old and nothing about it has changed. It is we who change as we learn to recognize what was formerly imperceptible.

J. M. Charcot

Cerebral infarction—the death of neurons, glia, and capillaries in a portion of the brain—is caused by a lack of oxygen, blood, or glucose. Each type of infarction (anoxic, ischemic, or hypoglycemic) has its own mode of onset, zones of predilection, histopathologic features, course, and resolution. The most common of the three is *ischemic* infarction, which is caused by a sudden interruption of the blood supply. *Anoxic* infarction results from a lack of oxygen in the blood (as in carbon monoxide poisoning), and *hypoglycemic* infarction occurs when the blood glucose falls below critical levels for a pro-

longed period; in both conditions the circulation of blood through the brain remains normal.

In this chapter consideration will be given only to brain infarction due to inadequate blood supply (ischemic infarction).

ETIOLOGY

The four major causes of ischemic infarction are aortocranial atherothrombosis; acute hypotension; emboli arising from a diseased heart, aortic arch, or artery in the neck; and vasospasm, which may be caused by hypertensive encephalopathy or occur secondary to ruptured intracranial berry aneurysm. Other causes are arteritis, compression of the brain with secondary ischemia, venous occlusion, and abnormalities in the blood itself. Most of these etiologic factors are considered in the appropriate chapters.

Cerebral infarcts caused by craniocervical atherosclerosis and those resulting from vasospasm secondary to ruptured intracranial aneurysms are pale in appearance. Hemorrhagic, or red, infarcts are usually seen (1) with venous occlusions or cerebral arterial emboli, (2) when intermittent compression of the posterior cerebral artery causes an infarct in the occipital lobe, (3) following repair of the carotid artery in a patient who has had a recent infarction, and (4) in patients who have been treated with anticoagulants.

PATHOLOGIC FINDINGS

Gross

The type and site of an infarct depend upon the underlying cause. In most cases, infarction is the result of arterial obstruction and follows the outline of the arterial bed distal to the point of occlusion. Infarction due to venous thrombosis affects the area normally drained by the occluded vein.

Infarction occurs earliest in the tissues that have the highest metabolic requirement for oxygen: the cell bodies of areas 3 to 5 of the cerebral cortex, the cells of the globus pallidus, Ammon's horns, and Purkinje cells of the cerebellum. Infarction confined to the cortical layers causes a characteristic picture known as cortical laminar necrosis.

The size of an infarct depends to some extent upon the size of the artery obstructed. Infarcts caused by obstruction of a penetrating artery (lacunes) may barely be visible; those resulting from interruption of the carotid arterial supply may destroy almost an entire hemisphere. The area of infarction is always sharply delineated

from the surrounding normal brain and can be identified by the grayish-white appearance and the soft, mushy consistency of the tissue (Fig. 14-1).

In the early stages of the infarct there may be a considerable amount of edema which may be extensive enough to act as a tumor. When the whole hemisphere is edematous, the gyri are flattened and the sulci obliterated, the brain may be displaced beneath the falx cerebri, and herniation of the hippocampal gyrus through the tentorium may compress the posterior cerebral artery against the sharp edge of the tentorium cerebelli, causing ischemic infarction in the occipital lobe. If blood flow is reestablished, the infarction becomes hemorrhagic. Furthermore, there may be displacement of the midbrain by the tissue herniating through the incisura. This may be of such degree that it compresses the midbrain against the sharp edge of the tentorium on the opposite side and results in secondary pyramidal tract signs. In extensive cases an indentation of the peduncle by the incisura can be seen at autopsy (Kernohan's notch).

In cases of massive infarction of the cerebellum, the structures in the posterior fossa are compressed and the cerebellum herniates up through the incisura and/or down through the foramen magnum. In such cases hydrocephalus occurs secondary to obstruction of the aqueduct.

Microscopic

An infarct 2 to 5 days old consists of necrotic nerve fibers with pyknotic glial nuclei and an accumulation of interstitial fluid. In sections stained with hematoxylin and eosin, the neurons appear shrunken and stained uniformly pink, glial nuclei are hyperchromatic, blood vessels are necrotic, and polymorphonuclear cells are seen invading the periphery of the lesion. At this stage there may be exfoliation of polymorphonuclear leukocytes, and rarely of brain tissue itself, into the cerebral spinal fluid.

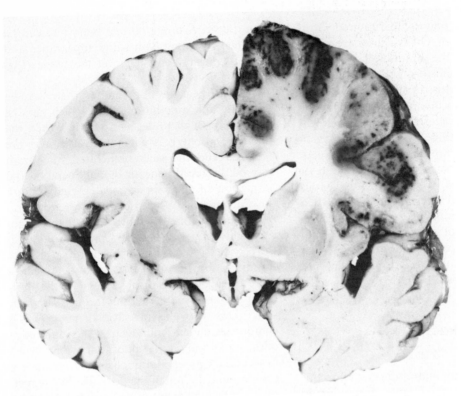

Figure 14-1 Hemorrhagic infarction (3 to 7 days old) in distribution of left anterior and middle cerebral arteries caused by thrombosis of the intracranial internal carotid artery (not shown). The gyri are edematous and there are confluent petechial hemorrhages. *(Courtesy of John Moossy, M.D., Department of Pathology, Bowman Gray School of Medicine.)*

After 5 to 6 days the neurons and fibers disintegrate; the polymorphonuclear reaction is replaced by a morphonuclear reaction which engulfs the cellular and fatty debris and thereby acquires the foamy cytoplasm of the granular macrophage. At about this same time, absorption of the interstitial fluid begins and new capillaries are formed.

After about 2 to 3 months the necrotic material is resorbed and a cavity is left. At the periphery there is proliferation of capillaries and swollen astrocytes, and the cavity itself is traversed by glial and fibrovascular elements. The overlying leptomeninges are thickened and in the later stages the cortex may be depressed and the adjoining ventricle dilated.

HEMORRHAGIC INFARCTION

In hemorrhagic infarction, diapedesis of red blood cells produces blotchy hemorrhages on the surface of the brain. Microscopically, hemorrhages are seen predominantly (1) in the gray matter, (2) distributed around the necrotic blood vessel, and (3) in association with phagocytes containing hemosiderin. In the late stages, the leptomeninges acquire a rusty brown color and the hemorrhage is seen as a cavity enclosed by a golden brown wall.

Unlike cerebral hemorrhage, which dissects between nerve fibers and along tracts, hemorrhagic infarct destroys all the tissue in the distribution of the involved artery or vein, including the nerve fibers. When the healing is complete, the walls of a hemorrhagic cavity are in close apposition; in contrast, those of a hemorrhagic infarct tend to be widely separated, and the cavity is spanned by strands of fibroglial tissue.

PATHOPHYSIOLOGY

The zones of predilection for infarction due to reduction in perfusion pressure (pump failure) can be explained by hydrodynamic principles. In a row of fields irrigated from a common source, the last field suffers most when the pumping pressure is inadequate. Similarly,

when cerebrovascular perfusion is inadequate, the maximal ischemia occurs in the neural tissues that are farthest from the source of supply (for example, when the middle cerebral artery is occluded, the infarct occurs in the area of its terminal distribution (Fig. 14-2).

Examples of infarction occurring between adjacent arterial trees are infarcts at the temporoparietooccipital junction in the most distal areas of perfusion of the anterior, middle, and posterior cerebral arteries and infarcts involving the putamen and the head of the caudate nucleus, which lie in the distal area between the striate branches of the anterior cerebral artery and

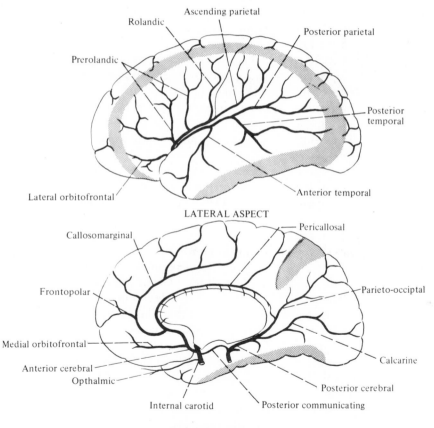

LATERAL ASPECT

MEDIAN SAGITTAL ASPECT

Figure 14-2 Zones of predilection for infarction in watershed areas. *(Courtesy of John Moossy, M.D., Department of Pathology, Bowman Gray School of Medicine.)*

Heubner's artery on the one side and the penetrating branches of the middle cerebral artery on the other.

The shape and size of the zone of infarction are dependent to some extent on the efficiency of collateral channels. When none are adequate, obliteration of a main artery will result in infarction of the entire area supplied by that artery. If collaterals develop, the infarct may shrink to a wedge shape in the center of the main field of distribution. On the other hand, if a main cerebral artery is occluded in association with stenosis of an adjacent main artery, the infarct will be massive because of the overlapping fields of ischemia.

In the initial stages of acute cerebral infarct, a considerable amount of the neurologic deficit may be due to edema, and as this edema resolves, the patient will recover function. An adequate circle of Willis and well-developed cerebral arteries, all free of atherosclerosis and with meningeal, choroidal, and capillary anastomoses, provide the conduits for supplying additional blood to the ischemic tissue. Blood supply to the ischemic zone is also provided by retrograde flow through microcirculatory anastomoses in vessels with a caliber of about 0.5 mm or less. This collateral circulation is responsible for the tumorlike blush seen on angiography in certain cases of cerebral infarction. The physiological factors (perfusion pressure, blood gases, tissue pH, and autoregulation) which are essential to the functional adequacy of the collateral channels have been described in Chap. 5.

In animal experiments, cerebral tissue is rendered nonviable after 4 to 8 min of ischemia. Recently, however, it has been demonstrated that maintenance of an adequate perfusion pressure during the recovery period can keep ischemic tissue viable for as long as 60 min, presumably by keeping the capillaries patent and also by washing away the local products of cellular metabolism, such as lactic acid.

It has been shown recently that the swelling of the endothelial and glial cells during or immediately after the ischemic insult causes a marked reduction in the lumen of the cerebral capillaries.

CLINICAL FEATURES

The clinical features of cerebral infarction are quite variable. Tiny infarcts in nonstrategic locations may not be detectable, whereas cerebral infarction with subsequent cerebral edema and swelling will mimic a cerebral neoplasm and may even cause death.

Atherothrombotic cerebral infarction usually occurs during repose or sleep, often in the early hours of the morning. It is not clear why this happens, but some think it may be the result of physiologic hypotension, hypoxemia, or mechanical factors and secondary constriction of arteries due to the position of the head on the neck. In some patients the underlying hypotensive episode is triggered by loss of blood, myocardial infarction, operation, or anesthesia. Often, there are no detectable precipitating factors.

Cerebral infarcts caused by embolus may occur at any time, whether the patient is awake or asleep. They may originate in pulmonary veins, cardiac valves or chambers, or ulcerated plaques in the aortic arch or the great vessels arising from it.

Neurologic examination following a cerebral infarct will reveal signs of focal neurologic deficit indicative of a lesion in an area of the brain supplied by either the internal carotid or the vertebral-basilar arteries. (Details are given in Chaps. 2, 10, and 11.)

Cerebellar infarct should be considered when a patient suspected of having an infarct in the distribution of the vertebral-basilar system has progressive intracranial hypertension and deteriorates suddenly. The condition is rare and requires prompt diagnosis and immediate operation. This clinical state is due to tonsillar herniation and acute obstructive hydrocephalus resulting from compression of the exit foramina of the fourth ventricle by the swollen cerebellum or by kinking of the aqueduct of Sylvius.

COURSE AND PROGNOSIS

In most instances, the neurologic deficit resulting from a cerebral infarct reaches its maximum within the first 72 hr. Old age, hypertension, coma, cardiorespiratory complications, anoxia, hypercapnia, and neurogenic hyperventilation are additional adverse prognostic factors, especially in the first 48 hr of a cerebral infarct. In rare instances the development of massive cerebral edema leads to progressive deterioration and sometimes death.

Some improvement may be apparent after the first 2 weeks, and by the end of 12 weeks the maximum recovery will be reached in most cases. With noticeably few exceptions, no further recovery should be expected after 6 to 9 months.

DIFFERENTIAL DIAGNOSIS

Severe headache and signs of meningeal irritation suggest a cause other than infarction—usually intracerebral hemorrhage. With subdural hematoma, the disturbance of consciousness is more striking than the hemiparesis, and the entire neurologic picture shows more daily or hourly fluctuation.

Differentiation of infarction from *brain tumor, intracerebral hemorrhage, chronic subdural hematoma,* or *abscess* is difficult, especially in cases in which an adequate history is lacking; in these instances, a negative brain scan at 2 to 4 hr during the first few days after onset helps to exclude cerebral infarct. In the absence of a reliable history, infarction can be differentiated from acute *postepileptic* or *postmigrainous hemiplegia* only by repeated neurologic examinations made over the ensuing 72 hr. *Herpes simplex*

encephalitis and *meningitis* can be excluded by examination of the spinal fluid.

Once diagnosis of infarction has been established, it is necessary to determine the underlying cause (cardiac dysrhythmia, hypotension, embolism, obstruction of neck arteries, arteritis, etc.) in order to institute appropriate specific therapy.

LABORATORY FINDINGS
Skull Films

X-rays of the skull are normal unless there is a massive cerebral hemispheric infarct, in which case the pineal shadow may be shifted to the opposite side.

Echoencephalogram

In cases of massive cerebral edema, the midline will be shifted to the opposite side. Dilatation of both lateral ventricles and of the third ventricle without any lateral displacement suggests an expanding lesion in the posterior fossa.

Electroencephalogram

A hemispheric infarction in the distribution of a major cerebral artery may cause voltage depression and a slow-wave focus. Unlike that seen in cases of cerebral neoplasm, this change is nonprogressive and will gradually resolve.

Lumbar Puncture

The cerebrospinal fluid is normal when infarcts are small or deeply placed; however, when an infarct approaches either the ventricular or the subarachnoid surface, there is often a polymorphonuclear response in the early stages that is sufficient to simulate that seen in cases of cerebral abscess. In such cases, lymphocytes appear before the fluid clears up completely. If the infarct is hemorrhagic, the fluid will be blood-stained.

The spinal fluid protein level is normal or mildly elevated in most cases, and although it may rise above 100 mg per 100 ml in the case of massive infarcts which extend into the ventricular or pial surfaces, such high levels should suggest a concomitant extraneural disorder such as diabetes mellitus or hypothroidism.

In cases of meningovascular syphilis there will be pleocytosis, an increase in protein content (especially the globulin fractions), and a positive test for syphilis.

Except in cases of intracranial hypertension associated with massive cerebral edema or of internal hydrocephalus caused by a cerebellar infarct, the cerebrospinal fluid pressure following brain infarction is within the normal range.

Brain Scan

Serial brain scans are valuable in differentiating an infarct from a cerebral neoplasm. About 75 percent of large cerebral infarcts appear on the brain scan at some time during their course; about 30 percent can be seen during the first week after the ictus. This is a poor prognostic sign for recovery of function. Arteriography may reveal slow emptying of local arteries or an avascular area where cerebral vessels are obstructed. If a primary vessel is occluded, emptying of collateral arterial channels is delayed; if a peripheral artery is blocked, slow filling to the point of the obstruction occurs in the proximal artery and filling remains into the venous phase (Fig. 14-3A and B).

Initial vasodilatation, manifested by an increase in the speed of circulation through the area of infarct, occurs within a few seconds after ischemia begins. This response to high CO_2 tension or to the lowering of pH lasts only a short time. *Persistent* vasodilatation appears in the infarct and/or the surrounding area in the first 10

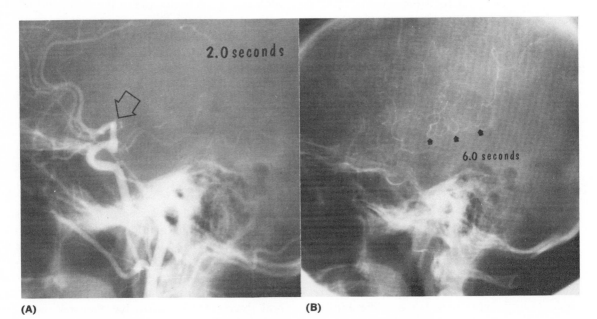

(A) **(B)**

Figure 14-3 Middle cerebral artery occlusion. (A) Arteriogram with nonfilling of the middle cerebral artery (arrow). (B) Later phase showing reversed filling through collateral channels (small arrows). *(Courtesy of Dr. F. Farrell, Department of Radiology, Bowman Gray School of Medicine.)*

days to 2 weeks after infarction, and the vessels remain dilated even after lysis of the clot. Early filling veins, which may be the only sign of vasodilatation, indicate an increase in the local circulatory rate (luxury-perfusion). A rapid passage of contrast material may be due to bypass of a blocked capillary bed with arteriovenous shunting. Slowing of the circulation time is common during the first week or two after the ictus and often affects the entire hemisphere.

Angiograms are normal in most cases in which recanalization has occurred following an infarct, indicating that spontaneous lysis of the clot has occurred. If occlusion was of a major vessel or of one of its branches, collateral circulation can be seen in the infarcted area.

Air Studies

Air studies are usually normal in the early stages of cerebral infarction except in cases in which the edematous area acts as an expanding lesion and displaces the lateral ventricles to the opposite side. In the late stages of a cerebral infarct, air study may show focal cortical atrophy, dilatation of the ipsilateral lateral ventricle, or a porencephalic cyst.

In cases of *cerebellar* infarct with massive cerebellar swelling, internal hydrocephalus will be seen, and the fourth ventricle either will not fill or will be displaced laterally.

MANAGEMENT

Medical

In general, a patient suffering from an acute cerebral infarct should be treated along the lines described in Chaps. 16 and 30. Specific treatment is indicated in cases associated with syphilis, tuberculosis, and the collagen group of diseases. Cardiac disorders giving rise to emboli should be treated by digitalization, cardioversion, or surgery.

Surgical

Operation is indicated only in the cases of acute cerebellar infarction leading to swelling and internal hydrocephalus. In such cases emergency posterior fossa bur holes with limited craniectomy should be followed by excision of the necrotic cerebellar tissue and the herniated cerebellar tonsils. This procedure is often lifesaving if carried out early enough.

Generally speaking, the repair of obstructed arteries in the neck in cases of established cerebral infarction is not wise. In some instances early revascularization of the devitalized cerebral tissue has converted it into a fatal hemorrhagic infarct.

In a very few instances, surgeons have successfully treated intracranial vascular obstructions by using microsurgical techniques to perform a thromboembolectomy or to insert a bypass graft. The successful management of cerebral infarcts by either intracranial or extracranial vascular surgical techniques is extremely rare, however, and no adequately studied control data are available as yet.

SUGGESTED READINGS

General

Acheson, J.: Factors affecting the natural history of "focal cerebral vascular disease," *Quart. J. Med.,* **40**:25, 1971.

———, and Hutchinson, E. C.: The natural history of "focal cerebral vascular disease," *Quart. J. Med.,* **40**:15, 1971.

Carter, A. B.: Cerebral Infarction, The Macmillan Company, New York, 1964.

Waltz, A. G.: Studies of the cerebral circulation: What have they taught us about stroke? *Mayo Clinic Proc.,* **46**:268, 1971.

Etiology

Adams, J. H.: Patterns of cerebral infarction: Some comments on their topography and pathogenesis, *Scottish Med. J.,* **12**:339, 1967.

Ames, A., III, Wright, R. L., Kowada, M., Thurston, J. M., and Majno, G.: Cerebral ischemia. II. The no-reflow phenomenon, *Am. J. Pathol.,* **52**:437, 1968.

Bergeron, R. T., and Wood, E. H.: Oral contraceptives and cerebrovascular complications, *Radiology,* **92**:231, 1969.

Dagenais, G. R., Barbeau, A., and Delorme, P.: Cryofibrinogenemia and cerebrovascular accident, *Can. Med. Assoc. J.,* **98**:475, 1968.

Danta, G.: Platelet adhesiveness in cerebrovascular disease, *Atherosclerosis,* **11**:223, 1970.

Friedman, G. D., Loveland, D. B., and Ehrlich, S. P., Jr.: Relationship of stroke to other cardiovascular disease, *Circulation,* **38**:533, 1968.

Hoogerverf, P. E.: Migraine and oral contraceptives, *Can. Med. Assoc. J.,* **97**:978, 1967.

Hossmann, K. A., and Sato, K.: Recovery of neuronal function after prolonged cerebral ischemia, *Science,* **168**:375, 1970.

Jennett, W. B., and Cross, J. N.: Influence of pregnancy and oral contraception on the incidence of strokes in women of childbearing age, *Lancet,* **1**:1019, 1967.

Jones, H. R., Jr., Siekert, R. G., and Geraci, J. E.: Neurologic manifestations of bacterial endocarditis, *Ann. Internal Med.,* **71**:21, 1969.

Jörgensen, L., and Torvik, A.: Ischaemic cerebrovascular diseases in an autopsy series. Part 2. Prevalence, location, pathogenesis, and clinical course of cerebral infarcts, *J. Neurol. Sci.,* **9**:285, 1969.

Kolodny, E. H., Rebeiz, J. J., Caviness, V. S., Jr., and Richardson, E. P., Jr.: Granulomatous angiitis of the central nervous system, *Arch. Neurol.,* **19**:510, 1968.

Landolt, A. M., and Millikan, C. H.: Pathogenesis of cerebral infarction secondary to mechanical carotid artery occlusion, *Stroke,* **1**:52, 1970.

Levine, J., and Swanson, P. D.: Nonatherosclerotic causes of stroke, *Ann. Internal Med.,* **70**:807, 1969.

Masi, A. T., and Dugdale, M: Cerebrovascular diseases associated with the use of oral contraceptives: A review in the English language literature, *Ann. Internal Med.,* **72**:111, 1970.

McDowell, F. H., Louis, S., and Monahan, K.: Seasonal variation of non-embolic cerebral infarction, *J. Chronic Diseases,* **23**:29, 1970.

Schneider, R. C., Kriss, F. C., and Falls, H. F.: Prechiasmal infarction associated with intrachiasmal and suprasellar tumors, *J. Neurosurg.,* **32**:197, 1970.

Schoenberg, B. S., Whisnant, J. P., Taylor, W. F., and Kempers, R. D.: Strokes in women of childbearing age; a population study, *Neurology,* **20**:181, 1970.

Pathologic Findings

Adams, J. H., Brierley, J. B., Connor, R. C. R., and Treip, C. S.: The effects of systemic hypotension upon the human brain. Clinical and neuropathological observations in 11 cases, *Brain,* **89**:235, 1966.

———, and Graham, D. I.: Twelve cases of fatal cerebral infarction due to arterial occlusion in the absence of atheromatous stenosis or embolism, *J. Neurol. Neurosurg. Psychiat.,* **30**:479, 1967.

Battacharji, S. K., Hutchinson, E. C., and McCall, A. J.: The circle of Willis—The incidence of developmental abnormalities in normal and infarcted brains, *Brain,* **90**:747, 1967.

———, ———, and ———: Stenosis and occlusion of vessels in cerebral infarction, *Brit. Med. J.,* **3**:270, 1967.

Blackwood, W., Hallpike, J. F., Kocen, R. S., and Mair, W. G. P.: Atheromatous disease of the carotid arterial system and embolism from the heart in cerebral infarction: A morbid anatomical study, *Brain,* **92**:897, 1969.

Brierley, J. B.: Brain damage complicating open-heart surgery: A neuropathological study of 46 patients, *Proc. Roy. Soc. Med.,* **60**:858, 1967.

Fisher, C. M.: Lacunes: Small, deep cerebral infarcts, *Neurology,* **15**:774, 1965.

Moossy, J.: Cerebral infarction and intracranial arterial thrombosis. Necropsy studies and clinical implications, *Arch. Neurol.,* **14**:119, 1966.

———: Cerebral infarcts and the lesions of intracranial and extracranial atherosclerosis, *Arch. Neurol.,* **14**:124, 1966.

Pickering, G.: Pathogenesis of myocardial and cerebral infarction: Nodular arteriosclerosis, *Brit. Med. J.,* **1**:517, 1964.

Romanul, F. C. A., and Abramowicz, A.: Changes in brain and pial vessels in arterial border zones. A study of 13 cases, *Arch. Neurol.,* **11**:40, 1964.

Vost, A., Wolochow, D. A., and Howell, D. A.: Incidence of infarcts of the brain in heart disease, *J. Pathol. Bacteriol.,* **88**:463, 1964.

Yates, P. O., and Hutchinson, E. C.: Cerebral infarction: The role of stenosis of the extracranial cerebral arteries, *Med. Res. Council Spec. Rept. (London),* **300**:1, 1961.

Zülch, K. J., and Kleihues, P.: "Neuropathology of cerebral infarction," in Thule International Symposium on Stroke, edited by A. Engel and T. Larsson, Nordiska Bokhandelns Forlag, Stockholm, 1967, pp. 57–75.

Pathophysiology

Cronqvist, S., and Laroche, F.: Transitory hyperaemia in focal cerebral vascular lesions studied by angiography and regional cerebral blood flow measurements, *Brit. J. Radiol.,* **40**:270, 1967.

Fieschi, C., Agnoli, A., Battistini, N., Bozzao, L., and Prencipe, M.: Derangement of regional cerebral blood flow and of its regulatory mechanisms in acute cerebrovascular lesions, *Neurology,* **18**:1166, 1968.

Høedt-Rasmussen, K., Skinhøj, E., Paulson, O., Ewald, T., Bjerrum, T. K., Fahrenkrug, A., and Lassen, N. A.: Regional cerebral blood flow in acute apoplexy: The "luxury perfusion syndrome" of brain tissue, *Arch. Neurol.,* **17**:271, 1967.

Ingvar, D. H.: The pathophysiology of occlusive cerebrovascular disorders related to neuroradiological findings, EEG and measurements of regional cerebral blood flow, *Acta neurol. scand.,* **43**(suppl. 31):93, 1967.

Jennett, W. B., Harper, A. M., and Gillespie, F. C.: Measurement of regional cerebral blood-flow during carotid ligation, *Lancet,* **2**:1162, 1966.

Johnson, H. D.: Critical closing pressure in blood vessels, *Nature,* **215**:858, 1967.

Lassen, N. A.: The luxury-perfusion syndrome and its possible relation to acute metabolic acidosis localised within the brain, *Lancet,* **2**:1113, 1966.

McHenry, L. C., Jr.: Cerebral blood flow studies in middle cerebral and internal carotid artery occlusion, *Neurology,* **16**:1145, 1966.

Meyer, J. S., Gotoh, F., and Tomita, M.: Cerebral metabolism during arousal and mental activity in stroke patients, *J. Am. Geriat. Soc.,* **14**:986, 1966.

Obrist, W. D., Chivian, E., Cronqvist, S., and Ingvar, D. H.: Regional cerebral blood flow in senile and presenile dementia, *Neurology,* **20**:315, 1970.

Paulson, O. B.: Regional cerebral blood flow in apoplexy due to occlusion of the middle cerebral artery, *Neurology,* **20**:63, 1970.

———, Lassen, N. A., and Skinhøj, E.: Regional cerebral blood flow in apoplexy without arterial occlusion, *Neurology,* **20**:125, 1970.

Rees, J. E., Du Boulay, G. H., Bull, J. W. D., Marshall, J., Russell, R. W. R., and Symon, L.: Regional cerebral blood-flow in transient ischaemic attacks, *Lancet,* **2**:1210, 1970.

Simard, D., Olesen, J., Paulson, O. B., Lassen, N. A., and Skinhøj, E.: Regional cerebral blood flow and its regulation in dementia, *Brain,* **94**:273, 1971.

Skinhøj, E., Høedt-Rasmussen, K., Paulson, O. B., and Lassen, N. A.: Regional cerebral blood flow and its autoregulation in patients with transient focal cerebral ischemic attacks, *Neurology,* **20**:485, 1970.

Toole, J. F.: Nocturnal strokes and arterial hypotension, *Ann. Internal Med.,* **68**:1132, 1968.

Clinical Features

Faris, A. A.: Limbic system infarction. A report of two cases, *Neurology,* **19**:91, 1969.

Lehrich, J. R., Winkler, G. F., and Ojemann, R. G.: Cerebellar infarction with brain stem compression. Diagnosis and surgical treatment, *Arch. Neurol.,* **22**:490, 1970.

Lhermitte, F., Gautier, J.-C., Derouesné, C., and Guiraud, B.: Ischemic accidents in the middle cerebral artery territory. A study of the causes of 122 cases, *Arch. Neurol.,* **19**:248, 1968.

———, Gautier, J.-C., and Derouesné, C.: Nature of occlusions in the middle cerebral artery, *Neurology,* **20**:82, 1970.

Louis, S., and McDowell, F.: Epileptic seizures in nonembolic cerebral infarction. *Arch. Neurol.,* **17**:414, 1967.

Mohr, J. P., Leicester, J., Stoddard, L., and Sidman, M.: Right hemianopia with memory, color and tactile letter deficits in circumscribed left posterior cerebral artery territory infarction, *Neurology,* **20**:378, 1970.

Norris, J. W., Eisen, A. A., and Branch, C. L.: Problems in cerebellar hemorrhage and infarction, *Neurology*, **19**:1043, 1969.

Omae, T., Katsuki, S., Nishimaru, K., Yamaguchi, T., Takeya, Y., Fujishima, M., and Kato, M.: Clinical features of cerebral infarction in the Japanese, *J. Chronic Diseases*, **21**:585, 1969.

Patel, A. N.: Syndromes of callosal infarction, *Neurology (India)*, **17**:191, 1969.

Plum, F.: Hyperpnea, hyperventilation, and brain dysfunction, *Ann. Internal Med.*, **76**:328, 1972.

Prineas, J., and Marshall, J.: Hypertension and cerebral infarction, *Brit. Med. J.*, **1**:14, 1966.

Tichy, F.: Syndromes of the cerebral arteries, *Arch. Pathol.*, **48**:475, 1949.

Van Trotsenburg, L., and Vinken, P. J.: Fatal cerebral infarction simulating an acute expanding lesion, *J. Neurol. Neurosurg. Psychiat.*, **29**:241, 1966.

Waddington, M. M., and Ring, B. A.: Syndromes of occlusion of middle cerebral artery branches. Angiographic and clinical correlation, *Brain*, **91**:685, 1968.

Wood, M. W., and Murphey, F.: Obstructive hydrocephalus due to infarction of a cerebellar hemisphere, *J. Neurosurg.;* **30**:260, 1969.

Course and Prognosis

Baker, R. N., Schwartz, W. S., and Ramseyer, J. C.: Prognosis among survivors of ischemic stroke, *Neurology*, **18**:933, 1968.

Cantu, R. C., and Ames, A., III: Distribution of vascular lesions caused by cerebral ischemia. Relation to survival, *Neurology*, **19**:128, 1969.

David, N. J., and Heyman, A.: Factors influencing the prognosis of cerebral thrombosis and infarction due to atherosclerosis, *J. Chronic Diseases*, **11**:394, 1960.

Ford, A. B., and Katz, S.: Prognosis after strokes. Part I: A critical review, *Medicine*, **45**:223, 1966.

Robinson, R. W., Demirel, M., and Lebeau, R. J.: Natural history of cerebral thrombosis: Nine to nineteen year follow-up, *J. Chronic Diseases*, **21**:221, 1968.

Differential Diagnosis

Aring, C. D.: Differential diagnosis of cerebrovascular stroke, *Arch. Internal Med.*, **113**:195, 1964.

————, and Merritt, H. H.: Differential diagnosis between cerebral hemorrhage and cerebral thrombosis: A clinical and pathologic study of 245 cases, *Arch. Internal Med.*, **56**:435, 1935.

Meyer, J. S., and Portnoy, H. D.: Localized cerebral hypoglycemia simulating stroke. A clinical and experimental study, *Neurology*, **8**:601, 1958.

Raskind, R.: Frontal lobe abscess simulating "stroke" in two women, one pregnant, *Angiology*, **17**:264, 1966.

Van Trotsenburg, L., and Vinken, P. J.: Fatal cerebral infarction simulating an acute expanding lesion, *J. Neurol. Neurosurg. Psychiat.*, **29**:241, 1966.

Weintraub, M. I., and Glaser, G. H.: Nocardial brain abscess and pure motor hemiplegia, *N. Y. State J. Med.*, **70**(2):2717, 1970.

Wise, G. R., and Farmer, T. W.: Bacterial cerebral vasculitis, *Neurology*, **21**:195, 1971.

Laboratory Findings

Einsen, A. A., and Sherwin, A. L.: Serum creatine phosphokinase activity in cerebral infarction, *Neurology*, **18**:263, 1968.

Lavy, S., Stern, S., Herishianu, Y., and Carmon, A.: Electrocardiographic changes in ischaemic stroke, *J. Neurol. Sci.*, **7**:409, 1968.

Tomkin, G., Coe, R. P. K., and Marshall, J.: Electrocardiographic abnormalities in patients presenting with strokes, *J. Neurol. Neurosurg. Psychiat.*, **31**:250, 1968.

Echoencephalogram, Ultrasonic Scanning and Flow Measurement

Achar, V. S., Coe, R. P. K., and Marshall, J.: Echoencephalography in the differential diagnosis of cerebral haemorrhage and infarction, *Lancet*, **1**:161, 1966.

Campbell, J. K., Clark, J., Jenkins, C., and White, D.: Ultrasonic studies of brain movements, *Neurology*, **20**:418, 1970.

Maroon, J. C., Campbell, R. L., and Dyken, M. L.: Internal carotid artery occlusion diagnosed by Doppler ultrasound, *Stroke*, **1**:122, 1970.

————, Pieroni, D. W., and Campbell, R. L.: Ophthalmosonometry. An ultrasonic method for assessing carotid blood flow, *J. Neurosurg.*, **30**:238, 1969.

Nichols, R. A., Whisnant, J. P., and Baker, H. L., Jr.: A-mode echoencephalography: Its value and limitations and report of 200 verified cases, *Mayo Clinic Proc.*, **43**:36, 1968.

Olinger, C. P.: Ultrasonic carotid echoarteriography, *Am. J. Roentgenol.*, **106**:282, 1969.

Electroencephalogram

Loeb, C.: Electro-encephalographic and pathological findings during the early stages of cerebral ischemia, *Europ. Neurol.*, **2**:31, 1969.

Silverman, D.: Serial electroencephalography in brain tumors and cerebrovascular accidents, *Arch. Neurol.*, **2**:122, 1960.

Brain Scan

Fish, M. B., Pollycove, M., O'Reilly, S., Khentigan, A., and Kock, R. L.: Vascular characterization of brain lesions by rapid sequential cranial scintiphotography, *J. Nucl. Med.*, **9**:249, 1968.

Glasgow, J. L., Currier, R. D., Goodrich, J. K., and Tutor, F. T.: Brain scans at varied intervals following C.V.A., *J. Nucl. Med.*, **6**:902, 1965.

Gutterman, P., and Shenkin, H. A.: Cerebral scans in completed strokes. Value in prognosis of clinical course, *J.A.M.A.*, **207**:145, 1969.

Marshall, J., and Popham, M. G.: Radioactive brain scanning in the management of cerebrovascular disease, *J. Neurol. Neurosurg. Psychiat.*, **33**:201, 1970.

Maynard, C. D., Witcofski, R. L., Janeway, R., and Cowan, R. J.: "Radioisotope arteriography" as an adjunct to the brain scan, *Radiology*, **92**:908, 1969.

―――, and Janeway, R.: "Radioisotope studies in neurodiagnosis," in Special Techniques for Neurologic Diagnosis (Contemporary Neurology Series, 3), edited by J. F. Toole, F. A. Davis Company, Philadelphia, 1969, pp. 71-91.

Molinari, G. F., Pircher, F., and Heyman, A.: Serial brain scanning using technetium$_{99m}$ in patients with cerebral infarction, *Neurology*, **17**:627, 1967.

Usher, M. S., and Quinn, J. L., III: Serial brain scanning with technetium$_{99m}$ pertechnetate in cerebral infarction, *Am. J. Roentgenol.*, **105**:728, 1969.

Wang, Y., Shea, F. J., and Rosen, J. A.: Comparison of the accuracy of brain scanning and other procedures used for brain tumor detection, *Neurology*, **15**:1117, 1965.

Waxman, H. J., Ziegler, D. K., and Rubin, S.: Brain scans in diagnosis of cerebrovascular disease, *J.A.M.A.*, **192**:453, 1965.

Thermography

Mawdsley, C., Samuel, E., Sumerling, M. D., and Young, G. B.: Thermography in occlusive cerebrovascular disease, *Brit. Med. J.*, **3**:521, 1968.

Cerebral Angiography

Cronqvist, S., and Laroche, F.: Transitory hyperaemia in focal cerebral vascular lesions studied by angiography and regional cerebral blood flow measurements, *Brit. J. Radiol.*, **40**:270, 1967.

Gabrielsen, T. O., and Greitz, T.: Normal size of the internal carotid, middle cerebral and anterior cerebral arteries, *Acta radiol. (diagn.)*, **10**:1, 1970.

Geraud, J., Rascol, A., Bes, A., Manelfe, C., Guiraud, B., David, J., Caussanel, J.-P., Geraud, G., and Croquennec, Y.: La méthode de Ring dans le diagnostic des occlusions des branches de l'artère cérébrale moyenne, Étude neuro-radiologique. Corrélations radio-clinique, *Rev. neurol.*, **123**:387, 1970.

Glickman, M. G., Mainzer, F., and Gletne, J. S.: Early venous opacification in cerebral contusion, *Radiology*, **100**:615, 1971.

Hass, W. K., Fields, W. S., North, R. R., Kricheff, I. I., Chase, N. E., and Bauer, R. B.: Joint study of extracranial arterial occlusion: II. Arteriography, techniques, sites, and complications, *J.A.M.A.*, **203**:961, 1968.

Hinck, V. C., and Dotter, C. T.: Appraisal of current techniques for cerebral angiography, *Am. J. Roentgenol.*, **107**:626, 1969.

―――, and Tanabe, C. T.: Comprehensive selective angiography in cerebrovascular insufficiency, *Surg. Gynecol. Obstet.*, **129**:519, 1969.

Jørgensen, J., Sigurdsson, J., and Ovesen, N.: Complications of vertebral arteriography by the Seldinger technique. A survey of 619 cases, *Danish Med. Bull.*, **17**:132, 1970.

Ring, B. A.: The Neglected Cause of Stroke; Occlusion of the Smaller Intracranial Arteries and Their Diagnosis by Cerebral Angiography, Warren H. Green, Inc., St. Louis, 1969.

Silverstein, A.: Arteriography of stroke. II. Factors relating to the normal angiogram, *Arch. Neurol.*, **13**:441, 1965.

Sindermann, F., Dichgans, J., and Bergleiter, R.: Occlusion of the middle cerebral artery and its branches: Angiographic and clinical correlates, *Brain,* **92**:607, 1969.

Taveras, J. M., Gilson, J. M., Davis, D. O., Kilgore, B., and Rumbaugh, C. L.: Angiography in cerebral infarction, *Radiology,* **93**:549, 1969.

———, and Wood, E. H.: Diagnostic Neuroradiology, The Williams & Wilkins Company, Baltimore, 1964.

Weibel, J., and Fields, W. S.: Atlas of Arteriography in Occlusive Cerebrovascular Disease, W. B. Saunders Company, Philadelphia, 1969.

Whitley, J. E., and Whitley, N. O'N.: Angiography: Techniques and Procedures, Warren H. Green, Inc., St. Louis, 1971.

Wilson, McC.: Angiography in cerebrovascular occlusive disease, *Am. J. Med. Sci.,* **250**:554, 1965.

Wise, G. R.: Vasopressor-drug therapy for complications of cerebral arteriography, *New Engl. J. Med.,* **282**:610, 1970.

Air Studies

Engeset, A., and Lønnum, A.: Pneumoencephalographic findings after occlusion of the carotid or middle cerebral arteries, *Europ. Neurol.,* **1**:85, 1968.

Management

Medical

Browne, T. R., III, and Poskanzer, D. C.: Treatment of strokes (in two parts), *New Engl. J. Med.,* **281**:594 and **281**:650, 1969.

Farhat, S. M., and Schneider, R. C.: Observations on the effect of systemic blood pressure on intracranial circulation in patients with cerebrovascular insufficiency, *J. Neurosurg.,* **27**:441, 1967.

Meyer, J. S., Sawada, T., Kitamura, A., and Toyoda, M.: Cerebral oxygen, glucose, lactate, and pyruvate metabolism in stroke. Therapeutic considerations, *Circulation,* **37**:1036, 1968.

———, Charney, J. Z., Rivera, V. M., and Mathew, N. T.: Treatment with glycerol of cerebral oedema due to acute cerebral infarction, *Lancet,* **2**:993, 1971.

Surgical

Donaghy, R. M. P., and Yaşargil, M. G. (eds.): Micro-vascular Surgery, Report of First Conference, October 6-7, 1966, The C. V. Mosby Company, St. Louis, 1967.

Greenwood, J., Jr.: Acute brain infarctions with high intracranial pressure: Surgical indications, *Johns Hopkins Med. Bull.,* **122**:254, 1968.

Hardy, J. D.: On the reversibility of strokes: Case of carotid artery repair with prompt recovery after hemiplegia and coma for two days, *Ann. Surg.,* **158**:1035, 1963.

Rob, C. G.: Operation for acute completed stroke due to thrombosis of the internal carotid artery, *Surgery,* **65**:862, 1969.

Wylie, E. J., Hein, M. F., and Adams, J. E.: Intracranial hemorrhage following surgical revascularization for treatment of acute strokes, *J. Neurosurg.,* **21**:212, 1964.

Yasargil, M. G., Krayenbühl, H. A., and Jacobson, J. H., II: Microneurosurgical arterial reconstruction, *Surgery,* **67**:221, 1970.

Additional References

McDowell, F. H., Louis, S., and Monahan, K.: Seasonal variation of nonembolic cerebral infarction, *J. Chron. Dis.,* **23**:29, 1970.

Patten, B. M., Mendell, J., Brunn, B., Curtin, W., and Carter, S.: Double blind study of the effects of dexamethasone on acute stroke, *Neurology,* **22**:377, 1972.

Schaafsma, S.: On the differential diagnosis between cerebral hemorrhage and infarction, *J. Neurol. Sci.,* **7**:83, 1968.

Sörnäs, R., Östlund, H., and Müller, R.: Cerebrospinal fluid cytology after stroke, *Arch. Neurol.,* **26**:489, 1972.

Stehbens, W. E.: Pathology of the Cerebral Blood Vessels, The C. V. Mosby Company, St. Louis, 1972.

Recurrent Episodes of Focal Neurologic Deficit (Transient Ischemic Attacks)

The fact that no two blades of grass are precisely alike, still less two cases of disease, is the fallacy of all statistics which relegates them to the place of secondary or confirmatory evidence. The precise study of single cases is, in my opinion, of much greater value.

W. Sampson Hadley

Ah, my dear Watson, there we come to the realms of conjecture where the most logical mind may be at fault. Each may form his own hypothesis upon the present evidence, and yours is as likely to be correct as mine.

Arthur Conan Doyle
The Empty House

Although physicians have been aware of the syndrome of recurrent short-lived episodes of focal neurologic deficit for years, the etiology, natural history, and management of these attacks are still matters of debate. The episodes are commonly called transient ischemic attacks (TIAs) and are customarily divided into two categories on the basis of the circulatory system involved (carotid or vertebral-basilar; see Chaps. 10 and 11).

The division of these cases into two groups is not always easy—partly because the attacks seldom occur at a time and location when a physician is available to examine the patient. Consequently, data concerning these attacks are based, for the most part, on historical information gathered from patients and their families. As might be expected, this may be inaccurate because the family is usually excited and the patient's mental acuity, insight, judgment, and memory may be impaired during the attack. Furthermore, there are no laboratory tests which can give an objective measure of these attacks and because (by definition) they are short-lived, postmortem material is not available to confirm clinical suspicions. Microinfarctions have been found at autopsy in some patients subject to transient ischemic attacks, but their relationship to the attacks is debatable.

Although all clinicians agree that TIAs have many causes, a relationship between the attacks and atherosclerosis is generally accepted because the episodes occur most commonly in patients who have aortocranial atherosclerosis. Microemboli of fibrin platelets or cholesterol have been seen in the optic fundi during transient ischemic attacks, and it is assumed that similar microemboli occurring in the cranial arterioles are responsible for the cerebral components of the episodes. An almost identical clinical syndrome, however, can be produced by acute bouts of hypoglycemia, extreme degrees of hypertension or hypotension, focal motor epilepsy with Todd's paralysis, Ménière's disease, hyperventilation, and abnormalities in the blood itself. Conditions which increase blood viscosity and lead to sludging (consumption coagulopathies, thrombocytosis, and dysproteinemias, for example) can cause ischemic attacks if the microcirculation in the brain becomes plugged by cellular aggregates. Vasospasm occurring as the result of an acute migraine attack or of hypertension is also a likely cause of TIAs.

PATHOGENESIS

There are many triggering mechanisms, and one must consider the probability that many factors contribute to each individual attack.

The ultimate cause of these episodes, however, is a temporary discrepancy between the metabolic needs of neural tissue and the available supply of blood containing oxygen and/or other nutrients. There is no evidence that attacks are in any way related to the accumulation of products of neuronal metabolism or to excessive activity of nerve cells. Although this discrepancy most often becomes apparent when atherosclerosis decreases the cerebrovascular reserve, it is probable (though not proved) that TIAs are related to the pial arteries or the microcirculation, where a small irritating lesion in a regional vascular bed leads to a reaction in the distal and adjacent vascular beds. This point of view is supported by those instances in which no disease of the large vessels is apparent—e.g., TIAs secondary to abnormalities in the blood. Conceivably, such attacks are the result of focal hypoxia in the arteriolar-capillary bed caused by occlusion of the penetrating arteries or arterioles.

If this theory is correct, TIAs represent malfunction of a protective mechanism designed to change vasomotor tone and thus protect the underlying nerve tissue from damage by abnormalities of the blood constituents or by foreign bodies in the blood (e.g., microemboli).

Whatever the cause, these attacks result from a deficiency in collateral channels upon which is superimposed one or more of the following triggering mechanisms.

Vasospasm

For years neurologists have debated the significance of spasm in the cerebral arteries. In order to consider the question logically, several facts must be kept in mind:

1 The reactivity of the leptomeningeal arteries and the larger arteries in the neck and in the circle of Willis is quite different from that of the penetrating arteries and arterioles comprising the microcirculation.

2 Vasospasm may be segmental or diffuse.

3 Vasospasm may result from different causes which themselves may produce varying effects upon the cerebral circulation.

Spasm in the Larger Arteries The evidence for spasm in these vessels is derived from angiography, although there are some pathologists who believe that antemortem vasospasm can be identified at the autopsy table.

One must keep in mind three conditions which may lead to an arteriographic picture simulating vasospasm:

1 When segmental narrowing of arteries in the neck is seen at angiography, it is usually attributable to the trauma caused by the procedure itself.

2 At times intracranial pressure is increased to the point that it exceeds intraluminal pressure within the arteries; the result is stagnation of the blood column and settling of the contrast material, which produces a spurious appearance of vasospasm.

3 A dissecting hematoma which reduces the lumen of the artery may also give the impression of spasm where none exists.

In some patients, usually young women, the vessels seem to be hyperreactive, and vasospasm causes a reduction in the lumen. In these patients Raynaud's phenomenon may be visible in the hands.

There can be no doubt that vasospasm does occur in the circle of Willis. A remarkable reduction in the caliber of the arteries has been seen by neurosurgeons when the large vessels at

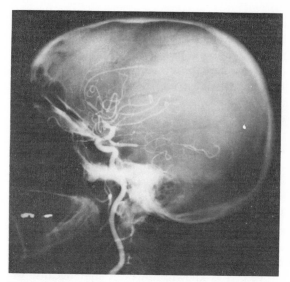

Figure 15-1 Carotid arteriogram showing attenuation of the middle cerebral artery and focal beading of the anterior cerebral and posterior communicating arteries (in a patient with recent subarachnoid hemorrhage).

the base of the brain are manipulated during operation. This vasospasm occurs in response to (1) abnormalities such as emboli within the lumen of the artery, (2) rupture of an aneurysm, (3) physical manipulation of the vessel, (4) vasoconstrictor substances in the blood, or (5) trauma to the vessel secondary to closed cranial injuries. In the case of subarachnoid hemorrhage due to rupture of an aneurysm, this spasm is segmental and may save the patient's life by helping to stop the flow of blood (Fig. 15-1).

Some authorities believe that constrictions in these large arteries result in reversible neurologic deficit; but there has been no good evidence to support this contention.

Arteriolar Spasm Spasm in the penetrating arteries and arterioles has been likened to the beading, sausage-shaped segmental spasm which can be seen in the retinal arterioles of patients suffering with grade II hypertensive retinopathy. This is thought to be a reversible process which is not accompanied by a decrease in cerebral blood flow. When arteriolar spasm is more intense and prolonged, it involves the entire circumference and length of the vessel and may be associated with focal hypoxia of neural tissue and may lead first to transudates and then exudates similar to those found in grades III and IV hypertensive retinopathy. Spasm of this degree is always secondary to some other primary process such as sustained severe hypertension, a vasoconstrictor agent, or irritation of the arteriolar bed by local trauma—possibly an embolus lodged within the lumen.

Most clinicians believe that migraine is a vasospastic disease involving the arteriolar vascular bed, although this hypothesis has not been proved. It is known, however, that because of an unusually high rate of complication arteriograms should not be made during attacks of migraine. Presumably this is because vessels that are already in spasm become hyperreactive in response to the irritating contrast material.

Hypotension

A sudden reduction of systemic blood pressure is sometimes associated with local or generalized cerebral dysfunction. Some authorities believe that hypotension can be the genesis of TIAs if segments of cerebral arteries have already been constricted by atherosclerosis. Few clinicians, however, have observed their patients to be hypotensive during an episode; nor have investigators been able to reproduce attacks by lowering the blood pressure in patients who have had spontaneous TIAs.

Hematologic Causes

Even when the arteries, arterioles, capillaries, and veins are apparently normal, abnormalities in the constituents of the blood can cause transient ischemic attacks. These abnormalities can be divided into as many groups as there are constituents of the blood:

1 Disorders of the red blood cells (e.g., erythrocytosis, polycythemia vera, and sickle-cell disease) can cause sludging or aggregation of red blood cells in the cerebral microcirculation. Severe anemia can cause TIA by reducing the ability of the blood to oxygenate neurons.
2 Myeloproliferative disorders such as leukemia can lead to episodes of neurologic dysfunction, either by causing cellular clumping in the lumen or by infiltrating the walls of the arterioles.
3 Thrombocytosis may cause micro-occlusions if platelet counts are above 500,000 per cu mm or if the platelets are unusually large or adhesive.
4 Dysproteinemias and abnormal globulins (e.g., macroglobulins, cryoglobulins, and those associated with multiple myeloma) may also reduce cerebral blood flow and cause TIAs.

Attacks related to hematologic abnormalities are relieved if the abnormality can be corrected. In some cases dramatic improvement occurs after venesection for polycythemia and the use of heparin for thrombocytosis, x-ray therapy for myeloproliferative disorders, and plasmapheresis and adrenocortical steroids for dysproteinemias.

Head Movements

Rapid, extreme degrees of rotation or extension of the head on the neck, which sometimes occur in working overhead or backing a car, for example, may cause feelings of giddiness, imbalance, or light-headedness presumably secondary to alterations in blood flow through the carotid or vertebral-basilar arteries. This effect is compounded in individuals with atherosclerosis and/or kinking of the vessels in the neck and is especially noticeable in patients with congenital craniovertebral anomalies or osteoarthritis of the cervical spine. In the waking state this insufficiency may be episodic because of continued head movements. During sleep, however, head rotation may be maintained for prolonged periods and may possibly be a cause of some cerebral infarctions.

Hyperlipoproteinemia

Patients with hyperlipoproteinemia have an accelerated development of atherosclerosis and are consequently predisposed to cerebrovascular insufficiency. Although there is no specific syndrome associated with the hyperlipoproteinemias, there is an unusually high incidence of Bell's palsy (which can mimic stroke). Consequently, a careful search should be made for xanthomatous deposits around the elbows and in the Achilles tendons of patients with Bell's palsy.

Postprandial hyperlipemia (lactescence) is thought to be a cause of angina pectoris, and some neurologists suspect that a similar mechanism can cause episodes of focal neural deficit.

Reversal of Cephalic Blood Flow

Lesions of the subclavian or brachiocephalic artery, the aortic arch, or even the carotid artery may invert the normal pressure gradients and cause blood to flow away from the brain into the upper limbs, depriving the brain of some of its blood supply. In such cases the brain is influenced to a certain degree by factors which affect the blood flow to the arms (Chap. 12).

Microembolism

Friable thrombi or cholesterol crystals within atherosclerotic carotid and vertebral arteries sometimes become dislodged and cause embolization of intracranial arteries (Chap. 18). By blocking local circulation, these microemboli produce symptoms of focal cerebral ischemia. If they than disintegrate or pass to more distal areas, circulation is restored and the neural deficit disappears. The occurrence of stereotyped clinical attacks is said to be due to the fact that laminar flow carries emboli to the same cerebral artery time after time.

When the first edition of this book was written, all the statements made in the preceding paragraph were based on conjecture because emboli had very rarely been found at autopsy. At that time it was generally held that microembolism was a comparative rarity and that a positive diagnosis of this condition could be made only if one were fortunate enough to see a microembolus in the optic fundus. Now angiog-

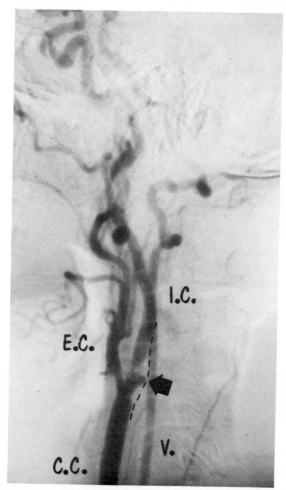

Figure 15-2 Subtraction of a carotid arteriogram. Arrow points to the ulcerated plaque. E.C.: external carotid; I.C.: internal carotid. *(Courtesy of Dr. F. Farrell, Department of Radiology, Bowman Gray School of Medicine.)*

raphers can demonstrate ulcerated plaques in the extracranial portions of the internal carotid artery, and it has been proved that removal of such plaques can stop transient ischemic attacks permanently (Fig. 15-2). At operation, surgeons sometimes see thrombi adherent to these ulcerated plaques, and pathologists have shown at autopsy that emboli composed of cholesterol and fibrin platelets are a common cause of transient ischemic attacks in patients suffering with symptomatic aortocervical-cranial atherosclerosis.

Hypercoagulable States

Normally blood platelets are disk-shaped and do not adhere to one another or to the endothelial wall. Certain states, however, cause them to swell and sometimes rupture, releasing their contents of histamine, lysosomal enzymes, serotonin, adenosine triphosphate (ATP), and adenosine diphosphate (ADP). ADP causes platelets to become sticky, and this increased adhesiveness, together with calcium ion present in the plasma, leads to an aggregation of platelets which is independent of the blood-coagulating mechanism. These conglomerations of platelets usually occur in response to vascular injury in diseased arteries and arterioles and lead to the formation of small thrombi. Although this process is reversible, a clotting reaction will occur if phospholipids are released from the platelet membrane to initiate the conversion of fibrinogen to fibrin. Fibrin enmeshes cellular elements, and a clot begins to form. By injuring the endothelium and causing a local vasculitis, the lysosomal enzyme released from the ruptured platelets accelerates the deposition of platelets and furthers thrombus formation.

Antigen-antibody complexes, endotoxins, and viral and bacterial invaders are among the stimuli which precipitate this platelet response. Medications which reverse the process are acetylsalicylic acid, dipyridamole, prostaglandin, and heparin.

Abnormalities of Cardiac Function

Transitory neurologic deficits which result from diseases of the heart can be classified as follows:

1 Valvular disorders
2 Abnormalities of rhythm due to conduction defects
3 Myocardial infarction
4 Inflammatory diseases (myocarditis or bacterial endocarditis)
5 Surgical manipulation of the heart and great vessels producing emboli (air, antifoaming agents, fat, or calcium)
6 Atrial myxoma, with tumor emboli to the cranial arteries
7 Heart failure, leading to stasis, thrombosis, and emboli from pulmonary veins

Intermittent cardiac dysrhythmia is difficult to diagnose because the electrocardiogram may be normal between attacks. Continuous cardiac monitoring may be required for 36 to 48 hr with the patient asleep and awake, preferably ambulatory in his natural environment, and under the stresses and strains of his customary business and social activities.

Decrease in cardiac output which results from borderline myocardial function is not customarily noted on physical examination and can also be difficult to detect. Cardiac output is the product of stroke volume and heart rate and is not related to arterial pulse pressure. Consequently, the functional state of the myocardial pump can be determined only by a ballistocardiogram or by direct measurement of the cardiac output.

Onset of the Attacks

Although there are many varieties of TIAs, episodes are usually rather stereotyped in the same individual. The patient suddenly becomes aware that a portion of his normal neural function is lost. Most commonly there is a loss of power in distal musculature (a hand or a foot), which rapidly progresses in an ascending fashion to involve the whole extremity and then perhaps the entire side of the body. Most patients describe a numbness or peculiar sensation which is not akin to any previously experienced, although some compare it to the lack of feeling that follows a nerve block for dental anesthesia.

In other cases, the attacks may be characterized by partial or complete blindness of one eye or both, diplopia, transitory dysphasia, dysarthria, vertigo, deafness, or drop attacks. The exact sequence of events and the symptoms which occur depend upon whether the vertebral-basilar or the carotid circulation is involved (Chaps. 10 and 11).

Episodic change in personality or memory may conceivably be a manifestation of focal neurologic deficit, and there may even be no recognized clinical symptoms or signs of recurrent focal dysfunction because of the area of the brain involved or because the patient denies illness.

Duration of the Attacks

The attacks usually last less than 12 hr and rarely more than 24 hr before full recovery. Generally speaking, the time taken from the moment when the attack is first noted until the height of the episode is less than the time taken for recovery to occur after symptoms begin to diminish.

It is a good general rule that episodes which last longer than 24 hr signify infarction or some other pathologic process; but there are occasional cases which take days after the initial ictus before complete recovery occurs. Although the pathogenetic mechanism of these prolonged attacks may be the same as those of short duration, they are usually classified as infarction with recovery.

Frequency of the Attacks

Some patients suffer as many as 12 to 20 very brief attacks in one day, but in most cases there are fewer than one or two attacks a week, and occasionally less than one a month. No statistics have been compiled to give further information on this subject.

Neurologic Examination

The results of a neurologic examination performed between attacks are normal. If a patient is seen during an episode, his symptoms and signs will be indistinguishable from those of evolving cerebral infarction.

DIFFERENTIAL DIAGNOSIS

A clinical diagnosis of recurrent episodes of focal neurologic deficit secondary to aortocranial atherosclerosis should be made only if the following diagnostic criteria are met:

1 The neural dysfunction must have a clear anatomic location.
2 The duration of the attack must not exceed 24 hr; it is usually less than 30 min.
3 The patient must have no abnormal neurologic signs between the attacks.
4 The patient should have evidence of aortocervical atherosclerosis.
5 The patient must have no clinical evidence of increased intracranial pressure.

Even if these criteria are met, it is not always possible to eliminate disorders such as Ménière's syndrome, epilepsy, syncope, psychophysiologic reactions, and migraine. Recurrent short-lived episodes without lasting deficit sometimes occur in patients with intracranial arterial occlusions and occasionally in those with brain neoplasms (Fig. 15-3). In such cases the brain scan and arteriographic examination are indispensable.

Sometimes one encounters patients with TIAs in whom a full evaluation including prolonged ECG monitoring and arteriographic examination fails to reveal any abnormality. In

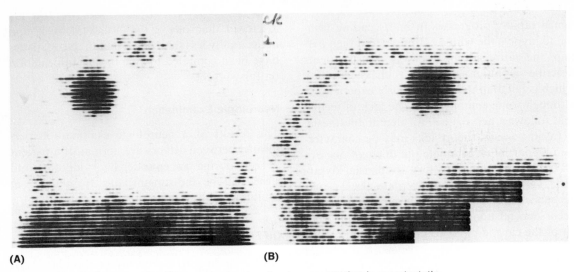

(A)

(B)

Figure 15-3 Brain scan using 99m$_{\text{Tc}}$, showing localized concentration in a metastatic lesion. (A) Posterior view. (B) Right lateral view.

these cases it is suspected that the causative lesion lies in the microcirculation which, although it makes up 80 to 90 percent of the vascular bed, cannot be visualized by arteriography.

COURSE AND PROGNOSIS

It is estimated that about one-third of those who suffer recurrent neurologic deficit will continue to have attacks without developing permanent disability; another third will eventually have cerebral infarction, and in the remainder the attacks will cease spontaneously. Unfortunately, we have no way to predict the group into which an individual patient will fall, but there is some indication that the natural history of attacks secondary to vertebral-basilar insufficiency is more benign than that associated with carotid artery syndrome.

MANAGEMENT

The treatment of every patient with recurrent neurologic deficit must be individualized. The key to therapy is removal or treatment of a trig-

gering mechanism (see appropriate sections of this book). When all systemic triggering mechanisms have been excluded and still the attacks continue, one must consider microembolism, for which anticoagulants may be used (Chap. 16), or stenosis of vessels, for which surgery may be indicated (Chap. 17).

SUGGESTED READINGS

General

Alajouanine, T., Lhermitte, F., and Gautier, J.-C.: Transient cerebral ischemia in atherosclerosis, *Neurology,* **10**:906, 1960.

Alvarez, W. C.: Little Strokes, J. B. Lippincott Company, Philadelphia, 1966.

Fisher, C. M.: Concerning recurrent transient cerebral ischemic attacks, *Can. Med. Assoc. J.,* **86**:1091, 1962.

Freidman, G. D., Wilson, S., Mosier, J. M., Collandrier, M. A., and Nichermon, N. Z.: Transient ischemic attacks in a community, *J.A.M.A.,* **210**:1428, 1969.

Kuhn, R. A.: Cerebral circulation and "cerebral ischemia": Blood flow through cervical arteries, *World Neurol.,* **3**:740, 1962.

Millikan, C. H.: The pathogenesis of transient focal cerebral ischemia, The Lewis A. Connor Memorial Lecture, *Circulation,* **32**:438, 1965.

Natural History

Acheson, J., and Hutchinson, E. C.: Observations on the natural history of transient cerebral ischemia, *Lancet,* **2**:871, 1964.

Brain, W. R.: Some unsolved problems of cervical spondylosis, *Brit. Med. J.,* **1**:771, 1963.

Marshall, J.: The natural history of transient ischaemic cerebrovascular attacks, *Quart. J. Med.,* **33**:309, 1964.

Mori, K., Goto, Y., Hasegawa, T., Araki, G., Hirai, S., Murakami, K., Sato, N., Yushida, K., Kato, M., and Tatsuzawa, Y.: A clinical evaluation of transient focal cerebral ischemia with some comments on its concept, *Japan Circulation J.,* **29**:847, 1965.

Pathogenesis

Darmody, W. R., Thomas, L. M., and Gurdjian, E. S.: Postirradiation vascular insufficiency syndrome: Case report, *Neurology,* **17**:1190, 1967.

Fisher, C. M.: "Intermittent cerebral ischemia," in Cerebral Vascular Diseases, Transactions of the Second Princeton Conference, edited by C. H. Millikan, Grune & Stratton, Inc., New York, 1958, pp. 81-97.

Foley, J. M.: "Precipitating factors in focal cerebral ischemia," in Modern Neurology: Papers in Tribute to Derek Denny-Brown, edited by S. Locke, Little, Brown and Company, Boston, 1969, pp. 491-496.

Fowler, N. O., Fenton, J. C., and Conway, G. F.: Syncope and cerebral dysfunction caused by bradycardia without atrioventricular block, *Am. Heart J.,* **80**:303, 1970.

Gurdjian, E. S., Darmody, W. R., and Thomas, L. M.: Recurrent strokes due to occlusive disease of extracranial vessels, *Arch. Neurol.,* **21**:447, 1969.

Levine, J., and Swanson, P. D.: Nonatherosclerotic causes of stroke, *Ann. Internal Med.,* **70**:807, 1969.

Moore, W. S., and Hall, A. D.: Ulcerated atheroma of the carotid artery. A cause of transient cerebral ischemia, *Am. J. Surg.,* **116**:237, 1968.

Vasospasm

Bickerstaff, E. R.: Ophthalmoplegic migraine, *Rev. neurol.,* **110**:582, 1964.

Bradshaw, P., and Parsons, M.: Hemiplegic migraine, a clinical study, *Quart. J. Med.,* **34**:65, 1965.

Buckle, R. M., Du Boulay, G., and Smith, B.: Death due to cerebral vasospasm, *J. Neurol. Neurosurg. Psychiat.,* **27**:440, 1964.

Dukes, H. T., and Vieth, R. G.: Cerebral arteriography during migraine prodrome and headache, *Neurology,* **14**:636, 1964.

Gurdjian, E. S., and Thomas, L. M.: Cerebral vasospasm, *Surg. Gynecol. Obstet.,* **129**:931, 1969.

Pool, J. L.: Cerebral vasospasm, *New Engl. J. Med.,* **259**:1259, 1958.

Potter, J. M.: Cerebral arterial spasm: A short review, *World Neurol.,* **2**:576, 1961.

Salatich, J. S.: Cerebral symptoms due to cigarette smoking, *J. Louisiana Med. Soc.,* **117**:227, 1965.

Hypotension

Editorial: Hypotension and cerebral ischemia, *J.A.M.A.,* **187**:450, 1964.

Fazekas, J. F., and Alman, R. W.: The role of hypotension in transitory focal cerebral ischemia, *Am. J. Med. Sci.,* **248**:567, 1964.

Johnson, R. H., Smith, A. C., Spalding, J. M. K., and Wollner, L.: Effect of posture on blood pressure in elderly patients, *Lancet,* **1**:731, 1965.

Kendall, R. E., and Marshall, J.: Role of hypotension in the genesis of transient focal cerebral ischaemic attacks, *Brit. Med. J.,* **2**:344, 1963.

Hematologic Causes

Levine, J., and Swanson, P. D.: Idiopathic thrombocytosis: A treatable cause of transient ischemic attacks, *Neurology,* **18**:711, 1968.

Millikan, C. H., Siekert, R. G., and Whisnant, J. P.: Intermittent carotid and vertebral-basilar insufficiency associated with polycythemia, *Neurology,* **10**:188, 1960.

Montgomery, B. M., and Pinner, C. A.: Transient hypoglycemic hemiplegia, *Arch. Internal Med.,* **114**:680, 1964.

Olivarius, B. de F.: Cerebral manifestations in thrombocythemia, *Acta psychiat. neurol.,* **32**:77, 1957.

Siekert, R. G., Whisnant, J. P., and Millikan, C. H.: Anemia and intermittent focal cerebral arterial insufficiency, *Arch. Neurol.,* **3**:386, 1960.

Swank, R. L.: Blood viscosity in cerebrovascular disease: Effects of low fat diet and heparin, *Neurology,* **9**:553, 1959.

Weber, M. D.: The neurological complications of consumption coagulopathies, *Neurology,* **18**:185, 1968.

Head Movements

Eiseman, B., Spencer, F., and Dachi, S. F.: The role of the dentist in the diagnosis and prevention of cerebrovascular accidents, *Oral Surg.,* **16**:1174, 1963.

Toole, J. F., and Tucker, S. H.: Influence of head position upon cerebral circulation, *Arch. Neurol.,* **2**:616, 1960.

Reversal of Cephalic Blood Flow

Patel, A., and Toole, J. F.: Subclavian steal syndrome—Reversal of cephalic blood flow, *Medicine,* **44**:289, 1965.

Microembolism

David, N. J., Klintworth, G. K., Friedberg, S. J., and Dillon, M.: Fatal atheromatous cerebral embolism associated with bright plaques in the retinal arterioles: Report of a case, *Neurology,* **13**:708, 1963.

Editorial: Atheromatous embolization to the brain, *J.A.M.A.,* **191**:44, 1965.

Fisher, C. M.: Observations of the fundus oculi in transient monocular blindness, *Neurology,* **9**:333, 1959.

Gunning, A. J., Pickering, G. W., Robb-Smith, A. H., and Russell, R. R.: Mural thrombosis of the internal carotid artery and subsequent embolism, *Quart. J. Med.,* **33**:155, 1964.

Hollenhorst, R. W.: Significance of bright plaques in the retinal arterioles, *J.A.M.A.,* **178**:23, 1961.

Horn, P., and Genovese, P. D.: The association of calcific valvular disease and retinal embolization, *J. Indiana Med. Assoc.,* **57**:227, 1964.

McBrien, D. J., Bradley, R. D., and Ashton, N.: The nature of retinal emboli in stenosis of the internal carotid artery, *Lancet,* **1**:697, 1963.

Russell, R. W. R.: Observations on the retinal blood-vessels in monocular blindness, *Lancet,* **2**:1422, 1961.

Abnormalities of Cardiac Function

Hutchinson, E. C., and Stock, J. P. P.: Paroxysmal cerebral ischaemia in rheumatic heart disease, *Lancet,* **2**:653, 1963.

Lavy, S., and Stern, S.: Transient neurological manifestations in cardiac arrhythmias, *J. Neurol. Sci.,* **9**:97, 1969

Walter, P. F., Reid, S. D., and Wenger, N. K.: Arrhythmia-induced cerebral ischemia, *Neurology,* **20**:418, 1970.

———,———, and ———: Transient cerebral ischemia due to arrhythmia, *Ann. Internal Med.,* **72**:471, 1970.

Yarnell, P. R., Spann, J. F., Dougherty, J., and Mason, D. T.: Episodic central nervous system ischemia of undetermined cause: Relation to occult left atrial myxoma, *Stroke,* **2**:35, 1971.

Clinical Features

Hutchinson, E. C.: Little strokes, *Brit. Med. J.,* **4**:32, 1969.

Patel, A. N.: Transient ischemic attacks, *Am. Family Physician,* **4**(4):96, 1971.

Zülch, K. J.: "Reconsiderations of the clinical problem of cerebrovascular insufficiency," in Research on the Cerebral Circulation, Third International Salzburg Conference, 1966, compiled and edited by J. S. Meyer, H. Lechner, and O. Eichhorn, Charles C Thomas, Publisher, Springfield, Ill., 1969, pp. 1–41.

Differential Diagnosis

Daly, D. D., Svien, H. J., and Yoss, R. E.: Intermittent cerebral symptoms with meningiomas, *Arch. Neurol.,* **5**:287, 1961.

Espir, M. L. E., Watkins, S. M., and Smith, H. V.: Paroxysmal dysarthria and other transient neurological disturbances in disseminated sclerosis, *J. Neurol. Neurosurg. Psychiat.,* **29**:323, 1966.

Faris, A. A., and Poser, C. M.: Experimental production of focal neurologic deficit by systemic hyponatremia, *Neurology,* **14**:206, 1964.

Gilbert, G. J.: Cluster headache and cluster vertigo, *Headache,* **9**:195, 1970.

Heron, J. R.: Migraine and cerebrovascular disease, *Neurology,* **16**:1097, 1966.

Marshall, J.: The differential diagnosis of "little strokes," *Postgrad. Med. J.,* **44**:543, 1968.

Okihiro, M. M., Daly, D., and Yoss, R. E.: Intermittent aphasia due to mass intracranial lesions, *Proc. Staff Meetings Mayo Clinic,* **36**:525, 1961.

Sarkari, N. B. S., and Bickerstaff, E. R.: Relapses and remissions in brain stem tumours, *Brit. Med. J.,* **2**:21, 1969.

Whitty, C. W. M.: Migraine without headache, *Lancet,* **2**:283, 1967.

Course and Prognosis

Goldner, J. C., Whisnant, J. P., and Taylor, W. F.: Long-term prognosis of transient cerebral ischemic attacks, *Stroke,* **2**:160, 1971.

Whisnant, J. P., Goldner, J. C., and Taylor, W. F.: "Natural history of transient ischemic attacks," in Cerebral Vascular Diseases, Transactions of the Seventh Princeton Conference, edited by J. Moossy and R. Janeway, Grune & Stratton, Inc., New York, 1971, pp. 161–165.

Laboratory Studies

Burrows, E. H., and Marshall, J.: Angiographic investigation of patients with transient ischaemic attacks, *J. Neurol. Neurosurg. Psychiat.,* **28**:533, 1965.

Capistrant, T. D., and Gumnit, R. J.: Thermography following a carotid transient ischemic episode, *J.A.M.A.,* **211**:656, 1970.

Cronqvist, S.: Total angiography in evaluation of cerebrovascular disease: A correlative study of aortocervical and selective cerebral angiography, *Brit. J. Radiol.,* **39**:805, 1966.

Drake, W. E., and Drake, M. A. L.: Clinical and angiographic correlates of cerebrovascular insufficiency, *Am. J. Med.,* **45**:253, 1968.

Kreindler, A., Poilici, I., and Marinchescu, C.: Electroencephalographic study of cerebral transient ischemic attacks, *Confinia neurol.,* **28**:385, 1966.

Poser, C. M., Zosa, A. M., Gomez, A. J., and Hardin, C. A.: Cervicocephalic angiography for cerebrovascular insufficiency, *Acta neurol. scand.,* **40**:321, 1964.

Sutton, D., and Davies, E. R.: Arch aortography and cerebrovascular insufficiency, *Clin. Radiol.,* **17**:330, 1966.

Tharp, B. R.: The electroencephalogram in transient global amnesia, *Electroencephalog. Clin. Neurophysiol.,* **26**:96, 1969.

Wood, E. H., and Correll, J. W.: Atheromatous ulceration in major neck vessels as a cause of cerebral embolism, *Acta radiol. (diagn.),* **9**:520, 1969.

Management

Browne, T. R., III, and Poskanzer, D. C.: Treatment of strokes (in two parts), *New. Engl. J. Med.,* **281**:594 and **281**:650, 1969.

Denny-Brown, D.: Symposium on specific methods of treatment; the treatment of recurrent cerebrovascular symptoms and the question of "vasospasm," *Med. Clin. N. Am.,* **35**:1457, 1951.

Leading article: Anticoagulants for cerebral arteriosclerosis, *Lancet,* **1**:34, 1965.

McAllen, P. M., and Marshall, J.: Cardiac dysrhythmia and transient cerebral ischaemic attacks, *Lancet,* **1**:1212, 1973.

Pearce, J. M. S., Gubbay, S. S., and Walton, J. N.: Long-term anticoagulant therapy in transient cerebral ischaemic attacks, *Lancet,* **1**:6, 1965.

Reed, R. L., Siekert, R. G., and Merideth, J.: Rarity of transient focal cerebral ischemia in cardiac dysrhythmia, *J.A.M.A.,* **223**:893, 1973.

Siekert, R. G., Millikan, C. H., and Whisnant, J. P.: Anticoagulant therapy in intermittent cerebrovascular insufficiency: Follow-up data, *J.A.M.A.,* **176**:19, 1961.

Chapter 16

Medical Management of Cerebrovascular Insufficiency and Infarction

. . . Accuracy is occasionally impossible; we can only be right in nineteen cases by being wrong in the twentieth. It is well to realize this. But remember that in practice we have to treat that which is only probable as if it were certain. We could not treat two thirds of our cases properly without doing this.

W. R. Gowers

The prelude to management of any disease is accurate diagnosis. When the history and the clinical findings suggest a vascular disorder, the physician must consider its pathogenesis and triggering mechanisms (detailed in Chap. 15) before concluding that his patient is suffering with atherothrombotic disease. Even if atherosclerosis is the probable cause, he must school himself to ask what precipitated the attack. The following are some of the possibilities.

1 Systemic disease

a Hypotension such as that resulting from acute blood loss, myocardial infarction, hypotensive medications, or hypersensitivity of the carotid sinus reflex.

b Intracranial embolism from pulmonary veins, heart valves, or mural thrombus of the endocardium.

c Hematologic disease such as polycythemia, iron-deficiency anemia, or sickle-cell anemia.

d Intoxication from barbiturates, alcohol, narcotics, or phenothiazines.

e Endocrine disorders such as diabetes mellitus or thyroid disease.

f Hypoglycemia.

2 Intracranial disease

a Cerebral hemorrhage. It should be remembered that about 10 percent of such hemorrhages remain encapsulated and cause no bleeding into the spinal fluid.

b Subdural hematoma. A head injury that appears trivial to the patient and his family may produce a subdural hematoma. Such a sequel to trauma is most likely to occur in the elderly and in patients who have been given anticoagulants.

c Brain tumor. Both benign and malignant neoplasms occasionally cause sudden loss of neurologic function and simulate vascular episodes.

d Epilepsy. Convulsions are sometimes followed by short-lived focal neurologic deficit (postictal paralysis).

e Ménière's syndrome. This may simulate vertebral-basilar insufficiency.

These possibilities must be eliminated before one can confidently assume that the neurologic episode is due to occlusive disease. Then one must distinguish clearly between disease of the intracranial arteries, which is usually managed medically, and atherosclerosis, arteritis, or embolism from the cervical arteries, all of which can be treated surgically. *The findings that point to aortocervical obstruction are abnormal pulsations in an extracranial vessel, a thoracic or cervical bruit, or unequal ophthalmic or brachial blood pressures.* If any of these are present, one may wish to carry out arteriography with a view toward reconstructive surgery. This procedure, as well as the possibilities for surgical intervention, is considered in the next chapter.

ACCESSORY CLINICAL STUDIES

Certain procedures are mandatory for all patients who suffer a sudden neurologic deficit. These are:

1 Urinalysis.

2 Blood studies including hematocrit; complete blood-cell count; serologic tests for syphilis; and determination of the levels of blood sugar (preferably 2 hr after a full meal), erythrocyte sedimentation rate, and urea nitrogen. In addition it is wise to ascertain the prothrombin time, protein concentration, and albumin/globulin ratio, and to make blood viscosity determinations.

3 X-ray of the chest, to reveal the heart size and to rule out passive hyperemia or carcinoma of the lung. (About 16 percent of lung cancers present clinically with an intracranial metastasis.)

4 X-rays of the skull, to delineate the position of the pineal gland and evidences of increased pressure such as demineralization of the posterior clinoid processes.

5 Cervical x-rays. (About half of the patients who have advanced atherosclerosis of the carotid bifurcation will have calcification visible in cervical x-rays. If this calcification is more than 1 cm in length, there is probably a stenotic lesion.)

6 Isotope flow study of the cervicocranial arteries to demonstrate delayed arrival of the bolus, suggesting arterial obstruction or early filling as in an arteriovenous malformation.

7 Radioisotopic brain scan. This procedure may give a clue to subdural hematoma, arteriovenous malformations, brain abscesses, and most vascular neoplasms (particularly meningiomas, malignant gliomas, and many metastatic tumors).

Because brain scans made within 2 hr of injection of the radioisotope $99m_{Tc}$ are almost always normal in the early stages of infarction and hemorrhage, an abnormal scan obtained within the first 48 hr after the appearance of a neurologic deficit suggests another cause. However, delayed scans performed 6 hr after injection may be positive within hours of the ictus. Furthermore, large infarctions such as those sometimes produced by occlusion of the internal carotid or middle cerebral may show uptake within 48 hr. In general, however, increased uptake due to infarction becomes visible only after several days; once developed, it may remain for months. Consequently, a scan that is negative at 24 hr but positive when repeated 7 to 10 days later strongly suggests an evolving infarction with neovascularization.

A most important use for this procedure is in screening patients in whom neurologic deficit appears some weeks following head injury; a negative brain scan strongly suggests that there is no chronic supratentorial subdural hematoma.

8 Lumbar puncture. A properly performed lumbar puncture is an invaluable diagnostic aid in patients suffering a cerebral vascular episode of any kind. It should be performed with the patient in the lateral recumbent position. The pressure must be measured before removal of any fluid. If it is elevated above 180 mm, a second measurement must be made after an attempt to eliminate any physiologic cause for the elevation by extending the patient's legs, putting the head in neutral position, having him breathe normally through his mouth, and allowing time for him to relax. Samples of fluid are then withdrawn and examined according to the procedure detailed in Chap. 24.

9 Serial electroencephalograms, to help differentiate infarctions from tumors.

10 Echoencephalograms, to reveal any shift of midline structures in cases where the pineal gland cannot be visualized on x-ray.

MEDICAL MANAGEMENT

The patient should be kept at complete bed rest with his face front as much as possible until the process has stabilized. If he can tolerate elevation of the foot of the bed, it should be about 4 in. higher than the head. General measures applicable to the care of most patients with neurologic deficit are considered in Chap. 30.

Anticoagulant Therapy

Even though the first articles on the use of anticoagulant therapy for cerebral infarction and embolism were published in 1950, there is still much disagreement concerning its indications and limitations. While the statistics accumulated thus far do not afford proof satisfactory to all investigators, the weight of evidence favors the administration of anticoagulants in adequate dosage to the following groups of patients: (1) those with evolving cerebral infarction, in an effort to halt progression except when the infarction is caused by cerebral embolus; (2) those with episodes of focal neurologic deficit which may be a prelude to cerebral infarction; (3) patients who are predisposed to recurrent cerebral emboli (see Chap. 18); (4) bedridden patients with neurologic deficit, in order to prevent phlebothrombosis and pulmonary embolism.

The incidence of hemorrhagic complications in patients on long-term anticoagulant therapy for prevention of further cerebral vascular episodes is approximately 3 percent per year—hence the importance of carefully selecting patients and of maintaining rigid laboratory controls, with skillful adjustment of dosage in order to keep the prothrombin time within the therapeutic range. A program which we have found to be satisfactory is outlined below.

Typical Regimen for Anticoagulant Therapy

1 Determine the clotting and prothrombin times before beginning anticoagulant therapy.

2 Administer concentrated heparin sodium subdermally in repository form 200 to 400 mg as soon as possible and then daily at 9 A.M. and 9 P.M. Determine the clotting time less than 1 hr before each dose and adjust the dosage so as to maintain the Lee-White clotting time between 20 and 30 min.

3 Give a coumarin compound such as warfarin sodium or bishydroxycoumarin orally each evening between 6 and 8 P.M., the dosage depending on the prothrombin time obtained daily at 8 A.M..

4 Give sufficient coumarin compound to reduce prothrombin time to 20 to 30 percent of control values. Continue use of heparin therapy until prothrombin time has reached these levels.

5 Many physicians omit the coumarin compound entirely and continue intermittent doses of concentrated (repository) heparin indefinitely because of its lipid-clearing effects on the blood. The chief disadvantages of this method are the necessity of using needle and syringe and the possibility of developing osteoporosis.

6 Most physicians dispense vitamin K_1 oxide for emergency use in case of bleeding and provide the patient with a medical identification card stating that he is taking anticoagulants.

7 Caution the patient to avoid the excessive use of salicylates and alcohol, to be alert for melena or hematuria, and to seek medical advice before undergoing dental extractions.

8 Continue the use of a coumarin compound or repository heparin until the patient has been without attacks for about 1 year.

Once it has been decided to use anticoagulants, the desired increase in clotting or prothrombin time should be achieved as rapidly as possible—if necessary, by administering medication intravenously in the initial phases. On the other hand, if it seems advisable to discontinue anticoagulants after a patient has been taking them for any length of time, the dose should be tapered off very gradually over a period of weeks, in order to avoid hypercoagulability—the so-called "rebound effect." Even if the clotting or prothrombin time is found to be unduly prolonged as the result of an overdose of the medication, it is usually wise to administer at most a very small dose of vitamin K_1 oxide (or protamine sulfate, if the patient is receiving heparin), in order to return the prothrombin time *toward* normal rather than *to* normal. Unless hemorrhage has occurred, a prolonged prothrombin time is not an emergency.

It has been found that the amount of anticoagulant medication required by a given patient varies according to the climate—the warmer the weather, the larger the dose required to achieve

the same effect. Other factors that may affect the prothrombin time and the required dosage of anticoagulant are medications such as salicylates, Dilantin, barbiturates, phenylbutazone, and antibiotics; vitamin K ingested in food and multiple-vitamin mixtures; consumption of alcohol; intercurrent illnesses (especially gastroenteritis); and the use of organic solvents in the patient's hobby or occupation. In the rare pregnant patient who requires anticoagulants, heparin rather than coumarin should be used.

The most common complication of anticoagulant therapy is bleeding from any one of a number of sites even though the prothrombin time may be within the therapeutic range. If bleeding from the gastrointestinal or urinary tract occurs when the prothrombin time is within the range of therapeutic effect, one should suspect a focal lesion such as carcinoma, ulcer, stone, or cystitis. Hemoptysis or epistaxis is rarely a problem, and hemarthrosis or bleeding into the muscles after minor trauma is even more infrequent.

Patients with ischemic brain disease who are maintained on anticoagulants may develop subdural or epidural hematomata within the calvaria or spinal canal. These may be insidious, and the symptoms and signs may be attributed to progression of the cerebrovascular process rather than to the hematoma.

Vasodilating Agents

There is no convincing evidence that vasodilating agents such as nylidrin hydrochloride and nicotinic acid have any significant effect on the cerebral blood flow. Carbon dioxide is a potent dilator of normal cerebral arterioles, but its use is contraindicated in patients with evolving infarction because dilatation of healthy arterioles may exceed that of arterioles in the damaged area and may actually shunt blood away from the infarcting area. Some authorities administer papaverine 500 mg every 12 hr in an intravenous infusion for 5 days. Long-acting papaverine 150 mg orally is continued twice daily for years.

Hypotensive Medications

Patients with hypertension should be given hypotensive medications during the acute stage of cerebral infarction only if they have been receiving maintenance doses for several weeks before the onset of the episode. However, as soon as the episode stabilizes, pressure should be reduced gradually to normotensive levels and maintained.

Low-Molecular-Weight Dextran

The antisludging properties of low-molecular-weight dextran have been recognized for many years. In addition, this material has an anticoagulant effect and reduces cerebral edema.

There has been recent interest in utilizing these properties for the prevention of cerebral thromboembolism and the treatment of evolving cerebral infarction; 500 ml is infused every 12 hr for several days. Urinary output must be followed carefully, and the drug discontinued if oliguria develops. Furthermore, intravenous infusion can produce local phlebitis.

Despite 10 years of use, the efficacy of this form of treatment has not been proved.

Salicylates

There is good evidence that platelet adhesiveness can be reduced dramatically by acetylsalicylic acid, dipyridamole, or phenylbutazone. Because this is a prelude to clot formation it has been suggested that these be employed also for prevention of TIAs and as treatment for evolving infarction. This form of therapy is being actively investigated at the time of this writing.

Cerebral Stimulants

Pentylenetetrazol (Metrazol) does not improve cerebral circulation or brain metabolism, and aminophylline causes cerebral vasoconstriction.

SUGGESTED READINGS

General

Browne, T. R., III, and Poskanzer, D. C.: Treatment of strokes (in two parts), *New Engl. J. Med.*, **281**:594 and **281**:650, 1969.

Fazekas, J. F., Alman, R. W., and Sullivan, J. F.: Prognostic uncertainties in cerebral vascular disease, *Ann. Internal Med.*, **58**:93, 1963.

Fisher, C. M.: Diagnosis and management of cerebrovascular disease, *Postgrad. Med.*, **38**:130, 1965.

Heron, J. R., and Anderson, E. G.: Concomitant cerebral and cardiac ischaemia, *Lancet*, **2**:405, 1965.

Hurwitz, L. J.: Management of major strokes, *Brit. Med. J.*, **3**:699, 1969.

Leading article: Management of strokes, *Brit. Med. J.*, **2**:446, 1968.

Marshall, J.: Management of Cerebrovascular Disease, 2d ed., The Williams & Wilkins Company, Baltimore, 1968.

Accessory Clinical Studies

Hansen, O. E.: Hyperuricemia in cerebral infarction, *Acta neurol. scand.*, **41**(suppl. 13, part 1):357, 1965.

Louis, S., and McDowell, F.: Epileptic seizures in nonembolic cerebral infarction, *Arch. Neurol.*, **17**:414, 1967.

Medical Management

Anticoagulant Therapy

Acheson, J., Danta, G., and Hutchinson, E. C.: Controlled trial of dipyridamole in cerebral vascular disease, *Brit. Med. J.*, **1**:614, 1969.

Aggeler, P. M., O'Reilly, R. A., Leong, L., and Kowitz, P. E.: Potentiation of anticoagulant effect of warfarin by phenylbutazone, *New Engl. J. Med.*, **276**:496, 1967.

Barron, K. D., and Ferguson, G.: Intracranial hemorrhage as a complication of anticoagulant therapy, *Neurology*, **9**:447, 1959.

Deykin, D.: The use of heparin, *New Engl. J. Med.*, **280**:937, 1969.

————: Warfarin therapy (in two parts), *New Engl. J. Med.*, **283**:691 and **283**:801, 1970.

Enger, E., and Bøyesen, S.: Long-term anticoagulant therapy in patients with cerebral infarction: A controlled clinical study, *Acta med. scand.*, **178** (suppl. 438), 1965.

Fields, W. S., and Hass, W. K. (eds.): Aspirin, platelets and stroke. Background for a clinical trial, Warren H. Green, Inc., St. Louis, Mo., 1971.

Flannery, E. P., MacDonald, B. S., O'Leary, D. S., and McGinty, J. M.: Japanese-restaurant syndrome, *New Engl. J. Med.*, **285**:414, 1971.

Foley, W. D., and Wright, I. S.: The treatment of cerebral thrombosis and embolism with anticoagulant drugs: Preliminary observations, *Med. Clin. N. Am.*, **34**:909, 1950.

Heyman, A.: Prolonged anticoagulation for cerebrovascular insufficiency, *J.A.M.A.*, **210**:1769, 1969.

Hirsch, J., Cade, J. F., and O'Sullivan, E. F.: Clinical experience with anticoagulant therapy during pregnancy, *Brit. Med. J.*, **1**:270, 1970.

Koch-Weser, J., and Sellers, E. M.: Drug interactions with coumarin anticoagulants (in two parts), *New Engl. J. Med.*, **285**:487 and **285**:547, 1971.

Kravitz, A. R., and Thomas, D. P.: Emotional reactions to long-term anticoagulant therapy, *Arch. Internal Med.*, **114**:663, 1964.

Leading article: Anticoagulants and cerebral infarction, *Lancet*, **1**:245, 1966.

MacDonald, M. G., and Robinson, D. S.: Clinical observations of possible barbiturate interference with anticoagulation, *J.A.M.A.*, **204**:97, 1968.

Marshall, J., and Reynolds, E. H.: Withdrawal of anticoagulants from patients with transient ischaemic cerebrovascular attacks, *Lancet*, **1**:5, 1965.

Mayne, E. E., Bridges, J. M., and Weaver, J. A.: The effect of dipyridamole on increased levels of platelet adhesiveness. Report of a controlled clinical trial, *J. Atheroscler. Res.*, **9**:335, 1969.

Millikan, C. H.: "Anticoagulant therapy in cerebrovascular disease," in Cerebrovascular Survey Report for Joint Council Subcommittee on Cerebrovascular Disease, National Institute of Neurological Diseases and Stroke, and National Heart and Lung Institute, edited by R. G. Siekert, National Institutes of Health, Bethesda, Md., 1970, pp. 218-227.

O'Reilly, R. A., and Aggeler, P. M.: Determinants of the response to oral anticoagulant drugs in men, *Pharmacol. Rev.*, **22**:35, 1970.

————, ————, Hoag, M. S., Leong, L. S., and Kropatkin, M. L.: Hereditary transmission of exceptional resistance to coumarin anticoagulant drugs, *New Engl. J. Med.*, **271**:809, 1964.

Richards, R. L., and Begg, T. B.: Long-term anticoagulant therapy in atherosclerotic peripheral arterial disease, *Vascular Diseases*, **4**:27, 1967.

Robinson, D. S., and Sylwester, D.: Interaction of commonly prescribed drugs and warfarin, *Ann. Internal Med.*, **72**:853, 1970.

Vasodilating Agents

McDowell, H. A., Jr., Clark, L. C., Jr., and Galbraith, J. G.: Prevention of cerebral ischemia during carotid occlusion by acetazolamide, *South. Med. J.*, **60**:940, 1967.

McHenry, L. C., Jr., Jaffe, M. E., Kawamura, J., and Goldberg, H. I.: Effect of papaverine on regional blood flow in focal vascular disease of the brain, *New Engl. J. Med.*, **282**:1167, 1970.

Skinhøj, E., and Paulson, O. B.: The mechanism of action of aminophylline upon cerebral vascular disorders, *Acta neurol. scand.*, **46**:129, 1970.

To-day's Drugs: Cerebral vasodilators, *Brit. Med. J.*, **2**:702, 1971.

Hypotensive Medications

Balow, J., Alter, M., and Resch, J. A.: Cerebral thromboembolism: A clinical appraisal of 100 cases, *Neurology*, **16**:559, 1966.

Carter, A. B.: Hypotensive therapy in stroke survivors, *Lancet*, **1**:485, 1970.

Douglas, R. M.: Hypertensive cerebrovascular disease: Considered in relation to treatment with hypotensive drugs, *Med. J. Australia*, **2**:525, 1964.

Hamilton, M., and Kellett, R. J.: The effect of antihypertensive therapy on the course of cerebral vascular disease, *Bull. N. Y. Acad. Med.*, **45**:933, 1969.

Low-Molecular-Weight Dextran

Foster, J. H., Killen, D. A., Jolly, P. C., and Kirtley, J. H.: Low molecular weight dextran in vascular surgery: Prevention of thrombosis following arterial reconstruction in 85 cases, *Ann. Surg.,* **163**:764, 1966.

Gonzalez, D., Gurjian, E. S., and Thomas, L. M.: Dextran 40: Anaphylaxis and stroke: A case report, *Neurology,* **20**:1139, 1970.

Salicylates

Evans, G.: "Effect of platelet-suppressive agents on the incidence of amaurosis fugax and transient cerebral ischemia," in Cerebral Vascular Disorders, Transactions of the Eighth Princeton Conference, edited by F. D. McDowell and W. Brennon, Grune & Stratton, Inc., New York, 1973, p. 297.

MacMillan, D. C.: Effect of salicylates on human platelets, *Lancet,* **1**:1151, 1968.

Additional References

McHenry, L. C., Jr.: Cerebral vasodilator therapy in stroke, *Stroke,* **3**:686, 1972.

Mundall, J., Quintero, P., von Kaulla, K. N., Harmon, R., and Austin, J.: Transient monocular blindness and increased platelet aggregability treated with aspirin. A case report, *Neurology,* **22**:280, 1972.

Toole, J. F., Truscott, B. L., Anderson, W. W., Aronson, P. R., et al. (Clinical Management Study Group): Report of the joint committee for stroke facilities VII. Medical and surgical management of stroke, *Stroke,* **4**:269, 1973.

Surgical Management of Aortocervical Atherosclerosis

No man can be a good physician who has no knowledge of operative surgery, and a surgeon is nothing if ignorant of medicine; a knowledge of both branches is essential.

Lanfranchi

Since the first successful repair of stenosis of the internal carotid artery in the neck was reported in 1954, the surgical management of patients with aortocervical occlusive disease has been the subject of numerous articles describing indications, techniques, and results. Since the publication of the first edition of this book, the results of the Cooperative Study of Surgery for Extracranial Vascular Diseases have been published. All of the material reported by this group has been sifted and, with modifications, forms the basis for this chapter. Surprisingly enough, despite the overwhelming number of cases and procedures from which the statistics have been drawn, there is still room for disagreement with the conclusions of the cooperative group. Among the reasons for this is the fact that the diagnostic and therapeutic skills of the individuals within the participating groups varied, so that in one institution the complication rate from angiography and surgery was high, whereas in another it was low. Furthermore, population groups and case selection varied. Recognizing such inherent defects, we compared these results with those of others who drew their patients from a more uniform population and in which one neurovascular team performed all procedures.

The most revealing product of this study is the fact that about 75 percent of patients with ischemic stroke syndromes were found to have one or more stenoses or occlusions in a surgically accessible site in the neck or chest—the vast majority being in the region of the carotid bifurcation.

In the experience of most surgeons, the surgical mortality associated with attempts at vascular reconstruction on patients with evolving infarction has been as high as 40 to 50 percent. Consequently, except in rare instances, surgery for ischemic brain disease is a prophylactic measure which should never be considered until 30 days after the process has stabilized.

SELECTION OF CANDIDATES FOR SURGERY

In addition, the importance of a team approach has been more than proved. Careful selection of appropriate patients, angiographic visualization of the carotid arteries throughout their entire lengths, skillful surgical and anesthetic techniques, and intensive postoperative care are the steps in what must be an unbroken chain for surgical management of occlusive disorders. If one link is weak or missing, the patient suffers.

The rationale for reconstructive vascular surgery is:

1 To prevent stenosis from progressing to occlusion

2 To establish normal pressures, volume, and direction of flow in patients such as those with high degrees of stenosis or those who have one of the steal syndromes

Surgery may be considered in the following cases:

1 Patients with recurrent episodes of focal neurologic deficit (TIAs) due to microemboli or stenosis; in these instances surgery must be performed after the attack has subsided completely

2 Rarely, patients with recent stabilized infarction and only minimal deficit

3 Asymptomatic patients with over 50 percent stenosis of the cervical carotid artery if surgery is to be performed for other disorders

4 In rare instances for removal of emboli lodged in the thoracic or cervical segments of the aortocranial arteries

As a general rule, patients with TIAs thought to be due to extracranial arterial lesions should be considered for surgery, while those with intracranial lesions should not. Patients with a combination of extracranial and intracranial arterial lesions are not ideal candidates but can be considered for extracranial reconstruction under some circumstances. Experimental attempts are being made to bypass obstruction of intracranial arteries by using microsurgical techniques to anastomose the superficial temporal artery to the middle cerebral artery.

The following physical findings suggest the presence of extracranial obstructions:

1 Bruit over a cervical artery (Chap. 6)

2 Unequal pressures in the ophthalmic or brachial arteries (Chap. 6)

3 Diminished pulsations in the common carotid artery or abnormally reduced or increased in the external carotid branches such as the facial, angular, or superficial temporal arteries

4 Pulse delay in one of the brachial arteries, together with other symptoms suggestive of subclavian steal (Chap. 12)

5 Typical internal carotid artery syndrome, with amaurosis fugax (Chap. 10)

6 Positive carotid artery compression test (Chap. 8)

These abnormalities on the neurovascular examination are, of course, only clues which suggest the need for a more complete evaluation before making a decision concerning medical or surgical management.

Even in the presence of a valid indication for surgery, one must consider the patient's physiological age, the presence of other life-threatening or limiting diseases, the skills of the surgeon, the facilities available for complete evaluation and management of the problem, and any emergencies that might arise.

Because of the risk involved in angiography (1 to 2 percent incidence of permanent neurologic deficit or death) and the surgical procedure itself (see page 211), removal of extracranial arterial obstructions, even when seemingly accessible, is a very serious undertaking, and except in the most unusual circumstances should not be prescribed for asymptomatic patients.

EVALUATION OF PATIENTS FOR POSSIBLE SURGICAL RECONSTRUCTION

A variety of diagnostic procedures common to the evaluation of all patients suspected of having a neurologic disorder, possibly cerebrovascular in nature, must precede consideration of surgery. If the patient is having recurrent attacks, it is wise to begin therapeutic doses of heparin during the preoperative evaluation and to continue this medication until 4 to 6 hr prior to surgery. If a bruit disappears or shows a marked change in intensity during the evaluation, one must consider emergency surgery because of the possibility that further stenosis or even occlusion of the artery is taking place.

Some clinicians also perform a *carotid compression test* (Chap. 8) to evaluate the patient's cerebrovascular reserve. Symptoms or signs of cerebrovascular insufficiency resulting from compression of either carotid artery for 30 sec would be considered a positive indication for arteriography and for the use of a shunt if subsequent repair is to be performed.

Repeated measurements of *ophthalmic artery pressures,* with the patient first erect and then recumbent, are particularly important in patients who are to have carotid reconstruction. The base-line information thus provided is important for the postoperative assessment of the result of surgery.

Arteriography is essential in arriving at a decision concerning the advisability of reconstructive surgery. The origins of the aortocranial arteries from the arch, the proximal, subclavian, and vertebral arteries, and the carotid bifurcation are of particular importance because they can be repaired by the surgeon. The visualization is best accomplished by threading a catheter into the ascending aorta from the right brachial or a femoral artery. Whichever method is chosen, the object is to thrust a large bolus of contrast material into the aortocranial circulation by injecting it under high pressure into the ascending aorta. Although a great deal of this material will flow down the thoracic aorta, enough will enter the brachiocephalic, the left common carotid, and the left subclavian arteries to opacify them and their branches up to the base of the skull. Rapid serial exposures of x-ray film will then allow one to assess the dynamics of the aortocervical circulation and to locate stenoses and occlusions.

No matter which of the methods for filling the aortic arch is used, only the extracranial segments of the aortocranial vessels can be seen consistently with techniques available at present. However, the use of an arterial catheter allows one to see the entire length of any artery by placing the tip in its ostium and injecting it separately. In addition, the catheter method allows pressure measurements to be taken and gradients to be determined.

Unfortunately, the catheter technique requires a degree of skill that many physicians do not have, and many succumb to the temptation to inject the contrast material by needle directly into the artery through a puncture in the neck. This technique is to be condemned for two reasons: (1) it allows visualization only of the segment distal to the puncture, not of the entire length, and (2) more important, it traumatizes diseased arteries. In most series the morbidity associated with puncture of the carotid artery in the neck is about 3 percent, and the mortality nearly 1 percent. Retrograde arteriography of the aortic arch, even though it is more expensive and time-consuming, is associated with fewer complications, and provides more complete information concerning the extracranial portion of the circulation. However, even the retrograde catheter techniques can be dangerous in inexperienced hands.

Depending upon one's school of thought, the following list of abnormalities, visible by angiography, are considered remediable by surgery.

1 Stenosis greater than 50 percent
2 Plaques with thrombus formation or ulcerations
3 Atherosclerotic or embolic obstruction
4 Kinks
5 Loops
6 Fascial bands constricting an artery
7 Osteophytes compressing an artery

Stenosis Greater than 50 Percent

Obstruction of greater than 50 percent to the cross-sectional area of a vessel lumen causes a reduction in pressure in the distal artery and its branches (Fig. 17-1). Volume of flow is reduced when the luminal diameter has been reduced by 90 percent. Consequently, lesions greater than 50 percent should be considered for operation. However, the lesion must be in an accessible location and the patient must have symptoms attributable to the lesion.

When lesions are found, the patient's symptoms can usually be related to the artery supplying the ischemic area. Removal of the lesion prevents further episodes. There are times, however, when stenosis or occlusion of three or rarely four arteries does not result in symptoms of cerebrovascular insufficiency. In other in-

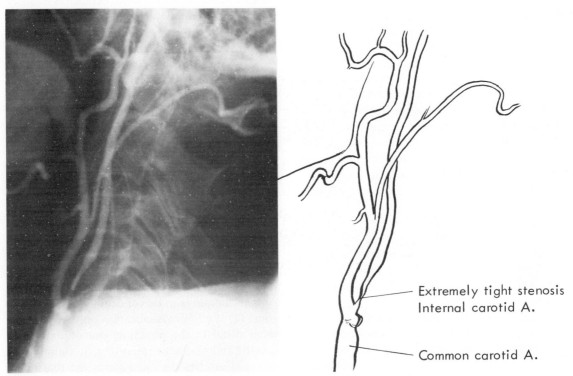

Extremely tight stenosis
Internal carotid A.

Common carotid A.

Figure 17-1 "Slim sign" of carotid stenosis which can be mistaken for hypoplasia of the artery. *(Courtesy of Dr. F. Farrell, Department of Radiology, Bowman Gray School of Medicine.)*

stances, carotid artery obstruction causes symptoms of vertebral-basilar insufficiency. The reverse case of vertebral obstructions causing abnormality in areas normally supplied by the carotid artery also occurs, though less frequently. Surgery should be directed at the offending lesion even if it is not in the artery normally supplying the involved territory.

Stenosis at One Carotid Bifurcation These patients are the ideal candidates for reconstructive surgery. Yet, even in this group lasting neurologic deficit or mortality approaches 2 percent. (Fig. 17-2).

Stenosis of Both Carotids at Their Bifurcations The more arteries repaired, the greater the op-

erative risk. The conservative approach is to repair only the symptomatic artery, although some surgeons advocate reconstruction of the more markedly stenotic artery (whether symptomatic or not) and a second operation 10 days later on the other artery.

Multiple Stenoses of One Carotid These so-called tandem lesions are found usually (1) at the carotid bifurcation in the neck and (2) intracranially at the siphon. Repair of the accessible cervical stenosis depends upon the condition of the inaccessible lesion. If the intracranial stenosis compromises the lumen by more than 80 percent, reconstruction of the cervical lesions is not justifiable because flow through the distal segment would not be increased.

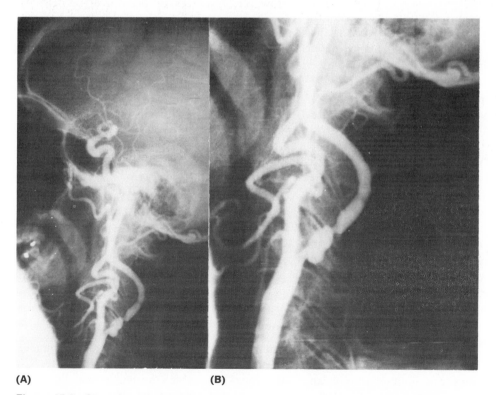

(A) **(B)**

Figure 17-2 Stenosis and ulceration of internal carotid artery near its origin. (B) Enlargement of (A) *(Courtesy of Dr. F. Farrell, Department of Radiology, Bowman Gray School of Medicine.)*

Stenosis of One and Occlusion of the Other Carotid It is estimated that symptoms are related to the occluded carotid in 30 percent of patients, to the carotid stenosis in 10 percent, and to both carotids in 50 percent. In the remaining 10 percent symptoms are attributable to the vertebral-basilar system.

The occluded artery should be explored if the appearance of the angiogram leads one to suspect a recent occlusion because, in a small percentage of cases, flow can be restored even after several weeks of apparent occlusion. Two weeks thereafter the stenotic carotid should be repaired.

Occlusion of One Cervical Carotid Artery Because flow can be reestablished in some cases, exploration is recommended if it is suspected that the occlusion occurred within the preceding month. There must be no signs of evolving infarction, and the patient's condition must have been stabilized for 3 weeks before operation.

Subclavian-Vertebral Artery Stenosis or Occlusion Operative results for such lesions are difficult to assess. When stenosis of one vertebral is associated with obstruction of the other due to anomaly or disease, the patient probably should be treated medically. When these lesions coexist with carotid abnormalities, repair of the carotid is the procedure of choice.

Intrathoracic Arterial Lesions Except in cases of Takayasu's disease and the subclavian steal syndrome, very few surgeons attempt arterial reconstruction for cerebrovascular insufficiency. (See appropriate chapters.)

Plaques with Thrombus Formation or Ulcerations

Ulcerations in plaques seen on angiography can be the source for microembolism and should be treated surgically by removal or medically with anticoagulants. These modes of treatment are discussed more fully in Chap. 16.

Atherosclerotic or Embolic Obstruction

As a general rule occlusions should not be operated upon for 3 weeks unless the patient has minimal deficit. The reason for this is the very real danger of converting an ischemic infarction into a hemorrhagic lesion when pressure is restored in the distal arterial tree. The mortality following operations on patients with evolving infarction of large size approaches 50 percent. The percentage of successful reestablishment of back flow in a chronically occluded carotid artery is estimated to be less than 20 percent. Some surgeons have used a Fogarty catheter to extract intracranial extension of the thrombus. However, instances of postoperative development of caroticocavernous fistula have been reported. Most physicians recommend the use of anticoagulants in such patients to reduce propagation of clot and to maintain the patient until flow can be restored safely 3 weeks after the neurologic status has stabilized.

Kinks

When an artery becomes sclerotic it elongates and becomes stiff. Because the carotid artery is mobile in the neck, elongation forces the normal segment to kink or buckle. Kinks rarely occur in the subclavian-vertebral system.

The effects of these kinks on pressure and flow through the artery can vary with change of position of the head on the neck and at times can almost completely obstruct flow. In these cases the kink should be removed.

Loops

These are considered to be congenital anomalies in an artery which is unusually long. Because the vessel is pliable, the coil is usually gentle and does not impair flow. They should not be repaired.

Fascial Bands Constricting an Artery

When these constrict an artery and cause symptoms, they should be removed.

Osteophytes Compressing an Artery

Osteophytes compress cervical segments of the vertebral arteries and at times seem to cause symptoms related to the position of the head on the neck. Few surgeons are enthusiastic about removing them, however.

SURGICAL PROCEDURES AND TECHNIQUES

The available surgical procedures range from the most conservative (endarterectomy with removal of the offending plaque) to radical operations in which large segments of stenotic and occluded arteries are bypassed with Dacron grafts attached to the arch of the aorta and to the distal segments of the vessels. In some cases dissection of the artery by CO_2 under pressure is favored. Most surgeons have a natural preference for the more conservative operations, such as endarterectomy followed by patch-grafting either with vein or with Dacron. These procedures are quite satisfactory, and clotting in the vessel operated upon is not a frequent problem, particularly if the patient is started on heparin as soon as the artery is sutured. Furthermore, the arteries usually remain patent and in many cases follow-up angiograms as long as 15 years after surgery have demonstrated no recurrence of stenosis.

Some surgeons perform operations on the carotid artery under local anesthesia, so that they can be warned of cerebral complications by the patient's failure to respond appropriately to commands. Others monitor their patients with electroencephalography or measurements of oxygen tension in the internal jugular vein. The carotid artery supplying the nondominant hemisphere should be repaired first, followed by repair of the other carotid and the subclavian or vertebral artery. This sequence is intended to protect the critical areas of brain, but because of the vagaries of the circle of Willis and of the collateral circulation of the brain, it does not always succeed.

Some surgeons operate with the patient in a state of controlled *hypertension* induced by methoxamine hydrochloride (Vasoxyl) or phenylephrine hydrochloride (Neo-Synephrine); their theory is that elevation of the systemic blood pressure increases cerebral perfusion. Others have the anesthesiologist administer 5 percent carbon dioxide in the gas mixture during the critical portion of the operation, in order to obtain maximum cerebral vasodilatation and flow through the cerebral vessels while the diseased carotid is occluded by clamps.

It is wise to put an internal shunt in the artery in order to maintain distal perfusion throughout the operation. Such shunts are harmless, can be inserted and removed easily, and add little extra time to the procedure.

Many surgeons measure the arterial pressure proximal and distal to the lesion before and after surgery, in order to obtain objective evidence that flow is reduced and a pressure gradient exists and has been corrected by the operation. Others sever the afferent nerves of the carotid sinus (Hering's nerve) to prevent the possibility of future hypersensitive reaction of the sinus, and still others denervate the sinus and cut the cervical sympathetic chain.

POSTOPERATIVE EVALUATION AND CARE

Anticoagulants such as heparin, aspirin, and coumarin, or antisludging agents such as low-molecular-weight dextran are often given for at least a week following surgery on any of the carotid, subclavian, or vertebral arteries. Many authorities continue use of anticoagulants for at least a month. Following carotid surgery particularly, measurements of pressure in the ophthalmic arteries and palpation of pulses in the

superficial temporal arteries must begin immediately and continue at very frequent intervals
for the first week, with a gradual lengthening of
the interval between determinations thereafter.
Time and again, a sudden reduction in ophthalmic pressure is the first indication of a clot at
the operative site in the internal carotid. Hypopulsation in the superficial temporal artery pres-
ages similar events in the external carotid system. If either of these signs appears or if the
patient's neurologic status deteriorates, the
wound should be reopened immediately, with
the expectation of performing a thrombectomy.
In equivocal cases there may be time to perform
an angiogram first.

Bilateral determination of the brachial blood
pressures is the only diagnostic test that will
give similar information about the subclavian-
vertebral system; this should be done at frequent intervals. At the same time one should
listen for bruits over the chest, neck, head, and
orbits. Although such bruits sometimes afford a
clue to recurrent stenosis or occlusion, we have
found them to be rather unreliable in the postoperative period and recommend a repetition of
angiography if the need arises.

SURGICAL MORBIDITY AND FOLLOW-UP

Operative mortality varies from 1 to 10 percent.
This, coupled with the morbidity (3 percent)
and mortality (0.7 percent) associated with preoperative arteriography, makes many physicians hesitant to suggest remedial surgery for
any patient with symptoms of aortocranial disease. However, surgeons with broad experience
have reduced their operative mortality to about
1 percent. Nevertheless, the complication rates
remain high (about 5 percent in most series are
made worse by the operation). Despite these
dangers, it is our opinion that for a young patient with recurrent episodes of dysfunction due
to carotid lesion, the prospect of a lifetime of
anticoagulant therapy or the danger of a perma-

nent neurologic deficit makes remedial surgery
imperative. For those with vertebral-basilar insufficiency secondary to plaques situated near
the origins of the vertebrals, the justification for
surgery seems tenuous. Patients suffering with
one of the "steal" syndromes should have surgical repair if attacks of insufficiency are frequent
or prolonged.

SUGGESTED READINGS

General

Crawford, E. S., DeBakey, M. E., Morris, G. C., and
Howell, J. F.: Surgical treatment of occlusion of
the innominate, common carotid, and subclavian
arteries: A 10 year experience, Surgery, 65:17,
1969.
Julian, O. C., and Javid, H.: Surgical management of
cerebral arterial insufficiency, Current Problems
Surg., March 1971.

Selection of Candidates for Surgery

Blaisdell, W. F., Clauss, R. H., Galbraith, J. G., Imparato, A. M., and Wylie, E. J.: Joint study of extracranial arterial occlusion. IV. A review of surgical considerations, J.A.M.A., 209:1889, 1969.
Dickinson, C. J.: Functional efficiency of the circle of
Willis: Implications for reconstructive surgery of
main cerebral arteries, Brit. Med. J., 1:858, 1961.
Gurdjian, E. S., Portnoy, H. D., Hardy, W. G., Lindner, D. W., and Thomas, L. M.: Evaluation of tortuosity of extracranial vessels, Angiology, 15:261,
1964.
Labauge, R., Thévenet, A., Crouzet, G., and Nivolas,
M.: Les insuffisances vertébro-basilaires d'incidence chirurgicale. (À propos de 87 malades
opérés), Rev. neurol., 117:373, 1967.
Rob, C. G.: Operation for acute completed stroke
due to thrombosis of the internal carotid artery,
Surgery, 65:862, 1969.
Thompson, J. E.: Surgery for Cerebrovascular Insufficiency (Stroke); with Special Emphasis on Carotid Endarterectomy, Charles C Thomas, Publisher, Springfield, Ill., 1968.
———, Austin, D. J., and Patman, R. D.:
Endarterectomy of the totally occluded carotid ar-

tery for stroke; Results in 100 operations, *Arch. Surg.,* **95**:791, 1967.

Wise, G. R.: Vasopressor-drug therapy for complications of cerebral arteriography, *New Engl. J. Med.,* **282**:610, 1970.

Evaluation and Preparation of the Patient for Surgery

Acheson, J., Boyd, W. N., Hugh, A. E., and Hutchinson, E. C.: Cerebral angiography in ischemic cerebrovascular disease, *Arch. Neurol.,* **20**:527, 1969.

Alexander, S. C., and Lassen, N. A.: Cerebral circulatory response to acute brain disease: Implications for anesthetic practice, *Anesthesiology,* **32**:60, 1970.

Bergström, K., and Lodin, H.: Arteriovenous fistula as a complication of cerebral angiography: Report of three cases, *Brit. J. Radiol.,* **39**:263, 1966.

Brinkman, C. A.: Brain scanning as an aid to surgery for strokes, *Am. J. Surg.,* **119**:452, 1970.

Galbraith, J. G.: Safeguards in carotid surgery, *Surgery,* **63**:1019, 1968.

Gurdjian, E. S., Lindner, D. W., Hardy, W. G., and Thomas, L. M.: Incidence of surgically treatable lesions in cases studied angiographically, *Neurology,* **11**(4)(part 2):150, 1961.

———, and Thomas, L. M.: Evaluation and indications for surgery in extracranial cerebrovascular disease, *J. Neurosurg.,* **26**:235, 1967.

McCleery, W. N. C., and Lewtas, N. A.: Subarachnoid injection of contrast medium: A complication of vertebral angiography, *Brit. J. Radiol.,* **39**:112, 1966.

McLean, C. E., Clason, W. P. C., and Stoughton, P. V.: The peripheral pulse as a diagnostic tool, *Angiology,* **15**:221, 1964.

Shenkin, H. A., Haft, H., and Somach, F. M.: Prognostic significance of arteriography in non-hemorrhagic strokes, *J.A.M.A.,* **194**:612, 1965.

White, C. W., Jr., Allarde, R. R., and McDowell, H. A.: Anesthetic management for carotid artery surgery, *J.A.M.A.,* **202**:1023, 1967.

Surgical Procedures and Techniques

Annotation: Restitution of internal carotid artery, *Lancet,* **1**:813, 1961.

Bakay, L., and Leslie, E. V.: Surgical treatment of vertebral artery insufficiency caused by cervical spondylosis, *J. Neurosurg.,* **23**:596, 1965.

Decker, K.: Komplikationen bei Angiographien der Hirngefässe—eine Übersicht nach 24,000 Untersuchungen, *Zentbl. Neurochir.,* **30**:299, 1969.

Eastcott, H. H. G., Pickering, G. W., and Rob, C. G.: Reconstruction of the internal carotid artery in a patient with intermittent attacks of hemiplegia, *Lancet,* **2**:994, 1954.

Hardin, C. A.: Operative treatment of extracranial artery occlusion: Results of 224 cases, *Arch. Surg.,* **91**:180, 1965.

Hass, W. K., Fields, W. S., North, R. R., Kricheff, I. I., Chase, N. E., and Bauer, R. B.: Joint study of extracranial arterial occlusion. II. Arteriography, techniques, sites, and complications, *J.A.M.A.,* **203**:961, 1968.

Humphries, A. W., Young, J. R., Beven, E. G., LeFevre, F. A., and deWolfe, V. G.: Relief of vertebrobasilar symptoms by carotid endarterectomy, *Surgery,* **57**:48, 1965.

Nagashima, C.: Surgical treatment of vertebral artery insufficiency caused by cervical spondylosis, *J. Neurosurg.,* **32**:512, 1970.

Sobel, S., Kaplitt, M. J., Reingold, M., and Sawyer, P. N.: Gas endarterectomy, *Surgery,* **59**:517, 1966.

Thompson, J. E.: Cerebral protection during carotid endarterectomy, *J.A.M.A.,* **202**:1046, 1967.

Postoperative Evaluation and Care

Adams, J. E., Smith, M. C., and Wylie, E. J.: Cerebral blood flow and hemodynamics in extracranial vascular disease: Effect of endarterectomy, *Surgery,* **53**:449, 1963.

Bauer, R. B., Boulos, R. S., and Meyer, J. S.: Natural history and surgical treatment of occlusive cerebrovascular disease evaluated by serial arteriography, *Am. J. Roentgenol.,* **104**:1, 1968.

Goldstein, S. S., Kleinknecht, R. A., and Gallo, A. E., Jr.: Neuropsychological changes associated with carotid endarterectomy, *Cortex,* **6**:308, 1970.

Hardy, J. D.: On the reversibility of strokes: Case of carotid artery repair with prompt recovery after hemiplegia and coma for two days, *Ann. Surg.,* **158**:1035, 1963.

Powers, S. R., Drislane, T. M., and Iandoli, E. W.:

The surgical treatment of vertebral artery insufficiency: Successes and failures, *Arch. Surg.*, **86**:60, 1963.

Schutz, H., Fleming, J. F. R., and Awerbuck, B.: Arteriographic assessment of carotid endarterectomy, *Ann. Surg.*, **171**:509, 1970.

Surgical Morbidity and Follow-up

Barker, W. F., Stern, W. E., Krayenbühl, H., and Senning, A.: Carotid endarterectomy complicated by carotid cavernous sinus fistula, *Ann. Surg.*, **167**:568, 1968.

Bauer, R. B., Meyer, J. S., Fields, W. S., Remington, R., Macdonald, M. C., and Callen, P.: Joint study of extracranial arterial occlusion. III. Progress report of controlled study of long-term survival in patients with and without operation, *J.A.M.A.*, **208**:509, 1969.

Bland, J. E., Chapman, R. D., and Wylie, E. J.: Neurological complications of carotid artery surgery, *Ann. Surg.*, **171**:459, 1970.

Boysen, G.: Cerebral hemodynamics in carotid surgery, *Acta. neurol. scand.*, **49** (suppl. 52), 1973.

Calo, A. A.: Sinus tachycardia and electrocardiographic changes following bilateral carotid artery occlusion and endarterectomy, *Angiology*, **19**:408, 1968.

Greenstone, S. M., Massell, T. B., and Heringmen, E. C.: Hazards and complications of retrograde aortography and arteriography, *Angiology*, **16**:93, 1965.

Heyman, A., Young, W. G., Jr., Brown, I. W., Jr., and Grimson, K. S.: Long-term results of endarterectomy of the internal carotid artery for cerebral ischemia and infarction, *Circulation*, **36**:212, 1967.

Maddison, F. E.: Arteriographic evaluation of carotid artery surgery, *Am. J. Roentgenol.*, **109**:121, 1970.

Murphey, F., and Maccubbin, D. A.: Carotid endarterectomy: A long-term follow-up study, *J. Neurosurg.*, **23**:156, 1965.

Silverman, S. M., Bergman, P. S., and Bender, M. B.: The dynamics of transient cerebral blindness: Report of nine episodes following vertebral angiography, *Arch. Neurol.*, **4**:333, 1961.

Silverstein, A.: Arteriography of stroke: III. Complications, *Arch. Neurol.*, **15**:206, 1966.

Wylie, E. J., Hein, M. F., and Adams, J. F.: Intracranial hemorrhage following revascularization for treatment of acute strokes, *J. Neurosurg.*, **21**:212, 1964.

Additional References

Javid, H., Ostermiller, W. E., Hengesh, J. W., Dye, W. S., Hunter, J. A., Najafi, H., and Julian, O. C.: Carotid endarterectomy for asymptomatic patients, *Arch. Surg.*, **102**:389, 1971.

Najafi, H., Javid, H., Dye, W. S., Hunter, J. A., Wideman, F. E., and Julian, O. C.: Emergency carotid thromboendarterectomy. Surgical indications and results, *Arch. Surg.*, **103**:610, 1971.

Vakkur, G. J.: Extracranial arterial occlusion, *J.A.M.A.*, **214**:374, 1970.

Cerebral Embolism

It is with anticoagulation as with love: rather easy to do, but difficult to understand.

Anonymous

In the adult the cerebrovascular bed strains a maximum of 20 percent of circulating blood, yet almost 50 percent of all symptom-producing arterial emboli lodge in the brain, accounting for 5 to 15 percent of strokes. Consequently, neurologic deficit is often an initial manifestation of multiple emboli to many parts of the body.

There are probably two reasons for the frequency of clinical signs of cerebral embolism:

1 Much of the brain is exquisitely sensitive to obstruction of its blood flow. A 1-mm speck of obstructing material lodged in an artery of the brainstem can produce a disastrous neurologic deficit, but if lodged in another organ of the body or in the extremities it will be asymptomatic.

2 The great vessels arise from the aortic arch in such a way that solid material expelled from the left ventricle tends to enter the brachiocephalic artery and the left common carotid, so that it goes to the brain instead of rounding the arch.

The vast majority of intracranial emboli lodge in the cerebral hemispheres, undoubtedly because the amount of blood traversing the carotid (more than 300 ml per min) is far greater than that carried by the vertebral artery (less than 100 ml per min), and also because of the circuitous route which foreign bodies must take in order to enter the vertebral system from the subclavian arteries. Because the middle cerebral artery is a direct continuation of the internal carotid, and because nearly 80 percent of the blood traveling through the internal carotid perfuses the area supplied by the middle cerebral, emboli that reach either internal carotid traverse the direct route into the trunk of the middle cerebral and lodge in one of its branches, often the ascending frontal. Consequently, recurring emboli have a tendency to lodge in the same cerebral artery.

The spinal cord is so rarely involved by embolus that some authorities would categorically state that embolus to a spinal artery never occurs, but an embolus lodged in the abdominal aorta can obstruct perfusion of the cord and cause neurologic deficit.

ETIOLOGY

The type of embolus (Fig. 18-1) varies with the age of the patient. Emboli subsequent to rheumatic valvular heart disease tend to occur in younger adults; those secondary to cholesterol plaques are seen most often in older patients.

Blood Clot

The most frequent cause of cerebral embolism is a blood clot from the heart—the result of valvular or endocardial disease. Clots form most frequently on cusps damaged by rheumatic fever, on the mural endocardium of the left atrium, and on the damaged left ventricular endocardium after myocardial infarction. When they become large enough, the continued movement of the beating heart throws them off into the systemic circulation. Atrial fibrillation increases this possibility enormously.

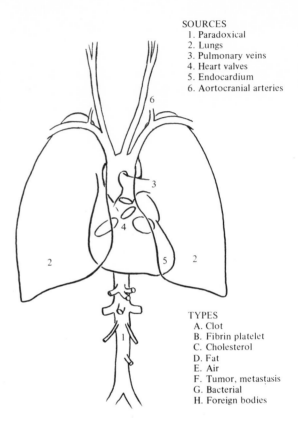

SOURCES
1. Paradoxical
2. Lungs
3. Pulmonary veins
4. Heart valves
5. Endocardium
6. Aortocranial arteries

TYPES
A. Clot
B. Fibrin platelet
C. Cholesterol
D. Fat
E. Air
F. Tumor, metastasis
G. Bacterial
H. Foreign bodies

Figure 18-1 Sources and types of cerebral emboli.

The eight cardiac conditions that may lead to cerebral emboli are:

1 Active rheumatic endocarditis; cerebral emboli are found in almost all fatal cases.
2 Postrheumatic valvular disease; 50 percent of emboli from rheumatic valves are intracranial.
3 Bacterial endocarditis, either acute or subacute.
4 Myocardial infarction with a mural thrombus; cerebral embolus may be the first sign of an otherwise silent infarction.
5 Congenital heart disease.
6 Cardiac surgery.
7 Prosthetic valves.

8 Marantic endocarditis in patients with carcinomatosis or collagen vascular disease.

The second most frequent source of blood clot emboli is the pulmonary veins. Cardiac decompensation, by increasing venous pressure and impairing the circulation of blood from the pulmonary veins, leads to formation of the clot.

A paradoxical embolus from the veins of the legs, the pelvic plexus, or even the liver may circumvent the pulmonary circulation, pass into the left atrium through a patent foramen ovale if the right atrial pressure is higher than the left, and continue into the cerebral circulation. This inverted pressure gradient occurs in cases of cardiac decompensation and tricuspid atresia. In patients with tetrad of Fallot who have a high pressure in the right ventricle and a patent interventricular septum, a similar situation exists without the cardiac decompensation. This unusual situation is stressed in medical teaching solely because of the interplay of embryology, anatomy, and pathophysiology required to understand its cause. In the fetus and newborn infant, however, the patent ductus arteriosus normally functions as a shunt from venous to arterial systems, and paradoxical emboli may occur more often, perhaps even from the umbilical vein following its ligation at birth.

Cholesterol and Fibrin Platelet

Probably ranking third as causes of cerebral embolism are emboli made up of cholesterol crystals which are thrown off from atheromatous plaques situated on the carotid and vertebral-basilar arteries. It is suspected that these plaques form slowly over the years and that if they become ulcerated they may discharge cholesterol crystals which obstruct distal arteries and produce infarctions. In other cases, the plaques may accumulate platelets and stringy clots of fibrin, which may be dislodged into the arterial stream by trauma to the arteries during compression, arteriography, or ligation.

Metastatic Deposits

Carcinomas of the lung, breast, stomach, kidney, and thyroid, as well as malignant melanomas, tend to lodge their metastatic deposits in the brain. The seeds of these neoplasms are carried in the bloodstream, usually as very small aggregates of cells that are asymptomatic until they take root in the brain and grow sufficiently to exert their influence as tumors. Some tumors, such as myxomas of the heart and certain lung neoplasms, occasionally send off metastatic emboli that are large enough to obstruct an artery and produce immediate neurologic deficit. In occasional cases, the primary tumor is so small that it is not detectable; neurologic signs caused by the embolus are then the first manifestations of the neoplasm.

Parasites and Ova

Various parasites—*Trichinella spiralis, Entamoeba histolytica,* cysticercus, and *Plasmodium falciparum* among others—may lodge and encyst in the small arteries of the brain.

Septic Emboli

Septic emboli, in addition to producing the same effects as those which are sterile, contain organisms that may proliferate to cause endarteritis, mycotic aneurysm, perforation of the artery, cerebritis, and brain abscess, or any combination of these conditions. Bacterial endocarditis is the most frequent cause of this chain of events. Pulmonary thrombophlebitis caused by bronchiectasis, lung abscess, or pneumonia can also be a source of septic emboli. Addicts who are not careful with intravenous medications are especially susceptible.

Emboli Caused by Trauma

Air and Foreign Bodies Trauma to systemic veins, the heart, lungs, or aortocranial arteries can introduce air or solid foreign bodies which move to the brain. Among the agents that have been inadvertently or maliciously introduced into the arterial tree are bullets, air, calcium from the heart valves, antifoaming agents, talcum crystals, cotton, and even catheters. All these obstruct arteries and can produce neurologic deficit. Air is particularly dangerous because it mixes so well with blood and is so widely distributed within the cerebral arterial circulation. The most common causes of this disaster are surgical procedures involving the dural sinuses or veins of the head, neck, and chest, and operations on the heart, both those utilizing bypass pump oxygenators and those done with the closed approach.

Fat Fat embolism is an occasional complication of trauma to long bones, especially those which contain marrow. Several days following crushing injury or fracture the patient develops signs secondary to obstruction of myriads of pulmonary, cerebral, and renal capillaries by fat globules.

There are two theories as to the source of these globules: (1) the crushed adipose cells of the marrow release fat into the marrow veins; (2) the normally emulsified chylomicra of the bloodstream aggregate into large globules which cannot pass through capillary beds.

Nitrogen Bubbles (Caisson Disease)

In persons who are subjected to rapid changes in atmospheric pressure, such as submariners and aviators, embolism caused by bubbles of nitrogen is the most frequent cause of neurologic abnormality. These bubbles form from inert nitrogen normally dissolved in the blood when atmospheric pressure is normal or high. When pressure is suddenly reduced, bubbles form, much as carbon dioxide foam forms when the cap is removed from a warm bottle of beer. They act as a vapor lock which plugs myriads of small arterioles and capillaries, producing tissue anoxia.

PATHOLOGIC PHYSIOLOGY

A blood clot is the most common cause of embolism. However, any solid, liquid, or gaseous foreign material can obstruct the flow of blood through an artery and produce anoxia in the tissue distal to the obstruction. In addition to obstruction, the foreign material may act as an irritant, causing vasospasm locally in the segment wherein it lodges or diffusely in an entire arterial bed. Therefore, not only the artery it obstructs but also the effect it has upon the vascular tree determines the neurologic abnormalities which occur. First and foremost, the syndrome produced depends on the vessel obstructed. An embolus large enough to lodge in the common carotid artery and obliterate all distal blood flow produces a different set of symptoms from one that lodges in a terminal branch of the middle cerebral artery, unless the latter causes massive vasospasm. This interplay between the branch occluded and the response of the vascular tree varies from person to person, some patients responding with intense spasm to a small embolus and others tolerating a large one with little or no spasm. Spasm seems to occur more frequently in younger patients, perhaps because their arteries are not sclerotic.

An embolus dislodged into the aortocranial circulation may or may not enter an artery destined for the eye or the brain. The flow through the internal carotid is about three times that of the external, and although fragments tend more often to travel into the internal carotid, some foreign material in the common carotid may be swept into the external carotid system to the mucous membranes and skin rather than traversing the internal carotid to the brain.

The initial obstruction generally occurs at the bifurcation of a vessel, because the lumens of the branches are smaller than those of the parent artery. In this location an embolus may obstruct one or both of the branches, to produce hypoxia of distal tissue. Stasis of the blood column leads to rouleaux formation and to clumping and settling of the formed elements along the inferior surface of the lumen, proximally as well as distally. As tissue metabolism continues, carbon dioxide accumulates locally, causing maximal dilatation of arteries, capillaries, and veins in the area. Neuron function ceases within seconds, and if collateral channels do not take over immediately, capillary diapedesis and necrosis of the supportive structures begin soon thereafter. If the embolus moves on into distal branches before irreversible changes begin, neuron function is promptly restored.

When, as usually happens, an embolus which initially has lodged for some time at a bifurcation breaks up, the pieces traverse branches through which the whole embolus could not pass. As they proceed distally into the necrosing area, the flow of blood through the now-weakened arterial system is reestablished, changing what had been a bloodless area into a hemorrhagic one. Consequently, in patients with cerebral embolism, hemorrhagic infarctions frequently exist side by side with anemic infarctions (Fig. 18-2). This situation is unusual in cases of nonembolic cerebral infarction.

In contrast to the local dilatation produced by carbon dioxide, spasm may occur in a large portion of the regional arterial bed as soon as the foreign material has entered it. The result is ischemia and perhaps infarction in areas remote from the embolus itself.

PATHOLOGIC FINDINGS

In many cases with a clinical picture typical of cerebral embolism, emboli may not be found at autopsy, even when the vessels are laid out and dissected millimeter by millimeter. Many explanations for this apparent lack of clinicopathologic correlation have been offered. The most plausible are as follows:

1 Massive vasospasm may occur in response to a very small embolus, so that a large deficit is produced by a small foreign body.
2 The original large embolus may divide into smaller and smaller fragments, which lodge in

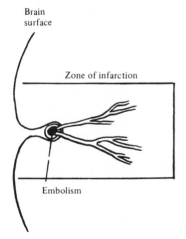
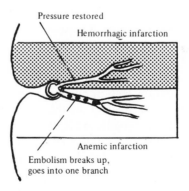

Figure 18-2 Possible pathogenesis of hemorrhagic infarction in cerebral embolism.

distal arterioles and thus are not visible at autopsy.

3 Alcohol used to fix the brain may dissolve emboli such as cholesterol.

4 Blood clots temporarily obstructing the cerebral circulation may be dissolved by normal fibrinolysis.

Despite the failure to demonstrate emboli in many cases, anatomic characteristics of cerebral embolism are such that the presence of emboli may be suspected even when they are not demonstrated.

Hemorrhagic cerebral infarction is the typical lesion produced by obstruction of one of the larger cerebral arteries, such as a leptomeningeal branch. In such cases the uncut brain usually shows edema over a large area, which is often stippled with multiple petechial hemorrhages. The gyri are swollen and purplish brown. A section made through the lesion shows it to involve primarily the cortex and subcortical white matter. Microscopic study shows varying amounts of disintegration of neurons, myelin sheaths, and neuroglia, together with perivascular hemorrhages.

Septic emboli have a similar distribution but frequently lead to suppuration and abscess formation. Metastatic emboli may also result in acute infarction at times. Parasites blocking the cerebral capillaries produce ischemia, hemorrhage, and a fibroglial response or granulomatous masses; often calcification is seen in association with parasitic lesions.

In patients dying of fat embolism, the lungs and kidneys as well as the brain are involved. The brain is edematous, and on section numerous petechial hemorrhages are evident in the white matter with little if any involvement of the gray matter. In microscopic examination sudanophilic granules are seen equally distributed throughout the gray and white matter, but the rich capillary anastomotic arrangement of the gray matter causes it to be free of hemorrhage and microinfarction.

In contrast to the above picture, there are no characteristic changes in the brain of a patient dying with air embolism. The arteries supplying it may show bubbles of air, and there may be large quantities of air in the right atrium and ventricle which bubble out if the organ is opened under water.

Even when the embolus itself cannot be found, its source can usually be demonstrated. This is most often the pulmonary veins, the left atrium or its auricular appendage, the mitral valve, or the endocardium of the left ventricle; the aortic valve is rarely a source of emboli. In the presence of chronic pulmonary infection, one must always consider the possibility that the cause of neurologic deficit was septic embolus.

Occasionally, but not often, a thrombus is dislodged so completely that no remaining clot can be found at the primary site. When this occurs, the massive embolus from the pulmonary veins, the left atrium, or the auricular appendage may produce an acute obstruction of the orifice of the mitral valve (with resulting sudden anoxia); or it may pass through the left ventricle to lodge in the ostium of one of the great vessels coming off the arch. Such massive emboli can always be found.

Emboli which originate or lodge in the cervical arteries are seldom searched for. The standard autopsy technique does not include examination of the length of the carotid, the subclavian, and the vertebral arteries. These are terra incognita as far as postmortem correlation of clinical findings is concerned. Yet emboli can lodge in these arteries, and their atheromatous plaques do serve as nidi for clots which may be cast off as emboli to the brain. Therefore whenever the heart and lungs do not reveal the source of an embolus to the brain, it is important to dissect out the cervical segments of the aortocranial arteries.

CLINICAL FEATURES

Almost without exception, a single nonseptic embolus to the nervous system announces itself with sudden loss of neurologic function. Although headache is not always a symptom, it often develops on the side where the embolus is lodged. Consciousness is preserved, and no disturbance of vital functions results unless, as rarely happens, a large clot obstructs a major vessel such as the carotid, or a shower of emboli is distributed simultaneously through many vessels, including the brainstem. Then delirium, stupor, or coma may occur, and signs of cerebral edema with elevated intracranial pressure may ensue. Ischemic brain tissue may cause focal seizures in a few patients, but the usual deficit is abrupt hemiplegia or a visual field defect. If the dominant hemisphere is involved, aphasia often occurs as well.

Sometimes the mode of onset does not suggest the diagnosis of embolus, and the true nature of the problem is understood only after the past history has been carefully reviewed. Emboli may strike during rest or physical exertion, when the patient is awake or asleep. In patients with symptoms suggestive of long-standing valvular heart disease or of a chronic lung infection such as bronchiectasis or abscess, the probability of embolism is high. A past history of sudden pain in the abdomen or flanks suggests a previous embolus to an abdominal organ or to a kidney.

When seen soon after onset of an attack, the patient may be aphasic, hemiplegic, or hemianoptic. He is usually alert and comprehends commands. Agitation and psychosis are unusual and occur most often in patients with cardiac decompensation, which at times is the sole manifestation of embolus. When these manifestations occur, a large embolus obstructing the carotid or vertebral-basilar system or a shower of emboli diffusely distributed to the brain should be considered.

Since sterile emboli seldom, if ever, lead to bleeding into the brain substance or spinal fluid, the neck is supple and the vital signs are normal. Neither fever nor leukocytosis is present unless the patient has a systemic illness such as subacute bacterial endocarditis or chronic lung abscess, or unless the obstruction is due to fat embolism. On the other hand, subarachnoid hemorrhage may occasionally be the presenting manifestation of septic microembolism.

Although the general examination yields many clues, no neurologic signs are pathognomonic for embolus. Systematic palpation of the peripheral arteries may yield evidence of emboli to arteries supplying the extremities. In a young person absence of any pulse suggests embolus. Petechiae in the skin, nail beds of fingers and toes, conjunctivae, and mucous membranes of the mouth must be sought with particular care. The presence of many small (1 mm), brownish petechiae in the skin of the thorax and axillae is highly suggestive of fat embolism. The lungs must be skillfully auscultated for abnormal breath sounds, and the heart and great vessels for murmurs. Myxoma of the heart may be silent, but valvular heart disease usually announces itself with the appropriate murmur.

A careful ophthalmoscopic examination with detailed attention to each of the retinal arterioles is vital. Abnormality seen in the vessels can suggest not only the source of the neurologic deficit but also its nature if cholesterol, fat, or fibrin platelets are found. If carotid obstruction is even the remotest possibility, pressures in the ophthalmic arteries must be measured by ophthalmodynamometry (see Chap. 7).

DIFFERENTIAL DIAGNOSIS

The diagnosis of embolism is usually made by inference. Only in some cases can obstruction of an artery be found on examination or by arteriography. The triad of findings which points strongly to the diagnosis of embolism is (1) acute onset, (2) the presence of a source for emboli, and (3) evidence of other peripheral emboli, especially in the retina.

Especially in the acute phases of the illness, other diagnostic possibilities that may be confused with embolus are hemiplegic migraine, intracranial neoplasm, aortocranial atherosclerosis with infarction, and localized cerebral hemorrhage. When skull x-rays, EEG, cerebrospinal fluid pressure and contents, and brain scan with radioactive material are all normal and systemic hypertension is absent, cerebral hemorrhage and intracranial neoplasm are unlikely. In patients who have no evidence of rheumatic heart disease, the differential diagnosis usually lies between embolus and infarction secondary to aortocranial arteriosclerosis. It is important to distinguish between them whenever possible, since the therapy of the two conditions may differ. The likelihood of embolus is increased in patients with atrial fibrillation, especially if the fibrillation is secondary to valvular heart disease rather than to thyrotoxicosis. The presence of murmurs about the head, neck, or orbits favors the diagnosis of atherosclerosis and secondary infarction.

LABORATORY FINDINGS

There is no laboratory test which provides proof of embolism. Chest x-ray may show a cardiac silhouette suggestive of rheumatic heart disease, and the urine may contain microscopic hematuria suggestive of an embolus lodged in the kidneys, but both are only supportive evidence for cerebral embolism. Fat globules found in profusion in urine, sputum, or spinal fluid are diagnostic of fat embolism. Initially the blood count and spinal fluid examination will be normal, and in most cases skull x-ray, radioactive brain scans, and echoencephalograms are also normal. The electroencephalogram may show a focal disturbance that may help to localize the abnormality, but it will not provide an etiologic diagnosis. Arteriography probably should not be performed if an embolus is suspected to have lodged in an intracranial artery. If it is done, however, arterial obstruction may be demonstrated.

In addition to chest and skull x-rays, an electrocardiogram must be done on all patients with cerebral episodes. The latter may reveal cardiac arrhythmias that have not been diagnosed clinically and in rare cases may show an unsuspected myocardial infarction which has been the source for embolus.

In a young person with an apparent cerebral embolus for which no source can be found, cardiac myxoma should be considered. Angiography may reveal a mass within the cardiac chamber, or microscopic examination of the embolic material (if it can be removed) may disclose tumor cells.

Later in the course of the illness results of tests which had initially been normal may change. Because some emboli produce tissue anoxia and infarction that may eventually become hemorrhagic, repeat examination of the spinal fluid may show red blood cells, xanthochromia, or elevated protein level. The brain scan may also show an abnormal degree of uptake of the material in the region of the infarction. In some patients secondary cerebral edema causes the midline structures to shift, displacing the pineal gland.

PROGNOSIS AND CLINICAL COURSE

Most patients recover from cerebral embolism. In some the recovery is complete, but others may have major neurologic deficits. Death is most often due to the effects of secondary cerebral edema. Improvement may begin within hours of the onset of cerebral embolism, perhaps because of disappearance of vasospasm, and remarkable return of neurologic function may occur. In some of these cases an embolus lodged in a large artery may move into smaller distal branches as arterial spasm diminishes. In still other cases, collateral circulation may account for the rapid return of function. Whatever the cause, this rapid improvement may be difficult to distinguish from the sequence of events in patients with other types of neurologic deficit.

MANAGEMENT

The aim of therapy is twofold: (1) management of the cerebral embolism and (2) prevention of recurrences by treatment of the systemic abnormality that produced it.

Management of the Embolism

If a clinical examination indicates that the embolus might have lodged in the extracranial circulation, angiography must be carried out immediately, because removal of an obstruction in the carotids or the brachiocephalic or subclavian artery is an emergency procedure.

When the obstruction is within the intracranial arteries, surgery has little to offer. If angiography shows an intracranial embolus lodged in the carotid arterial tree and if the patient is young, presumably with supple arteries, cervical sympathetic block may be tried as a measure to combat vasospasm. (It should be noted that such blocks are useless in patients with nonembolic infarcts.)

In the acute phases of cerebral embolism, the inhalation of oxygen (50 to 95 percent) mixed with carbon dioxide (5 percent) may be used in an attempt to combat spasm. It is theorized that the carbon dioxide may counteract to some degree any element of spasm that may be present, and that it may cause generalized cerebral vasodilatation, so that the embolus will move distally into smaller vessels.

Thrombolytic agents have not proved useful in restoring blood flow through arteries obstructed by clot. Although patency has been reestablished in some cases, the therapeutic effect has been too slow to restore neurologic function. In addition, the agents currently available are considered to be unsafe because of their high incidence of undesirable reactions.

If the heart is the source of the embolus, the patient should be kept at absolute bed rest during the acute phase of cerebral embolism, in the hope of minimizing the danger of further embolus by keeping the cardiac rate slow. Patients with cerebral embolism from any other source may walk at once. While the patient is in bed, the limbs should be exercised actively and passively in order to prevent contractures and venous thrombosis.

Prevention of Recurrences

In theory, every patient who has an embolus suspected of being a blood clot should be given anticoagulants in doses sufficient to prevent the formation of a new clot that might serve as the source for recurrent emboli. Although anticoagulants given in the acute stages of embolism sometimes cause the infarct to become hemorrhagic, many clinicians believe that the danger of recurrent embolus outweighs this risk and, provided the initial lumbar puncture contains no blood, initiate anticoagulant therapy immediately. For patients with short-lived attacks that do not cause residual damage, anticoagulant therapy is imperative and must be initiated as rapidly as possible. Once anticoagulants are started, they should probably be given indefinitely, unless the source of the embolus is removed. See Chap. 16 for regimen.

Only recently has it been recognized that arteriosclerotic plaques on the aortocranial arteries, particularly in the region of the carotid bifurcation, may serve as a source of emboli to the brain. Anticoagulants may prevent further propagation of fibrin platelet clots which are thrown into the distal circulation from this site. Some clinicians advocate surgery to remove the source of emboli in such cases. This subject is discussed further in Chap. 17.

Measures for controlling heart rate and rhythm and for treating subacute bacterial endocarditis are outside the scope of this text. Most clinicians, however, believe that the rhythm of the fibrillating heart should be reverted to normal as soon as possible.

Cerebral embolus is sometimes the initial

manifestation of previously undiagnosed valvular heart disease. In such cases corrective surgery may be indicated as an emergency measure, particularly if embolization of other arteries takes place. The use of the heart-lung machine, however, requires massive doses of anticoagulants, and the neurologic status may be a limiting factor in this type of therapy. Whenever possible, therefore, it seems prudent to wait for at least a month after cerebral embolism before undertaking such surgery.

SUGGESTED READINGS

General

Breutsch, W. C., and Williams, C. L.: Embolic cerebral sequel in rheumatic mitral stenosis precipitating senile mental deterioration, *Am. J. Psychiat.,* **116**:364, 1959.

Cogan, D. G., Kuwabara, T., and Moser, H.: Fat emboli in the retina following angiography, *Arch. Ophthalmol.,* **71**:308, 1964.

Fisher, C. M., and Adams, R. D.: Observations on brain embolism with special reference to the mechanism of hemorrhagic infarction, *J. Neuropathol. Exptl. Neurol.,* **10**:92, 1951.

Gulkin, T. A., and Asbury, A. K.: Fragment of great-vessel wall causing cerebral embolism, *New Engl. J. Med.,* **277**:751, 1967.

Ide, C. H., Almond, C. H., Hart, W. M., Simmons, E. M., and Wilson, R. J.: Hematogenous dissemination of microemboli. Eye findings in a patient with Starr-Edwards aortic prosthesis, *Arch. Ophthalmol.,* **85**:614, 1971.

Javid, H., Tufo, H. M., Najafi, H., Dye, W. S., Hunter, J. A., and Julian, O. C.: Neurological abnormalities following open-heart surgery, *J. Thoracic Cardiovascular Surg.,* **58**:502, 1969.

Maroon, J. C., and Campbell, R. L.: Atrial myxoma: A treatable cause of stroke, *J. Neurol. Neurosurg. Psychiat.,* **32**:129, 1969.

Meyer, J. S., Gotoh, F., and Tazaki, Y.: Circulation and metabolism following experimental cerebral embolism, *J. Neuropathol. Exptl. Neurol.,* **21**:4, 1962.

New, P. F. J.: Myxomatous emboli in brain, *New Engl. J. Med.,* **282**:396, 1970.

———, Price, D. L., and Carter, B.: Cerebral angiography in cardiac myxoma. Correlation of angiographic and histopathological findings, *Radiology,* **96**:335, 1970.

Penry, J. K., and Netsky, M. G.: Experimental embolic occlusion of a single leptomeningeal artery, *Arch. Neurol.,* **3**:391, 1960.

Russell, R. R.: Cerebral and retinal embolism, *Am. Heart J.,* **69**:142, 1965.

Sisel, R. J., Parker, B. M., and Bahl, O. P.: Cerebral symptoms in pulmonary arteriovenous fistula. A result of paradoxical emboli,? *Circulation,* **41**:123, 1970.

Swank, R. L., and Hain, R. F.: The effect of different sized emboli on the vascular system and parenchyma of the brain, *J. Neuropathol. Exptl. Neurol.,* **11**:280, 1952.

VanGilder, J. C., and Coxe, W. S.: Shotgun pellet embolus of the middle cerebral artery, *J. Neurosurg.,* **32**:711, 1970.

Vost, A., Wolochow, D. A., and Howell, D. A.: Incidence of infarcts of the brain in heart disease, *J. Pathol. Bacteriol.,* **88**:463, 1964.

Etiology

Cholesterol and Fibrin Platelet

Eliot, R. S., Kanjuh, V. I., and Edwards, J. E.: Atheromatous embolism, *Circulation,* **30**:611, 1964.

Harder, H. I., and Brown, A. F.: Embolization of basilar artery by myocardial fragment. Report of a case, *Arch. Internal Med.,* **95**:587, 1955.

Haygood, T. A., Fessel, J., and Strange, D. A.: Atheromatous micro-embolism simulating polymyositis, *J.A.M.A.,* **203**:423, 1968.

Russell, R. W. R.: Atheromatous retinal embolism, *Lancet,* **2**:1354, 1963.

Soloway, H. B., and Aronson, S. M.: Atheromatous emboli to central nervous system: Report of 16 cases, *Arch. Neurol.,* **11**:657, 1964.

Wood, E. H., and Correll, J. W.: Atheromatous ulceration in major neck vessels as a cause of cerebral embolism, *Acta radiol. (diagn.),* **9**:520, 1969.

Metastatic Deposits

Aguayo, A. J.: Cerebral thrombo-embolism in malignancy, *Arch. Neurol.,* **11**:500, 1964.

Joynt, R. J., Zimmerman, G., and Khalifeh, R.: Cerebral emboli from cardiac tumors, *Arch. Neurol.,* **12**:84, 1965.

Neufeld, H. N., Cadman, N. L., Miller, A. W., and Edwards, J. E.: Embolism from marantic endocarditis as a manifestation of occult carcinoma, *Proc. Staff Meetings Mayo Clinic,* **35**:292, 1960.

Septic Emboli

Case Records of the Massachusetts General Hospital: Case 45212, *New Engl. J. Med.,* **260**:1085, 1959.

Air and Foreign Body Emboli

Chason, J. L., Landers, J. W., and Swanson, R. E.: Cotton fiber embolism: A frequent complication of cerebral angiography, *Neurology,* **13**:558, 1963.

Gilman, S.: Cerebral disorders after open-heart operations, *New Engl. J. Med.,* **272**:489, 1965.

Gottlieb, J. D., Ericsson, J. A., and Sweet, R. B.: Venous air embolism: Review, *Anesth. Analg. Current Res.,* **44**:773, 1965.

Kornfeld, D. S., Zimberg, S., and Malm, J. R.: Psychiatric complications of open-heart surgery, *New. Engl. J. Med.,* **273**:287, 1965.

Landew, M. L., Bowles, L. T., Gelman, S., Lowenfels, A. B., Tepper, R., and Lord, J. W., Jr.: Effects of intraarterial microbubbles, *Am. J. Physiol.,* **199**:485, 1960.

Lee, J. C., and Olszewski, J.: Effect of air embolism on permeability of cerebral blood vessels, *Neurology,* **9**:619, 1959.

Penry, J. K., Cordell, A. R., Johnston, F. R., and Netsky, M. G.: Cerebral embolism by antifoam A in a bubble oxygenatory system: An experimental and clinical study, *Surgery,* **47**:784, 1960.

Fat Emboli

Cross, H. E.: Examination of CSF in fat embolism, *Arch. Internal Med.,* **115**:470, 1965.

Sevitt, S.: The significance and classification of fat-embolism, *Lancet,* **2**:825, 1960.

Nitrogen Bubble Emboli (Caisson Disease)

Flinn, D. E., and Womack, G. J.: Neurological manifestations of dysbarism: A review and report of a case with multiple episodes, *Aerospace Med.,* **34**:956, 1963.

Haymaker, W., and Johnston, A. D.: Pathology of decompression sickness. A comparison of the lesions in airmen with those in caisson workers and divers, *Milit. Med.,* **117**:285, 1955.

Clinical Features

Babcock, R. H., and Netsky, M. G.: Respiratory and cardiovascular responses to experimental cerebral emboli, *Trans. Am. Neurol. Assoc.,* **84**:85, 1959.

Berkman, N., Amstutz, P., and Vic-Dupont, V.: Les manifestations oculaires des embolies graisseuses, *Presse med.,* **78**:491, 1970.

David, N. J., Klintworth, G. K., Friedberg, S. J., and Dillon, M.: Fatal atheromatous cerebral embolism associated with bright plaques in the retinal arterioles, *Neurology,* **13**:708, 1963.

Fisher, C. M., and Pearlman, A.: The nonsudden onset of cerebral embolism, *Neurology,* **17**:1025, 1967.

Gazzaniga, A. B., and Dallen, J. E.: Paradoxical embolism: Its pathophysiology and clinical recognition, *Ann. Surg.,* **171**:137, 1970.

Gillen, H. W.: Symptomatology of cerebral gas embolism, *Neurology,* **18**:507, 1968.

Kilpatrick, Z. M., Greenberg, P. A., and Sanford, J. P.: Splinter hemorrhages—Their clinical significance, *Arch. Internal Med.,* **115**:730, 1965.

McDonald, W. I.: Recurrent cholesterol embolism as a cause of fluctuating cerebral symptoms, *J. Neurol. Neurosurg. Psychiat.,* **30**:489, 1967.

Wells, C. E.: Premonitory symptoms of cerebral embolism, *Arch. Neurol.,* **5**:490, 1961.

Differential Diagnosis

Bickerstaff, E. R.: Aetiology of acute hemiplegia in childhood, *Brit. Med. J.,* **2**:82, 1964.

Evarts, C. M.: The fat embolism syndrome: A review, *Surg. Clin. N. Am.,* **50**(2):493, 1970.

Jones, H. R., Jr., Siekert, R. G., and Geraci, J. E.: Neurologic manifestations of bacterial endocarditis, *Ann. Internal Med.,* **71**:21, 1969.

Jordan, F. A., Gleason, I. O., and Feld, M.: Atrial myxoma manifested as cerebral vascular disease, *Calif. Med.,* **112**(3):20, 1970.

Kane, W. C., and Aronson, S. M.: Cardiac disorders predisposing to embolic stroke, *Stroke,* **1**:164, 1970.

Patrick, J., and Whitty, C. W.: Recurrent cerebral emboli and diagnosis of focal epilepsy, *Lancet,* **1**:1291, 1965.

Rennie, A. M.: Fat embolism, *Can. J. Surg.,* **13**:41, 1970.

Ziment, I.: Nervous system complications in bacterial endocarditis, *Am. J. Med.,* **47**:593, 1969.

Laboratory Findings

Bladin, P. F.: A radiologic and pathologic study of embolism of the internal carotid-middle cerebral arterial axis, *Radiology,* **82**:615, 1964.

Dalal, P. M., Shah, P. M., and Aiyar, R. R.: Arteriographic study of cerebral embolism, *Lancet,* **2**:358, 1965.

———, ———, Sheth, S. C., and Deshpande, C. K.: Cerebral embolism—Angiographic observations on spontaneous clot lysis, *Lancet,* **1**:61, 1965.

———, ———, Deshpande, C. K., and Sheth, S. C.: Recanalization after cerebral embolism, *Lancet,* **2**:495, 1966.

Ferris, E. J., Rudikoff, J. C., and Shapiro, J. H.: Cerebral angiography of bacterial infection, *Radiology,* **90**:727, 1968.

Maroon, J. C., Edmonds-Seal, J., and Campbell, R. L.: An ultrasonic method for detecting air embolism, *J. Neurosurg.,* **31**:196, 1969.

Prognosis and Clinical Course

Carter, A. B.: Prognosis of cerebral embolism, *Lancet,* **2**:514, 1965.

Rosenblum, J. A., and O'Connor, R. A.: Late seizures as a sequela of open heart surgery, *Angiology,* **18**:655, 1967.

Wells, C. E.: Cerebral embolism: The natural history, prognostic signs and effects of anticoagulation, *Arch. Neurol. Psychiat.,* **81**:667, 1959.

Management

Ashbaugh, D. G., and Petty, T. L.: The use of corticosteroids in the treatment of respiratory failure associated with massive fat embolism, *Surg. Gynecol. Obstet.,* **123**:493, 1966.

Carter, A. B.: The immediate treatment of cerebral embolism, *Quart. J. Med.,* **26**:335, 1957.

Chou, S. N.: Embolectomy of middle cerebral artery: Report of a case, *J. Neurosurg.,* **20**:161, 1963.

Kleaveland, R. N.: Internal-carotid-artery embolectomy, *New Engl. J. Med.,* **264**:759, 1961.

Lougheed, W. M., Gunton, R. W., and Barnett, H. J. M.: Embolectomy of internal carotid, middle and anterior cerebral arteries: Report of a case, *J. Neurosurg.,* **22**:607, 1965.

Additional References

Calkins, R. A.: Cerebral embolism; review and current perspectives, *Arch. Internal Med.,* **130**:430, 1972.

Halsey, J. H., Jr.: Cerebral embolism, *Current Concepts Cerebrovascular Dis.—Stroke,* **6**:23, 1971.

Meyer, J. S., Charney, J. Z., Rivera, V. M., and Mathew, N. T.: Cerebral embolization: Prospective clinical analysis of 42 cases, *Stroke,* **2**:541, 1971.

Mundall, J., Quintero, P., von Kaulla, K. N., Harmon, R., and Austin, J.: Transient monocular blindness and increased platelet aggregability treated with aspirin. A case report, *Neurology,* **22**:280, 1972.

Williams, I. M.: Intravascular changes in retina during open-heart surgery, *Lancet,* **2**:688, 1971.

Winter, P. M., Alvis, H. J., and Gage, A. A.: Hyperbaric treatment of cerebral air embolism during cardiopulmonary bypass, *J.A.M.A.,* **215**:1786, 1971.

Chapter 19

Hypertensive Vascular Disease

Even ambrosia becomes as harmful as a poison, a weapon, or a thunderbolt if prescribed by an ignorant physician and should be equally avoided.

Susruta

Arterial blood pressure fluctuates in a diurnal rhythm with the nadir occurring during sleep and the zenith during daytime activities. Superimposed upon this circadian cycle are abrupt, short-lived elevations and reductions which result from vasomotor readjustments to stresses such as emotion, exertion, and changes in posture. With each passing year blood pressure tends to increase gradually from the normal childhood range of 80 to 110 mm Hg systolic and 50 to 70 mm Hg diastolic to adult levels which in the United States are commonly accepted as 100 plus one's chronologic age systolic and up to 90 mm Hg diastolic.

Despite these variations, pressure in the arteriolar-capillary network of the brain remains constant. When arterial blood pressure increases, the cerebral arterioles constrict, the degree depending upon the pressure elevation. If this is of short duration and the pressure is not too high, there is no apparent harm, but if pressure is sustained at even moderate elevations for months or years, hyalinization of the muscularis occurs, and the caliber of the lumen becomes fixed. This is a dangerous situation because it means that the cerebral arterioles can no longer dilate or constrict in order to compensate for fluctuations in systemic pressure. A fall in arterial pressure may then lead to inadequate perfusion of the brain and consequent tissue ischemia, and an increase in systemic arterial pressure may cause excessive perfusion pressure in the capillary bed, with resultant hyperemia, edema, and possibly hemorrhage.

LACUNAR STATE (*ÉTAT LACUNAIRE*)

Sustained hypertension also accelerates atherosclerosis, which leads to added dangers. Small arteries and arterioles already thickened as a result of hypertension may become occluded with thrombus, while others may be plugged with emboli from atherosclerotic plaques in larger arteries upstream. The microinfarctions which result are called "lacunes" (lakes). A multiplicity of lacunes is called the "lacunar state" *(état lacunaire)* (Fig. 19-1).

Lacunes are the most common cerebrovascular lesions found in elderly hypertensive patients at autopsy. They appear as multiple, irregular cavities, ranging in size from 0.5 to 15.0 mm, and are distributed in such strategic locations as the putamen, pons, thalamus, caudate nucleus, internal capsule, corona radiata, and cerebellar white matter, roughly in that order of frequency. They are conspicuously absent in the spinal cord and cerebral cortex.

Although in most patients these lesions apparently do not cause recognizable symptoms and signs, four characteristic syndromes have been described:

1 Homolateral cerebellar ataxia with pyramidal tract signs in which the ataxia and weakness involve the leg more than the arm. It is thought that the responsible lesion lies where the corona

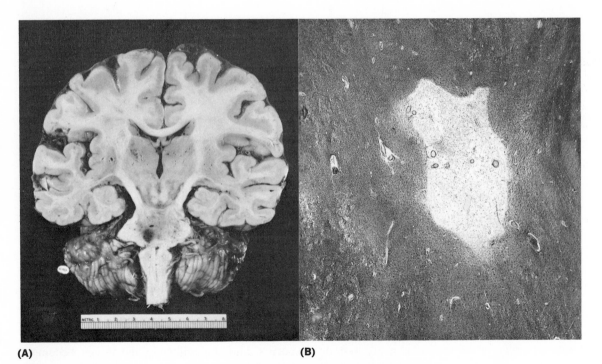

(A)   **(B)**

Figure 19-1   (A) Coronal section of the brain showing small cystlike formations (*état lacunaire,* or "lacunar state") in the basal ganglia and pons. (B) Old, small cavitary infarct, "lacune." (magnification × 100)

radiata funnels into the internal capsule. In spite of its name, the ataxia is probably *not* due to involvement of the cerebellum but to damage to the corticopontine pathways.

2 Hemiplegia unaccompanied by sensory deficit, visual field defect, or aphasia. This syndrome results from infarction in the internal capsule more commonly than in the basis pontis. In either case the lesion is on the side opposite the hemiplegia.

3 "Dysarthria-clumsy hand syndrome," in which there is a sudden onset of moderate to severe dysarthria, central facial weakness, deviation of the tongue on protrusion, slight dysphagia, clumsiness and slowness in fine manipulations of the affected hand, and some weakness and ataxia on the finger-to-nose test. The patient experiences mild imbalance on walking, and some corticospinal tract signs are present without associated symptoms. The lesion responsible is probably in the pons.

4 Pure sensory stroke involving the face, arm, and leg, with parasthesias described as numbness, sleeping sensations, tingling, stiffness, pressing sensation, or a dead feeling. The affected side may feel distorted in size or compressed as in a vise. This condition is probably the result of a lacune in the posteroventral nucleus of the thalamus.

Because these lesions are usually bilateral and located in the basal ganglia and brainstem, patients suffering from them are commonly misdiagnosed as having Parkinson's disease particularly since they may eventually become quite rigid and have a small-stepped gait. The patient does not, however, develop tremor at rest.

Lacunes are seldom the result of any process other than end-stage hypertensive vascular disease, although in rare cases a small cholesterol embolus, such as may occur from an ulcerated atherosclerotic plaque, may result in a picture identical with a lacunar infarct. Lacunes are not related specifically to disease of the internal carotid artery or to diabetes mellitus.

The pseudobulbar palsy seen in association with the lacunar state is described in Chap. 13.

When one of these lacunar syndromes can be diagnosed clinically, angiography is not needed. Anticoagulants are potentially harmful because the patients are hypertensive (see Chap. 16). The treatment of choice is gradual reduction of systemic arterial blood pressure to levels which are nearly normotensive for the patient's age.

MILIARY ANEURYSMS

Charcot and Bouchard, in 1868, described microaneurysms of the penetrating arteries and arterioles in patients with long-standing hypertension. They depicted them as outpouchings of endothelium through areas of weakened media (Fig. 19-2).

Since this initial description, it has been confirmed that these lesions are confined to the brain and are found only in hypertensive patients. For a long time many pathologists thought that these lesions were small dissecting hematomas; it has been shown that they are aneurysms. Their importance lies in the fact that their rupture is thought to be the underlying cause of intracerebral hemorrhage in hypertensive patients (see Chap. 27).

"CONGENITAL" BERRY ANEURYSMS

The pathogenesis of this variety of aneurysm, arising most frequently near the circle of Willis, is a controversial topic. Because of their rarity in infancy, when blood pressure is low, it is hypothesized that as blood pressure increases with age there are herniations of the intima through weakened places in the media (see Chap. 25).

ACUTE HYPERTENSIVE ENCEPHALOPATHY

The term *hypertensive encephalopathy* was first used in 1928 by Oppenheimer and Fishberg to

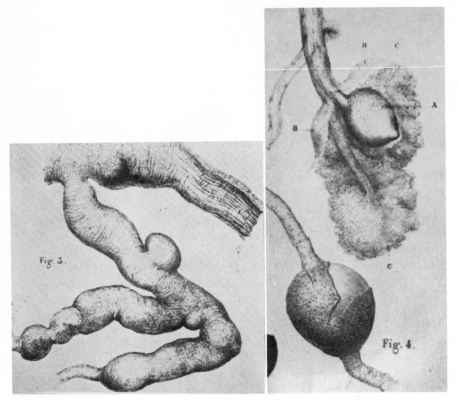

Figure 19-2 "Miliary" aneurysms illustrated by Messrs. Charcot and Bouchard.

describe a group of acute and usually transient neurologic phenomena occurring in patients with high systemic blood pressure. These authors found the brains of patients who died with the syndrome to be pale on gross inspection. Because no microscopic studies were made, they attributed the abnormality to intense cerebral arteriospasm with resultant cerebral edema. The term quickly became a catchall for a variety of intracranial catastrophes occurring in patients with persistent hypertension, thus making it difficult to define a clear-cut syndrome that excludes the possibility of multifocal cerebral hemorrhages and microinfarctions. If the diagnosis is restricted to reversible cerebral disorders associated with marked or sudden rise in blood pressure in the absence of any evidence of uremia, cerebral infarction, or cerebral hemor-

rhage, it is found that hypertensive encephalopathy is very infrequent.

Etiology and Pathogenesis

The cerebral effects of hypertensive encephalopathy are believed to be due to arterial or arteriolar spasm occurring in response to extreme elevation of the systemic blood pressure. It is suspected that the key factors are the mean arterial blood pressure (the diastolic pressure plus one-half of the pulse pressure) and the rate of increase in pressure. *Sustained* arterial hypertension can be tolerated, but *rapid* elevation of the mean pressure to levels of 150 mm Hg or above may result in an exaggerated autoregulatory response to the cerebral arterioles. The diffuse vasospasm leads to reduced flow into the capillary bed and causes capillary and neuronal ischemia. The end result is transudation of fluid into the extracellular space (cerebral edema), rupture of capillaries (petechial hemorrhages), and tissue necrosis (ischemic microinfarction). Even though the process is generalized, the sequence of events listed above is multifocal, and a constellation of neurologic deficits develops.

Encephalopathy may be secondary to malignant hypertension from any cause or to uncontrolled hypertension produced by aldosteronism, glomerulonephritis, pheochromocytoma, or eclampsia. Of these, acute nephritis and toxemia of pregnancy are the most frequent offenders. Recently some features of hypertensive encephalopathy have been noted in patients receiving certain monoamine oxidase (MAO) inhibitors as antidepressants. In these patients the hypertensive crises have sometimes been precipitated by the ingestion of food containing tyramine. All types of cheeses except cream and cottage cheese contain tyramine, but the highest concentration (1,416 μg per Gm) has been found in New York cheddar cheese. Most beers and wines have rather small amounts of tyramine, but Chianti contains about 25 μg per ml.

Pathology

The brain is usually swollen and pale, with flattening of the gyri and obliteration of the sulci. Signs of increased pressure (incisural and transforaminal herniation) are apparent. Petechiae may be noted over the surface, and on cut section, slit hemorrhages and lacunae are visible, but large infarcts and hemorrhages are not part of the picture of hypertensive encephalopathy.

In addition to neuronal swelling and degeneration secondary to ischemia, necrotizing arteriolitis and microinfarcts with glial scars can often be found.

Clinical Features

The initial symptom of encephalopathy is usually the subacute onset of generalized or suboc-

cipital headache, which increases gradually in intensity and is usually aggravated by coughing and straining (Valsalva's maneuver). In contrast to the more benign causes of headaches, those of hypertension are said to occur in the early-morning hours and may be accompanied by vomiting. Transient attacks of blindness, paresis, and generalized or focal convulsions are common. After a variable interval, somnolence, disorientation, confusion, delirium, stupor, and coma occur to complete the triad of headaches, convulsions, and altered consciousness.

On physical examination the diastolic pressure is usually above 120 mm Hg, and the mean arterial pressure is often 150 to 200 mm Hg. However, in women with toxemia of pregnancy and in children with acute glomerulonephritis, encephalopathy may occur when arterial pressure is no higher than 180 mm Hg systolic and 110 mm Hg diastolic. Furthermore, patients with other abnormalities which can result in diffuse cerebral disease, for example, uremia, have a lower threshold for hypertensive encephalopathy. Examination of the optic fundus usually shows grades III to IV hypertensive retinopathy. There are cases in which the fundus shows only severe retinal arteriolar spasm without hemorrhages, exudates, or papilledema. Patients with long-standing hypertension will show evidence of left ventricular enlargement and often have a diastolic gallop rhythm which suggests incipient cardiac decompensation.

Neurologic examination in the early stages shows the patient to be confused and often hyperirritable. The irritability of his nervous system may be reflected in focal twitching and myoclonic movements of his extremities. Hemiparesis, cortical blindness, hemianopia, aphasia, or some other evidence of focal neurologic dysfunction is often present.

Differential Diagnosis

The occurrence of fleeting neurologic signs in hypertensive patients with markedly elevated

Table 19-1 Antihypertensive Drugs for Parenteral Administration in Managing Hypertensive Encephalopathy

Drugs	Dosage			Side effects	Onset of action	Remarks
	Intramuscular*	Single dose	Intravenous infusion†			
Diazoxide (Hyperstat)		300–600 mg (rapid injection essential)		Nausea, vomiting, flushing, hyperglycemia	3–5 min	Prompt response and standard dosage will make this the drug of choice.
Sodium nitroprusside			50–100 mg/L	Nausea, vomiting, muscle twitching, sweating, apprehension, thiocyanate intoxication	Instantaneous	Not commercially available but can be prepared easily. It requires constant supervision. Thiocyanate blood levels must be assessed.
Ganglion-blocking agents:						Usually effective, but large doses are often necessary to reduce supine blood pressure since the effect is primarily orthostatic. Repeated doses usually lead to atony of bowel and bladder.
Pentolinium	1–20 mg	10 mg‡	20–200 mg/L	Urinary retention, paralytic ileus	I.M.: 30 min I.V.: 5–10 min	
Trimethaphan camsylate (Arfonad)			1,000 mg/L		I.V.: 5–10 min	

Hydralazine	10–50 mg	10 mg‡	I.M.: 30 min I.V.: 10 min	Tachycardia, palpitations, flushing, headache, vomiting	More effective in acute glomerulonephritis and eclampsia than in essential hypertension. Contraindicated in heart failure or coronary insufficiency.
Reserpine	1–5 mg		2–3 hr	Drowsiness, stupor, parkinsonian rigidity	Delayed effect and somnolence are major disadvantages.
Methyldopate	250–500 mg§		2–3 hr	Drowsiness	Same disadvantages as reserpine and is less likely to be effective.

* Start with the smallest dose shown. Subsequent doses and intervals of administration should be adjusted according to the response of the blood pressure.

† Start the infusion slowly and adjust the rate according to the response of the blood pressure. Constant surveillance is mandatory. The concentration of the solution can be adjusted to the patient's fluid requirements.

‡ The total dose should be contained in a volume of at least 20 ml, and the solution should be administered from a 20- or 50-ml syringe. The blood pressure should be monitored continuously while the injection is being made. The rate of injection should not exceed 0.5 ml per min, and in order to avoid hypotension the injection should be stopped frequently when the blood pressure is falling.

§ Administered in 100 ml of a 5 percent solution of dextrose in distilled water over a period of 30 to 60 min.

Source: R. W. Gifford, Jr., and N. G. Richards, Hypertensive encephalopathy: I. Etiology, pathology, and clinical findings, *Current Concepts Cerebrovascular Dis.—Stroke,* **5**:43, 1970; by permission of The American Heart Association, Inc.

diastolic pressure and grades III to IV retinopathy, especially when accompanied by severe headache, vomiting, drowsiness, and focal or generalized seizures, should suggest the possibility of hypertensive encephalopathy. Although the absence of signs of meningeal irritation helps to exclude subarachnoid hemorrhage, a cerebral infarct or encapsulated cerebral hemorrhage must still be considered. The absence of albuminuria, renal casts, or elevated blood urea nitrogen level helps to exclude *uremic encephalopathy.*

In patients with no previous history of hypertension, it is sometimes difficult to rule out the possibility of *brain tumor.* The appearance of the optic fundus usually gives the clue, however. Hemorrhages and exudates diffusely distributed through the retina and only mild to moderate papilledema are seen in patients with hypertensive encephalopathy, whereas in those with *brain tumor* the papilledema is pronounced and hemorrhages and exudates are confined to the peripapillary region.

Hypertensive encephalopathy in a child suffering from acute glomerulonephritis may be mistaken for *acute lead encephalopathy.* Urine examination will reveal albuminuria, hematuria, and renal casts in cases of glomerulonephritis. On the other hand, lead encephalopathy simulates hypertensive encephalopathy so closely that at times the elevated cerebrospinal fluid protein level may be the first clue to suggest lead intoxication. Basophilic stippling and x-ray evidence of lead lines will also reveal lead intoxication.

At times *systemic lupus erythematosus, acute angiitis,* and *acute anxiety* with labile hypertension can simulate hypertensive encephalopathy.

The best diagnostic criterion is response to reduction of blood pressure. When the clinical picture is due to hypertensive encephalopathy, adequate reduction in blood pressure results in a sometimes dramatic recovery with disappearance of headache, vomiting, somnolence, and neurologic deficit. If prompt recovery does not occur, the physician must conclude that either his diagnosis is in error or there is an associated complicating process such as cerebral hemorrhage, uremia, or drug intoxication.

Laboratory Findings

In an emergency situation, when a patient's condition is rapidly deteriorating, reduction of blood pressure should precede time-consuming laboratory tests.

Spinal fluid contents are usually normal, and the cerebrospinal fluid pressure may be either normal or elevated. Patients who have been examined electroencephalographically show focal abnormalities and bilaterally synchronous sharp and slow waves, at times rhythmic.

Appropriate tests often show accompanying cardiac and renal damage. Radiographic studies using contrast medium may be contraindicated and should be reserved for instances in which encapsulated hemorrhage or brain tumor cannot be excluded on clinical grounds. Radioisotopic brain scans will show normal results.

Course of the Disease

Recurring, self-limited episodes of confusion, lethargy, and seizures are sometimes seen in patients with uncontrolled severe hypertension. The ultimate outlook is dependent primarily, not on the initial neurologic process, but on the extent to which the blood pressure can be controlled and on the severity of the accompanying hypertensive cardiac and renal disease.

Management

The primary treatment is rapid reduction of the blood pressure to a level low enough to reverse the arteriospasm without precipitating cerebral, myocardial, or renal insufficiency. The danger of such complication is especially great in patients whose cerebral, coronary, and renal arterial perfusion pressures have adjusted to higher levels. Of the various medications used for a rapid hypotensive effect (Table 19-1), we prefer Diazoxide, since it is relatively safe and effective. Furthermore it is very rapid in its action.

Patients with hypertensive encephalopathy should be treated in an intensive care unit.

Increased intracranial pressure is reduced when the systemic blood pressure is lowered, and does not require specific treatment. Repeated lumbar punctures to reduce cerebrospinal fluid pressure may precipitate herniation of the brain, and hence should not be done.

Seizures should be controlled by the usual anticonvulsants (Chap. 30). Cardiac decompensation, when present, should be managed by the usual methods.

Once the acute crisis is controlled, the underlying cause of the patient's hypertension should be sought. If a specifically remediable cause is not found, well-controlled, long-term management with oral hypotensive medications will be needed.

SUGGESTED READINGS

General

Baker, A. B., Resch, J. A., and Loewenson, R. B.: Hypertension and cerebral atherosclerosis, *Circulation,* **39**:701, 1969.

Cole, F. M., and Yates, P. O.: Comparative incidence of cerebrovascular lesions in normotensive and hypertensive patients, *Neurology,* **18**:255, 1968.

Harmsen, P., Kjaerulff, J., and Skinøj, E.: Acute controlled hypotension and EEG in patients with hypertension and cerebrovascular disease, *J. Neurol. Neurosurg. Psychiat.,* **34**:300, 1971.

Merrett, J. D., and Adams, G. F.: Comparison of mortality rates in elderly hypertensive and normotensive hemiplegic patients, *Brit. Med. J.,* **2**:802, 1966.

Miall, W. E., and Lovell, H. G.: Relation between change of blood pressure and age, *Brit. Med. J.,* **2**:660, 1967.

Pickering, G. W.: High Blood Pressure, 2d ed., Grune & Stratton, Inc., New York, 1968.

Zülch, K. J.: Pathological aspects of cerebral accidents in arterial hypertension, *Acta neurol. psychiat. belg.,* **71**:196, 1971.

Lacunar State

Fisher, C. M.: The arterial lesions underlying lacunes, *Acta neuropathol. (Berlin),* **12**:1, 1969.

————: A lacunar stroke. The dysarthria-clumsy hand syndrome, *Neurology,* **17**:614, 1967.

————: Lacunes: Small, deep cerebral infarcts, *Neurology,* **15**:774, 1965.

————: Pure sensory stroke involving face, arm, and leg, *Neurology,* **15**:76, 1965.

————, and Caplan, L. R.: Basilar artery branch occlusion: A cause of pontine infarction, *Neurology,* **21**:900, 1971.

————, and Cole, M.: Homolateral ataxia and crural paresis: A vascular syndrome, *J. Neurol. Neurosurg. Psychiat.,* **28**:48, 1965.

————, and Curry, H. B.: Pure motor hemiplegia of vascular origin, *Arch. Neurol.,* **13**:30, 1965.

Hughes, W.: Origin of lacunes, *Lancet,* **2**:19, 1965.

Leading article: Lacunes, *Brit. Med. J.,* **1**:251, 1970.

Miliary Aneurysms

Cole, F. M., and Yates, P.: Intracerebral microaneurysms and small cerebrovascular lesions, *Brain,* **90**:759, 1967.

Acute Hypertensive Encephalopathy

Gifford, R. W., Jr., and Richards, N. G.: Hypertensive encephalopathy. I: Etiology, pathology, and clinical findings, *Current Concepts Cerebrovascular Dis.—Stroke,* **5**:43, 1970.

Oppenheimer, B. S., and Fishberg, A. M.: Hypertensive encephalopathy, *Arch. Internal Med.,* **41**:264, 1928.

Ziegler, D. K., Zosa, A., and Zileli, T.: Hypertensive encephalopathy, *Arch. Neurol.,* **12**:472, 1965.

Etiology and Pathogenesis

Bercovici, J. P., and Collin de l'Hortet, G.: Hypertension and the pill, *Lancet,* **2**:1300, 1969.

Byrom, F. B.: The Hypertensive Vascular Crisis, William Heinemann, Ltd., London, 1969.

―――: Vascular lesions in malignant hypertension, *Lancet,* **2**:495, 1969.

―――: The calibre of the cerebral arteries in experimental hypertension, *Proc. Roy. Soc. Med.,* **61**:605, 1968.

Leading article: Pressor attacks during treatment with monoamine-oxidase inhibitors, *Lancet,* **1**:945, 1965.

Meyer, J. S., Waltz, A. G., and Gotoh, F.: Pathogenesis of cerebral vasospasm in hypertensive encephalopathy: I. Effects of acute increases in intraluminal blood pressure on pial blood flow; II. The nature of increased irritability of smooth muscle of pial arterioles in renal hypertension, *Neurology,* **10**:735 and **10**:859, 1960.

Pathology

Adachi, M., Rosenblum, W. I., and Feigin, I.: Hypertensive disease and cerebral edema, *J. Neurol. Neurosurg. Psychiat.,* **29**:451, 1966.

Kung, P. C., Lee, J. C., and Bakay, L.: Electron microscopic study of experimental acute hypertensive encephalopathy, *Acta neuropath. (Berlin),* **10**:263, 1968.

Rodda, R., and Denny-Brown, D.: The cerebral arterioles in experimental hypertension. II. The development of arteriolonecrosis, *Am. J. Pathol.,* **49**:365, 1966.

Clinical Features

Breslin, D. J.: Hypertensive crisis, *Med. Clin. N. Am.,* **53**(2):351, 1969.

Clarke, E., and Murphy, E. A.: Neurological manifestations of malignant hypertension, *Brit. Med. J.,* **2**:1319, 1956.

Freis, E. D.: Hypertensive crisis, *J.A.M.A.,* **208**:338, 1969.

Jellinek, E. H., Painter, M., Prineas, J., and Russell, R. R.: Hypertensive encephalopathy with cortical disorders of vision, *Quart. J. Med.,* **33**:239, 1964.

Rosenberg, R. S., Mitchell, A. M., and Lester, H. A.: Transient visual cortical defects associated with paroxysmal hypertension; in patients with traumatic spinal cord transections, *Arch. Ophthalmol.,* **81**:325, 1969.

Differential Diagnosis

Cameron, S. J., and Doig, A.: Cerebellar tumours presenting with clinical features of phaeochromocytoma, *Lancet,* **1**:492, 1970.

Godtfredsen, E.: Choked disc or hypertensive retinopathy IV? *Acta ophthalmol.,* **42**:387, 1964.

Jefferson, A.: Hypertensive cerebral vascular disease and intracranial tumor; study in diagnosis, *Quart. J. Med.,* **24**:245, 1955.

Morris, C. E., Heyman, A., and Pozefsky, T.: Lead encephalopathy caused by ingestion of illicitly distilled whiskey, *Neurology,* **14**:493, 1964.

Thomas, J. E., Rooke, E. D., and Kvale, W. F.: The neurologist's experience with pheochromocytoma: A review of 100 cases, *J.A.M.A.,* **197**:754, 1966.

Laboratory Findings

Ananthachari, M. D., and Saroja, D.: Relationship between cerebrospinal fluid and blood pressure in hypertensive patients, *J. Indian Med. Assoc.,* **52**:20, 1969.

Management

Dollery, C. T.: Hypertension in the elderly, *Brit. Med. J.,* **2**:33, 1966.

Freis, E. D.: The chemotherapy of hypertension, *J.A.M.A.,* **218**:1009, 1971.

Gifford, R. W., Jr., and Richards, R. G.: Hypertensive encephalopathy. Part II: Differential diagnosis and treatment, *Current Concepts Cerebrovascular Dis.—Stroke,* **5**:47, 1970.

Moser, M.: Treatment of "hypertensive encephalopathy" (accelerated hypertension), Part II, *Am. Heart J.,* **77**:704, 1969.

VA Cooperative Study Group on Antihypertensive Agents: Effects of treatment of morbidity in hypertension. Results in patients with diastolic blood pressures averaging 115 through 129 mm Hg, *J.A.M.A.,* **202**:1028, 1967.

Additional References

Fang, H. C. H.: Lacunar infarction: A clinico-pathologic correlation study, *J. Neuropathol. Exptl. Neurol.,* **31**:212, 1972.

Finnerty, F. A., Jr.: Hypertensive encephalopathy, *Am. J. Med.,* **52**:672, 1972.

Skinhøf, E., and Strandgaard, S.: Pathogenesis of hypertensive encephalopathy, *Lancet,* **1**:461, 1973.

Cerebrovascular Manifestations of Syphilis

The Lord may forgive us our sins—but the nervous system never does.

William James

Who served the gods die young—Venus, Bacchus and Vulcan send in no bills in the seventh decade.

Sir William Osler

Forty years ago, syphilis ranked fourth as a cause of death in the United States and was one of the leading forms of cerebrovascular disease. Although penicillin has been responsible for a sharp decline in its incidence and death rate here, the disease remains the most important public health problem in many countries where the incidence approaches 25 percent of the population. Recently there has been a resurgence of syphilis in the continental United States. Among the factors chiefly responsible are extensive travel, which increases the difficulty of locating contacts, increased promiscuity, and inadequate treatment, which suppresses the initial lesion without eradicating the organism.

In this chapter we will consider only central nervous system manifestations of syphilis, since it is one of those few cerebrovascular diseases for which medical treatment can effect a cure.

The most important aspect of therapy is early recognition of infection, for which the prerequisite is an understanding of the various disguises of *Treponema pallidum.*

ETIOLOGY AND PATHOGENESIS

It has been recognized for centuries that the syphilitic chancre is usually followed, after about 4 to 6 weeks, by a generalized mucocutaneous eruption, subsequent to which it is asymptomatic for 5 to 15 years before tertiary manifestations of cardiovascular or nervous system involvement become apparent.

In 1905, Schaudinn isolated *T. pallidum* from a chancre; and a few years later Noguchi demonstrated the same organism in paretic brains. During the years following these discoveries, Koch's postulates have been fulfilled, and the epidemiology and natural history of the disease have been extremely well documented.

After initial contact with a person who has exudative lesions, or with contaminated blood or utensils, the organisms penetrate the intact skin or mucous membranes, form a raised ulcer (chancre), and cause a local lymphadenitis (hard bubo). The spirochetes are then disseminated by the bloodstream, and mucocutaneous eruption (secondary syphilis) appears within 4 weeks. At the same time organisms lodge in many areas, including the aorta and the brain and its meninges, sometimes producing signs of acute inflammation such as syphilitic meningitis. Once developed, the rash and other secondary manifestations disappear in about 3 weeks, and there follows an asymptomatic period of 5 to 15 years before the tertiary stage begins. During the latent interval the only clues to syphilis are an accurate history, the scar left by chancre, and a reactive serum or spinal fluid. Even though spirochetes can be eradicated at any stage by appropriate therapy, the tertiary stage can cause irreversible damage to the brain or heart that may cripple or kill the patient despite

his "cure." Consequently it is during the first two stages that syphilis must be identified and treated.

PATHOLOGIC FINDINGS

Of the various tertiary manifestations, the meningovascular form is most likely to be confused with other forms of cerebrovascular episodes. For this reason, the description of the pathologic findings will be limited to this form of the disease. The leptomeninges and the blood vessels of the brain and spinal cord are affected simultaneously but to varying degrees in different patients.

When meningeal involvement predominates, diffuse low-grade leptomeningitis surrounds the arteries and cranial nerves at the base of the brain, eventually constricting them and obliterating the subarachnoid space. In later stages, organization and fibrosis of the exudate can obstruct the foramina of Luschka and Magendie and produce internal hydrocephalus. In occasional cases the adhesive process extends up over the convexity, especially in the frontal and parietal regions.

When involvement is predominantly vascular, there is circumscribed thickening of segments of the carotid and vertebral-basilar systems, the circle of Willis, and the cortical veins. Histologic examination shows intimal proliferation with endarteritis obliterans and round-cell infiltration of the outer coats of the artery. The smaller arteries present a similar histologic picture, with varying amounts of leptomeningeal reaction surrounding them. When the lumen of one of these vessels is narrowed or obliterated by thrombus, brain infarction is produced in its area of irrigation. In other areas perivascular aggregations of lymphocytes and local edema of the brain are conspicuous. Except in a large artery like the basilar, syphilis rarely, if ever, produces an intracranial aneurysm.

CLINICAL FEATURES

The clinical features of neurosyphilis vary according to the site and extent of vascular involvement, as indicated in the following outline:

I Primary—no neurologic phenomena
II Secondary—syphilitic meningitis (rare)
III Tertiary
    A Extracranial
        1 aortocervical syndrome (aneurysm and/or endarteritis)
    B Intracranial
        1 Meningovascular (infarction)
        2 Paretic (general paralysis of the insane)
        3 Gummatous
        4 Optic atrophy

Except for aneurysms and luetic valvulitis, the *aortocervical syndrome* does not differ greatly from that produced by aortocranial atherosclerosis, and the neurologic symptoms resemble those of carotid or vertebral-basilar disease.

Meningovascular syphilis appears in early and late forms. The early type (syphilitic meningitis) presents usually within 3 to 6 weeks of primary infection. The patient has fever, severe headache, vomiting, photophobia, and neck stiffness. Somnolence, delirium, psychosis, and focal signs such as hemiplegia, seizures, aphasia, and cranial nerve palsies may occur alone or as a group. At times intracranial pressure is elevated and papilledema develops. The course of the illness is self-limited, but the acute meningitis must be treated as soon as the cause has been established.

The late form of meningovascular syphilis has so many guises that it is known as "the great mimic." The endarteritis may affect any aortocranial artery but is usually confined to the intracerebral penetrating branches. Here it produces signs of focal cerebral insufficiency or infarction, the manifestations depending on the artery involved.

Chronic low-grade basilar meningitis does not cause signs of meningeal irritation and is so insidious that the first manifestation of a long-standing meningitis may be entrapment of cranial nerves, hydrocephalus produced by acute obstruction of the subarachnoid pathways, or vascular obstruction. This arachnoiditis sometimes affects the region of the foramen magnum and the cervical spinal cord, producing spastic paraplegia.

Paresis (general paralysis of the insane, GPI) occurs when the brain parenchyma itself is the locus of the infection by the spirochete. The usual picture is that of a slowly progressive dementia and gradual onset of psychosis. In about 10 percent of cases the presenting abnormality is a convulsion or sudden focal neurologic deficit. On examination the patient may have impaired intellectual function, delusions, hallucinations, or all three. At times a circumoral tremor, which is strongly suggestive of *paresis*, may be the only clue to the presence of cerebral syphilis. Pupillary reactions may be normal to light, but in most instances they are unequal in size, eccentric in contour, and usually sluggish in their response to light because of involvement of the region of the Edinger-Westphal nucleus.

DIFFERENTIAL DIAGNOSIS

Central nervous system syphilis must be distinguished by its mode of clinical presentation from meningitis, occlusive vascular diseases, epilepsy, brain tumor, and various psychiatric disorders. In meningovascular syphilis, the pupils vary from normal to the classical Argyll-Robertson pupils (bilateral, irregular, small pupils reacting to accommodation but not to light and with poor response to atropine). True Argyll-Robertson pupils, quite frequent in paresis, are less common in meningovascular syphilis, but when present they are almost pathognomonic of neurosyphilis.

LABORATORY FINDINGS

A positive serum reaction for syphilis does not necessarily mean that a patient has syphilis or that syphilis is the cause of his neurologic deficit. Collagen vascular diseases, as well as treated syphilis, can cause reactive serum. Antinuclear antibody tests can distinguish between the two.

On the other hand, reactive cerebrospinal fluid is practically pathognomonic of neurosyphilis, which may or may not be active. Pleocytosis signifies activity, and in its presence antisyphilitic therapy is mandatory. *Because 10 to 15 percent of patients with active neurosyphilis have nonreactive serum, the spinal fluid must be tested in all cases of neurologic disease where syphilis is even remotely possible.*

The usual CSF findings in patients with active neurosyphilis are normal pressure, 10 to more than 1,000 lymphocytes, elevated protein level, and increased amount of globulin with a first- or second-zone colloidal-gold curve.

With treatment, the cells disappear within 6 weeks and protein tends to diminish to a normal level by the end of 6 months, although its concentration may remain elevated for as long as 2 years after eradication of the infection. However, the elevated globulins often persist for several years; during this interval titers of quantitative tests usually decline slowly.

Patients with "burned-out" syphilis may have either positive or negative reactions in both blood and spinal fluid. If these reactions are negative, the *T. pallidum* immobilization or complement-fixation test or fluorescent-antibody absorption test will provide the only proof of neurosyphilis.

COURSE OF THE DISEASE

The loss of function caused by meningovascular syphilis sometimes improves without treatment but results in episodes of reversible neurologic deficit due in part to acute endarteritis with perivascular encephalitis and perhaps edema. Because these episodes may subside spontaneously, further attacks may not appear until obliteration of the artery causes infarction. The manifestations then depend on the vessel involved. Intellectual deterioration is not as prominent a feature as it is in the syndrome of paresis.

Patients with meningovascular syphilis often respond well to antisyphilitic treatment, and the course of the illness may be arrested or reversed. Long-standing phenomena such as headaches and convulsions are common residua and are little affected by therapy.

Paresis usually has an insidious onset and in most untreated patients leads eventually to psychic manifestations, dementia, and convulsions. Progress of the disorder can be arrested by therapy, but residual damage is great if the disease is not caught early, and many patients end their days in a mental institution.

There is a growing suspicion that neurosyphilis may progress despite reversion of cerebrospinal fluid contents to normal by penicillin therapy. Some authorities assert that in these cases spirochetes remain viable in loculated foci such as the anterior chambers of the eye and within the parenchyma of the brain.

MANAGEMENT

The currently accepted method of treating all forms of active syphilis is by repository penicillin. Five intramuscular injections of benzathine penicillin, 2.4 million units each, are given at weekly intervals. A broad-spectrum antibiotic such as tetracycline, when given in 500-mg doses four times a day for 20 days, is equally effective for patients who have hypersensitivity reactions and for those instances of penicillin resistance.

The most serious untoward effect of therapy is the rare Jarisch-Herxheimer reaction, which begins within 24 hr of the first dose of the antibiotic with high fever, agitation, and at times seizures, but rarely lasts longer than a day. It has been suggested that a preliminary course of iodides or bismuth or a low initial dose of penicillin may prevent this sometimes serious complication, but the general belief is that there is no effective way of either predicting or forestalling the reaction. When it does occur, it should be managed symptomatically.

SUGGESTED READINGS

General

Brown, W. J., Donohue, J. F., Axnick, N. W., Blount, J. H., Ewen, N. H., and Jones, O. G.: Syphilis and Other Venereal Diseases, Harvard University Press, Cambridge, Mass., 1970.

Dewhurst, K.: The neurosyphilitic psychoses today. A survey of 91 cases, *Brit. J. Psychiat.*, **115**:31, 1969.

Joffe, R., Black, M. M., and Floyd, M.: Changing clinical picture of neurosyphilis: Report of seven unusual cases, *Brit. Med. J.*, **1**:211, 1968.

Leading article: Jarisch-Herxheimer reaction, *Brit. Med. J.*, **1**:384, 1967.

Merritt, H. H., Adams, R. D., and Soloman, H. C.: Neurosyphilis, Oxford University Press, Fair Lawn, N. J., 1946.

Rockwell, D. H., Yobs, A. R., and Moore, M. B., Jr.: The Tuskegee study of untreated syphilis: The 30th year of observation, *Arch. Internal Med.*, **114**:792, 1964.

Smith, J. L.: Spirochetes in Late Seronegative Syphilis, Penicillin Notwithstanding, Charles C Thomas, Publisher, Springfield, Ill., 1969.

———, Israel, C. W., and Harner, R. E.: Syphilitic temporal arteritis, *Arch. Ophthalmol.*, **78**:284, 1967.

Thomas, E. W.: Some aspects of neurosyphilis, *Med. Clin. N. Am.*, **48**(3):699, 1964.

Clinical Features

Wetherill, J. H., Webb, H. E., and Catterall, R. D.: Syphilis presenting as an acute neurological illness, *Brit. Med. J.*, **1**:1157, 1965.

Differential Diagnosis

Galbraith, A. J., and Meyer, A.: Lissauer's dementia paralytica: Contribution to the study of its diagnosis and pathogenesis, *J. Neurol. Neurosurg. Psychiat.*, **5**:22, 1942.

Géraud, J., Rascol, A., Bénazet, J., Arbus, L., and Bés, A.: Thrombose vertébro-basilaire par méningo-artérite syphilitique (Étude clinique-angiographique et hémodynamique d'une observation avec survie), *Rev. neurol.*, **109**:461, 1963.

Laboratory Findings

Cole, M.: "Examination of the cerebrospinal fluid," in Special Techniques for Neurologic Diagnosis (Contemporary Neurology Series, 3), edited by J. F. Toole, F. A. Davis Company, Philadelphia, 1969, pp. 29–47.

Dewhurst, K.: Atypical serology in neurosyphilis, *J. Neurol. Neurosurg. Psychiat.*, **31**:496, 1968.

Kellogg, D. S., and Mothershed, S. M.: Immunofluorescent detection of *Treponema pallidum*. A review, *J.A.M.A.*, **207**:938, 1969.

Mackey, D. M., Price, E. V., Knox, J. M., and Scotti, A.: Specificity of the FTA-ABS test for syphilis: An evaluation, *J.A.M.A.*, **207**:1683, 1969.

Oxelius, V.-A., Rorsman, H., and Laurell, A.-B.: Immunoglobulins of cerebrospinal fluid in syphilis, *Brit. J. Vener. Dis.*, **45**:121, 1969.

Smith, J. L.: The false-negative *Treponema pallidum* immobilization test in syphilis. Pseudobiologic false-positive syndrome, *J.A.M.A.*, **199**:128, 1967.

Zellmann, H. E., and Lutz, W. B.: The Treponema pallidum immobilization test in the cerebrospinal fluid: With a discussion of the phenomenon of chronic biologic false positivity in the cerebrospinal fluid, *J. Chronic Diseases*, **3**:390, 1956.

Course of the Disease

Cannefax, G. R.: Immunity in syphilis, *Brit. J. Vener. Dis.*, **41**:260, 1965.

Dowzenko, A., and Krysztofiak, B.: Relapses in the cerebrospinal fluid and acquired resistance to penicillin in cases of neurosyphilis, *J. Neurol. Sci.*, **2**:197, 1965.

Wilner, E., and Brody, J. A.: Prognosis of general paresis after treatment, *Lancet*, **2**:1370, 1968.

Management

Fiumara, N. J.: The treatment of syphilis, *New Engl. J. Med.,* **270**:1185, 1964.

Additional References

Ch'ien, L., Hathaway, B. M., and Israel, C. W.: Seronegative dementia paralytica: Report of a case, *J. Neurol. Neurosurg. Psychiat.,* **33**:376, 1970.

Fiumara, N. J.: (Editorial) A laboratory test is not a diagnosis, *J.A.M.A.,* **217**:71, 1971.

Goldman, N. N., and Lantz, M. A.: FTA-ABS and VDRL slide test reactivity in a population of nuns, *J.A.M.A.,* **217**:53, 1971.

Hooshmand, H., Escobar, M. R., and Kopf, S. W.: Neurosyphilis. A study of 241 patients, *J.A.M.A.,* **219**:726, 1972.

Izzat, N. N., Bartruff, J. K., Glicksman, J. M., Holder, W. R., and Knox, J. M.: Validity of the VDRL test on cerebrospinal fluid contaminated by blood, *Brit. J. Vener. Dis.,* **47**:162, 1971.

Kostant, G. H.: Familial chronic biologic false-positive seroreactions for syphilis. Report of two families, one with three generations affected, *J.A.M.A.,* **219**:45, 1972.

O'Neill, P., and Nicol, C. S.: IgM class antitreponemal antibody in treated and untreated syphilis, *Brit. J. Vener. Dis.,* **48**:460, 1972.

Sparling, P. F.: Diagnosis and treatment of syphilis, *New Engl. J. Med.,* **284**:642, 1971.

Diseases of Intracranial Veins and Venous Sinuses

The greater the ignorance the greater the dogmatism.

Sir William Osler

Diseases of the intracranial veins and venous sinuses produce effects by obstructing the vein lumen or by causing inflammation of surrounding brain parenchyma. Occlusion by thrombus is the commonest by far and may be caused by dehydration, trauma, sickle-cell crisis, infection, or postpartum thrombophlebitis. Recently the oral contraceptives (progestational hormones) have been blamed for some thromboses. Less frequent abnormalities are occlusion of veins by primary or metastatic neoplasm.

CORTICAL THROMBOPHLEBITIS

Pathogenesis

The lumen of the vein may be stenosed or occluded by septic or sterile thrombus. Although the source of infection may lie far from the brain within the thoracic or abdominal cavity, the most common sources are the middle ear, mastoid air cells, and paranasal sinuses. The venous interconnections between these and the intracranial veins are such that infection can spread to the brain from any one of them.

The rich interconnections between the superficial veins and the lack of valves allow almost instantaneous local shunting of blood from one area to another. The potentialities of these venous anastomoses are so great that experimental production of cerebral infarction by occlusion of cerebral veins or sinuses is extremely difficult. When deficit does develop, recovery may be rapid because of the recanalization of the vein and establishment of collateral channels.

Pathology

At autopsy, the involved veins are thrombosed. The underlying brain parenchyma may be edematous, with or without hemorrhagic infarction in the area normally drained by the thrombosed veins. An infarction resulting from venous occlusion usually involves the cortex and the subjacent white matter and is hemorrhagic, in contrast to infarction resulting from arterial occlusion, which is usually wedge-shaped and bloodless. In cases with infection there may be evidence of leptomeningitis and abscess.

Clinical Features

When the superior group of superficial veins is involved, contralateral focal motor or sensory seizures are seen predominantly in the leg. Central facial palsy, focal seizures about the face, and aphasia occur when the middle cerebral group is occluded. Occlusion in the inferior group commonly originates in the middle ear and extends via emissary veins to the superficial veins of the temporal lobe, resulting in temporal lobe seizures. Signs of intracranial hypertension do not develop unless one of the sagittal sinuses becomes involved or massive cerebral edema develops.

Differential Diagnosis

Acute onset of headaches, focal seizures, or paralysis in an individual with sinusitis or otitis media should alert one to the possibility of cortical thrombophlebitis, meningitis, or intracranial abscess. Focal signs accompanied by severe headaches, stupor, or lateralizing signs suggest abscess. Absence of focal signs in a patient with high fever and neck stiffness favors meningitis. However, cortical thrombophlebitis may present in any of these ways, and at times differentiation cannot be made on clinical grounds alone.

In patients without discernible predisposing

cause, the distinction between a venous thrombosis and an arterial occlusion may be difficult. Predominant weakness of the leg, in contrast to the arm, suggests either the anterior cerebral artery or the superior cerebral group of veins. With the latter, plastic-type rigidity is said to be typical and the motor and sensory disturbances show considerable hour-to-hour and day-to-day variation. Focal convulsions are also more common with the venous than with the arterial disorder. In many cases recovery is virtually complete within a few days, and even in patients with severe paralysis, complete recovery is possible after weeks or months.

DURAL SINUS OCCLUSION

Superior Sagittal Sinus Thrombosis

This is probably the most commonly occluded sinus. Dehydration in infants, head injury, and extension of thrombosis from cortical thrombophlebitis or the transverse sinus are frequent causes. Occlusion may sometimes be asymptomatic if the most anterior portions are occluded, but it may cause severe deficit if the parietooccipital region is affected. Because this sinus drains spinal fluid as well as venous blood, occlusion may produce elevation of intracranial pressure, with headaches, vomiting, somnolence, and diplopia due to abducens palsy. Papilledema with retinal hemorrhages may develop.

Occlusion of the sinus at or behind the entrance of the Rolandic veins frequently progresses to involve the cortical veins bilaterally. Flaccid paraparesis is later replaced by severe spasticity. Involvement of veins draining the parietal lobes will result in contralateral sensory deficit, particularly in the leg. When the arm is involved, its proximal portion is the more severely affected, since representation on the sensory cortex is closer to the superior sagittal sinus. Focal seizures and paralysis may occur, and bladder and bowel incontinence may result from disturbance of function of the parietal lobules.

Transverse Sinus Thrombosis

Mastoid infection and otitis media are the most frequent causes of this lesion. Occlusion per se usually causes no symptoms. In patients with a congenital anomaly of the confluens sinuum or opposite transverse sinus and in those in whom the thrombosis propagates to involve the superior sagittal or the opposite transverse sinus, progressive cerebral edema develops.

Rarely the thrombus extends downward to involve the superior bulb of the internal jugular vein, resulting in compression and loss of function of the ninth, tenth, and eleventh cranial nerves (jugular foramen syndrome).

Inferior Petrosal Sinus Thrombosis

This is frequently associated with infection of the middle ear. The abducens nerve travels across the petrous bone in the canal of Dorello and is involved by the distended and thrombosed sinus to produce ipsilateral abducens palsy and facial pain (Gradenigo's syndrome).

Superior Petrosal Sinus Thrombosis

This results from middle-ear infection through the thin tegmen tympani or as a result of spread from cavernous sinus or inferior petrosal sinus thrombosis. Ipsilateral facial pain is frequent because of the proximity of the trigeminal ganglion. Thrombophlebitis may spread to involve veins of the temporal lobe and can cause local scarring which may serve as a focus for epileptic discharge in the future.

Cavernous Sinus Thrombosis

Localized infection of the area around the mouth, the nostrils, and the frontal sinuses is the usual source of cavernous thrombophlebitis.

Usually the onset is explosive, but when the infective nidus is in the orbit or pharynx, the clinical picture may be subacute and insidious. Headache, high fever, toxemia, unilateral proptosis, conjunctival injection, and chemosis are always present. Involvement of the trigeminal nerve produces facial pain. One pupil is frequently fixed and dilated, and vision is impaired. Ophthalmoscopic examination reveals papilledema with hemorrhages due to involvement of the ophthalmic veins. Shortly thereafter, the other eye may be involved as well. In contrast with caroticocavernous fistula, cavernous sinus thrombosis almost never produces an ocular bruit. At times thrombosis of the veins draining the pituitary gland results in pituitary necrosis and hypopituitarism.

THROMBOSIS OF THE GALENIC SYSTEM

This may precipitate coma with decerebrate rigidity, hyperpyrexia, tachycardia, tachypnea, and death. In the few survivors, a clinical picture of bilateral choreoathetosis is seen because of infarction of the basal ganglia. Birth trauma and neonatal infection are the most frequent culprits.

LABORATORY FINDINGS

Results of laboratory investigations of patients with cortical thrombophlebitis or dural thrombosis are quite similar. The patient is usually febrile and has leukocytosis. In Negroes one should search for sickle cells and make an electrophoretic pattern for abnormal hemoglobin.

Lumbar Puncture

Manometric Tests The initial pressure may be either normal or elevated. It is a dictum in neurology that jugular compression should never be performed if an intracranial process is suspected. This is because the test provides no information of value and may precipitate acute transtentorial or transforaminal herniation by the acute increase in venous pressure which it creates. Perhaps the only exception to this rule occurs when transverse sinus thrombosis is suspected. In this instance the jugular vein is compressed, first on one side and then on the other. If one sinus is occluded, the normal rise and fall of the cerebrospinal fluid pressure may be absent on that side. If the transverse sinuses or the confluens sinuum is anomalous or if the thrombus does not completely occlude the vein, this test may give misleading results.

A few cells and increased proteins are common in nonseptic thrombosis, but with infection polymorphonuclear cells are found. Smear and culture of the fluid must be done whenever thrombosis of a sinus or cerebral vein is suspected. If hemorrhagic infarction has occurred, the fluid may be bloodstained.

Roentgenologic Studies

Special roentgenologic views of the skull are needed to detect infection of the mastoid process or of the paranasal sinuses.

Venography This is usually performed by taking serial x-ray films after an injection of contrast medium into the carotid artery. The later films generally show the superficial and deep venous systems slightly earlier than the dural sinuses. At times, contrast medium is injected directly into the superior sagittal sinus after a hole has been drilled into the skull; in infants the material can be injected into the sinus through the anterior fontanelle. Alternatively, a catheter can be threaded from the jugular vein up into the transverse sinus, and positive contrast material injected to outline the dural sinuses.

Electroencephalography

The electroencephalogram in the majority of patients with cortical thrombophlebitis is nor-mal or shows mild, nonspecific changes. In instances of superior sagittal sinus thrombosis, bilateral slowing is sometimes seen.

COURSE AND PROGNOSIS

Except for patients with cavernous sinus thrombosis, those suffering with intracranial veno-occlusive diseases usually recover. With good supportive measures and antibiotic therapy for the primary infection, a patient's recovery of function is often rapid in spite of the extent of the initial deficit. Some patients have no residua, but others are left with persisting paralysis, mental changes, seizures, or choreoathetosis. Those who die succumb to septicemia or brain abscess. An ominous sign in this unusual group is falling temperature with accelerating pulse—the so-called cross of death.

Some patients with transverse sinus thrombosis, especially those with extension to the confluens sinuum or superior sagittal sinus, may develop the clinical picture of benign intracranial hypertension or "pseudotumor cerebri."

MANAGEMENT

Appropriate antibiotics should be administered to patients with infection until it is eradicated. Once phlebitis has been controlled, abscess in the sinus or mastoid should be removed and brain abscess should be excised.

The idiopathic group of veno-occlusive diseases is best left alone, permitting spontaneous recanalization to occur. The temptation to use anticoagulants should be resisted if there is evidence of hemorrhagic infarction; but if spinal fluid is clear and there is no evidence of infarction, they may be used, especially if there is evidence of a venous thrombosis elsewhere in the body. Seizures should be managed with anticonvulsants.

If elevated cerebrospinal fluid pressure develops, the most important aspect of management is the preservation of function of the optic nerves. Increased pressure may result in papilledema and eventually in secondary optic atrophy. Consequently visual acuity and visual fields must be determined at least weekly, and if deterioration occurs, the elevated cerebrospinal fluid pressure must be reduced. Some neurologists prefer repeated lumbar puncture; others advocate a subtemporal decompression. Recently corticosteroids have been used, but their efficacy is not clear cut.

SUGGESTED READINGS

General

Carroll, J. D., Leak, D., and Lee, H. A.: Cerebral thrombophlebitis in pregnancy and the puerperium, *Quart. J. Med.,* **35**:347, 1966.

Landers, J. W., Chason, J. L., and Samuel, V. N.: Central pontine myelinolysis: A pathogenetic hypothesis, *Neurology,* **15**:968, 1965.

Lemmi, H., and Little, S. C.: Occlusion of intracranial venous structures: A consideration of the clinical and electroencephalographic findings, *Arch. Neurol.,* **3**:252, 1960.

Stuart, E. A., O'Brien, F. H., and McNally, W. J.: Cerebral venous thrombosis: Its occurrence; its localization; its sources and sequelae, *Ann. Otol. Rhinol. Laryngol.,* **60**:406, 1951.

Symonds, C.: Intracranial thrombophlebitis: Otolaryngology lecture, *Ann. Roy. Coll. Surg. Engl.,* **10**:347, 1952.

Walsh, F. B.: Ocular signs of thrombosis of the intracranial venous sinuses, *Arch. Ophthalmol.,* **17**:46, 1937.

Cortical Thrombophlebitis

Atkinson, E. A., Fairburn, B., and Heathfield, K. W. G.: Intracranial venous thrombosis as complication of oral contraception, *Lancet,* **1**:914, 1970.

Barnett, H. J. M., and Hyland, H. H.: Non-infective intracranial venous thrombosis, *Brain,* **76**:36, 1953.

Deshpande, D. H.: Puerperal intracranial venous thrombosis (an autopsy study of 7 cases), *Neurology (India),* **15**:164, 1967.

Endtz, L. J., van Rijn, J. M. L., van Beusekom, G. T., and Luyendijk, W.: Les obstructions veineuses cérébrales pendant la grossesse; thromboses ou phlébites? Revue de la littérature et présentation d'un cas, *Rev. neurol.,* **116**:43, 1967.

Kalbag, R. M., and Woolf, A. L.: Cerebral Venous Thrombosis, with Special Reference to Primary Aseptic Thrombosis, Oxford University Press, New York, 1967.

Kendall, D.: Thrombosis of intracranial veins, *Brain,* **71**:386, 1948.

Manterola, A., Towbin, A., and Yakovlev, P. I.: Cerebral infarction in the human fetus near term, *J. Neuropathol. Exptl. Neurol.,* **25**:479, 1966.

Martin, J. P., and Sheehan, H. L.: Primary thrombosis of cerebral veins (following childbirth), *Brit. Med. J.,* **1**:349, 1941.

Merwarth, H. R., and Relkin, R.: Thrombophlebitis migrans: With syndrome of rolandic vein occlusion, *New York State J. Med.,* **66**(part 1):876, 1966.

Moore, M. T., and Book, M. H.: Cerebral segmental nodular phlebitis, *J. Neuropathol. Exptl. Neurol.,* **25**:269, 1966.

Pathak, S. N., Dhar, P., Berry, K., and Kumar, S.: Venous and arterial thrombosis in 30 young Indian women, *Neurology, (India),* **14**:102, 1966.

Raskind, R., and Weiss, S. R.: Postpartum cortical venous thrombosis with unusual angiographic and operative findings, *Angiology,* **20**:102, 1969.

Vuia, O.: Necrotic leucoencephalopathy of venous origin, *Psychiat. Neurol. Neurochir.,* **71**:287, 1968.

Dural Sinus Occlusion

Amias, A. G.: Cerebral vascular disease in pregnancy. 2. Occlusion, *J. Obstet. Gynaec. Brit. Commonwealth,* **77**:312, 1970.

Bailey, O. T.: Results of long survival after thrombosis of the superior sagittal sinus, *Neurology,* **9**:741, 1959.

Buchanan, D. S., and Brazinsky, J. H.: Dural sinus and cerebral venous thrombosis. Incidence in young women receiving oral contraceptives, *Arch. Neurol.,* **22**:440, 1970.

Gabrielsen, T. O., and Heinz, E. R.: Spontaneous aseptic thrombosis of the superior sagittal sinus and cerebral veins, *Am. J. Roentgenol.,* **107**:579, 1969.

Greitz, T., and Link, H.: Aseptic thrombosis of intracranial sinuses, *Radiol. Clin.*, **35**:111, 1966.

Holmes, G., and Sargent, P.: Injuries of the superior longitudinal sinus, *Brit. Med. J.*, **2**:493, 1915.

Ivey, K. J., and Smith, H.: Hypopituitarism associated with cavernous sinus thrombosis. Report of a case, *J. Neurol. Neurosurg. Psychiat.*, **31**:187, 1968.

Krayenbühl, H. A.: Cerebral venous and sinus thrombosis, *Clin. Neurosurg.*, **14**:1, 1967.

Matthew, N. T., Abraham, J., Taori, G. M., and Iyer, G. V.: Internal carotid artery occlusion in cavernous sinus thrombosis, *Arch. Neurol.*, **24**:11, 1971.

Mones, R. J.: Increased intracranial pressure due to metastatic disease of venous sinuses: A report of six cases, *Neurology*, **15**:1000, 1965.

Movsas, S., and Movsas, I.: Carotico-cavernous fistula complicating cavernous sinus thrombophlebitis, *Clin. Radiol.*, **19**:90, 1968.

Thrombosis of the Galenic System

Bots, G. Th. A. M.: Thrombosis of the galenic system veins in the adult, *Acta neuropathol. (Berlin)*, **17**:227, 1971.

Laboratory Findings

Edwards, E. A.: Anatomic variations of the cranial venous sinuses; their relation to the effect of jugular compression in lumbar manometric tests, *Arch. Neurol. Psychiat.*, **26**:801, 1931.

Galligioni, F., Bernardi, R., Pellone, M., and Iraci, G.: The veins of the posterior cranial fossa: An angiographic study under pathologic conditions, *Am. J. Roentgenol.*, **110**:39, 1970.

Tobey, G. L., and Ayer, J. B.: Dynamic studies on the cerebrospinal fluid in the differential diagnosis of lateral sinus thrombosis, *Arch. Otolaryngol.*, **2**:50, 1925.

Vines, F.: Clinical radiologic correlates in cerebral venous occlusive disease, *Neurology*, **20**:375, 1970.

Vines, F. S., and Davis, D. O.: Clinical-radiological correlation in cerebral venous occlusive disease, *Radiology*, **98**:9, 1971.

Course and Prognosis

Merwarth, H. R.: The syndrome of Rolandic vein (hemiplegia of venous origin), *Am. J. Surg.*, **56**:526, 1942.

Management

Malik, S. R. K., Gupta, A. K., Singh, G., and Choudhry, S.: Pyrrolidinomethyl tetracycline in cavernous sinus thrombosis, *Brit. J. Ophthalmol.*, **54**:113, 1970.

Benign Intracranial Hypertension (Pseudotumor Cerebri)

Foley, J.: Benign forms of intracranial hypertension—"toxic" and "otitic" hydrocephalus, *Brain*, **78**:1, 1955.

Greer, M.: Benign intracranial hypertension: I. Mastoiditis and lateral sinus obstruction, *Neurology*, **12**:472, 1962.

Patterson, R., DePasquale, N., and Mann, S.: Pseudotumor cerebri, *Medicine*, **40**:85, 1961.

Additional Reference

Chazot, G., Dumas, R., Creyssel, R., and Girard, P.-F.: Cryofibrinogénémie comme facteur étiologique des trombophlébites cérébrales. A propos d'une observation, *Rev. neurol.*, **124**:269, 1971.

Johnsen, S., Greenwood, R., and Fishman, M. A.: Internal cerebral vein thrombosis, *Arch. Neurol.*, **28**:205, 1973.

Chapter 22

Spinovascular Diseases

Vascular disease of the spinal cord is the Cinderella of neurology.

Anonymous

OCCLUSION

An obstructive lesion causing spinal cord ischemia may be situated anywhere from the aortic origin of the segmental arteries to the intraspinal arterioles. Compared to the frequency of occlusive vascular disease of the brain, however, spinal cord vascular disease is very unusual in clinical practice. Yet symptomatic aortospinal atherosclerosis does occur, and cord infarction, as well as transient ischemia with reversible neurologic deficit, has been recognized. The rarity of their occurrence and recognition probably results from a combination of the following causes:

1 Unknown factors which render spinal vessels relatively resistant to atherosclerosis

2 The apparently greater tolerance of the spinal cord for hypoxia
3 Inadequate techniques for angiographic evaluation of spinal vessels
4 Failure to examine the spinal cord at autopsy, and lack of interest in the study of pathology of the vasculature of the cord

The obstructive arterial lesions which are most often responsible for spinal ischemia and infarction are listed in Table 22-1.

Clinical Features

Because it is supplied by terminal portions of the ascending and descending blood columns perfusing the spinal cord, the midthoracic region is particularly vulnerable to vascular insuf

Table 22-1 Obstructive Arterial Lesions Sometimes Responsible for Spinal Cord Infarction

Site	Causative factors
Aorta	Dissection (most frequent) Atherosclerosis Aneurysm, atherosclerotic or syphilitic Takayasu's disease Pressure applied to lumbar aorta to arrest uterine hemorrhage
Vertebral arteries	Fracture with dislocation of the spine Hyperextension injuries of the cervical spine Cervical spondylosis Vertebral arteriography
Intercostal arteries	Postoperative { thoracoplasty / dorsolumbar sympathectomy Coarctation of the aorta (enlarged intercostal arteries)
Medullary arteries	Ligation during surgery for replacement of thoracolumbar aorta Occlusion by malignant tumor, tuberculosis, psoas abscess Injection of contrast material during aortic arteriography Compression by osteoarthritis
Anterior median spinal artery	Atherosclerosis (rare) Diabetic arteriopathy Syphilitic arteritis Mechanical compression by cervical disk (?)
Sulcal arteries	Collagen diseases Endarteritis obliterans { syphilis / tuberculosis / sarcoidosis Air embolism Radiation myelopathy
Pial arteriolar network	Chronic adhesive arachnoiditis

ficiency. Clinically this is evidenced by weakness or paralysis in the legs while strength is preserved in the arms. This weakness may be intermittent, as in ischemia, or permanent if cord infarction occurs.

The diagnosis of intermittent ischemia of the thoracic or lumbar sections of the cord should be considered when weakness of the lower limbs is precipitated by physical effort, particularly if strength is rapidly restored by rest. During this weakness the patient experiences no pain, and pedal pulses remain palpable. However, if the causative lesion is in the abdominal aorta, exercise may also lead to pain in the hips (because of ischemia of gluteal muscles) and impotence (Leriche syndrome). Cervical cord ischemia, which is manifest as "drop attacks" and which is considered in detail in Chap. 11, may also occur.

Although obstruction of the anterior median spinal artery is not common, it produces a characteristic picture which one must recognize in order to institute appropriate measures yet avoid needless neurosurgical procedures. Occasionally infarction is preceded by intermittent episodes of weakness suggestive of ischemia, but most occlusions occur without warning in a predisposed person who has, for example, mechanical deformity of the spine.

The effects of infarction vary with the level at which the artery is occluded. In most instances obstruction is segmental, so that infarction occurs only in the areas supplied by the sulcal arteries and pial arteriolar plexus which spring from the occluded portion. Two distinctly different syndromes occur:

Occlusion of the Anterior Spinal Ramus Obstruction in the intracranial portion of the anterior spinal ramus on one side causes infarction of the homolateral pyramid, the medial lemniscus, and the hypoglossal nucleus and nerve—the ventral medullary syndrome. The results are manifest as contralateral spastic paralysis of the arm and leg, with ipsilateral loss of vibration, position, and light-touch perception, flaccid paralysis, and atrophy of the tongue; perception of pain and temperature is preserved. Occlusion of both anterior spinal rami results in tetraplegia and loss of vibration and position sense in all four limbs.

Occlusion of the Anterior Median Spinal Artery Obstruction in its cervical, thoracic, or lumbar portion is usually initiated by back pain, which may radiate in radicular fashion at the involved level.

Since infarction occurs most frequently in the midthoracic region, the pain radiates in girdle fashion around the thorax and perhaps into the upper part of the abdomen. There follows an acute flaccid paralysis of the lower extremities, associated with loss of pain and temperature sensations. Sphincter control is lost immediately, and there is often reflex ileus and abdominal distention secondary to acute interruption of sympathetic pathways. Because the posterior columns are not involved, perception of vibration, position, and light touch is preserved. This loss of spinothalamic function with preservation of posterior-column function—just the opposite of the proprioceptive loss produced by infarction at the medullary level—is the distinguishing characteristic of this syndrome.

The initial flaccidity and the loss of tendon reflexes result from spinal shock and are gradually replaced by spasticity in all muscles below the level of the lesion, with brisk tendon reflexes and extensor plantar responses. Because of necrosis of the anterior horn cells, however, the muscles at the level of occlusion (the intercostal or abdominal muscles) remain flaccid and become atrophic.

In the late stages of cervical cord lesion, the pattern of motor disability resembles that seen in amyotrophic lateral sclerosis; the small muscles of the hands become atrophied, and the lower limbs show evidence of corticospinal tract involvement as described above.

Etiology

Syphilitic arteritis, now a rarity, was once the most common cause of anterior median spinal artery occlusion. Now the most commonly listed causes are diabetic arteriopathy, cervical spondylosis, and collagen vascular disease, such as polyarteritis nodosa or systemic lupus erythematosus; occasionally caisson disease, a blood clot, or air embolus may be responsible for the syndrome. In many cases no primary cause can be discovered.

Differential Diagnosis

Infarction of the spinal cord may follow dissection or thrombosis of the aorta, trauma to the medullary arteries, or occlusion of the anterior median spinal artery or its branches. If posterior columns are involved, the abnormality is not a thrombosis of the anterior median spinal artery, but may be caused by any of a number of problems ranging from a neoplasm to multiple sclerosis. In all cases of acute loss of cord function, compression by tumor is the primary consideration, and elimination of this possibility must be foremost in the mind of the physician. To be certain, emergency myelography is usually necessary. As a prelude, the entire length of the spine must be examined by x-ray, which may reveal the collapse or erosion of a vertebra by neoplasm. The initial lumbar puncture should be performed as a prelude to the myelographic procedure. If the symptoms are caused by thrombosis of the anterior median spinal artery, the spinal fluid will be clear and will contain no cells; the results of the Queckenstedt test and the myelogram will be normal.

Treatment

Although there is no specific "cure" for infarction of the cord, rehabilitative measures should be initiated immediately after the condition is diagnosed (see Chap. 30). If the stage of "intermittent claudication of the spinal cord" can be correctly diagnosed, anticoagulant therapy may possibly prevent or postpone the development of infarction.

Occlusion of Posterior Arteriolar Plexus (Posterior Spinal Arteries)

Infarction of the cord in the area supplied by the posterior arteriolar plexus is rare because of the rich anastomoses present in the pial plexus. When infarction does occur, it results in interruption of posterior column and posterior horn function. At times portions of the lateral corticospinal tract may be involved as well.

Occlusion of the Great Anterior Medullary Artery (of Adamkiewicz)

Injury to this artery usually results from surgery which involves the lumbar aorta, such as resection of an abdominal aortic aneurysm or renal

arterial reconstruction. Occlusion of this medullary artery, which can arise at any level from T_{10} to L_3, may cause infarction of the anterior two-thirds of the lumbosacral cord, leading to flaccid paralysis and loss of pain and temperature sensations in both lower limbs. Sphincter control is also lost. Clinically this syndrome cannot be differentiated from anterior median spinal artery thrombosis.

OTHER CAUSES OF SPINAL CORD INFARCTION

Cervical Spondylosis, Herniated Nucleus Pulposus, and "Whiplash" Injuries

Spondylosis, particularly in the cervical region where the arteries enter the spinal canal through the vertebral foramina, may impair blood supply to the cord. Protrusion of a nucleus pulposus may compress the anterior median spinal artery or may displace the spinal cord posteriorly, thereby stretching dentate ligaments which suspend the cord in the spinal canal. This causes venous congestion and ischemia by squeezing the cord between these ligaments and the nucleus pulposus. Flexion-and-extension injuries of the cervical spine (whiplash injuries), in addition to causing acute concussion of the cord, may interrupt its blood supply by compressing the arteries or by stretching them, so that vasospasm of the vertebral arteries or of their branches results. At times this constriction persists long after the acute episode and results in persistent symptoms.

Acute Dissection of the Aortic Arch

Spontaneous or traumatic dissection of the thoracic or lumbar aorta can cause infarction of the spinal cord by occluding the ostia of the segmental arteries. Patients suffering this catastrophe have no pulse in the arteries below the abdominal aorta, and require emergency surgery to correct the dissection. Unfortunately, correction of the aortic lesion seldom restores cord function. (See Chap. 29.)

Chronic dissection of the aorta may lead to an insidious paraparesis with normal peripheral pulses. In such cases an aortogram may be the only method by which the diagnosis can be made.

Iatrogenic Myelopathy

Contrast medium inadvertently introduced into the aorta near the ostium of a segmental artery, usually the great anterior medullary artery, during the performance of a lumbar or renal aortogram may flood the spinal cord and cause infarction.

Radiation Myelopathy

Following therapeutic radiation of the thyroid, cervical lymph nodes, posterior part of the tongue, or upper part of the respiratory tract, radiation-induced damage to the small blood vessels of the spinal cord may cause infarction. Similar damage to the thoracic cord may follow radiation for bronchogenic carcinoma. Neural deficit becomes manifest only after a latent period of 1 to 2 years and is manifested by rapidly progressive neural deficit below the level of the radiation. The myelopathy usually runs a course of 1 to 2 months, sometimes leading to the loss of function in all tracts traversing the cord.

This complication of radiation therapy is very rare and is dependent on the total dose, on the technique and duration of therapy, and perhaps on individual sensitivity. Diagnosis should be made only after intraspinal metastasis has been excluded by myelographic examination.

VENOUS DISEASE

Subacute Necrotic Myelitis (Foix-Alajouanine Disease)

This rare disease most frequently affects middle-aged individuals. The clinical picture is that of progressive paraparesis extending over a period of a few months to 5 years. Both upper and lower motor neurons are involved and there is often a sensory loss below the mid- or lower thoracic region. Sphincteric involvement is also evident. The spinal fluid may show a few cells, with moderate or marked rise of protein level (albuminocytologic dissociation).

Pathologic examination reveals degeneration or necrosis of the spinal cord, with surface vessels appearing dilated and tortuous and often containing intraluminal thrombi. A few investigators believe this appearance to represent a primary thrombophlebitis of the superficial veins of the spinal cord with secondary vascular dilatation. Most consider the primary lesion to be an arteriovenous malformation in which secondary thrombosis of veins has developed.

ARACHNOIDITIS

This condition can be caused by trauma, infection, neoplasms, subarachnoid bleeding, or intrathecal administration of foreign substances, but often the cause is undetermined. There is evidence of root and/or cord involvement at multiple levels. Rarely arachnoiditis may lead to secondary cavitation within the substance of the spinal cord, simulating syringomyelia. Pathologic examination usually reveals an obliterative angiopathy with variable involvement of the vessels of the leptomeninges, roots, and spinal cord, accompanied by some inflammatory response.

SPINAL HEMORRHAGE

Spinal hemorrhage, like intracranial hemorrhage, may be epidural, subdural, subarachnoid, or intramedullary and may be spontaneous or traumatic in origin. Since aneurysms of spinal arteries are very rare, the anatomic abnormality most frequently responsible for spontaneous spinal hemorrhage is arteriovenous malformation. Such arteriovenous malformations of the spinal cord interconnect with the arteries and veins of the thorax and abdomen, and sometimes with the pelvic vessels. In the spinal cord, arteriovenous malformations may be intramedullary, meningeal, or a combination of the two types (Fig. 22-1). The presenting symptoms may be caused by compression myelopathy, intraspinal hemorrhage, or both; the hemorrhage may be subarachnoid, epidural, or intramedullary.

Some patients with compression myelopathy caused by an arteriovenous malformation give a history of remissions and relapses, radicular pain made worse upon standing up, and aggravations during pregnancy. Occasionally the presence of intraspinal vascular malformation is suggested by cutaneous nevus or a bruit at the appropriate level of the spine.

On the myelogram large arteriovenous malformations cause dilated, tortuous filling defects in the opaque column. Because vascular malformations are often located on the posterior as-

pect of the cord, they may be missed unless thoracic myelography is carried out with the patient supine as well as prone (Fig. 22-2).

Surgery is the only effective method of treatment; however, surgical removal of intramedullary angioma may lead to myelomalacia, producing a deficit worse than the original illness.

The anatomy of spinal angioma can be demonstrated vividly by vertebral or aortic angiography utilizing subtraction techniques. When more experience has been gained, this method should enable surgeons to visualize the anatomic ramifications of the malformation, so that arterial feeders to the malformation can be ligated, sparing the normal circulation to the rest of the cord.

Epidural and Subdural Hemorrhage

Epidural and subdural bleeding are usually traumatic in origin, but such hemorrhages also occur in patients who have been receiving anticoagulant medication or who have blood dys-

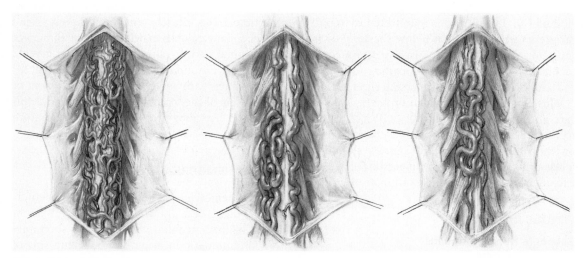

Figure 22-1 Artist's conception of various types of arteriovenous malformations of the spinal cord and canal.

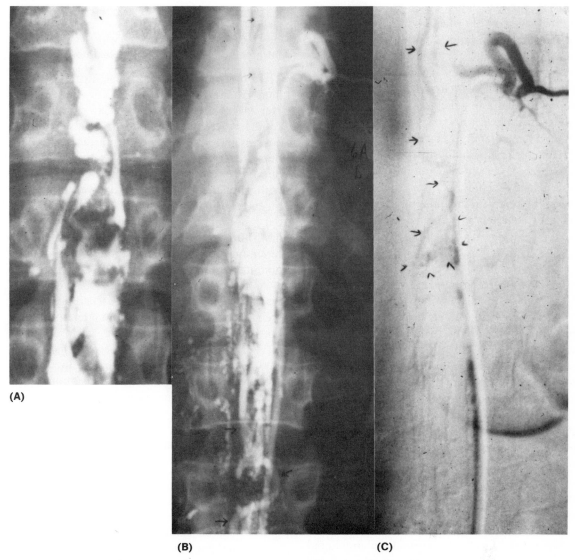

(A)

(B) **(C)**

Figure 22-2 (A) Myelographic defect showing enlarged cord and irregular outlines suggestive of dilated vessels. (B) Combined myelogram and angiogram demonstrating that the irregular myelographic defects are arteries and veins. (C) Subtraction film of spinal angiogram demonstrating the arteriovenous malformation. *(Courtesy of Dr. F. Farrell.)*

crasias. In these latter cases the defect in the clotting mechanism must be corrected immediately. At the same time, the patient should be observed carefully for signs of cord involvement, since emergency surgery is occasionally required to remove a clot which compresses the cord. Any acute spinal cord syndrome is a possible neurosurgical emergency and must be investigated immediately by myelography.

Hemangioma, usually involving the thoracic vertebrae, is an unusual but surgically remediable cause of epidural hemorrhage. X-rays of the spine reveal the telltale honeycomb appearance of a vertebra which might be collapsed.

Subarachnoid Hemorrhage

This may be traumatic or spontaneous. Subarachnoid hemorrhage following lumbar puncture is of no clinical consequence unless the bleeding is profuse, as it may be in rare cases where the patient has a blood dyscrasia or has been taking anticoagulant medication. Trauma to the back may sometimes cause spinal subarachnoid hemorrhage.

When a cause for spontaneous bleeding into the spinal subarachnoid space is found, it is usually rupture of an aneurysm in an arteriovenous malformation. Other causes include neoplasm of the spinal cord; blood dyscrasias such as hemophilia, thrombocytopenic purpura, and leukemia; and, rarely, the rupture of an atherosclerotic or inflamed artery.

Hemorrhage into the spinal subarachnoid space is usually manifested first by excruciating pain in the back, with radiation into the nerve roots. Opisthotonos, followed by temporary partial paralysis of the extremities, may occur. The abnormalities in the spinal fluid are described in Chap. 24.

Treatment consists of bed rest and the correction of any underlying deficit in the clotting mechanism. Extramedullary angiomas need surgical excision.

Intramedullary Hemorrhage (Hematomyelia)

Like subarachnoid hemorrhage, intramedullary hemorrhage may be traumatic or spontaneous. Hematomyelia may result from rupture of a capillary hemangioma following Valsalva's maneuver and may spread in any direction, producing a variety of clinical signs and symptoms. Sudden excruciating pain in the back, often with radicular radiation, is followed by an immediate loss of muscle tone below the level of the lesion. The results are paralysis (flaccid at first, but becoming spastic after several days), retention of urine and feces, and sometimes abdominal distention caused by reflex ileus.

As the blood clot accumulates in the cord, it displaces and compresses the ascending and descending tracts. When the more laterally placed portions of the spinothalamic tracts are preserved, as is often the case, the result is preservation of sensory perception in the sacral dermatomes even though sensory perception in the thoracic and lumbar regions is lost (sacral sparing).

Differential Diagnosis

Whenever there is sudden paraplegia with a sensory loss on the trunk, the primary consideration is acute compression of the spinal cord by extrinsic tumor; hence, the entire length of the spine must be examined roentgenographically as an emergency procedure. If tumor is present, films of the suspected area may reveal evidence of vertebral collapse or erosion of the pedicles. In any event, myelography must be done. When the lumbar puncture is performed, samples of fluid should be collected for cell count and protein determinations. If the myelogram demonstrates evidence of obstruction, immediate decompression of the canal is essential.

SUGGESTED READINGS

General

Corbin, J. L.: Anatomie et Pathologie Arterielles de la Moelle, Masson et Cie, Paris, 1961.

Gilles, F. H., and Nag, D.: Vulnerability of human spinal cord in transient cardiac arrest, *Neurology,* **21**:833, 1971.

Hughes, J. T., and Brownell, B.: Spinal cord ischemia due to arteriosclerosis, *Arch. Neurol.,* **15**:189, 1966.

Odom, G. L.: Vascular lesions of the spinal cord: Malformations, spinal subarachnoid and extradural hemorrhage, *Clin. Neurosurg.,* **8**:196, 1962.

Palleske, H., and Herrmann, H.-D.: Experimental investigations on the regulation of the blood flow of the spinal cord. I. Comparative study of the cerebral and spinal cord blood flow with heat clearance probes in pigs, *Acta neurochir.,* **19**:73, 1968.

———, Kivelitz, R., and Loew, F.: Experimental investigation on the control of spinal cord circulation. IV. The effect of spinal or cerebral compression on the blood flow of the spinal cord, *Acta neurochir.,* **22**:29, 1970.

Vuia, O., and Alexianu, M.: Arteriovenous shunt in the spinal cord circulation, *Acta neurol. scand.,* **45**:216, 1969.

Zülch, K. J., and Kurth-Schumacher, R.: The pathogenesis of "intermittent spinovascular insufficiency" ("spinal claudication of Dejerine") and other vascular syndromes of the spinal cord, *Vascular Surg.,* **4**:116, 1970.

Occlusion

Clinical Features

Davison, C.: Syndrome of anterior spinal artery of the medulla oblongata, *J. Neuropathol. Exptl. Neurol.,* **3**:73, 1944.

Dejerine, J.: Sur la claudication intermittente de la moelle, épinière, *Rev. neurol.,* **14**:341, 1906.

———: La claudication intermittente de la moelle épinière, *Presse med.,* **19**(95):981, 1911.

Deller, J. J., Jr., Scalettar, R., and Levens, A. J.: Pain as a manifestation of acute anterior-spinal-artery thrombosis, *New Engl. J. Med.,* **262**:1078, 1960.

Garland, H., Greenberg, J., and Harriman, D. G. F.: Infarction of the spinal cord, *Brain,* **89**:645, 1966.

Henson, R. A., and Parsons, M.: Ischaemic lesions of the spinal cord: An illustrated review, *Quart. J. Med.,* **36**:205, 1967.

Jellinger, K.: Spinal cord arteriosclerosis and progressive vascular myelopathy, *J. Neurol. Neurosurg. Psychiat.,* **30**:195, 1967.

Julian, H., Djindjian, R., Caron, J. P., and Houdart, R.: Syndrome d'ischémie médullaire par compression discale de l'artère due renflement lombaire, *Neuro-Chirurgie* **14**:163, 1968.

Mannen, T.: Vascular lesions in the spinal cord in the aged: A clinicopathological study, *Geriatrics,* **21**:151, 1966.

Peterman, A. F., Yoss, R. E., and Corbin, K. B.: The syndrome of occlusion of the anterior spinal artery, *Proc. Staff Meetings Mayo Clinic,* **33**:31, 1958.

Reichert, F. L., Rytand, D. A., and Bruck, E. L.: Arteriosclerosis of the lumbar segmental arteries producing ischemia of the spinal cord and consequent claudication of the thighs; Clinical syndrome with experimental confirmation, *Am. J. Med. Sci.,* **187**:794, 1934.

Wells, C. E. C.: Clinical aspects of spinovascular disease, *Proc. Roy. Soc. Med.,* **59**:790, 1966.

Yoss, R. E.: Vascular supply of the spinal cord: The production of vascular syndromes, *Univ. Michigan Med. Bull.,* **16**:333, 1950.

Etiology

Albert, M. L., Greer, W. E. R., and Kantrowitz, W.: Paraplegia secondary to hypotension and cardiac arrest in a patient who has had previous thoracic surgery, *Neurology,* **19**:915, 1969.

Chung, M.-F.: Thrombosis of the spinal vessels in sudden syphilitic paraplegia, *Arch. Neurol. Psychiat.,* **16**:761, 1926.

Coccagna, G., Poppi, M., and Lugaresi, E.: Sindrome dell'arteria spinale anteriore da trombosi dell'arteria vertebrale, *Sist. Nerv.,* **18**:39, 1966.

Djindjian, R., Hurth, M., and Houdar, R.: Artériographie et ischémie médullaire dorso-lombaire d'origine athérmateuse (a propos de 5 cas), *Rev. neurol.,* **122**:5, 1970.

Fieschi, C., Gottlieb, A., and De Carolis, V.: Ischaemic lacunae in the spinal cord of arteriosclerotic subjects, *J. Neurol. Neurosurg. Psychiat.,* **33**:138, 1970.

Jennings, G. H., and Newton, M. A.: Persistent paraplegia after repeated cardiac arrest, *Brit. Med. J.*, **3**:572, 1969.

Joffe, R., Appleby, A., and Arjona, V.: "Intermittent ischaemia" of the cauda equina due to stenosis of the lumbar canal, *J. Neurol. Neurosurg. Psychiat.*, **29**:315, 1966.

Toole, J. F.: Some vascular disorders affecting the spinal cord, *Current Concepts Cerebrovascular Dis.—Stroke*, **4**:11, 1969.

Wolman, L., and Bradshaw, P.: Spinal cord embolism, *J. Neurol. Neurosurg. Psychiat.*, **30**:446, 1967.

Differential Diagnosis

Di Chiro, G., and Doppman, J. L.: Differential angiographic features of hemangioblastomas and arteriovenous malformations of the spinal cord, *Radiology*, **93**:25, 1969.

Djindjian, R.: Arteriography of the spinal cord, *Am. J. Roentgenol.*, **107**:461, 1969.

———, Hurth, M., Houdart, R., Laborit, G., Julian, H., and Mamo, H.: Angiography of the Spinal Cord, University Park Press, Baltimore, 1970.

Doppman, J. L., Di Chiro, G., and Ommaya, A. K.: Selective Arteriography of the Spinal Cord, Warren H. Green, Inc., St. Louis, 1969.

Martin, J. P.: Amyotrophic meningo-myelitis (spinal progressive muscular atrophy of syphilitic origin), *Brain*, **48**:153, 1925.

Wilson, C. B.: Significance of the small lumbar spinal canal: Cauda equina compression syndromes due to spondylosis. Part 3: Intermittent claudication, *J. Neurosurg.*, **31**:499, 1969.

Occlusion of Posterior Arteriolar Plexus (Posterior Spinal Arteries)

Hughes, J. T.: Thrombosis of the posterior spinal arteries. A complication of intrathecal injection of phenol, *Neurology*, **20**:659, 1970.

Perier, O., Demanet, J.-C., Henneaux, J., and Vincente, A. N.: Existe-t-il un syndrome des artères spinales postérieures? A propos de deux observations anatomo-cliniques, *Rev. neurol.*, **103**:396, 1960.

Williamson, R. T.: Spinal softening limited to the parts supplied by the posterior arterial system of the cord, *Lancet*, **2**:520, 1895.

Other Causes of Spinal Cord Infarction

Feigin, I., Popoff, N., and Adachi, M.: Fibrocartilagenous venous emboli to the spinal cord with necrotic myelopathy, *J. Neuropathol. Exptl. Neurol.*, **24**:63, 1965.

Leading article: Spinal cord embolism, *Brit. Med. J.*, **1**:785, 1968.

Penn, A. S., and Rowan, A. J.: Myelopathy in systemic lupus erythematosus, *Arch. Neurol.*, **18**:337, 1968.

Rouges, L.: Les paraplégies cypho-scoliotiques: Révision critique, *Rev. neurol.*, **98**:358, 1958.

Cervical Spondylosis, Herniated Nucleus Pulposus, and Whiplash Injuries

Brieg, A.: Biomechanics of the Central Nervous System, Year Book Medical Publishers, Inc., Chicago, 1960.

Hughes, J. T., and Brownell, B.: Cervical spondylosis complicated by anterior spinal artery thrombosis, *Neurology*, **14**:1073, 1964.

Janes, J. M., and Hooshmand, H.: Severe extension-flexion injuries of the cervical spine, *Mayo Clinic Proc.*, **40**:353, 1965.

Schneider, R. C., and Crosby, E. C.: Vascular insufficiency of brain stem and spinal cord in spinal trauma, *Neurology*, **9**:643, 1959.

Stortebecker, T. P.: Disturbances of arterial blood supply to the spinal cord and brain stem caused by spondylosis, disc protrusions and root-sleeve fibrosis: A concept concerning factors eliciting amyotrophic lateral sclerosis, *Acta orthopaed. scand.*, **29**(suppl. 42):1, 1960.

Acute Dissection of the Aortic Arch

Barnett, W. E., Moorman, W. W., and Merrick, B. A.: Thrombotic obliteration of the abdominal aorta: A report of 6 cases, *Ann. Internal Med.*, **37**:944, 1952.

Kempinsky, W. H.: Paraparesis associated with atherosclerotic aneurysms of abdominal aorta, *Neurology*, **6**:368, 1956.

Mehrez, I. O., Nabseth, D. C., Hogan, E. L., and Deterling, R. A.: Paraplegia following resection of abdominal aortic aneurysm, *Ann. Surg.*, **156**:890, 1962.

Moersch, F. P., and Sayre, G. P.: Neurologic manifestations associated with dissecting aneurysm of the aorta, *J.A.M.A.,* **144**:1141, 1950.

Schwarz, G. A., Shorey, W. K., and Anderson, N. S.: Myelomalacia secondary to dissecting aneurysm of the aorta, *Arch. Neurol. Psychiat.,* **64**:401, 1950.

Thompson, G. B.: Dissecting aortic aneurysm with infarction of the spinal cord, *Brain,* **79**:111, 1956.

Iatrogenic Myelopathy

Adams, H. D., and Van Geertruyden, H. H.: Neurologic complications of aortic surgery, *Ann. Surg.,* **144**:574, 1956.

Adams, J. H., and Cameron, H. M.: Obstetrical paralysis due to ischaemia of the spinal cord, *Arch. Disease Childhood,* **40**:93, 1965.

Feigelson, H. H., and Ravin, H. A.: Transverse myelitis following selective bronchial arteriography, *Radiology,* **85**:663, 1965.

Hogan, E. L., and Romanul, F. C. A.: Spinal cord infarction occurring during insertion of aortic graft, *Neurology,* **16**:67, 1966.

Hughes, J. T., and Brownell, B.: Paraplegia following retrograde abdominal aortography: An example of toxic myelitis, *Arch. Neurol.,* **12**:650, 1965.

Levy, N. A., and Strauss, H. A.: Myelopathy following compression of abdominal aorta for postpartum hemorrhage; Report of a case, *Arch. Neurol. Psychiat.,* **48**:85, 1942.

Wikler, A., Marmor, J., and Hurst, A.: Air embolism of the spinal cord following attempted pneumothorax, *J.A.M.A.,* **109**:430, 1937.

Radiation Myelopathy

Boden, G.: Radiation myelitis of the cervical spinal cord, *Brit. J. Radiol.,* **21**:464, 1948.

Jones, A.: Transient radiation myelopathy (with reference to Lhermitte's sign of electrical paraesthesia), *Brit. J. Radiol.,* **37**:727, 1964.

Pallis, C. A., Louis, S., and Morgan, R. L.: Radiation myelopathy, *Brain,* **84**:460, 1961.

Venous Disease

Coman, D. R., and DeLong, R. P.: The role of the vertebral venous system in the metastasis of cancer to the spinal column: Experiments with tumor-cell suspensions in rats and rabbits, *Cancer,* **4**:610, 1951.

Di Chiro, G., and Doppman, J. L.: Endocranial drainage of spinal cord veins, *Radiology,* **95**:555, 1970.

Doppman, J. L., Wirth, F. P., Jr., et al.: Value of cutaneous angiomas in the arteriographic localization of spinal-cord arteriovenous malformations, *New Engl. J. Med.,* **281**:1440, 1969.

Gillilan, L. A.: Veins of the spinal cord. Anatomic details; suggested clinical applications, *Neurology,* **20**:860, 1970.

Gregorius, F. K., and Weingarten, S. M.: The natural history of vascular malformation of the spinal cord with a presentation of two cases and a review of the literature, *Bull. Los Angeles Neurol. Soc.,* **35**:25, 1970.

Hughes, J. T.: Venous infarction of the spinal cord, *Neurology,* **21**:794, 1971.

Jurkovič, I., and Eiben, E.: Fatal myelomalacia caused by massive fibrocartilaginous venous emboli from nucleus pulposus, *Acta neuropathol. (Berlin),* **15**:284, 1970.

Subacute Necrotic Myelitis

Flament, J., Vincente, A. N., Coërs, C., and Guazzi, G.: La myélomalacie angiodysgénétique (Foix-Alajouanine) et sa différentiation des nécroses spinales sur angiomatose intra-médullaire, *Rev. neurol.,* **103**:12, 1960.

Mair, W. G. P., and Folkerts, J. F.: Necrosis of spinal cord due to thrombophlebitis (subacute necrotic myelitis), *Brain,* **76**:563, 1953.

Arachnoiditis

Kramer, W.: Multiocular myelomalacia following adhesive arachnoiditis, *Neurology,* **6**:594, 1956.

Spinal Hemorrhage

Antoni, N.: Spinal vascular malformations (angiomas) and myelomalacia, *Neurology,* **12**:795, 1962.

Bidzinski, J.: Spontaneous spinal epidural hematoma during pregnancy, *J. Neurosurg.,* **24**:1017, 1966.

Bouzarth, W. P., and Gutterman, P.: Delayed traumatic spinal subarachnoid hemorrhage, *J.A.M.A.,* **205**:880, 1968.

Cloward, R. B., and Yuhl, E. T.: Spontaneous intra-spinal hemorrhage and paraplegia complicating dicumarol therapy, *Neurology, 5*:600, 1955.

Lougheed, W. M., and Hoffman, H. J.: Spontaneous spinal extradural hematoma, *Neurology, 10*:1059, 1960.

Newman, M. J.: Spinal angioma with symptoms in pregnancy, *J. Neurol. Neurosurg, Psychiat., 21*:38, 1958.

Rao, B. D., Rao, K. S., Subrahmanian, M. V., and Reddy, M. V. R.: Spinal epidural hemorrhage, *Brit. J. Surg., 53*:649, 1966.

Epidural and Subdural Hemorrhage

Cooper, D. W.: Spontaneous spinal epidural hematoma, *J. Neurosurg., 26*:343, 1967.

Harik, S. I., Raichle, M. E., and Reis, D. J.: Spontaneously remitting spinal epidural hematoma in a patient on anticoagulants, *New Engl. J. Med., 284*:1355, 1971.

Markham, J. W., Lynge, H. N., and Stahlman, G. E. B.: The syndrome of spontaneous spinal epidural hematoma, *J. Neurosurg., 26*:334, 1967.

Rebello, M. D., and Dastur, H. M.: Spinal epidural hemorrhage (a review and two case reports), *Neurology (India), 14*:135, 1966.

Subarachnoid Hemorrhage

Henson, R. A., and Croft, P. B.: Spontaneous spinal subarachnoid haemorrhage, *Quart. J. Med., 25*:53, 1956.

Janon, E. A.: Arteriographic demonstration of spontaneous spinal subarachnoid hemorrhage: Case report, *Radiology, 97*:385, 1970.

Nassar, S. I., and Correll, J. W.: Subarachnoid hemorrhage due to spinal cord tumors, *Neurology, 18*:87, 1968.

Plotkin, R., Ronthal, M., and Froman, C.: Spontaneous spinal subarachnoid haemorrhage. Report of 3 cases, *J. Neurosurg., 25*:443, 1966.

Watson, A. B.: Spinal subarachnoid haemorrhage in patient with coarctation of aorta, *Brit. Med. J., 4*:278, 1967.

Intramedullary Hemorrhage (Hematomyelia)

Dastur, D. K., Wada, N. H., Desai, A. D., and Sinh, G.: Medullospinal compression due to atlanto-axial dislocation and sudden haematomyelia during decompression. Pathology, pathogenesis and clinical correlations, *Brain, 88*:897, 1965.

Grossiord, A., Held, J. P., and Odivère, M.: A propos du syndrome hématomyélitique: Ses formes dites spontaneés. Étude critique, *Rev. neurol., 104*:265, 1961.

Perot, P., Feindel, W., and Lloyd-Smith, D.: Hematomyelia as a complication of syringomyelia: Gowers' syringal hemorrhage. Case report, *J. Neurosurg., 25*:447, 1966.

Richardson, J. C.: Spontaneous haematomyelia: A short review and a report of cases illustrating intramedullary angioma and syphilis of the spinal cord as possible causes, *Brain, 61*:17, 1938.

Spinal Angiomata

Bergstrand, A., Höök, O., and Lidvall, H.: Vertebral haemangiomas compressing the spinal cord, *Acta neurol. scand., 39*:59, 1963.

Brion, J., Netsky, M. G., and Zimmerman, H. M.: Vascular malformations of spinal cord, *Arch. Neurol. Psychiat., 68*:339, 1952.

Cross, G. O.: Subarachnoid cervical angioma with cutaneous hemangioma of a corresponding metamere: Report of a case and review of the literature, *Arch. Neurol. Psychiat., 58*:359, 1947.

Doppman, J. L., Di Chiro, G., and Glancy, D. L.: Collateral circulation through dilated spinal cord arteries in aortic coarctation and extraspinal arteriovenous shunts. An arteriographic study, *Clin. Radiol., 20*:192, 1969.

Greenberg, J.: Spontaneous arteriovenous malformations in the cervical area, *J. Neurol. Neurosurg. Psychiat., 33*:303, 1970.

Herdt, J. R., Di Chiro, G., and Doppman, J. L.: Combined arterial and arteriovenous aneurysms of the spinal cord, *Radiology, 99*:589, 1971.

Hopkins, C. A., Wilkie, F. L., and Voris, D. C.: Extramedullary aneurysm of the spinal cord. Case report, *J. Neurosurg., 24*:1021, 1966.

Kaufman, H. H., Ommaya, A. K., Di Chiro, G., and Doppman, J. L.: Compression vs. steal. The pathogenesis of symptoms in arteriovenous malformations of the spinal cord, *Arch. Neurol., 23*:173, 1970.

Krayenbühl, H., Yaşargil, M. G., and McClintock, H. G.: Treatment of spinal cord vascular malformations by surgical excision, *J. Neurosurg.*, **30**:427, 1969.

Lepoire, J., Tridon, P., Montaut, J., Hepner, H., Picard, L., and Weber, M.: Angio-réticulome récidivant au cours d'une maladie de Von Hippel-Lindau. Aspects cliniques et artériographiques, *Neuro-Chirurgie*, **15**:529, 1969.

Lombardi, G., and Migliavacca, F.: Angiomas of the spinal cord, *Brit. J. Radiol.*, **32**:810, 1951.

Matthews, W. B.: The spinal bruit, *Lancet*, **2**:1117, 1959.

Shephard, R. H.: Some new concepts in intradural spinal angioma, *Riv. Patol. Nerv. Ment.*, **86**:276, 1965.

Taylor, J. R., and Van Allen, M. W.: Vascular malformation of the cord with transient ischemic attacks. Case report, *J. Neurosurg.*, **31**:576, 1969.

Teng, P., and Papatheodorou, C.: Myelographic appearance of vascular anomalies of the spinal cord, *Brit. J. Radiol.*, **37**:358, 1964.

Additional References

Di Chiro, G.: Angiography of obstructive vascular disease of the spinal cord, *Radiology*, **100**:607, 1971.

———, Harrington, T., and Fried, L. C.: Microangiography of human fetal spinal cord, *Am. J. Roent.*, **118**:193, 1973.

Doppman, J. L.: The nidus concept of spinal cord arteriovenous malformations. A surgical recommendation based upon angiographic observations, *Brit. J. Radiol.*, **44**:758, 1971.

Henry, P., Castaigns, G., Hoerni, B., and Touchard, J.: La myélopathie progressive post-radiothérapeutique tardive, *J. Neurol. Sci.*, **14**:325, 1971.

Subdural and Extradural Hematoma

As no two faces, so no two cases are alike in all respects, and unfortunately it is not only the disease itself which is so varied, but the subjects themselves have peculiarities which modify its action.

Sir William Osler

There must be few conditions of which the pathology is so gross, for which our diagnostic criteria are so inadequate, yet which offer to diagnosis such an ample reward.

J. Purdon Martin

SUBDURAL HEMATOMA

The finding of trephine holes in the skulls of Neanderthal man and ancient Egyptians suggests that subdural hematomas may have been treated since prehistoric times (Fig. 23-1). Even today, many aboriginal tribes which have never been exposed to modern medicine practice the art. In man's never-ending battles, a blow to the head with a stick, stone, or club has always been a favorite method of disposing of the enemy, and many a patient with subdural hematoma caused by such a blow may have been cured by trephination. However, the first modern description of the condition was published in 1857 by Virchow, who believed chronic inflammation

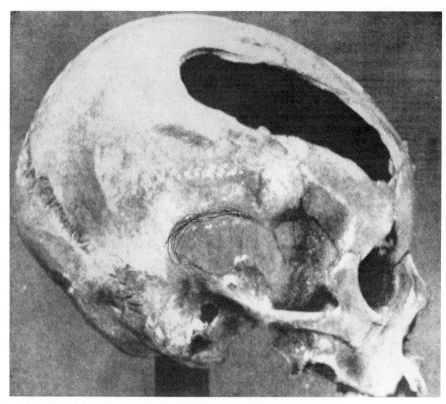

Figure 23-1 Peruvian skull in which cranioplasty had been practiced using a silver plate. *(From Gilbert Horrax, Neurosurgery: An Historical Sketch, 1952. Courtesy of Charles C Thomas, Publisher, Springfield, Ill.)*

of the dura caused rupture of veins, leading to hemorrhage between the meninges. The relationship between subdural hematoma and preceding trauma was shown by Wilfred Trotter.

Hematomas may be acute or chronic. Because the acute types follow head trauma, which is seldom treated by the general physician, only chronic hematoma will be discussed in this chapter.

Etiology and Pathogenesis

Situated between the dura mater and the piarachnoid membrane is a potential space (the subdural space), across which cortical (bridg-

ing) veins drain blood from the brain into the dural sinuses. If these veins rupture, blood dissecting between these membranes enlarges the space in all directions, and eventually a mass large enough to compress adjacent portions of the brain may be created (Fig. 23-2). If rupture of the piarachnoid membrane occurs as well, cerebrospinal fluid leaks into the mass from the subarachnoid space and adds to its bulk. In occasional cases, trauma tears the piarachnoid without rupturing the veins, so that a collection of cerebrospinal fluid forms in the subdural space (subdural hygroma). In other instances, the blood in a subdural hematoma is resorbed, leaving a yellow-tinged, clear effusion with a

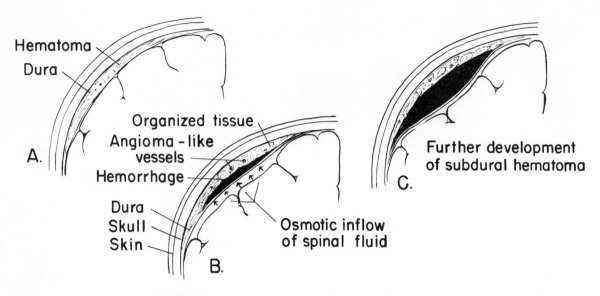

Hematoma
Dura

Organized tissue
Angioma-like
vessels
Hemorrhage

Dura
Skull
Skin

A.

B.

Osmotic inflow
of spinal fluid

Further development
of subdural hematoma

C.

Figure 23-2 Stages in the formation of subdural hematoma. *(From Klaus-Joachim Zulch, "Medical Causation" in The Late Effects of Head Injury, 1969. Courtesy of Charles C Thomas, Publisher, Springfield, Ill.)*

protein content much higher than that of normal cerebrospinal fluid.

Small subdural hematomas may be produced by intracranial surgery, but these rarely grow large enough to cause symptoms.

Closed head injury, with or without fracture, is responsible for the vast majority of subdural hematomas, although "spontaneous" hemorrhage, unrelated to known trauma, does occur. When the moving head suddenly strikes an object, or when the stationary head is displaced by a blow, the brain moves within the skull. One result may be rupture of the cortical veins that drain blood from the hemispheres into the intradural venous sinuses. The effect of displacement of the brain within the cranium is usually greatest in the parasagittal region, where these cortical draining veins are longest and have the least support.

The severity of injury necessary to produce subdural hematoma varies considerably. Severe injuries with skull fracture may not be associated with subdural hematoma, while chronic subdural hematoma may follow mild trauma to the head. The initial injury often does not cause loss of consciousness and is sometimes so trivial that the patient forgets the episode, which occurred long before symptoms appear. At times subdural hematomas are produced by minor injuries to the back, buttocks, or heels—injuries that merely jar the head. It is even possible that rupture of intracranial veins may occasionally result from an acute rise in venous pressure, such as that caused by vigorous coughing or straining. Patients taking anticoagulant medications for cardiac or cerebral vascular disease may develop subdural hematoma following minor head injury because of their abnormal clotting mechanisms. Another unusual cause of hematoma is stretching and rupture of veins by injection of air during pneumoencephalography.

Subdural hematoma is more common in older patients because the aging process is associated with brain shrinkage within the cranial cavity and the gap across which the bridging veins must travel is increased. Subdural hematoma is more common in males, perhaps because men receive more head injuries than women. Patients on long-term hemodialysis for chronic renal failure are predisposed to subdural hematoma.

Why does a subdural hematoma increase in size? The answer to this question is not definitely known. Many pathologists believe that the high protein content of the serum, augmented by protein released from degenerating cellular elements of the blood, draws cerebrospinal fluid into the subdural space through the semipermeable piarachnoid membrane. A more likely explanation is that oozing from the vascular membrane causes the progressive enlargement. Because of its relative avascularity and lack of lymphatic drainage, the piarachnoid membrane has little resorptive capacity, and the process of resorption takes place through the moderately vascularized dura mater. The rate of uptake is often so slow that fluid accumulates faster than it can be removed, and progressive enlargement occurs.

Pathologic Findings

Site Hematomas are most likely to develop where the veins crossing the subdural space are longest. The sites usually involved are:

1 The frontoparietal region of the brain (superior cerebral veins draining into the superior sagittal sinus). In 10 to 20 percent of patients, hematomas in this area are bilateral.
2 The tip of the temporal lobe (inferior cerebral veins draining into the sphenoparietal sinus).

Less commonly they may be found beneath the frontal or temporal lobes, and rarely they accumulate between the hemispheres or in the posterior fossa.

Gross Appearance When seen at surgery or autopsy, the dura overlying a hematoma has a bluish-green hue. Beneath the dura lies a glistening brown outer membrane. When this is stripped and the mass is removed, a shiny inner membrane stippled with petechial hemorrhages can be seen (Fig. 23-3). The mass composing a hematoma usually contains fluid (from a film to as much as 500 ml) surrounded by fibrin clot. It varies from yellow to black and does not clot because it contains no fibrinogen. The piarachnoid membrane usually lies free of the inner membrane, although in long-standing cases some adhesions may occur.

The portion of brain underlying the hematoma is usually compressed and is discolored by bilirubin. When the mass is very large, the underlying brain is compressed and displaced from its normal position, perhaps herniating through the tentorial notch. Eventually the tissue adjacent to the hematoma becomes atrophic.

Microscopic Appearance The outer membrane, 1 to 5 mm thick and adherent to the dura, is composed of granulation tissue containing fibroblasts, new blood vessels, histiocytes, pigment, and occasional red and white blood cells. A characteristic feature of this layer is the presence of thin-walled, sinus-like vessels; some pathologists believe that these contribute to the progressive enlargement of the hematoma by oozing fresh blood into the cavity. The inner membrane, which is almost completely avascular, consists of a layer of mesothelial cells lying on a sheet of connective tissue. The fluid portion of the hematoma, supported in a fibrin network, contains red blood cells in various stages of disintegration.

Although hematomas are usually well developed after 4 to 6 weeks, the time required for the formation of the encapsulating membranes varies from about 2 to 7 weeks.

Clinical Features

The manifestations of subdural hematoma differ with the age of the patient.

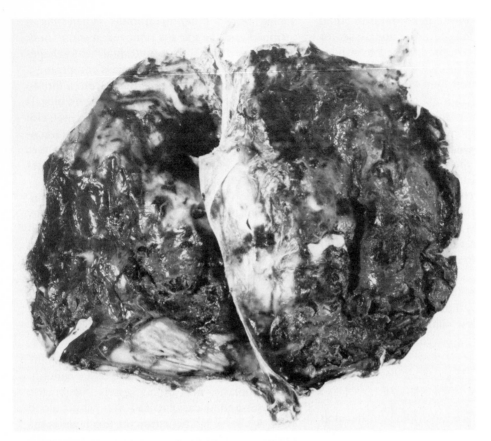

Figure 23-3 Top view of the falx cerebri showing bilateral subdural hematomas on inner surface of the dura mater; there is partial encapsulation by "membranes," i.e., granulation tissue. *(Courtesy of John Moossy, M.D., Department of Pathology, Bowman Gray School of Medicine.)*

In Infants Hematomas become symptomatic most commonly in infants between the ages of 2 and 4 months; they are bilateral in about 80 percent of cases, compared with 10 to 20 percent in adults. In many instances no history of trauma is obtainable. Traumatic delivery is often blamed, but the evidence supporting this hypothesis is inconclusive. Abnormal presentation and permaturity seem to have no predisposing effect. Blood dyscrasias and dehydration must be considered, and some authorities believe that primary inflammation of the dura is a common cause of hematomas during infancy. As in

adults, head trauma can cause hematoma; in infants with hematoma following such trauma, the "battered-baby" syndrome should be considered.

Symptoms depend partly on the stage of evolution of the process. About half of these cases are characterized by nonspecific symptoms such as feeding problems, vomiting, irritability, and failure to thrive; many infants have associated respiratory or intestinal infections resulting in fever. In others, clues such as generalized or focal convulsions suggest brain irritation. Stupor occurs in about 25 percent of these cases and hemiparesis or brisk reflexes with mild spasticity in about 15 percent.

Enlargement of the head, at times manifested only by an increase in biparietal diameter, is noted in about 25 percent of infants with subdural hematoma. The anterior fontanelle is usually tense and bulging unless the infant is dehydrated. Transillumination of the head may reveal an underlying subdural hygroma. When present, retinal hemorrhages without papilledema are characteristic of long-standing hematoma. Blood loss and low serum protein levels result in progressive anemia in about one-third to one-half of infants with chronic hematoma. Skull x-rays reveal separation of the sutures. The cerebrospinal fluid is under increased pressure and may contain red blood cells, white blood cells, and abnormal amounts of protein. A positive diagnosis can often be made on the basis of bilateral subdural taps.

In Children Clinical features are similar to those seen in adults, except that mental symptoms are rare. The youngster may have manifestations suggestive of an intracranial tumor, or he may be brought to the physician because of painless progressive bulging of the temporal bone.

Skull x-rays may show expansion of one side of the middle cranial fossa and thinning of the inner table (a finding not seen in adults). The expansion of the middle fossa, as well as the proptosis and bulging of the temporal region, is caused by a forward and upward displacement of the sphenoid bone.

In Adults Subdural hematomas produce local effects related to their site, and general effects secondary to their mass. Headache is the most prominent symptom in more than 80 percent of patients. It is usually agonizing and incapacitating; may be diffuse or localized over the site of the hematoma; and is often exacerbated by coughing, stooping, or straining. At the height of the headache, nausea and vomiting are common.

In the early stages it is notoriously difficult to locate or even lateralize a subdural hematoma on the basis of clinical evidence. Subdural hematomas developing in the most common location (the central or postcentral region) cause recurrent headache which may be localized to the side of the collection. As the hematoma enlarges, the headaches become more severe and signs of neurologic dysfunction develop. The latter usually consist of mild paresis of the contralateral arm and leg, together with speech difficulty if the hematoma lies over the dominant hemisphere. Convulsion, either focal or generalized, may occur.

In more than 90 percent of all cases, lateralizing signs have developed before the diagnosis is made. These include:

1 Brisk tendon reflexes and an extensor plantar response on the contralateral side.
2 Homolateral hemiparesis, due to compression of the opposite cerebral peduncle against the sharp free edge of the tentorium. The same mechanism sometimes produces homolateral or bilateral signs of corticospinal tract involvement.
3 Dysphasia, indicating that the lesion is on the dominant side.
4 Paresis of the ipsilateral oculomotor nerve due to compression by the displaced brain. The pupil is first dilated and later becomes unresponsive to light and accommodation.
5 Homonymous hemianopia due to pressure of the hematoma on the optic radiations or, rarely, compression of the posterior cerebral vessels against the free edge of the tentorium.

The later stages of subdural hematoma are often characterized by drowsiness, inability to concentrate, deterioration of memory, confusion, and disorientation. These changes, which are often more noticeable to friends and relatives than to the patient, may be followed by stupor or coma.

Signs of increased intracranial pressure occurring in the late stages include papilledema, slowing of the pulse and respiration, and elevation of the blood pressure.

In the Elderly The cerebral atrophy usually present to some degree in old age causes widening of the subdural space and makes the bridging veins more susceptible to rupture. The progressive friability of the veins that occurs with advancing age further increases the hazard of rupture.

In the elderly, the mental deterioration that often dominates the clinical picture with hematoma may be attributed incorrectly to senility. Neurologic abnormalities, if present, are usually thought to be the result of a "stroke" or "cerebral" atherosclerosis.

When a patient develops signs of cerebral damage concomitant with head injury, it is often difficult to determine whether the neural deficit is due to the injury or whether the head injury resulted from a fall following a spontaneous (nontraumatic) cerebrovascular episode. In cases where a subdural hematoma may be present, the only way to answer this vexing question may be to use a brain scan, a contrast study, or diagnostic bur holes.

Acute "Spontaneous" Subdural Hemorrhage

Recently, attention has been drawn to a newly recognized cause of subdural hemorrhage—the rupture of a small artery on the convexity of the cerebrum. The pathogenesis is as yet unclear, but it has been postulated that at the time of head injury, a small asymptomatic venous subdural hematoma is formed. Following absorption of this subdural blood, adhesions develop between the dura mater and the cortical surface, entrapping a small cortical artery. Later, these adhesions bind the artery and in a subsequent blow to the head, the brain is displaced and the artery torn, resulting in an acute subdural hemorrhage.

In such instances, patients present with an abrupt onset of headache, vomiting, progressive deterioration in consciousness, and signs of meningeal irritation. On examination, the patient usually has a dilated pupil and *ipsilateral* hemiparesis due to displacement of the brain with compression of the peduncle against the incisura. At times, ipsilateral hemisensory loss and ipsilateral homonymous hemianopia caused by compression of the posterior cerebral artery against the incisura of the opposite side are seen. In some cases papilledema is evident.

The diagnosis of acute subdural hematoma caused by arterial bleeding is confirmed by carotid angiography, and the lesion is treated by evacuating the subdural blood and clipping the spurting artery.

Differential Diagnosis

Errors in the diagnosis of subdural hematoma are legion. Symptoms produced by subdural hematoma that are often erroneously attributed to other conditions include changes in the psyche occurring in elderly patients, repeated seizures in epileptics, behavior problems in young people, and symptoms suggestive of inebriation in alcoholics. Other conditions frequently confused with subdural hematoma are intracranial neoplasms and cerebrovascular episodes. Because subdural hematoma is one of the few reversible causes of dementia, correct diagnosis is of paramount importance.

Aside from the history of preceding head injury, three clinical signs should strongly suggest a diagnosis of subdural hematoma: (1) daily or even hourly fluctuations in the symptoms, especially those of drowsiness, confusion, and headache; (2) signs of hemispheric involvement, such as motor weakness, sensory changes, and aphasia; and (3) the prominence of mental aberration in comparison to signs related to the corticospinal tract. Unfortunately, these differentiating features are not always reliable.

In infants the diagnosis is frequently made

still more difficult by the absence of specific manifestations. A history of birth injury followed by failure to thrive, seizures, or progressive enlargement of the head should suggest subdural hematoma.

Laboratory Findings

Lumbar Puncture The spinal fluid pressure may be raised, normal, or low; a pressure of 180 to 200 mm is a common finding, but pressures below 50 mm are sometimes associated with subdural hematoma, particularly in older patients. Although the fluid is xanthochromic in about half the patients, an entirely normal cerebrospinal fluid does not exclude subdural hematoma. The protein content may be normal or elevated.

Skull X-ray If the pineal gland is calcified, it is almost always displaced away from a unilateral hematoma of the convexity; with bilateral hematomas, however, it may remain in the midline because of equal compression of the brain from the two sides. Furthermore, pineal displacement may not occur if the collection consists of less than 100 ml of fluid, or if it is subfrontal or temporal or infratentorial in location. Calcification of the inner wall of the hematoma is seen rarely in long-standing cases.

The changes in the bony wall in juvenile cases have already been described.

Echoencephalogram A unilateral lesion may cause a shift of midline structures to the opposite side (Fig. 23-4). In addition, a group of abnormal echoes is sometimes reflected from the hematoma walls.

Electroencephalogram Suppression of the electrical activity in the region of the hematoma has been stated to be the typical feature of the EEG, particularly when the lesion is situated in the parietal area. Theoretically, the fluid de-

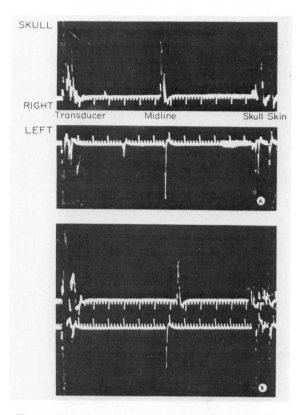

Figure 23-4 Echoencephalograms. (Above) Normal reflections from the midline structures. The ultrasonic beam is directed from the right to the left. (Below) Displacement of midline structures to the left by a right-sided lesion.

creases the amplitude of brain waves by insulating the recording electrodes from the brain. This insulating effect is overcome as blood accumulates and compresses the brain, and, in addition to more nonspecific slowing of brain rhythms which results from increased intracranial pressure, delta waves are seen over the hematoma. This EEG abnormality is the one most often seen in patients with subdural hematoma.

Brain Scan Radioactive brain scan is one of the most valuable diagnostic methods available for the detection of chronic subdural hematoma and should be done on all patients who might conceivably harbor such a lesion. With the use of technetium 99m, few chronic hematomas of a size sufficient to cause symptoms will be overlooked; on the other hand, the scan may be normal in patients with acute hematoma or a posterior fossa accumulation. The hematoma appears as a zone of increased isotope uptake which is evident in the posterior and anterior view but not in the lateral scan.

In some instances the initial brain scan may be normal, but a second one taken 4 to 6 hr after the injection of the radioactive isotope will show areas of increased uptake (Fig. 23-5).

(A)
(C)

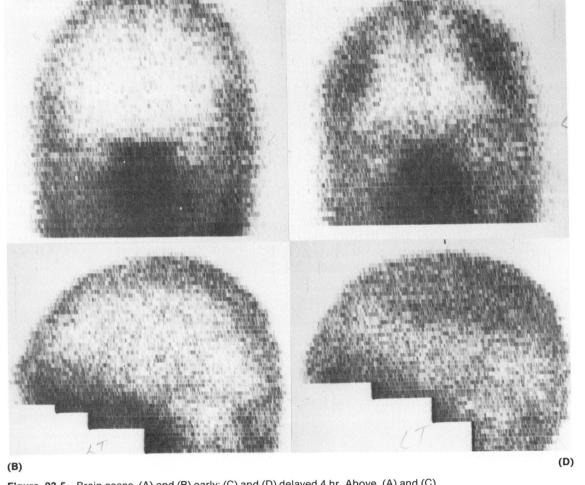

(B)
(D)

Figure 23-5 Brain scans. (A) and (B) early; (C) and (D) delayed 4 hr. Above, (A) and (C) are anteroposterior views. Upper left normal; upper right delayed scan shows abnormal uptake of radioisotope. Below, (B) and (D) are lateral views. Left is normal; right shows abnormal uptake of isotope.

Carotid Arteriography The pathognomonic sign of a subdural collection of fluid is an avascular area beneath the inner table of the skull, caused by a shift of the brain and its vessels away from the periphery (Fig. 23-6). During its first 2 weeks, the hematoma spreads evenly and conforms to the contour of the underlying brain. Thereafter, it shows signs of expansion, and from the fourth week onward the typical biconvex-lens-shaped avascular area, deform-ing the underlying brain, is often seen best on tangential projections.

The anterior cerebral artery and deep veins are frequently pushed across the midline, unless the hematoma is quite small or unless another hematoma is exerting pressure from the other side.

Because of the frequency of bilateral subdural hematomas, both carotid trees must be visualized in every case.

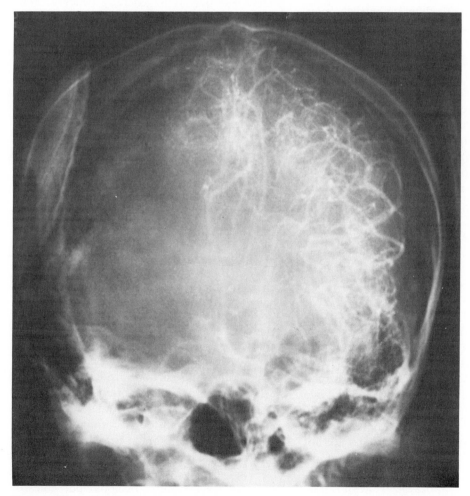

Figure 23-6 Left carotid arteriogram showing an avascular area between the calvarium and the vessels of the convexity of hemisphere—findings typical of subdural hematoma. Minimal displacement of the anterior cerebral artery strongly suggests the possibility of an associated hematoma on the right side as well.

Air Study   Because of the accuracy of radioactive brain scan in diagnosing subdural hematoma, pneumoencephalography has become less important and may soon be abandoned altogether as a method of diagnosis for this condition. Air studies are frequently performed, however, in elderly patients whose presenting symptom is progressive mental deterioration and in patients suspected of harboring a posterior fossa hematoma.

In the presence of a chronic subdural hematoma of the convexity, the lateral ventricles may be shifted to the opposite side. The contralateral ventricle may be dilated and have a high roof. The ipsilateral ventricle is either unaltered or smaller than normal, with a flattened roof and a concave lateral border. The ipsilateral temporal horn may be displaced medially.

These changes are produced by a large disklike lesion overlying the cerebral hemisphere and must be differentiated from convexity meningioma, abscess, or brain neoplasm.

When some air manages to enter the subarachnoid space, as it does in rare cases, a pathognomonic clear zone can be seen between the subdural hematoma and the underlying brain.

Diagnostic Bur Holes   The old maxim that no patient should die of undiagnosed coma without having had exploratory bur holes performed still applies to elderly hypertensive individuals *in extremis* (since bur holes can be performed more quickly and safely than bilateral carotid angiography, and echoencephalography and rapid brain scanning are not yet available in most institutions), and to persons with emergency conditions when a tentorial pressure cone is present and facilities for angiography are not available. Except in these special situations, brain scan and bilateral carotid angiography should always precede surgical exploration. These methods will not only reveal hematomas located beneath the frontal or temporal lobes, but may also provide the clue to the diagnosis of some unsuspected intracranial lesion such as aneurysm or arteriovenous malformation.

Course and Prognosis

In spite of their frequency, the natural history of chronic subdural hematomas is not fully known. Many are diagnosed and removed surgically; others are not suspected until they are found as incidental abnormalities at autopsy. Some become quiescent and calcify; still others are completely resorbed. It is generally believed, however, that the majority of chronic subdural hematomas ultimately produce signs of an expanding intracranial lesion, with or without collapse of the underlying brain. Left untreated, they may cause intellectual deterioration, hemiparesis, seizures, or a combination of these conditions, and ultimately coma and death from compression of the midbrain (from herniation of the hippocampus through the incisura of the tentorium cerebelli). A fluctuating downhill course is said to be typical and is probably related to alterations in the volume of fluid within the membranes. In some patients sudden, unexplained death occurs. Even if the hematoma stabilizes, mental deterioration, headache, and recurrent convulsions may persist.

Treatment

The fact that a few patients may live for years with a chronic subdural hematoma does not diminish the importance of prompt diagnosis and therapy. In some cases treatment consists of draining the fluid portion through bur holes, or through the fontanelles in infants; in other cases the solid portions of the clot and the membranes must be removed through craniotomy. If bur holes are used, they should be placed bilaterally even when the lesion is thought to be unilateral. The rare case of a subdural hematoma in the posterior fossa requires occipital bur holes on each side or a suboccipital craniectomy.

For infants, the treatment of choice is the daily removal of 10 to 14 ml of fluid from first one and then the other side on alternate days if the condition of the patient permits the elective approach. Only in emergencies should greater volumes be removed simultaneously from the two sides. Generally speaking, as much of the membranes as possible should be removed through small-flap craniectomies.

If hemoglobin and hematocrit values are low, a transfusion may be required.

In most cases prompt removal of the subdural hematoma is a therapeutic triumph, and the patient's prompt return to consciousness after removal of the clot is probably the most dramatic and gratifying experience in the entire realm of neurosurgical practice. At times when the underlying brain fails to expand, the results are not so dramatic. In such instances some neurosurgeons inject normal saline solution into the lumbar theca or into the contralateral ventricle to promote reexpansion of the brain. Mental aberrations, seizures, and hemiparesis, due either to a late diagnosis or to an atrophic or unexpanded brain, are at times noted postoperatively.

EXTRADURAL HEMATOMA

Extradural hematoma—an accumulation of blood between the dura mater and the inner table of the skull—is almost always the result of bleeding from a meningeal artery or vein or venous sinus following head injury. Spontaneous extradural hematomas caused by congenital aneurysms of the meningeal artery or by hemorrhagic disorders are very rare.

Pathogenesis and Pathologic Findings

The vast majority of extradural hematomas accumulate in the temporal region, where the calvarium is thin and the middle meningeal artery and vein and their branches can be torn if the skull is fractured. In occasional cases, hematomas collect in the frontal, parietal, or occipital region.

Extradural hematomas can be associated with head injuries which lacerate the skin but which do not perforate the skull. Their rarity in penetrating wounds is explained by the fact that blood can drain freely and hence does not dissect between the dura and the inner table of the skull.

A blow forceful enough to indent the skull may perhaps loosen the dura from the inner table of the skull, so that bleeding from vessel rupture can dissect between them, creating a hematoma. At times the inner table of the skull is fractured by the displacement while the outer table remains intact. Occasionally rupture of the underlying artery or vein occurs without fracture of either table.

As the hematoma increases in size, local compression of the underlying brain causes signs of focal deficit. Further enlargement pushes the brain toward the opposite side and down into the tentorial notch. In addition to causing displacement and compression of the midbrain, this impaction of the medial aspect of the homolateral temporal lobe puts pressure on the oculomotor nerve and on the homolateral posterior cerebral artery and veins (Fig. 23-7).

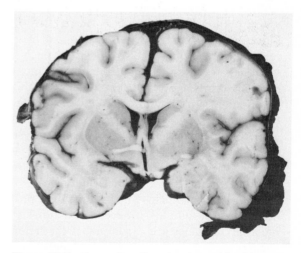

Figure 23-7 Coronal section showing epidural hematoma in association with subdural and subarachnoid hemorrhage.

Trauma to the occipital region may produce an extradural hematoma located in the posterior fossa, leading to compression of the lower cranial nerves, the cerebellum, and the brainstem.

Clinical Features

The clinical features depend on three variables: (1) the site of the initial injury, (2) the presence or absence of concussion and coma caused by the original blow, and (3) the rate at which the hematoma accumulates. Arterial bleeding can produce a hematoma large enough to cause compression of the brain within the hour of injury. If the initial blow caused a severe concussion, consciousness may not return during this interval. With bleeding from a small artery or a vein, the clot may accumulate more slowly, so that a lucid interval is common. In rare cases venous hemorrhages cease spontaneously and the presence of a chronic extradural hematoma may not be suspected for weeks after the injury.

Because of these variables, four general patterns may occur: (1) initial unconsciousness from the injury with return of consciousness and the development of focal neurologic abnormalities; (2) initial coma from the injury followed by a variable period of lucidity before return of coma; (3) coma uninterrupted by a return of consciousness; (4) no initial unconsciousness from the blow but the gradual onset of coma as hematoma accumulates. Of this group initial unconsciousness followed by a lucid interval and gradual return of coma is said to be the typical pattern, but it occurs in only 30 percent of the cases (Fig. 23-8).

Headache of a throbbing nature is frequent in those patients who recover consciousness.

The neurologic deficits most commonly produced by pressure on adjacent structures as blood accumulates are dysphasia (if the lesion overlies the dominant hemisphere), hemiparesis, and hemianoptic field defects. The occurrence of focal or generalized convulsions is unusual.

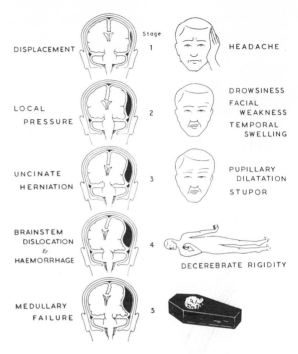

Figure 23-8 Stages in the development of the clinical picture in middle fossa epidural hemorrhage. *(Courtesy of R. Hooper, Brit. J. Surg., 47:71, 1959. Reproduced by kind permission of the British Journal of Surgery.)*

Displacement of the brain and herniation of the temporal lobe may produce signs of oculomotor nerve compression, beginning usually with dilatation of the pupil. When it occurs, the homolateral pupil is dilated in about 90 percent of cases and the contralateral in the remainder.

Increasing intracranial pressure, sometimes manifested by papilledema, causes vomiting, slowing of the pulse rate, slow and stertorous respiration, and elevation of the systolic blood pressure.

Many authorities believe that the site of scalp injury, often revealed by the presence of a palpable hematoma or a visible contusion or laceration, is as reliable a clue to the site of hematoma as is the location of the skull fracture. For adequate inspection of the area, it may be necessary to shave part of the head. Injuries to the frontal region are most often associated with hematoma of the anterior fossa; injuries of the temporal area, with hematoma of the middle fossa; and blows to the occipital area, with hematoma of the posterior fossa.

Differential Diagnosis

The typical case of extradural hematoma poses no problems in diagnosis, but atypical ones may be difficult to distinguish from subarachnoid hemorrhage, cerebral contusion, or laceration of the brain. Evidence of impact over the site of the middle meningeal artery and the history of a "lucid interval" following injury are features favoring extradural hematoma.

The early diagnosis of extradural hemorrhage depends to a large extent on suspicion, and it is well to keep in mind the possibility that extradural hematoma may follow any head injury. Many patients who die might be saved by appropriate studies for subdural and extradural hematoma—including, in many cases, diagnostic bur holes over the site of the injury.

Laboratory Findings

Skull X-ray A linear fracture is seen in 85 to 90 percent of adults with extradural hematoma. The most common site is over the grooves in which lie the middle meningeal vessels or their branches. If the pineal gland is calcified, it is often shifted from the midline.

Angiography Carotid arteriograms usually reveal displacement of the arteries and veins away from the side of the lesion. Characteristically, the superior sagittal sinus is displaced from the vault, and the distance between the inner table of the skull and the visualized cortical vessels is increased.

Air Study Ventriculograms should be done in cases of suspected extradural hematoma only if bur holes do not reveal the cause for the neurologic deficit. In such cases the air study may demonstrate the presence of a hematoma in an unusual location—e.g., beneath the frontal lobe or in the posterior cranial fossa.

Echoencephalography The echoencephalogram may reveal a shift of the midline structures away from the lesion, as well as abnormal echoes from the region of the inner table of the skull.

Radioactive Brain Scan Conclusions cannot be drawn from the small number of cases reported to date. In most cases studied by this method, it has been impossible to discriminate between the increased uptake in the contused scalp and muscle and the uptake in the hematoma. In chronic subdural hematoma, on the other hand, radioactive brain scan is a most valuable diagnostic aid.

Lumbar Puncture Because of the danger of precipitating transtentorial or transforaminal herniation, it is unwise to perform lumbar puncture in cases where extradural hematoma is suspected. In cases where this procedure is mistakenly carried out, cerebrospinal fluid is clear unless there is an associated subarachnoid hemorrhage. The pressure may be either normal or raised, depending on the stage of evolution of the hematoma.

Course and Prognosis

With very few exceptions, the patient will die if the hematoma is not removed. The degree of ultimate recovery may depend on early diagnosis and prompt operation to remove clot and stop further bleeding. The longer the pressure remains on the brain, the more serious the sequelae. The chances of satisfactory recovery are also related inversely to the age of the patient, the degree of cerebral compression, and the depth of the coma.

The overall mortality from extradural hematoma approaches 30 to 50 percent. This high figure does not reflect the difficulties of surgery but indicates the rapidity with which this disorder can cause fatal compression of the brain.

Treatment

The management of extradural hematoma can be summarized in one sentence: "Remove the clot and stop the bleeding at once." A high index of suspicion should lead to early diagnosis, and early diagnosis to immediate surgical intervention. In many instances it is unwise to delay surgery even for the performance of such routine diagnostic studies as blood counts, blood chemistry determinations, and x-rays of the skull and chest. Exploratory bur holes over the site of the external injury may save the patient's life by allowing drainage of the hematoma. If these reveal the presence of blood, the surgical field can then be enlarged for complete evacuation of the hematoma and the achievement of hemostasis after the lifesaving drainage has been done.

SUGGESTED READINGS

Subdural Hematoma

General

Gortvai, P., and Anagnostopoulos, D. I.: Subdural haematoma simulating primary subarachnoid haemorrhage, *Brit. Med. J.*, **1**:323, 1971.

McKissock, W., Richardson, A., and Bloom, W. H.: Subdural haematoma: A review of 389 cases, *Lancet*, **1**:1365, 1960.

Trotter, W.: Chronic subdural haemorrhage of traumatic origin and its relation to pachymeningitis haemorrhagica interna, *Brit. J. Surg.*, **2**:271, 1914.

Etiology and Pathogenesis

Arieff, A. J., and Wetzel, N.: Subdural hematoma following epileptic convulsion, *Neurology*, **14**:731, 1964.

Capistrant, T., Goldberg, R., Shibasaki, H., and Castle, D.: Posterior fossa subdural haematoma associated with anticoagulant therapy, *J. Neurol. Neurosurg. Psychiat.*, **34**:82, 1971.

Ciembroniewicz, J. E.: Subdural hematoma of the posterior fossa. Review of the literature with addition of three cases, *J. Neurosurg.*, **22**:465, 1965.

Clark, E., and Walton, J. N.: Subdural haematoma complicating intracranial aneurysms and angioma, *Brain*, **76**:378, 1953.

Clein, L. J., and Bolton, C. F.: Interhemispheric subdural hematoma: A case report, *J. Neurol. Neurosurg. Psychiat.*, **32**:389, 1969.

German, W. J., Flanigan, S., and Davey, L. M.: Remarks on subdural hematoma and aphasia, *Clin. Neurosurg.*, **12**:344, 1966.

Goodell, C. L., and Mealey, J., Jr.: Pathogenesis of chronic subdural hematoma: Experimental studies, *Arch. Neurol.*, **8**:429, 1963.

Guiterrez-Luque, A. G., MacCarty, C. S., and Klass, D. W.: Head injury with suspected subdural hematoma: Effect on EEG, *Arch. Neurol.*, **15**:437, 1966.

Illingworth, R. D.: Subdural haematoma after the treatment of chronic hydrocephalus by ventriculocaval shunts, *J. Neurol. Neurosurg. Psychiat.*, **33**:95, 1970.

Ommaya, A. K., and Yarnell, P.: Subdural haematoma after whiplash injury, *Lancet*, **2**:237, 1969.

Russell, D. S., and Cairns, H.: Subdural false membrane or haematoma (pachymeningitis interna haemorrhagica) in carcinomatosis and sarcomatosis of the dura matter, *Brain*, **57**:32, 1934.

Talalla, A., Halbrook, H., Barbour, B. H., and Kurze, T.: Subdural hematoma associated with long-term hemodialysis for chronic renal disease, *J.A.M.A.*, **212**:1847, 1970.

Weir, B.: The osmolality of subdural hematoma fluid, *J. Neurosurg.*, **34**:528, 1971.

Wright, R. L.: Traumatic hematomas of the posterior cranial fossa, *J. Neurosurg.*, **25**:402, 1966.

Pathologic Findings

Christensen, E.: Studies on chronic subdural hematoma, *Acta psychiat. scand.*, **19**:69, 1944.

Friede, R. L.: Incidence and distribution of neomembranes of dura mater, *J. Neurol. Neurosurg. Psychiat.*, **34**:439, 1971.

Munro, D., and Merritt, H. H.: Surgical pathology of subdural hematoma; based on a study of one hundred and five cases, *Arch. Neurol. Psychiat.*, **35**:64, 1936.

Clinical Features

Allen, A. M., Moore, M., and Daly, B. B.: Subdural hemorrhage in patients with mental disease; statistical study, *New Engl. J. Med.,* **223**:324, 1940.

Arseni, C., and Stanciu, M.: Particular clinical aspects of chronic subdural haematoma in adults, *Europ. neurol.,* **2**:109, 1969.

Bortnick, R. J., and Murphey, J. P.: Paraparesis with incontinence of bowel and bladder: A syndrome of bilateral subdural hematomas, *J. Neurosurg.,* **20**:352, 1963.

Cole, M., and Spatz, E.: Seizures in chronic subdural hematoma, *New Engl. J. Med.,* **265**:628, 1961.

Hoyt, W. F.: Vascular lesions of the visual cortex with brain herniation through the tentorial incisura: Neuro-ophthalmologic considerations, *Arch. Ophthalmol.,* **64**:44, 1960.

Maroon, J. C., and Campbell, R. L.: Subdural hematoma with inappropriate antidiuretic hormone secretion, *Arch. Neurol.,* **22**:234, 1970.

Pevehouse, B. C., Bloom, W. H., and McKissock, W.: Ophthalmologic aspects of diagnosis and localization of subdural hematoma: An analysis of 389 cases and review of the literature, *Neurology,* **10**:1037, 1960.

Sunderland, S.: The tentorial notch and complications produced by herniations of the brain through that aperture, *Brit. J. Surg.,* **45**:422, 1958.

Walker, A. E.: The syndromes of the tentorial notch, *J. Nervous Mental Disease,* **136**:118, 1965.

Clinical Features in Infants

Christensen, E., and Husby, J.: Chronic subdural hematoma in infancy, *Acta neurol. scand.,* **39**(suppl. 4):323, 1963.

Govan, C. D., Jr., and Walsh, F. B.: Symptomatology of subdural hematoma in infants and in adults: Comparative study with particular reference to ocular signs; observation concerning pathogenesis of subdural hematoma, *Arch. Ophthalmol.,* **37**:701, 1947.

Hollenhorst, R. W., Stein, H. A., Keith, H. M., and MacCarty, C. S.: Subdural hematoma, subdural hygroma and subarachnoid hemorrhage among infants and children, *Neurology,* **7**:813, 1957.

Ingraham, F. D., and Matson, D. D.: Subdural hematoma in infancy, *J. Pediat.,* **24**:1, 1944.

McLaurin, R. L., Issacs, E., and Lewis, H. P.: Results of nonoperative treatment in 15 cases of infantile subdural hematoma, *J. Neurosurg.,* **34**:753, 1971.

Russell, P. A.: Subdural haematoma in infancy, *Brit. Med. J.,* **2**:446, 1965.

Clinical Features in Children

Davidoff, L. M., and Dyke, C. G.: Relapsing juvenile chronic subdural hematoma; A clinical and roentgenographic study, *Bull. Neurol. Inst. N. Y.,* **7**:95, 1938.

Shulman, K., and Ransohoff, J.: Subdural hematoma in children: The fate of children with retained membranes, *J. Neurosurg.,* **18**:175, 1961.

Watts, C. C., and Acosta, C.: Pertussis and bilateral subdural hematomas, *Am. J. Diseases Children,* **118**:518, 1969.

Clinical Features in the Elderly

Perlmutter, I.: Subdural hematoma in older patients, *J.A.M.A.,* **176**:212, 1961.

Stuteville, P., and Welch, K.: Subdural hematoma in the elderly person, *J.A.M.A.,* **168**:1445, 1958.

Electroencephalography

Jaffe, R., Librot, I. E., and Bender, M. B.: Serial EEG studies in unoperated subdural hematoma, *Arch. Neurol.,* **19**:325, 1968.

Radiology

Bull, J. W. D.: The radiological diagnosis of chronic subdural haematoma, *Proc. Roy. Soc. Med.,* **33**(part 1):203, 1940.

————: The diagnosis of chronic subdural haematoma in children and adolescents, *Brit. J. Radiol.,* **22**:68, 1949.

Ferris, E. J., Lehrer, H., and Shapiro, J. H.: Pseudosubdural hematoma, *Radiology,* **88**:75, 1967.

Heiser, W. J., Quinn, J. L., III, and Mollihan, W. V.: The crescent pattern of increased radioactivity in brain scanning, *Radiology,* **87**:483, 1966.

Rothman, J., Shatsky, S., Kricheff, I., and Chase, N.: Ultrasonic diagnosis of subdural hematomas, *Am. J. Roentgenol.,* **105**:413, 1969.

Angiography

McLaurin, R. L.: Contributions of angiography to the pathophysiology of subdural hematoma, *Neurology*, **15**:866, 1965.

Zingesser, L. H., Schechter, M. M., and Rayport, M.: Truths and untruths concerning the angiographic findings in extracerebral hematomas, *Brit. J. Radiol.*, **38**:835, 1965.

Air Study

Calkins, R. A., Van Allen, M. W., and Sahs, A. L.: Subdural hematoma following pneumoencephalography: Case report, *J. Neurosurg.*, **27**:56, 1967.

Dyke, C. G.: A pathognomonic encephalographic sign of subdural hematoma, *Bull. Neurol. Inst, N. Y.*, **5**:135, 1936.

Natural History and Prognosis

Afra, D.: Ossification of subdural hematoma: Report of two cases, *J. Neurosurg.*, **18**:393, 1961.

Ambrosetto, C.: Post-traumatic subdural hematoma: Further observations on nonsurgical treatment, *Arch. Neurol.*, **6**:287, 1962.

Bender, M. B.: Recovery from subdural hematoma without surgery, *J. Mt. Sinai Hosp. N. Y.*, **27**:52, 1960.

Gannon, W. E., Cook, A. W., and Browder, E. J.: Resolving subdural collections, *J. Neurosurg.*, **19**:865, 1962.

MacLean, J. A., and Levy, L. F.: Calcified subdural hematoma, *Neurology*, **5**:520, 1955.

Mosberg, W. H., Jr., and Smith, G. W.: Calcified solid subdural hematoma; review of literature and report of an unusual case, *J. Nervous Mental Disease*, **115**:163, 1952.

Treatment

Hancock, D. O.: Cerebral collapse associated with chronic subdural haematoma in adults: A comparison of two methods of treatment, *Lancet*, **1**:633, 1965.

LaLonde, A. A., and Gardner, W. J.: Chronic subdural hematoma; expansion of compressed cerebral hemisphere and relief of hypotension by spinal injection of physiologic saline solution, *New Engl. J. Med.*, **239**:493, 1948.

Prager, D., and Kowalyshyn, T.: Subdural haematoma and anticoagulant treatment, *Lancet*, **2**:800, 1969.

Rosenbluth, P. R., Arias, B., Quartetti, E. V., and Carney, A. L.: Current management of subdural hematoma: Analysis of 100 consecutive cases, *J.A.M.A.*, **179**:759, 1962.

Suzuki, J., and Takaku, A.: Nonsurgical treatment of chronic subdural hematoma, *J. Neurosurg.*, **33**:548, 1970.

Yashon, D., Jane, J. A., White, R. J., and Sugar, O.: Traumatic subdural hematoma of infancy. Long-term follow-up of 92 patients, *Arch. Neurol.*, **18**:370, 1968.

Acute Spontaneous Subdural Hemorrhage

Talalla, A., and McKissock, W.: Acute "spontaneous" subdural hemorrhage. An unusual form of cerebrovascular accident, *Neurology*, **21**:19, 1971.

Extradural Hematoma

Pathogenesis and Pathologic Findings

Columella, F., Gaist, G., Piazza, G., and Caraffa, T.: Extradural haematoma at the vertex, *J. Neurol. Neurosurg. Psychiat.*, **31**:315, 1968.

Ford, L. E., and McLaurin, R. L.: Mechanisms of extradural hematomas, *J. Neurosurg.*, **20**:760, 1963.

Gallagher, J. P., and Browder, E. J.: Extradural hematoma. Experience with 167 patients, *J. Neurosurg.*, **29**:1, 1968.

Hooper, R.: Observations on extradural haemorrhage, *Brit. J. Surg.*, **47**:71, 1959.

Jacobson, W. H. A.: On middle meningeal haemorrhage, *Guy's Hosp. Rept.*, **43**:147, 1886.

Jamieson, K. G., and Yelland, J. D. N.: Extradural hematoma. Report of 167 cases, *J. Neurosurg.*, **29**:13, 1968.

Kosary, I. Z., Goldhammer, Y., and Lerner, M. A.: Acute extradural hematoma of the posterior fossa, *J. Neurosurg.*, **24**:1007, 1966.

Kuhn, R. A., and Kugler, H.: False aneurysms of the middle meningeal artery, *J. Neurosurg.*, **21**:92, 1964.

Margulies, M. E.: Concerning unusual etiologic factors in the production of extradural hemorrhage, *Angiology*, **14**:564, 1963.

McKissock, W., Taylor, J. C., Bloom, W. H., and Till, K.: Extradural haematoma: Observations on 125 cases, *Lancet*, **2**:167, 1960.

Oblu, N., and Sandulescu, G.: L'hématome extradural préfrontal (fronto-orbitaire), *Acta neurol. psychiat. belg.,* **69**:249, 1969.

Stevenson, G. C., Brown, H. A., and Hoyt, W. F.: Chronic venous epidural hematoma at the vertex, *J. Neurosurg.,* **21**:887, 1964.

Clinical Features

Hayashi, H., Hollin, S. A., and Gross, S. W.: Massive parasagittal epidural hematoma of venous origin, *J. Mt. Sinai Hosp. N. Y.,* **33**:125, 1966.

Phillips, D. G., and Azariah, R. G.: Acute intracranial haematoma from head injury; a study in prognosis, *Brit. J. Surg.,* **52**:218, 1965.

Troupp, H., Heiskanen, O., Tarkkanen, A., Koivusalo, P., Aho, J., and Tarkkanen, J.: The neurological deficit after extradural haematoma, *Lancet,* **2**:891, 1964.

Laboratory Findings

Ferris, E. J., Kirch, R. L. A., and Shapiro, J. H.: Epidural hematomas; varied angiographic signs, *Am. J. Roentgenol.,* **101**:100, 1967.

Koch, R. L., and Glickman, M. G.: The angiographic diagnosis of extradural hematoma of the posterior fossa, *Am. J. Roentgenol.,* **112**:289, 1971.

Kramer, S., and Rovit, R. L.: The value of Hg^{203} brain scans in patients with intracranial hematomas, *Radiology,* **83**:902, 1964.

Perlmutter, I., Dooley, D. M., and Auld, A. W.: Vertebral angiography in the presence of extradural hematoma of the posterior fossa, *South Med. J.,* **64**:245, 1971.

Weinman, D. F., and Jayamanne, D.: The role of angiography in the diagnosis of extradural haematomas, *Brit. J. Radiol.,* **39**:350, 1966.

Additional References

Apfelaum, R. I., Newman, S. A., and Zingesser, L. H.: Dynamics of technetium scanning of subdural hematomas, *Radiology,* **107**:571, 1973.

Galbraith, S. L.: Age distribution of extradural hemorrhage without skull fracture, *Lancet,* **1**:1217, 1973.

Holloway, W., El Gammal, T., and Pool, W. H., Jr.: Doughnut sign in subdural hematomas, *J. Nucl. Med.,* **13**:630, 1972.

Iwakuma, T., and Brunngraber, C. V.: Chronic extradural hematomas. A study of 21 cases, *J. Neurosurg.,* **38**:488, 1973.

Jain, K. K., and Schober, B.: Diagnosis of extradural hematoma by brain scan, *Can. Med. Assoc. J.,* **107**:218, 1972.

Radcliffe, W. B., Guinto, F. C., Jr., Adcock, D. F., and Krigman, M. R.: Subdural hematoma shape: New look at an old concept, *Am. J. Roentgenol.,* **115**:72, 1972.

Seshia, S. S.: Subdural haematoma: A complication of lumbar pneumoencephalography, *Neurology (India),* **19**:207, 1971.

Subarachnoid Hemorrhage

Diagnoses are missed not because of lack of knowledge on the part of the examiner, but rather because of lack of examination.

Sir William Osler

Subarachnoid hemorrhage (SAH) occurs when blood leaks into the subarachnoid space, either from a ruptured artery or vein *(primary subarachnoid hemorrhage)* or from an intracerebral hemorrhage that dissects through the parenchyma to the surface of the brain or into the ventricles *(secondary subarachnoid hemorrhage).* These hemorrhages are called *spontaneous* if there is no apparent cause and *traumatic* if there has been injury. Because patients suffering traumatic hemorrhage are best managed by the neurosurgeon, traumatic SAH, the most common type, will not be discussed in this volume.

ETIOLOGY AND PATHOGENESIS

Probably because of case selection, the incidence of the etiologic factors involved in subarachnoid hemorrhage varies from one report to another. Radiologists report aneurysms in as many as 90 percent of patients with subarachnoid hemorrhage; pathologists find aneurysms in about 30 percent. Cases of hemorrhage secondary to blood dyscrasia would probably not be seen by the radiologist for angiography but would be included in postmortem statistical analyses. In occasional cases, SAH is the presenting feature of an intracranial neoplasm such as ependymoma or meningioma, or a malignant lesion such as glioblastoma multiforme, hypernephroma, or melanoma. Occasionally systemic disease such as leukemia, blood dyscrasia, or angiopathy causes subarachnoid hemorrhage. Cortical thrombophlebitis and bacterial meningitis are rare causes of secondary subarachnoid hemorrhage.

In some patients with spontaneous subarachnoid hemorrhage, no cause can be found, even at autopsy. In some of these, an aneurysm or a small arteriovenous malformation may have burst, disappearing without a trace in the mass of blood over the surface of the brain. Moreover, most autopsies do not include examination of the spinal subarachnoid space, and yet hemorrhage may originate there and spread into the skull.

Factors Precipitating Rupture of an Intracranial Aneurysm

Among the factors that have been suspected of initiating dilatation or precipitating rupture of an aneurysm are head injury and hypertension. Transient hypertension occurring during strenuous exercise, excitement, sexual intercourse, and the Valsalva maneuver (performed unconsciously with defecation, sneezing, coughing, or lifting heavy loads) has also been regarded as a precipitating factor. It is probable that any of them can cause a rupture if the vascular abnormality is already ballooned out with a thin wall; but they are only the straws that break the camel's back, not the primary etiologic agents. In a third instance, no provoking factor can be discovered, the rupture occurring in a patient with a normal blood pressure while he is at rest or is apparently sleeping placidly.

CLINICAL FEATURES

Although there is no close relationship between headaches and subsequent subarachnoid hem-

orrhage, recurrent headache, monotonous in its location and characteristics (so-called unilateral migraine), can indicate an underlying vascular lesion, perhaps an arteriovenous malformation or an aneurysm. A change in the frequency, duration, or intensity of such headaches may presage rupture. However, the vast majority of so-called vascular headaches (migraine, histamine cephalalgia, or "cluster" headache) are not associated with any demonstrable intracranial vascular lesion and have no relation to SAH.

Careful inquiry will sometimes uncover a history of previous attacks of bleeding in other parts of the body, or some other evidence of blood dyscrasias; in other cases the use of anticoagulants may be a factor.

Present Illness

Although in the vast majority of individuals, subarachnoid hemorrhage strikes instantaneously, like a bolt from the blue, a carefully elicited study reveals a history of headaches, giddiness, diplopia, blurred vision, or neck stiffness in the preceding fortnight in about 30 to 40 percent of the cases. The patient may think that something has struck him on the head, or he may feel something "pop" or snap inside his skull. As a rule he is seized by excruciating headache, more severe than any he has ever experienced before. Although the ache may begin focally in any part of the head or behind the eye, in most cases it rapidly becomes generalized over the entire calvarium and suboccipital region, radiating into the nape of the neck. In cases of anteriorly placed aneurysms, however, it may remain confined to the ipsilateral forehead and orbit. The ache or pain is aggravated by flexion of the neck, movements of the head, and Valsalva's maneuver, as well as by sound and light. The patient seeks relief by lying quietly.

In occasional cases the patient may have only a trivial headache, so transient that he may seek no medical attention unless, as sometimes happens, a second, more massive hemorrhage occurs. In other cases, the headache is less troublesome than signs secondary to "chemical" meningitis: vomiting, fever, and clouding of consciousness. Such a clinical picture suggests bacterial meningitis, and only a lumbar puncture will reveal the true nature of the problem.

Once in a while the presenting symptom is back pain, which may radiate down one or both legs and may be accompanied by motor and sensory paresis of the lower limbs with acute retention of urine. These signs as the initial manifestation suggest primary spinal subarachnoid hemorrhage.

Sometimes SAH causes acute confusion and disorientation, irritability, irrelevant speech, and violent behavior, apparently without any headache whatsoever. It is possible that, in such instances, the hemorrhage remains encapsulated, as in rupture of an aneurysm of the anterior communicating artery between the two hemispheres or of the middle cerebral artery in the Sylvian fissure. Subtle signs of meningeal irritation may be overlooked because of the overwhelming psychiatric abnormalities.

EXAMINATION OF THE PATIENT

The signs present on examination are caused by the subarachnoid hemorrhage and by the underlying lesion whose rupture created it. Most often this lesion is silent, causing neither symptoms nor signs. The signs directly related to the leakage of blood depend on the origin of the rupture, the quantity of blood sprayed into the subarachnoid space, and the rate at which it accumulates. Arterial blood spurting under high pressure from an aneurysm of the anterior communicating artery produces findings that are very different from those caused by venous blood oozing from an arteriovenous malformation of the parietal lobe. Another factor that may contribute greatly to the clinical picture is

spasm of arteries in the vascular tree on which the aneurysm is located.

In the hours following the onset of hemorrhage, the patient's level of consciousness varies from normal to deeply comatose. If coma is to occur, it usually develops immediately or soon after the rupture. Disorientation, amnesia, delirium, and confabulation are common in the acute stages but usually clear within a week; although late recovery may occur, confusion persisting longer than several weeks is an ominous sign, suggesting the possibility of permanent intellectual deficit.

Headache gradually subsides but can be initiated again by sudden movement or the Valsalva maneuver. Hyporeflexia or areflexia is common; both plantar responses are often extensor within an hour of the ictus. Signs of meningeal irritation, such as resistance to neck flexion, usually develop within the first 24 hr. Less frequently, examination elicits a positive Kernig's sign (pain in the back and spasm in the hamstring muscles elicited by flexing the thigh on the abdomen and then extending the leg at the knee). Both these signs of meningeal irritation may be less marked or absent in patients who are deeply comatose.

Fever (100 to 102°F) and leukocytosis commonly develop within hours of onset and may persist for several days. This reaction to a sterile or chemical meningitis is caused by irritant hemoglobin or plasma in the subarachnoid space. Reappearance of these signs is often an indication of recurrent bleeding.

At times transient hypertension occurring as a result of acutely increased intracranial pressure or of stimulation of vasopressor reflexes can suggest hypertensive encephalopathy.

Almost any cranial nerve may be affected by SAH. Those close to arteries which rupture frequently (e.g., the oculomotor nerve) and those most vulnerable to an increase in intracranial pressure (e.g., the abducens nerve) are affected most often. Abnormalities of the abducens nerve are of little localizing value, but involvement of the oculomotor nerve, when present, points to the junction of the posterior communicating and internal carotid arteries as the site of the aneurysm. Of the many signs of oculomotor dysfunction, the first to appear is usually pupillary dilatation; consequently, the size, shape, and reaction of the pupils should be noted repeatedly during the course of the patient's illness.

Papilledema may develop within an hour of rupture and persist for some weeks, but is more often absent than present. It may be accompanied by flame-shaped or round hemorrhages in the retina. Subhyaloid (preretinal) hemorrhages may be present within an hour of the ictus. Although they are characteristic of subarachnoid hemorrhage, they are not pathognomonic, since they may be caused by any acute rise in intracranial pressure (Fig. 24-1).

Hemiplegia, hemianesthesia, hemianopia, or aphasia suggests concomitant involvement of the cerebral hemisphere but gives little clue to the cause of the cerebral deficit. These and other deficits may result from (1) the jet of arterial blood gushing from a ruptured aneurysm, (2) spasm in the neighboring or distant arteries which can cause cerebral infarction, (3) intracerebral hemorrhage, (4) pressure on the brain from subarachnoid hematoma, or (5) cerebral edema.

Convulsions, focal or generalized, may occur at the time of the ictus or immediately thereafter. They often signify direct involvement of the brain substance but are occasionally seen in subarachnoid hemorrhage without concomitant brain damage. A past history of convulsions suggests the possibility of other underlying brain disease such as arteriovenous malformation or tumor. Convulsions occurring after the ictus are more suggestive of brain damage due to bleeding.

When auscultation of the skull reveals a *bruit,* the possibility of an underlying arteriovenous malformation must be considered, because saccular aneurysms rarely produce bruits. It has been noted, however, that regardless of etiology intracranial murmurs are often absent during the phase of active bleeding, perhaps because of vasospasm or temporarily slowed cerebral circulation. It is therefore necessary to perform repeated auscultations during the illness in order to ascertain if a bruit becomes audible or changes its characteristics.

DIFFERENTIAL DIAGNOSIS

In patients with the classical picture of SAH, the diagnosis is not difficult. Since the presenting manifestations are not always typical, however, errors in diagnosis are common. When papilledema and retinal hemorrhages are seen in a patient with clouded consciousness, the clinical picture may suggest hypertensive encephalopathy or acute intracranial hypertension without hemorrhage. Bacterial meningitis causes signs and symptoms closely resembling those of SAH.

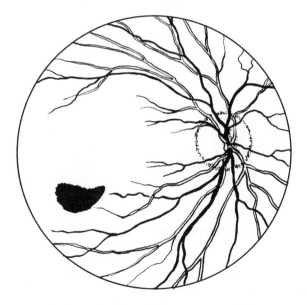

Figure 24-1 Illustration of optic fundus with subhyaloid (preretinal) hemorrhage.

If the patient is pregnant, eclampsia might be considered.

Unless one fears impending transtentorial or transforaminal herniation, diagnostic lumbar puncture should always be performed on any patient who has a history of an abrupt onset of headache, whose level of consciousness or cerebration is disturbed, and who presents evidence of meningeal irritation. If the spinal fluid contains blood, one is dealing with a traumatic puncture, or with primary or secondary subarachnoid hemorrhage.

If not due to trauma, bloodstained fluid signifies primary subarachnoid hemorrhage or intracerebral hemorrhage that has ruptured into the subarachnoid space. At times it may be impossible to distinguish between the two conditions. In cerebral hemorrhage, neurologic deficits develop over a period of several hours as blood oozes into the brain—the time required being dependent, of course, on the initial site and degree of the hemorrhage. There may be no headache at the onset, but as blood and cerebral edema begin to stretch or cause pressure on pain-sensitive structures, gradually increasing headache develops. The spinal fluid contains blood only if the hemorrhage ruptures through the surface of the brain or into the ventricles. When this happens, headache becomes excruciating and the patient often loses consciousness. Unless the brainstem is the site of the initial hemorrhage, consciousness is usually preserved during the initial stages of cerebral hemorrhage and may be lost with primary SAH. There are exceptions to this rule, however.

Clear spinal fluid usually means either that the patient has not had subarachnoid bleeding or that a cerebral hemorrhage has remained encapsulated. In very rare cases, fluid may remain clear when an intracranial aneurysm ruptures directly into the subdural space or intracerebrally, when a hemorrhage remains loculated in the subarachnoid space because of previous ad-

hesions, or when the lumbar puncture has been performed within 2 hr of SAH.

ETIOLOGIC DIAGNOSIS

Once the diagnosis of SAH has been established, its cause remains to be determined. In patients between 20 and 60 years of age who have never had neurologic symptoms before the bleeding episode, saccular aneurysm or intracerebral hemorrhage secondary to hypertension are likely causes. If the patient's blood pressure is not unusually elevated, aneurysm is probable. Arteriovenous malformations are sometimes associated with recurrent "migraine," or with focal sensory or motor seizures, and a cranial bruit is sometimes present. Rarely, rupture of a vessel is the initial manifestation of a cerebellar hemangioblastoma, tuberculous or fungal meningitis, a pituitary adenoma, an ependymoma, metastases from the lung or kidney, or a glioma. When this occurs, only the brain scan or angiogram may reveal the underlying disease.

When a patient has had a subarachnoid hemorrhage, it is always necessary to consider systemic disease such as carcinoma and blood dyscrasia. Special studies to rule out coagulation defects, leukemia, and thrombocytopenic purpura are not needed as routine procedures unless there is an appropriate history of bleeding or a family history of dyscrasia. Since subarachnoid hemorrhage is seldom the initial and only manifestation of blood dyscrasia, the patient should be examined for petechiae or purpura in the skin and for evidences of internal bleeding.

LABORATORY FINDINGS

A WBC count of 15,000 to 20,000 cells per cu mm, predominantly neutrophils, is common. When leukemia or thrombocytopenia is present, characteristic forms will be seen on smears of the blood and bone marrow. The erythrocyte sedimentation rate shows a mild to moderate rise, in keeping with the degree of fever and leukocytosis. When a blood dyscrasia is suspected or the patient has been receiving anticoagulants, bleeding and clotting times and other appropriate tests must be done.

During the acute phase, the urine may occasionally contain casts or large amounts of albumin, or both. Glycosuria may be present if the blood-sugar level is elevated or if the renal threshold is low, and dehydration or protracted vomiting may lead to ketosuria.

Examination of the Spinal Fluid

Lumbar puncture is essential whenever signs of meningitis are present or subarachnoid hemorrhage is suspected, and the quantity of fluid removed should be sufficient to yield definitive information as to the cause of the meningitis (bacterial, fungal, viral, or hemorrhagic). According to a long-held belief, removal of more than a few drops of fluid may lead to herniation of the parafloccular lobules of the cerebellum (cerebellar tonsils), especially in patients with papilledema or suspected intracerebral hematoma. This danger has been greatly overemphasized and at times has caused indecision actually detrimental to the patient. We believe that adequate samples can safely be withdrawn unless there are signs pointing to involvement of the brainstem and cerebellum. Even if the spinal fluid pressure is above the upper normal limit of 180 mm, there is little or no danger in removing up to 6 ml of fluid for cell count and determinations of the glucose and protein content. Pressure under 100 mm suggests the possibility of a partial block at the foramen magnum, and in such cases only the fluid contained in the manometer should be taken for microscopic examination and microdetermination of sugar and protein content.

The lumbar tap should be performed carefully with a fine-bore needle. Even with the best technique, however, insertion of the needle occasionally traumatizes a vein in the lumbar theca, causing it to bleed into the spinal subarachnoid space. This iatrogenic hemorrhage must be differentiated from spontaneous subarachnoid hemorrhage by the following test:

Collect spinal fluid in three sterile test tubes, allowing 3 ml to flow into the first, 2 ml into the second, and 1 ml into the third. One can then readily determine the order in which the samples were collected by the amount of fluid contained in each tube. Do a cell count on the first and last samples. In SAH the RBC are evenly distributed. In traumatic hemorrhage there will usually be more RBC in the first specimen than the last. *Crenated RBC do not help in distinguishing between traumatic and spontaneous subarachnoid hemorrhage.*

Centrifuge one sample and compare the color and clarity of the supernatant fluid with a sample of water in a similar tube. This examination should be made in good light (preferably daylight) against a white background. Xanthochromia is an indication that the bleeding occurred more than 2 hr previously. This xanthochromia is due to oxyhemoglobin, which is released into the cerebrospinal fluid by the breakdown of red blood cell membranes. Leptomeningeal metabolism begins immediately to change orange oxyhemoglobin to the darker brown-yellow of bilirubin. After 3 to 4 days, this process is complete and the fluid gives a positive indirect van den Bergh reaction.

Successive specimens of spinal fluid may be compared, either visually or photometrically, for changes in the degree of xanthochromia. The breakdown process is arrested when the fluid is removed from the subarachnoid space, so that the specimen undergoes no further change in color and can be saved for visual comparison with subsequent specimens. Macroscopic blood disappears from the cerebrospinal fluid between the seventh and the fourteenth day after SAH, and xanthochromia clears up in about 3 weeks.

Even in grossly bloody fluid, a white blood cell count must be performed after laking of the red blood cells has been produced with glacial acetic acid. In the early stages of SAH, the white blood cells are proportional to their number in the peripheral blood, but soon the neutrophil count in the spinal fluid may exceed this ratio. The neutrophils are gradually replaced by lymphocytes, and the cell count returns to normal within 2 to 3 days after xanthochromia is no longer evident. This leukocytosis is not due to infection but results from chemical irritation of the leptomeninges by subarachnoid blood.

The protein content of the cerebrospinal fluid is invariably increased after a subarchnoid hemorrhage, partly because of blood in the fluid and partly because of exudation. It is calculated that for each increase of 10,000 per cu mm in the red blood cell count there is a concomitant rise of 15 mg per 100 ml in the CSF protein. A disproportionate elevation of protein in the early stages may be due to hemodialysis. The protein content tends to return to normal about the time that the white blood cells disappear.

In most cases spinal fluid glucose is not affected by SAH. If it is low, infection should be suspected and a specimen of fluid should be obtained for examination by smear and culture. Both bacteria and fungi should be sought. However, in about 10 percent of cases low CSF glucose can be found in spite of a sterile spinal fluid.

Electroencephalogram

This test, which is of limited value in this condition, usually shows diffuse slow activity. Focal delta waves or unilateral voltage depression may sometimes be of help in detecting an underlying tumor or intracranial hematoma. Serial EEGs do not aid materially.

X-ray Examinations

X-ray examination of the skull may occasionally reveal curvilinear calcification in an aneurysmal wall or a calcified arteriovenous malformation. Demineralization of the posterior clinoid processes gives evidence of local or generalized intracranial hypertension and is suggestive of an intracranial tumor. Displacement of a calcified pineal body from the midline is suggestive of neoplasm, blood clot, or edema. In patients without a calcified pineal gland, a shift of the midline structures may be detected by means of an echoencephalogram.

The chest x-ray is usually normal in patients with subarachnoid hemorrhage unless they have aspirated. Occasionally signs of pulmonary congestion with increased bronchovascular markings will be found, usually the result of myocardial damage and acute left ventricular decompensation. A chest film is a routine part of the evaluation and may reveal a latent bronchogenic carcinoma or the presence of multiple metastases.

Electrocardiogram

Patients with SAH may have striking changes in their cardiac rate and rhythm. The rate may be slowed to such a degree that a diagnosis of heart block is entertained clinically, and changes in the T waves and S-T segments on the ECG may be so profound that myocardial ischemia and infarction are considered probable. These changes may develop within an hour of the onset of the hemorrhage, at which time nuchal rigidity is not apparent and the patient may be unconscious and unable to complain of headache.

The mechanism producing these changes is not understood. It is thought by some physicians that damage to the subfrontal cortex is associated with an unusually high incidence of electrocardiographic changes, perhaps by setting up reflex vasospasm in the coronary arteries. Irritation in the posterior fossa may stimulate cardioinhibition or vasodepression by triggering the terminal portions of the glossopharyngeal nerve or the dorsal motor nucleus of the vagus, and traction on the circle of Willis can have similar effects. These effects may result in myocardial infarction and pulmonary edema.

Radioactive Brain Scan

Next to angiography, a brain scan using technetium 99m is the most useful procedure for detecting the source of SAH. Although it will not locate small aneurysms, it is very helpful in detecting malignant gliomas, metastases, arteriovenous malformations, and complications associated with aneurysmal rupture (e.g., intracerebral or chronic subdural hematomas).

Angiography

Just as lumbar tap is mandatory for the diagnosis of subarachnoid hemorrhage, so is an angiographic examination essential to locate the type and site of the offending lesion, particularly for defining the location, size, shape, direction of pointing, multiplicity, and complications of aneurysmal rupture. Until recently, there has been fierce debate regarding the optimal time to perform angiography; now it is generally agreed that if the patient is a potential candidate for surgery and if adequate radiologic facilities and an experienced surgical team are available, cerebral angiography should be carried out as soon as possible after a diagnosis of SAH has been established. Some authorities consider this to be an emergency undertaking. The more conservative believe it should be done within 14 days of the ictus.

There are at least three reasons for performing angiography soon after a subarachnoid hemorrhage:

1 Angiographic findings aid in planning the best approach (medical or surgical) to an individual case.
2 In almost half the cases, ruptured aneurysms bleed again some time within the first 6 weeks, the majority within the first 3 weeks. Hence any aneurysm that may be present and can be operated on should be corrected by remedial surgery within the first 3 weeks.
3 When done by experienced physicians, angiography seldom has an adverse effect on the patient's clinical status, and the value of the information gained far outweighs the risk involved.

It should be emphasized, however, that angiography is contraindicated in patients whose SAH was caused by a systemic disease, and is justified only if the patient is potentially a candidate for remedial surgery in the event that a lesion is found. Hence a neurosurgeon should always be called into consultation before angiography is performed.

Salient Features of Angiographic Technique in Patients with Intracranial Subarachnoid Hemorrhage Although the details of the procedure vary from one center to another, depending primarily on the judgment of the chief of service, the following points are worthy of mention:

1 Every patient must have a bilateral visualization of the carotid arteries and vertebral-basilar system in the lateral and Towne projections.
2 Biplane rapid seriographic studies are preferable to single-film exposures. Oblique projections may be necessary to display coiled and superimposed vessels, in order to distinguish artifacts, and to reveal concealed aneurysms.
3 Displaying the entire cerebrovascular tree on one injection (panangiography), while theoretically ideal, is impractical at present, because injection of contrast material into the aortic arch does not produce adequate visualization of

intracerebral vessels. The best procedures seem
to be the retrofemoral catheter approach to the
carotid and vertebral arteries or to inject the
material into the left carotid and make a right
retrograde brachial angiogram to display the
right vertebral and basilar system along with
the right carotid system.

4 During injection of the left carotid, the
contralateral carotid artery may be compressed
in order to ascertain the degree of cross filling of
the opposite anterior and middle cerebral arteries. The extent of cross filling will help the surgeon to plan his approach.

5 The circulation time (transit time) should
be noted. If prolonged, it is an indication of increased intracranial pressure or diffuse vasospasm; if the time is short, arteriovenous malformation should be suspected.

Angiographic Findings in Ruptured Aneurysm
A "congenital" saccular aneurysm is found in
about 50 percent of the spontaneous (nontrau-
matic) subarachnoid hemorrhages studied by
adequate angiography; about 25 percent show
hypertensive intracerebral hemorrhage; and
about 5 percent, an arteriovenous malformation. In the remainder, a clot or spasm may prevent filling of an aneurysm or a small arteriovenous malformation. Then, too, a vein or an
arteriosclerotic arteriole may be too small to be
seen. It is extremely rare to visualize the contrast material actually coming from a ruptured
vessel. Arterial spasm is very commonly seen,
usually in the immediate neighborhood of the
ruptured aneurysm and occasionally in the carotids of both sides; rarely, diffuse spasm may
involve even the basilar arterial branches. The
incidence of spasm is highest in the first 3 weeks
after the ictus; it diminishes gradually thereafter.

From 10 to 20 percent of the cases of intracranial aneurysm are multiple. Although others
disagree, some authorities say that in 85 to 90
percent of such patients, rupture occurs in the
largest aneurysm. In addition, the following

roentgenologic signs may be helpful in indicating which of several aneurysms has ruptured:

1 Displacement and stretching of surrounding vessels, indicating the presence of a hematoma.

2 Localized arterial spasm. Visualization of
focal spasm, but no aneurysm, on films taken in
the week following SAH is presumptive evidence that the causative lesion lies near or on
the spastic vessel. Repetition of angiography a
week or 10 days later, after spasm has subsided,
may demonstrate the cause.

3 Irregular interior contour of the aneurysm.
This is supposedly due to blood clot but is not a
very reliable sign.

4 Escape of contrast material through the
aneurysmal sac. This very rare finding is pathognomonic of a ruptured aneurysm.

5 A nipplelike protrusion at the dome of the
ruptured aneurysm. Some authorities believe
this finding to be almost diagnostic of recent
rupture.

About 10 percent of patients in whom complete angiographic findings have been considered negative are found at autopsy to have had
an intracranial aneurysm. This error in diagnosis may be due to poor technique or to errone-
ous interpretation of the findings, or to (1) spontaneous thrombosis in an aneurysm, (2)
nonfilling caused by spasm of the parent artery,
or (3) extremely small size of the aneurysm (i.e.,
a diameter less than 2 mm). It is worth remembering that the prognosis following SAH is better in patients with normal angiograms than in
those in whom an aneurysm is demonstrated.

In addition to aneurysm, angiography may
reveal displacement of arteries or veins by blood
clot, neoplasm, or edema. Vasospasm can be detected only by angiography. Arteriovenous malformation, the usual cause of venous bleeding,
can also be demonstrated. In such cases, the arteries feeding and veins draining the malforma-

tion should be scrupulously traced out through serial films in multiple projections. Only in this manner can the true extent of the lesion and the feasibility of surgical correction be determined.

In seriously ill patients, especially those with signs of brainstem involvement, angiography may reveal cerebral circulatory arrest. In such cases the intracranial arteries fail to fill or fill very poorly, because of the marked elevation of intracranial pressure.

Air Study

In a few reported cases of SAH, air study has revealed a bleeding intraventricular or paraventricular neoplasm after angiographic examination has failed to disclose a lesion. This condition is so rare, however, that air study is seldom justified in patients with SAH.

Myelography

Occasionally a ruptured arteriovenous malformation or an ependymoma of the spinal cord can be demonstrated by a myelogram. See Chap. 22.

COURSE OF THE DISEASE

Subarachnoid hemorrhage is probably the only intracranial lesion capable of producing almost instantaneous death in an otherwise healthy individual (Fig. 24-2). (Patients usually survive at least 2 hr following intracerebral hemorrhage.) SAH carries the most uncertain prognosis of all intracranial lesions, and the outlook varies according to the underlying cause. Patients whose hemorrhage is due to leukemia have a much poorer prognosis than those with a ruptured aneurysm. Perhaps the most favorable prognosis is associated with arteriovenous malformation.

Although a second hemorrhage may occur as late as 20 years after rupture of an intracranial aneurysm, the danger is considerably lessened

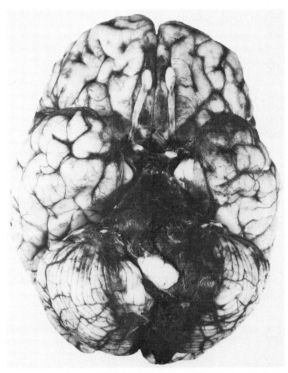

Figure 24-2 The base of the brain showing massive recent subarachnoid hemorrhage with clot in the basal cisterns. *(Courtesy of John Moossy, M.D., Department of Pathology, Bowman Gray School of Medicine.)*

after 3 to 6 months have passed. The mortality from succeeding attacks is probably no higher than that from the initial hemorrhage. The patient's age, sex, and occupation, as well as the severity of the initial attack, appear to have no bearing on the likelihood of recurrence, but hypertension perhaps increases the danger.

In about 20 percent of patients who have four-vessel arteriography no source of bleeding will be uncovered. In these cases the lesion may be too small to be visible, or the vessel involved may not fill because of spasm or occlusion by clot.

The mortality in such patients surviving the initial bleeding episode is only 6 percent, compared with about 40 percent in patients in whom an aneurysm is found.

In some patients the development of subarachnoid adhesions obstructs the free flow of cerebrospinal fluid and produces hydrocephalus.

MANAGEMENT

Management of spontaneous subarachnoid hemorrhage may be entirely medical or both medical and surgical.

Transportation of the Patient

All too often SAH begins in inappropriate places far from home, and the patient must be taken to the nearest hospital. He should be held and given medical therapy there until his condition seems stabilized, open airway is assured, and survival seems probable. Then he should be transported by ambulance or airplane to a center where complete facilities for diagnosis and surgical therapy are available. The patient should be heavily sedated for the trip, and he must be accompanied by a nurse who can maintain the open airway in case of vomiting or convulsions.

Medical Therapy

Medical therapy alone is indicated in the following situations:

1 When angiography reveals no aneurysm, neoplasm, or other surgical abnormality.
2 When the lesion is situated in an inaccessible site.
3 In the presence of multiple intracranial lesions, especially when these are bilateral and there are neither clinical nor angiographic clues as to which has ruptured. (Some surgeons advocate multiple approaches to these.)
4 In the presence of arteriosclerotic fusiform aneurysms, especially of the basilar artery.
5 When the patient is *in extremis* or is suffer-

ing from a major ailment that precludes surgery.
6 When the family or the patient refuses surgery.

Management of the Acute Phase Strict bed rest is usually enforced for a period of 4 to 6 weeks following hemorrhage until fibroblastic proliferation and wound repair become maximal. Constant attendance by a devoted nurse is probably the most essential part of the program of medical therapy. Only excellent nursing care can prevent respiratory and urinary complications and the development of bed sores. The patient should be kept almost flat in bed and not be permitted to feed himself. He should avoid all forms of straining, and the bowels should be kept open by means of mild laxatives. A low-residue diet will help reduce the frequency and bulk of the stools.

In most patients headache can be controlled with aspirin and codeine. Anxiety and restlessness may be controlled with barbiturates, chloral hydrate, or paraldehyde, given in doses sufficient to keep the patient quiet. No visitors other than the immediate family should be allowed, and radio or television should not be permitted; news and sports events are frequently upsetting or too exciting. No active exercises should be instituted for 3 weeks, but passive movement of all four extremities by the nurse or therapist several times daily is essential if the patient does not move spontaneously.

Induced Hypotension Reduction of blood pressure during the acute phase of the illness is the medical treatment of choice. Controlled hypotension sustained at levels just sufficient for coronary, renal, and cerebral perfusion reduces the number of fatalities that result from rebleeding. For nomotensive patients, this level is about 100 mm Hg systolic; the level for hypertensive patients is higher. Reduction is achieved by tilting the patient or by a variety of hypotensive medications. Apparently, the means is not as important as the degree of hypotension which can be sustained.

Control of Intracranial Pressure Because cerebral edema often contributes to a poor prognosis, many advocate the use of dexamethasone 6 to 10 mg every 6 hr. It is suggested also that this drug reduces the likelihood of arachnoidal adhesions with secondary hydrocephalus and consequent intracranial hypertension.

Some advocate placement of a ventricular catheter for constant cerebrospinal fluid drainage for patients with increased intracranial pressure. Others use the dehydrating agents mannitol, urea, or glycerol to reduce extracellular fluid volume and to control edema. The patient should be kept slightly dehydrated and have his head slightly elevated during the first few weeks after the ictus.

Control of Vasospasm Vasospasm occurring either as a result of blood in the subarachnoid space or a direct myogenic response to rupture can cause infarction unrelated to the original vascular rupture. Most clinicians have not treated the vasospastic element, but a possibly beneficial approach is aggressive management with vasodilators such as phenoxybenzamine or papaverine. Hemispheric blood flow is estimated by radioisotopic methods; if flow on one side is reduced substantially, a diffuse disturbance such as vasospasm is postulated.

Thrombogenic Agents Epsilon-aminocaproic acid in high doses has been used to prevent lysis of blood clot and to induce further clotting in the region of rupture.

Lumbar Puncture An initial lumbar tap is essential for diagnostic purposes. If the CSF is under increased pressure, fluid should be withdrawn gradually until the pressure is lowered to about 200 mm. Lumbar puncture should be re-

peated only if fresh signs or symptoms appear, or for the relief of persistent, severe headaches. A few neurologists advocate withdrawing spinal fluid at frequent intervals in order to reduce the CSF pressure. Their theory is that this procedure, in addition to preventing headaches, helps to drain off subarachnoid blood that might lead to subsequent adhesions and hydrocephalus. We believe that the latter consideration is highly theoretical and that the danger of causing a transtentorial or transforaminal herniation in cases associated with intracerebral hemorrhage or cerebral edema is very real.

SAH in Pregnancy The causes of SAH in pregnancy are the same as those described for the nonpregnant state, with the addition of eclampsia, which is diagnosed by the presence of hypertension, albuminuria, edema, and seizures. Intracranial aneurysms and arteriovenous malformations rupture most frequently during the twentieth to the thirtieth weeks of gestation. The criteria used to determine the diagnostic procedures (including angiography) and therapeutic measures that should be employed during pregnancy are the same as those given for nonpregnant patients.

If an aneurysm is demonstrated, appropriate neurosurgical treatment should be carried out immediately; if the patient is found to have an arteriovenous malformation, no attempt should be made to treat the lesion until after childbirth. Termination of pregnancy is not indicated in either case. Since the incidence of rebleeding from intracranial abnormalities is as high in patients delivered by cesarean section as in those allowed a normal labor, delivery at term should be through the vagina, with the use of low forceps to aid extraction of the head. Further pregnancies are not contraindicated for surgically treated patients; but if the vascular abnormality has not been corrected, it is advisable to postpone pregnancy for some years.

In cases where an arteriovenous malformation is demonstrated, no attempt should be made to treat the lesion until after childbirth. In those for whom surgery seems unwise, further pregnancies may carry some risk of rebleeding.

Convalescent Care In spite of the possible relationship between transient arterial hypertension and rupture of an aneurysm, it is best not to restrict the patient's activity too severely during the convalescent period. After the first 3 months are past, the patient may be permitted, even encouraged, to lead as normal a life as possible.

Prevention of Seizures Convulsions occur as sequelae of ruptured intracranial aneurysms in 10 to 14 percent of the cases. The incidence of seizures is highest in younger patients in whom rupture of an aneurysm in the middle cerebral artery is associated with intracerebral hematoma or evidence of residual brain damage. Anticonvulsants may be given prophylactically.

Surgical Management

It has to be emphasized that SAH in itself is not an indication for surgery. Complications produced by intracerebral or subdural hematomas acting as enlarging lesions must be treated by surgical removal of the clot, either through a bur hole or by craniotomy. Obstructive hydrocephalus following SAH may require shunting procedures later on.

When the source of SAH can be determined, its extirpation is a prophylactic measure aimed at preventing recurrence. Surgery is naturally more hazardous during the acute episode, and it is usually best to postpone the removal of arteriovenous malformations, gliomas, or metastases until the patient is in good condition. In cases of ruptured aneurysm, however, early surgery is justified by the high incidence of fatal recurring hemorrhage. The surgical management of aneurysm and arteriovenous malforma-

tions is discussed in more detail in Chaps. 25 and 26.

SUGGESTED READINGS

General

Fields, W. S., and Sahs, A. L. (eds.): Intracranial Aneurysms and Subarachnoid Hemorrhage, Charles C Thomas, Publisher, Springfield, Ill., 1965.

Walton, J. N.: Subarachnoid Hemorrhage, The Williams & Wilkins Company, Baltimore, 1956.

Etiology and Pathogenesis

Barron, K. D., and Fergusson, G.: Intracranial hemorrhage as a complication of anticoagulant therapy, *Neurology,* **9**:447, 1959.

Jain, K. K.: Mechanism of rupture of intracranial saccular aneurysms, *Surgery,* **54**:347, 1963.

Kerr, C. B.: Intracranial haemorrhage in haemophilia, *J. Neurol. Neurosurg. Psychiat.,* **27**:166, 1964.

Lombardo, L., Mateos, J. H., and Barroeta, F. F.: Subarachnoid hemorrhage due to endometriosis of the spinal canal, *Neurology,* **18**:423, 1968.

Nassar, S. I., and Correll, J. W.: Subarachnoid hemorrhage due to spinal cord tumors, *Neurology,* **18**:87, 1968.

Pakarinen, S.: Incidence, aetiology, and prognosis of primary subarachnoid haemorrhage. A study based on 589 cases diagnosed in a defined urban population during a defined period, *Acta neurol. scand.,* **43**(suppl. 29):9, 1967.

Petty, P. G.: Subarachnoid haemorrhage of undetermined aetiology, *Med. J. Australia,* **2**:1, 1966.

Quickel, K. E., Jr., and Whaley, R. J.: Subarachnoid hemorrhage in a patient with hereditary hemorrhagic telangiectasis, *Neurology,* **17**:716, 1967.

Ramamurthi, B.: Are subarachnoid haemorrhages uncommon in India? *Neurology (India),* **13**:42, 1965.

Sahs, A. L., Perret, G. E., Locksley, H. B., and Nishioka, H. (eds.): Intracranial Aneurysms and Subarachnoid Hemorrhage. A Cooperative Study, J. B. Lippincott Company, Philadelphia, 1969.

Symonds, C. P.: Spontaneous subarachnoid haemorrhage, *Quart J. Med.,* **18**:93, 1924.

Watson, A. B.: Spinal subarachnoid haemorrhage in patient with coarctation of aorta, *Brit. Med. J.,* 4:278, 1967.

Clinical Features

Calvert, J. M.: Premonitory symptoms and signs of subarachnoid haemorrhage, *Med. J. Australia,* 1:651, 1966.
Crompton, M. R.: Hypothalamic lesions following the rupture of cerebral berry aneurysms, *Brain,* 86:301, 1963.
Heck, A. F.: Manifestations of spontaneous subarachnoid hemorrhage in the orbit of bulbus oculi; report of previously undescribed hemorrhagic phenomena in the conjunctivae, *Neurology,* 11:701, 1961.
Money, R. A., and Vanderfield, G. K.: Premonitory symptoms and signs of subarachnoid haemorrhage, *Med. J. Australia,* 1:859, 1966.

Examination of the Patient

Fahmy, J. A., Knudsen, V., and Andersen, S. R.: Intraocular haemorrhage following subarachnoid haemorrhage, *Acta ophthalmol.,* 47:550, 1969.
Greenhoot, J. H., and Reichenbach, D. D.: Cardiac injury and subarachnoid hemorrhage. A clinical, pathological and physiological correlation, *J. Neurosurg.,* 30:521, 1969.
Wong, T. C., and Cooper, E. S.: Atrial fibrillation with ventricular slowing in a patient with spontaneous subarachnoid hemorrhage, *Am. J. Cardiol.,* 23:473, 1969.

Differential Diagnosis

Arena, J. M.: Cerebral vascular lesions accompanying sickle-cell anemia, *J. Pediat.,* 14:745, 1939.
Franklin, E. C., Powell, M. J., and Krueger, E. G.: Subarachnoid hemorrhage from an aneurysm in a patient with thrombocytopenic purpura, *Neurology,* 7:293, 1957.
Froman, C., and Smith, A. C.: Hyperventilation associated with low pH of cerebrospinal fluid after intracranial haemorrhage, *Lancet,* 1:780, 1966.
Glass, B., and Abbott, K. H.: Subarachnoid hemorrhage consequent to intracranial tumors; review of literature and report of seven cases, *Arch. Neurol. Psychiat.,* 73:369, 1955.
Goran, A., Ciminello, V. J., and Fisher, R. G.: Hemorrhage into meningiomas, *Arch. Neurol.,* 13:65, 1965.
Halpern, L., Feldman, S., and Peyser, E.: Subarachnoid hemorrhage with papilledema due to spinal neurofibroma, *Arch. Neurol. Psychiat.,* 79:138, 1958.
Huskisson, E. C., and Hart, F. D.: Fulminating meningococcal septicaemia presenting with subarachnoid haemorrhage, *Brit. Med. J.,* 2:231, 1969.
Morris, D. A., and Henkind, P.: Relationship of intracranial optic-nerve sheath and retinal hemorrhage, *Am. J. Ophthalmol.,* 64:853, 1967.
Ray, H., and Wahal, K. M.: Subarachnoid hemorrhage in subacute bacterial endocarditis, *Neurology,* 7:265, 1957.
Secher-Hansen, E.: Subarachnoid haemorrhage and sudden unexpected death: A medico-legal material, *Acta neurol. scand.,* 40:115, 1964.
Skultety, F. M.: Meningioma simulating ruptured aneurysm. Case report, *J. Neurosurg.,* 28:380, 1968.

Laboratory Findings

James, I. M.: Changes in cerebral blood flow and in systemic arterial pressure following spontaneous subarachnoid haemorrhage, *Clin. Sci.,* 35:11, 1968.
Uttley, A. H. C., and Buckell, M.: Biochemical changes after spontaneous subarachnoid haemorrhage. Part III. Coagulation and lysis with special reference to recurrent haemorrhage, *J. Neurol. Neurosurg. Psychiat.,* 31:621, 1968.

Examination of the Spinal Fluid

Barrows, L. J., Hunter, F. T., and Banker, B. Q.: The nature and clinical significance of pigments in the cerebrospinal fluid, *Brain,* 78:59, 1955.
Cole, M.: "Examination of the cerebrospinal fluid," in Special Techniques for Neurologic Diagnosis (Contemporary Neurology Series, 3), edited by J. F. Toole, F. A. Davis Company, Philadelphia, 1969, pp. 29–47.
Froman, C., and Smith, A.C.: Metabolic acidosis of the cerebrospinal fluid associated with subarachnoid haemorrhage, *Lancet,* 1:965, 1967.

McMenemey, W. H.: The significance of subarachnoid bleeding, *Proc. Roy. Soc. Med.*, **47**:701, 1954.

Tourtellotte, W. W., Metz, L. N., Bryan, E. R., and DeJong, R. N.: Spontaneous subarachnoid hemorrhage: Factors affecting the rate of clearing of the cerebrospinal fluid, *Neurology*, **14**:301, 1964.

Troost, B. T., Walker, J. E., and Cherington, M.: Hypoglycorrhachia associated with subarachnoid hemorrhage, *Arch. Neurol.*, **19**:438, 1968.

Van Der Meulen, J. P.: Cerebrospinal fluid xanthochromia: An objective index, *Neurology*, **16**:170, 1966.

X-ray Findings

Bjorkesten, G., and Halonen, V.: Incidence of intracranial vascular lesions in patients with subarachnoid hemorrhage investigated by four-vessel angiography, *J. Neurosurg.*, **23**:29, 1965.

du Boulay, G.: Distribution of spasm in the intracranial arteries after subarachnoid haemorrhage, *Acta radiol. diagn.*, **1**:257, 1963.

Heiskanen, O.: Cerebral circulatory arrest caused by acute increase in intracranial pressure: A clinical and roentgenological study of 25 cases, *Acta neurol. scand.*, **40**(suppl. 17):1, 1964.

Kak, V. K., and Taylor, A. R.: Cerebral blood-flow in subarachnoid haemorrhage, *Lancet*, **1**:875, 1967.

Kalbag, R. M.: Recurrent subarachnoid haemorrhage from paraventricular lesions with normal angiography, *J. Neurol. Neurosurg. Psychiat.*, **27**:435, 1964.

Mitchell, O. C., de la Torre, E., Alexander, E., Jr., and Davis, C. H., Jr.: The nonfilling phenomenon during angiography in acute intracranial hypertension: Report of 5 cases and experimental study, *J. Neurosurg.*, **19**:766, 1962.

Sutton, D., and Trickey, S. E.: Subarachnoid haemorrhage and total cerebral angiography, *Clin. Radiol.*, **13**:297, 1962.

Electroencephalography

Millar, J. H. D.: The electroencephalogram in cases of subarachnoid haemorrhage, *Electroencephalog. Clin. Neurophysiol.*, **5**:165, 1953.

Walton, J. N.: The electroencephalographic sequelae of spontaneous subarachnoid haemorrhage, *Electroencephalog. Clin. Neurophysiol.*, **5**:41, 1953.

Electrocardiography

Burch, G. E., Meyers, R., and Abildskov, J. A.: A new electrocardiographic pattern observed in cerebrovascular accidents, *Circulation*, **9**:719, 1954.

Cropp, G. J., and Manning, G. W.: Electrocardiographic changes simulating myocardial ischemia and infarction associated with spontaneous intracranial hemorrhage, *Circulation*, **22**:25, 1960.

Hoffbrand, B. I., and Morgan, B. D.: Electrocardiographic changes associated with subarachnoid haemorrhage, *Lancet*, **1**:844, 1965.

Course of the Disease

Arutiunov, A. I., Baron, M. A., and Majorova, N. A.: Experimental and clinical study of the development of spasm of the cerebral arteries related to subarachnoid hemorrhage, *J. Neurosurg.*, **32**:617, 1970.

Cronqvist, S.: Encephalographic changes following subarachnoid haemorrhage, *Brit. J. Radiol.*, **40**:38, 1967.

Editorial: Prognosis of subarachnoid haemorrhage, *Lancet*, **2**:590, 1960.

Ellington, E., and Margolis, G.: Block of arachnoid villus by subarachnoid hemorrhage, *J. Neurosurg.*, **30**:651, 1969.

Gurdjian, E. S., and Thomas, L. M.: Cerebral vasospasm, *Surg. Gynecol. Obstet.*, **129**:931, 1969.

Hammes, E. M., Jr.: Reaction of the meninges to blood, *Arch. Neurol. Psychiat.*, **52**:505, 1944.

Höök, O.: Prognosis in subarachnoid haemorrhages: A report of 152 acute cases, *Acta med. scand.*, **162**:475, 1958.

————: Subarachnoid haemorrhage: Prognosis when angiography reveals no aneurysm; a report of 138 cases, *Acta med. scand.*, **162**:493, 1958.

Hughes, J. T., and Oppenheimer, D. R.: Superficial siderosis of the central nervous system. A report on nine cases with autopsy, *Acta neuropath. (Berlin)*, **13**:56, 1969.

Katsiotis, P. A., and Taptas, J. N.: Embolism and spasm following subarachnoid hemorrhage, *Acta radiol. diagn.*, **7**:140, 1968.

Kibler, R. F., Couch, R. S., and Crompton, M. R.: Hydrocephalus in the adult following spontaneous subarachnoid haemorrhage, *Brain*, **84**:45, 1961.

Storey, P. B.: Psychiatric sequelae of subarachnoid haemorrhage, *Brit. Med. J.,* **3**:261, 1967.

Tappura, M.: Prognosis of subarachnoid haemorrhage: A study of 120 patients with unoperated intracranial arterial aneurysms and 267 patients without vascular lesions demonstrable in bilateral carotid angiograms, *Acta med. scand.,* **173**(suppl. 392):1, 1962.

Theander, S., and Granholm, L.: Sequelae after spontaneous subarachnoid haemorrhage, with special reference to hydrocephalus and Korsakoff's syndrome, *Acta neurol. scand.,* **43**:479, 1967.

Trumpy, J. H.: Subarachnoid haemorrhage. Time sequence of recurrences and their prognosis, *Acta neurol. scand.,* **43**:48, 1967.

Management

Medical Management

Ahmed, R. H., and Sedzimir, C. B.: Ruptured anterior communicating aneurysm. A comparison of medical and specific surgical treatment, *J. Neurosurg.,* **26**:213, 1967.

Cheatham, M. L., and Brackett, C. E.: Problems in management of subarachnoid hemorrhage in sickle cell anemia, *J. Neurosurg.,* **23**:488, 1965.

Copelan, E. L., and Mabon, R. F.: Spontaneous intracranial bleeding in pregnancy, *Obstet. Gynecol.,* **20**:373, 1962.

Dalsgaard-Nielsen, T.: The prognosis of unoperated cases of first attack of spontaneous, uncomplicated subarachnoid haemorrhage with or without detected aneurysm, *Acta neurol. scand.,* **44**:130, 1968.

Heiskanen, O., and Nikki, P.: Rupture of intracranial arterial aneurysm during pregnancy, *Acta neurol. scand.,* **39**:202, 1963.

Rose, F. C., and Sarner, M.: Epilepsy after ruptured intracranial aneurysm, *Brit. Med. J.,* **1**:18, 1965.

Singer, R. P., and Schneider, R. C.: The successful management of intracerebral and subarachnoid hemorrhage in hemophilic infant: A case report, *Neurology,* **12**:293, 1962.

Surgical Management

Shulman, K., Martin, B. F., Popoff, N., and Ransohoff, J.: Recognition and treatment of hydrocephalus following spontaneous subarachnoid hemorrhage, *J. Neurosurg.,* **20**:1040, 1963.

Stornelli, S. A., and French, J. D.: Subarachnoid hemorrhage—Factors in prognosis and management, *J. Neurosurg.,* **21**:769, 1964.

Richardson, A.: Subarachnoid haemorrhage, *Brit. Med. J.,* **4**:89, 1969.

Additional References

Harmsen, P., Kjaerulff, J., and Skinøj, E.: Acute controlled hypotension and EEG in patients with hypertension and cerebrovascular disease, *J. Neurol. Neurosurg. Psychiat.,* **34**:300, 1971.

Keller, A. Z.: Hypertension, age and residence in the survival with subarachnoid hemorrhage, *Am. J. Epidemiol.,* **91**:139, 1970.

Lin, J. P., and Kricheff, I. I.: Angiographic investigation of cerebral aneurysms. Technical aspects, *Radiology,* **105**:69, 1972.

Robinson, J. L., Hall, C. J., and Sedzimir, C. B.: Subarachnoid hemorrhage in pregnancy, *J. Neurosurg.,* **36**:27, 1972.

Wilkins, R. H., Wilkinson, R. H., and Odom, G. L.: Abnormal brain scans in patients with cerebral arterial spasm, *J. Neurosurg.,* **36**:133, 1972.

Intracranial Arterial Aneurysms

The diagnosis is, as a rule, impossible. The larger sacs produce the symptoms of tumor and their rupture is usually fatal.

W. Osler
The Principles and Practice of Medicine, 1920

An aneurysm is an abnormal localized dilatation of an arterial lumen. Aneurysmal dilatations must be distinguished from tortuosity or looping of vessels and from diffuse enlargements of the lumen. Arteriovenous and cirsoid aneurysms, usually included in discussions of arterial aneurysms, will be considered in Chap. 26.

There are four types of intracranial arterial aneurysms:

1 "Congenital" (berry or saccular), comprising over 90 percent of arterial aneurysms
2 Arteriosclerotic (fusiform), about 7 percent

3 Septic (mycotic), about 0.5 percent
4 Dissecting, about 0.5 percent

"CONGENITAL" (BERRY OR SACCULAR) ANEURYSMS

Etiology and Pathogenesis

Congenital aplasia or hypoplasia of the arterial muscularis, combined with the incessant pounding of arterial blood against these weak areas, is believed to be the most important factor in the genesis of intracranial aneurysms. Normally, the muscular coat of an artery develops from islands of mesenchyme which fuse with one another to form a continuous supporting and strengthening structure capable of dilating and constricting with ease. Imperfect fusion at bifurcations and incomplete resorption of embryonic branches provide potential sites for herniation of the intima and formation of a saccular aneurysm. Such defects, present at birth, are rarely associated with visible herniation. Only when the ravages of time lead to elevation of the systemic blood pressure and/or atherosclerosis is herniation thought to occur.

Since medial defects are found in at least 80 percent of supposedly normal cerebral arterial trees, it is reasonable to assume that aneurysmal formation is dependent on additional factors. Perhaps the most important of these is a strong head of pulsatile blood pressure beating against the weakened area. This situation is analogous

to the production of an inguinal hernia by chronic or oft-repeated transient increases in intraabdominal pressure pressing against a large inguinal ring.

Frequency

Unruptured, asymptomatic saccular aneurysms are incidental findings in 0.4 to 1.5 percent of autopsies. Postmortem examination reveals such aneurysms in about 30 to 40 percent of patients who died of spontaneous subarachnoid hemorrhage. In 10 to 20 percent of these, two or more aneurysms or an aneurysm combined with an arteriovenous malformation will be found.

Saccular aneurysms are very rarely found in infants and children. They usually develop in youth and become symptomatic during the fifth decade, 50 percent of the patients being past the

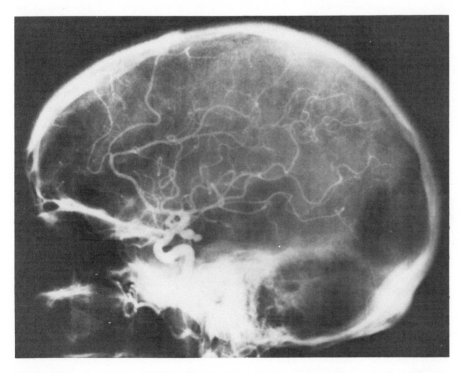

Figure 25-1 Carotid arteriogram showing bilocular aneurysm of the posterior communicating artery.

age of 40 when symptoms appear. Men and women are about equally affected, except that aneurysms in the intracavernous portion of the internal carotid are more common in middle-aged women.

Almost all saccular aneurysms are within or very close to bifurcations in the axil of arteries. About 75 percent of intracranial aneurysms are located in the anterior half of the circle of Willis on the internal carotid or its branches, or on the anterior communicating artery; the remainder are found in the posterior communicating or the vertebral-basilar system (Fig. 25-1). For a further breakdown of the sites of aneurysms see the following table.

Junction of anterior cerebral–anterior communicating arteries	30%
Junction of internal carotid–posterior communicating arteries	25%
Middle cerebral bifurcation	25%
Multiple sites	15%
Vertebral-basilar arteries	5%

Since most aneurysms occur at bifurcations, it is often difficult to decide which of the two arteries is the site of origin. The incidence given for different sites depends to some extent on whether the data were collected by a pathologist, a radiologist, or a surgeon. The important point to remember is that only 80 percent of the aneurysms causing subarachnoid hemorrhages are found in the carotid system. Therefore, bilateral carotid arteriography as well as vertebral-basilar angiography must be performed if all possible sources of bleeding are to be identified.

Pathologic Anatomy

Gross Appearance   Aneurysmal sacs are attached to the parent vessel by a stalk or neck, which may be quite narrow or even wider than the fundus (dome) of the aneurysm (Fig. 25-2A and B). Most ruptures occur in the fundus of the sac.

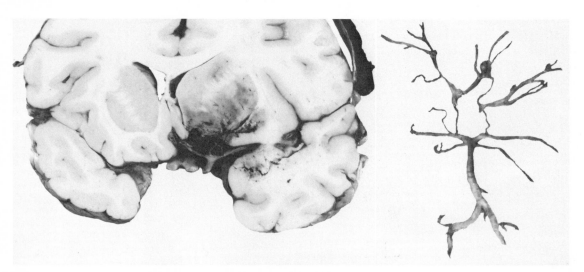

(A)   **(B)**

Figure 25-2 Morphological aspects of an aneurysm and its complications. (A) Coronal section of the brain showing a ruptured aneurysmal sac located at the bifurcation of the internal carotid artery. Note the subarachnoid hemorrhage and destruction of tissue at the base of the brain. (B) Arteries at the circle of Willis dissected to show an aneurysmal sac located at the junction of the anterior communicating artery and the left anterior cerebral artery. There are also outpouchings on the middle cerebral arteries at both sides.

Although most aneurysms are the size of a pea, they may be as small as a pinhead or as large as a walnut. Rarely, one reaches gigantic proportions, almost filling the entire middle or posterior cranial fossa. At autopsy or operation, large aneurysms are sometimes seen to be compressing the neighboring structures (the cranial nerves and the brain substance). At times, a tiny aneurysm appears to have healed.

Some sacs lying in the subarachnoid space enlarge with the passage of time; others, once developed, seem to remain static. The sac of a large aneurysm is often partially filled with laminated, organized, or organizing blood clot—a factor which may hinder progressive enlargement and subsequent rupture of the aneurysm. Calcification of the clot and of the wall is not uncommon. We find no reports of distal embolism from aneurysmal clots. Enlarging aneurysms may become bilocular or multilocular, the surface of the wall being studded with fragile blebs, caruncles, or "bubbles." Occasional aneurysms lie in the subdural space or are buried in the substance of the brain. These structures may provide some support and impede further enlargement. If rupture occurs, however, the symptoms and signs produced will differ from those associated with the rupture of an aneurysm in the subarachnoid space.

Atherosclerosis has a predilection for bifurcations, where it may weaken the wall and lead to further enlargement of a preexisting aneurysm. In such cases the wall of the sac is often translucent, consisting of thin fibrous tissue.

When autopsy or intracranial surgery is performed on a patient who has had an aneurysm rupture in the past, brownish pigmentation, fibrous thickening, and adhesions of surrounding tissues are found.

Microscopic Appearance   The muscular coat of the artery is seen to stop at the neck of the aneurysm, but the degenerated internal elastic membrane, similar to that seen in arteriosclerotic arteries, continues for at least a short distance into the sac. The wall of the sac is formed of fibrous tissue continuous with the intima and adventitia of the parent artery. In cases where bleeding has occurred previously, the sac is surrounded by phagocytes containing hemosiderin, some lymphocytic infiltration, and fibrous thickening.

Associated Congenital Anomalies

The incidence of congenital anomalies in the circle of Willis is about twice as great in patients with saccular aneurysms as in the rest of the population. This association lends support to the hypothesis that saccular aneurysms are congenital anomalies related to the incomplete disappearance of normal embryonic arteries.

Only in rare cases are extracranial aneurysms found in patients with aneurysms in the head. Coarctation of the aorta and polycystic kidneys are said to be found somewhat more commonly in patients with intracranial aneurysms than in the general population.

Natural History

The changes that may occur in a congenital (saccular) aneurysm once it has developed are:

1 Degeneration and disappearance—extremely rare
2 Thrombosis, partial or complete, with or without calcification—occasional
3 Progressive enlargement—common
4 Rupture—common

The course of any aneurysm is unpredictable, and the factors affecting it are largely unknown, although hypertension is thought to contribute to progressive enlargement. Whether aneurysms develop and subsequently disappear spontaneously is unknown.

Irrespective of size, saccular aneurysms may rupture and spill blood into the following:

1 Subarachnoid space
2 Surrounding brain
3 Ventricles
4 Subdural space
5 Two or more of the above areas

The clinical syndrome that results will depend on the location of the aneurysm and the amount of bleeding.

Clinical Features

Most intracranial aneurysms are asymptomatic until they rupture. Because of their size and strategic location, however, some of them do produce symptoms and signs prior to rupture. Most common are palsy of the oculomotor nerve and various defects in the visual fields. Aneurysms in the posterior fossa may be associated with brainstem signs and lower cranial nerve palsies. The only intracranial aneurysms likely to produce headaches prior to rupture are certain aneurysms of the posterior fossa which produce internal hydrocephalus, and aneurysms of the infraclinoid portions of the internal carotid artery, which may simulate tic douloureux along the ophthalmic or maxillary divisions of the trigeminal nerve. Contrary to commonly held opinion, headache is quite unusual as a symptom of aneurysm. When it does occur, it is usually unilateral and is located above or behind the orbit. At times focal transient episodes of neurologic deficit occur in the distribution of the aneurysmal artery and suggest transient cerebral ischemia. These may be a prelude to rupture of the aneurysm. Bruits are rarely heard in patients with aneurysm unless the lesion is in the cavernous sinus.

ANEURYSMAL SYNDROMES

The salient diagnostic features of intracranial aneurysms are described briefly in the following pages. It should be emphasized, however, that these descriptions are intended to serve only as guides to the anatomic location of intracranial aneurysms, since the clinical features of these lesions show a great deal of variation, depending on their size, shape, and type and the direction in which they enlarge.

Internal Carotid Artery

Aneurysms arising from the internal carotid are classified as infraclinoid or supraclinoid, depending on whether they arise inferior or superior to the anterior clinoid processes. Infraclinoid aneurysms are frequently located inside the cavernous sinus.

Infraclinoid   Intracavernous   Aneurysms

These aneurysms occur most frequently in middle-aged women, and it has been said that the wall of the carotid artery at this level affords the only anatomic evidence for the belief that the female is the weaker sex. The presenting symptom is pain over the eye and forehead, diplopia from partial or complete paralysis of the oculomotor nerve, and paralysis of the trochlear and abducens nerves. Since the abducens is closest to the internal carotid artery in the cavernous sinus, abducens palsy is an early sign. The pupil varies in size, being dilated and fixed if the pupilloconstrictor fibers in the oculomotor nerve are involved, and constricted if the pericarotid sympathetic plexus is compressed (Fig. 3-6).

The extent of the trigeminal nerve involvement depends on the exact location of the aneurysm in the sinus. Anterior lesions cause pain and hypalgesia restricted to the ophthalmic division; those located in the midportion of the sinus involve both the ophthalmic and the maxillary division; posteriorly placed or very large aneurysms may involve all three divisions of the trigeminal nerve. The patient sometimes hears a sound in his head, and the examiner may hear a soft systolic bruit over the ipsilateral eye, although this sign is present less frequently than in patients with caroticocavernous fistula. Very extensive aneurysms may simulate a pituitary neoplasm and produce signs of hypopituitarism. At times a curvilinear calcification is visible in the aneurysmal wall on plain x-ray films.

Because of their location in the dura, infraclinoid aneurysms are more likely to rupture into the cavernous sinus than into the subarachnoid space, thus saving the patient's life at the expense of vision. The caroticocavernous fistula so produced is discussed in Chap. 26.

Supraclinoid Aneurysms Aneurysms arising from the internal carotid after it emerges from the cavernous sinus may project in any direction and produce a variety of clinical signs. They rupture often. Since the internal carotid runs between the optic nerve and the optic chiasm medially and the oculomotor nerve laterally, supraclinoid aneurysms often produce a third-nerve palsy or variable defects in the visual fields. Pressure on the optic nerve produces a scotoma and, later, unilateral optic atrophy; pressure on the optic chiasm leads to visual field defects which may mimic pituitary adenoma. Binasal hemianopia may result from bilateral internal carotid aneurysms, although these are rare, or from sclerosis, dilatation, and tortuosity of both internal carotid arteries. Very large sacs occasionally produce unilateral anosmia.

Aneurysms of the terminal portion of the carotid are rare in adults (3 to 5 percent of the total incidence), but in those under 20 years of age the incidence is 35 percent.

Ophthalmic Artery

Aneurysms on this vessel are extremely unusual. They cause optic atrophy, progressive blindness, and enlargement, as well as erosion, of the optic foramen.

Middle Cerebral Artery

The first or second division of the middle cerebral artery within the depth of the Sylvian fissure is a very common site for intracranial aneurysm. Aneurysms in this location do not produce extraocular palsies. Their cardinal features are hemiplegia, dysphasia, visual field defects, and focal seizures. One or more of these signs may develop suddenly as a result of hemorrhage

or vasospasm of the arterial tree, or insidiously because of pressures on the adjacent cortex produced by slow expansion of the sac.

Anterior Cerebral Artery

Large aneurysms from the proximal portion of this artery produce unilateral amaurosis and anosmia, but most aneurysms of this artery are asymptomatic until they rupture. Suprachiasmatic pressure may rarely lead to altitudinal hemianopia affecting the lower half of both visual fields. Rupture into the frontal lobe can cause personality change and paralysis of the contralateral lower limb.

Anterior Communicating Artery

Aneurysms in this location are often silent until rupture occurs. Large lesions may simulate a basal meningioma by causing suprachiasmatic pressure, thus producing defects in the lower halves of both visual fields. Rupture produces immediate coma or profound mental symptoms with severe frontal headache and confusion. Akinetic mutism, which may be permanent, is a sequel of rupture and can also produce a Korsakoff's psychosis, either transient or permanent, following intracranial surgery. This complication is presumably due to infarction of the region of the septum, medial forebrain bundle, or fornix.

Posterior Communicating Artery

Aneurysms of this artery are most commonly found where this vessel joins the internal carotid and, very rarely, where it joins the posterior cerebral artery. An aneurysm in either location may result in palsy of the oculomotor and abducens nerves, and the location can be determined definitely only by arteriography.

Posterior Cerebral Artery

These very rare lesions may produce quadrantanopia. Large aneurysms may compress the brainstem, producing signs of bulbar involvement.

Basilar Artery

Aneurysms in this location may be fusiform or saccular. The former rarely rupture and are commonly atherosclerotic. They are tortuous, so that bilateral palsies of many cranial nerves and signs indicating involvement of the ascending or descending tracts or internal hydrocephalus may develop. Tic douloureux and hemifacial spasm may be the initial manifestations. Blockage of the cerebral aqueduct may cause internal hydrocephalus and progressive dementia. Since these aneurysms tend to calcify, they can sometimes be recognized on x-ray films of the skull. In their differential diagnosis one must consider tumor of the posterior fossa, demyelinating lesions, and brainstem encephalitis.

The rare saccular aneurysms of the basilar artery may rupture, causing severe suboccipital pain, decerebrate rigidity, and bulbar paralysis, which is often fatal.

Vertebral Artery

Aneurysms on this artery are unusual, and the symptoms they produce resemble those caused by aneurysms of the basilar artery. In addition they may lead to attacks of Ménière-like syndrome, ataxia, or signs of bulbar involvement. Some aneurysms of the vertebral artery protrude into the cervical canal, producing bulbar and spinal cord involvement (foramen magnum syndrome).

Cerebellar Arteries

Aneurysms of these vessels are rare. Palsy of the oculomotor and, at times, abducens nerve may be caused by aneurysms of the proximal portion of the superior cerebellar artery. Aneurysms of the anterior inferior cerebellar artery may explain a few cases of tic douloureux and Mé-

nière-like syndrome. Aneurysms of the posterior inferior cerebellar artery may simulate tumor of the foramen magnum. Some aneurysms of the cerebellar arteries produce no localizing signs other than those of an expanding, bleeding lesion in the posterior cranial fossa.

COURSE OF THE DISEASE

If an intracranial aneurysm ruptures, the signs, symptoms, and prognosis depend in large part on the following factors:

1 Location of the aneurysm; e.g., aneurysms of the anterior communicating artery are associated with a higher mortality than aneurysms of the posterior communicating artery.
2 Severity of the hemorrhage.
3 The development of arterial vasospasm, hematoma, cerebral edema, or infarction.
4 The presence of associated disease such as hypertension, diabetes, or arteriosclerosis.
5 Age of the patient.

The gloomy prognosis associated with rupture of a saccular aneurysm treated medically contrasts somewhat with the outlook for patients with venous bleeding from arteriovenous malformations who are treated the same way. Surgery, whenever it is feasible, is the preferred method of therapy for aneurysm.

ROENTGENOLOGIC FINDINGS

Skull x-rays rarely identify the lesion, and accurate localization usually depends on arteriography. Signs suggestive of partial or total aneurysmal thrombosis are:

1 Curvilinear calcification or local erosion of bone visible in skull x-rays
2 Displacement of arteries in the vicinity of the sac or prolonged retention of contrast medium inside the cavity of the fundus of the aneurysm

Junctional Dilatation (Infundibular Dilatations or Ectasia)

Approximately 10 percent of all bilateral carotid angiograms reveal a small arterial outpouching at the junction of the internal carotid with the posterior communicating artery. This ectasia is usually less than 2 mm in diameter, is round or conical in shape, and has no neck. There is no evidence of local vasospasm or displacement of neighboring structures. Although it is believed that these ectasias rarely rupture, a few may enlarge progressively and ultimately develop into saccular aneurysms. Most pathologists believe that they are of no clinical significance.

MANAGEMENT

Most saccular aneurysms cause no symptoms and signs until they rupture. Most of those which produce effects like those of a tumor by causing pressure on adjacent structures will eventually rupture. In such cases, if the patient presents a good operative risk, angiography should be undertaken after consultation with a neurosurgeon. If for any reason surgery cannot be carried out, one must make efforts to keep the patient's blood pressure normal. This includes the use of hypotensive medications and alteration of life-style.

Types of Surgical Procedures

Occlusion of the common or internal carotid artery in the neck reduces arterial pressure in the distal branches and may allow a clot to form in the sac. When intracranial collateral circulation is adequate, common carotid ligation is not likely to cause ischemia or infarction, and the external-internal carotid shunt which is formed prevents clot formation. Internal carotid ligation, on the other hand, causes stasis in the internal carotid artery, with clot formation. Rarely, these clots may embolize or propagate

to obstruct the entire carotid tree on the side of the ligation.

Other forms of intracranial surgery are designed to isolate the aneurysm or reduce arterial pressure within it, to strengthen its walls by spraying or wrapping material around it, or to promote thrombosis in it by injecting an irritant such as a horsehair (pilojection). Intracranial surgery is curative but is a much more delicate procedure than cervical carotid ligation and is attended by a higher mortality. Sometimes both these operations are performed on the same patient, the carotid occlusion being carried out in the acute stage of subarachnoid hemorrhage and the intracranial surgery being postponed until the patient's condition is optimum.

The number and variety of procedures for the surgical correction of aneurysm provide mute testimony that all leave something to be desired. Their relative merits cannot be decided until many more cases have been adequately studied and followed. Because even a tiny aneurysm is a smoldering volcano which may erupt again at any time, postoperative arteriography should probably be done to provide proof of successful surgery.

Timing of Surgery

The timing and mode of surgical approach vary with each school of neurosurgery, since improved or novel techniques are constantly being evolved. However, a few broad principles are generally accepted. Alert patients should be operated on as soon as angiography reveals a treatable lesion, unless it also shows severe diffuse spasm. If spasm is present, operation should be delayed 4 to 7 days, in the hope that it will subside. Since recurrent hemorrhage is most likely to occur 7 to 14 days after the initial rupture, it is advisable to wait no more than 7 days. Although surgical intervention after a delay of 3 to 4 weeks is associated with a much lower surgical mortality, the mortality from a second hemorrhage during the same period is quite high.

Extracranial Approach

Extracranial carotid occlusion is usually employed in patients who have aneurysm of the internal carotid artery situated close to the anterior clinoid process or at the origin of the anterior cerebral, middle cerebral, or posterior communicating artery. The operation may be done to occlude the common carotid alone, the common and external carotids, or the internal carotid alone; each of these procedures has its proponents. Occlusion may be sudden and complete, as by ligation of the artery, or it may be done gradually by means of a clamp which is tightened slowly over a period of hours or days. Ligation of the external carotid is then carried out later. Gradual occlusion is usually preferred, since the clamp can be released if complications develop. Some of the possible complications are:

1 Hemispheric ischemia or infarction due to inadequate collateral circulation. Some neurologists believe that repeated measurements of pressure in the ophthalmic artery by ophthalmodynamometry should be performed before and after occlusion for the dual purpose of determining the effectiveness of the procedure and possibly forestalling the development of ischemic infarction if pressure is reduced too much.

2 Cerebral vasospasm with cerebral ischemia or infarction.

3 Embolism from the site of cervical ligation to intracranial arteries, or the propagation of a thrombus into the intracranial arteries.

4 Hemispheric ischemia caused by the reversal of blood flow from the internal to the external carotid artery after occlusion of the common carotid. Because of this possibility, some surgeons occlude the external carotid artery along with the common carotid.

5 Aneurysm or rupture of the artery in the neck.

6 Hypotension or bradycardia due to a hyperreactive carotid sinus reflex. Carotid sinus massage and compression for about 10 min *must* be done before arteriography to give warning of the possibility of this complication and of cerebral vascular insufficiency.

The first two of the above-listed complications often can be prevented by appropriate preoperative tests, by choosing the common carotid artery for the initial occlusion, and by using a clamp for gradual occlusion. The third complication cannot be forestalled and is likely to have permanent effects.

Intracranial Approach

When a patient with an accessible lesion represents a good surgical risk, intracranial repair is the treatment of choice. It is the only satisfactory method for dealing with aneurysms situated distally on the anterior, middle, or posterior cerebral artery, and for certain aneurysms arising from the vertebral-basilar system. After the aneurysm is exposed, it may be (1) clipped at its neck; (2) isolated between two clips placed on the parent vessel; (3) wrapped carefully with muscle, fascia, or Gelfoam, or sprayed with plastic; (4) injected with a foreign body which acts as a nidus for clot formation.

The intracranial approach to aneurysms has been greatly simplified by the advent of anesthetic techniques for controlling respiration and inducing hypotension and hypothermia. The use of intravenous urea or mannitol to reduce intracranial pressure has made surgical approach easier. Yet the mortality remains high (about 20 percent), and precipitation of bleeding by manipulation of the aneurysm is a real danger. A few neurosurgeons have utilized deep hypothermia in an attempt to circumvent infarction by decreasing cerebral metabolic rate and spasm. To make the patient safe for delayed surgery, or early surgery safe for the acutely ill patient, some surgeons utilize microsurgery or stereotactic electrolysis through a bur hole.

MULTIPLE INTRACRANIAL ANEURYSMS

In instances of subarachnoid hemorrhage resulting from rupture of congenital aneurysms, about 15 percent of patients have multiple intracranial aneurysms (Fig. 25-3). Clinical, electroencephalographic, and angiographic findings are used to determine which aneurysm has ruptured. Of these the angiographic criteria are the most reliable and are described in Chap. 24. As a general rule, the largest of the multiple aneurysms is responsible for the initial bleeding as well as subsequent bleeding.

If the site of the bleeding can be identified definitely and is surgically accessible, then operation is advised. If only two aneurysms are

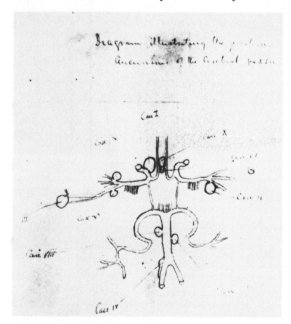

Figure 25-3 Sketch by William Osler showing sites of aneurysms on cerebral arteries in ten cases examined at Montreal General Hospital. *(Reproduced with permission from Feindel, W., Highlights of Neurosurgery in Canada, J.A.M.A. **200**:853–859, 1967; copyright 1967 by the American Medical Association.)*

present on the same side of the circle of Willis, then both lesions can be operated upon either by ipsilateral common carotid artery ligation or through a direct intracranial approach. If the offending aneurysm cannot be determined or more than two are found in different locations, the patient should be managed conservatively.

It is worth remembering that subarachnoid hemorrhage with multiple intracranial aneurysms has a mortality of 60 percent in the first 6 months, as compared to 40 percent over the same period in instances of single aneurysms.

OTHER FORMS OF ANEURYSM

Arteriosclerotic (Fusiform) Aneurysms

Whereas almost all saccular aneurysms are developmental in origin, most fusiform aneurysms are due to arteriosclerosis. Arteriosclerosis destroys the media and the internal elastic membrane, resulting in a spindle-shaped dilatation of the artery. The basilar artery, the internal carotids on both sides, and the vertebral arteries—the largest intracranial arteries—are the only vessels involved by arteriosclerotic aneurysms. In contrast to saccular aneurysms, which have a strong predilection for the carotid circulation, arteriosclerotic aneurysms are about equally distributed between the anterior and posterior circulations. Such aneurysms are usually asymptomatic and almost never rupture, but they sometimes compress, distort, or destroy neighboring structures such as cranial nerves, the brain parenchyma, or the bony skull. Since they are long and have no neck, they are inaccessible to a direct surgical approach.

Septic (Mycotic) Aneurysms

The term *mycotic* is a misnomer, since these aneurysms are not due to fungi but arise from infected emboli that lodge in the artery, causing arteritis and consequent dilatations of the vessel. Microscopic examination reveals an in-

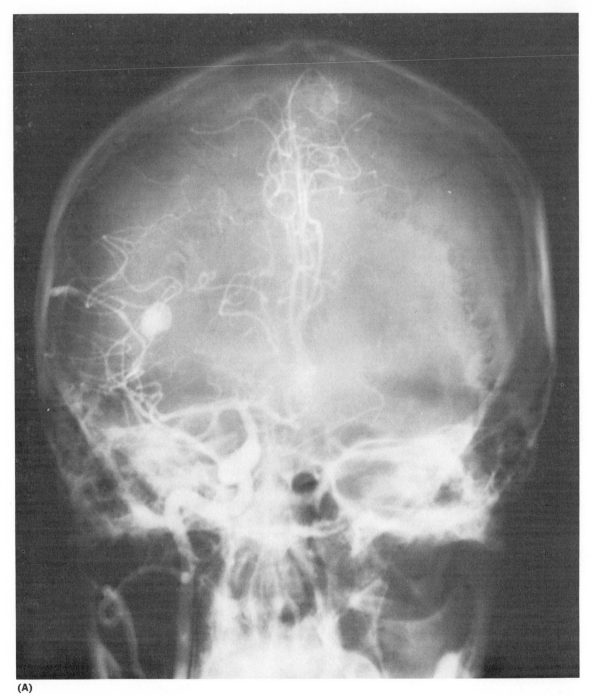

(A)

Figure 25-4 Carotid arteriograms showing a large mycotic aneurysm on the middle cerebral artery.

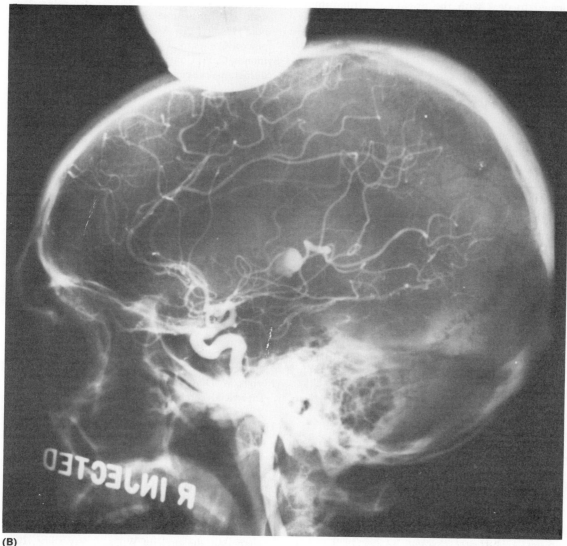

(B)

fected embolus adherent to the acutely inflamed and necrotic arterial wall. The organisms responsible for septic aneurysms are usually of low virulence, whereas those of high virulence tend to produce meningitis or brain abscess. Subacute bacterial endocarditis or suppurative disease of the bronchopulmonary tree is the common source of an embolus (Fig. 25-4A and B).

Septic aneurysms are found most often on the branches of the middle cerebral artery, either in the Sylvian fissure or distal to it; and they tend to be multiple. The embolus may cause ischemic necrosis in the area of the brain supplied by the artery. If the weakened arterial wall ruptures, hemorrhagic bacterial meningitis may result. The acute infection must be controlled by antibiotic therapy before intracranial surgery is performed to deal with the aneurysm. Inflammation of the artery without infection, as in polyarteritis nodosa, rarely results in aneurysm.

Dissecting Aneurysms

Dissection of the aortic arch and its consequences are discussed in Chap. 29 in the section on dissecting hematomas. Dissection initiating spontaneously in the cervical and cerebral arteries is rare, but trauma to the carotid artery in the neck from a blow or injection of material beneath the intima during arteriography is more common. Syphilis or a congenital defect of the media may initiate subintimal dissection, causing the internal elastic membrane to split and separate from the media, either spontaneously or following cranial trauma. Intracranial arteries, particularly the middle cerebral and the basilar arteries, may dissect spontaneously or after trauma. If dissections occur on the carotid artery in the neck, the intima can be sutured to the media to destroy the false channel. Rarely, intracranial dissecting aneurysms may also be amenable to surgical measures.

SUGGESTED READING

General

Fields, W. S., and Sahs, A. L. (eds.): Intracranial Aneurysms and Subarachnoid Hemorrhage, Charles C Thomas, Publisher, Springfield, Ill., 1965.

McDonald, C. A., and Korb, M.: Intracranial aneurysms, *Arch. Neurol. Psychiat.,* **42**:298, 1939.

Patel, A. N., and Richardson, A. E.: Ruptured intracranial aneurysms in the first two decades of life. A study of 58 patients, *J. Neurosurg.,* **35**:571, 1971.

Pool, J. L., and Potts, D. G.: Aneurysms and Arteriovenous Anomalies of the Brain: Diagnosis and Treatment, Harper & Row, Publishers, Incorporated, New York, 1965.

Richardson, J. C., and Hyland, H. H.: Intracranial aneurysms; clinical and pathological study of subarachnoid and intracerebral haemorrhage caused by berry aneurysms, *Medicine,* **20**:1, 1941.

Sahs, A. L., Perret, G. E., Locksley, H. B., and Nishioka, H.: Intracranial Aneurysms and Subarachnoid Hemorrhage. A Cooperative Study, J. B. Lippincott Company, Philadelphia, 1969.

Symonds, C. P.: Contributions to the clinical study of intracranial aneurysms, *Guy's Hosp. Rept.,* **73**:139, 1923.

"Congenital," Berry, or Saccular Aneurysms

Etiology and Pathogenesis

Bannerman, R. M., and Ingall, G. B.: The familial occurrence of intracranial aneurysms, *Neurology,* **20**:283, 1970.

Black, S. P., and German, W. J.: Observations on the relationship between the volume and the size of the orifice of experimental aneurysms, *J. Neurosurg.,* **17**:984, 1960.

Crawford, T.: Some observations on the pathogenesis and natural history of intracranial aneurysms, *J. Neurol. Neurosurg. Psychiat.,* **22**:259, 1959.

Crompton, M. R.: Mechanism of growth and rupture in cerebral berry aneurysms, *Brit. Med. J.,* **1**:1138, 1966.

————: The pathogenesis of cerebral aneurysms, *Brain,* **89**:797, 1966.

Forbus, W. D.: On the origin of miliary aneurysms of superficial cerebral arteries, *Bull. Johns Hopkins Hosp.,* **47**:239, 1930.

Hassler, O.: Morphological studies on the large cerebral arteries with reference to the aetiology of subarachnoid haemorrhage, *Acta psychiat. neurol. scand.,* **36**(suppl. 154):1, 1961.

————: Media defects in intracerebral arteries, *Acta neurol. scand.,* **38**:29, 1962.

————: Experimental carotid ligation followed by aneurysmal formation and other morphological changes in the circle of Willis, *J. Neurosurg.,* **20**:1, 1963.

Kak, V. K., Gleadhill, C. A., and Bailey, I. C.: The familial incidence of intracranial aneurysms, *J. Neurol. Neurosurg. Psychiat.,* **33**:29, 1970.

Leading article: Aetiology of intracranial aneurysms, *Brit. Med. J.,* **1**:60, 1966.

Pathologic Anatomy

Crompton, M. R.: The comparative pathology of cerebral aneurysms, *Brain,* **89**:789, 1966.

————: The pathology of ruptured middle-cerebral aneurysms with special reference to the differences between the sexes, *Lancet*, **2**:421, 1962.

Freytag, E.: Fatal rupture of intracranial aneurysms: Survey of 250 medicolegal cases, *Arch. Pathol.*, **81**:418, 1966.

Sharati, S.: An analysis of 213 intracranial aneurysms verified by autopsy, *Am. J. Pathol.*, **59**:15a, 1970.

Stehbens, W. E.: Histopathology of cerebral aneurysms, *Arch. Neurol.*, **8**:272, 1963.

Associated Congenital Anomalies

Riggs, H. E., and Rupp, C.: Miliary aneurysms: Relation of anomalies of the circle of Willis to formation of aneurysms, *Arch. Neurol. Psychiat.*, **49**:615, 1943.

Stehbens, W. E.: Cerebral aneurysms and congenital abnormalities, *Australas. Ann. Med.*, **11**:102, 1962.

Clinical Features

Arseni, C., Ghitescu, M., Cristescu, A., and Mihăilă, G.: Intrasellar aneurysms simulating hypophyseal tumors, *Europ. Neurol.*, **3**:321, 1970.

Bull, J.: Massive aneurysms at the base of the brain, *Brain*, **92**:535, 1969.

Frankel, K.: Relation of migraine to cerebral aneurysm, *Arch. Neurol. Psychiat.*, **63**:195, 1950.

Hyland, H. H., and Barnett, H. J. M.: The pathogenesis of cranial nerve palsies associated with intracranial aneurysms, *Proc. Roy. Soc. Med.*, **47**:141, 1954.

Miller, H. J., and Hinkley, C. M.: Berry aneurysms in pregnancy: A 10 year report, *South. Med. J.*, **63**:279, 1970.

Sarner, M., and Rose, F. C.: Clinical presentation of ruptured intracranial aneurysm, *J. Neurol. Neurosurg. Psychiat.*, **30**:67, 1967.

White, J. C., and Ballantine, H. T.: Intrasellar aneurysms simulating hypophyseal tumours, *J. Neurosurg.*, **18**:34, 1961.

Wilkins, R. H., Alexander, J. A., and Odom, G. L.: Intracranial arterial spasm: A clinical analysis, *J. Neurosurg.*, **29**:121, 1968.

Neuroophthalmic Features

Bird, A. C., Nolan, B., Gargano, F. P., and David, N. J.: Unruptured aneurysm of the supraclinoid carotid artery. A treatable cause of blindness, *Neurology*, **20**:445, 1970.

Cogan, D. G., and Mount, H. T.: Intracranial aneurysms causing ophthalmoplegia, *Arch. Ophthalmol.*, **70**:757, 1963.

Hepler, R. S., and Cantu, R. C.: Aneurysms and third nerve palsies. Ocular status of survivors, *Arch. Ophthalmol.*, **77**:604, 1967.

Odom, G. L.: "Ophthalmic involvement in neurological vascular lesions," in Neuro-ophthalmology Symposium, vol. 1, compiled and edited by J. L. Smith, Charles C Thomas, Publisher, Springfield, Ill., 1964, pp. 181–276.

Riise, R.: Ocular symptoms in saccular aneurysms of the internal carotid artery (a survey of 100 cases), *Acta ophthalmol.*, **47**:1012, 1969.

Walsh, F. B.: Visual field defects due to aneurysms at the circle of Willis, *Arch. Ophthalmol.*, **71**:15, 1964.

Aneurysmal Syndromes

Internal Carotid Artery

Davis, R. H., Daroff, R. B., and Hoyt, W. F.: Hemicrania, oculosympathetic paresis, and subcranial carotid aneurysm: Raeder's paratrigeminal syndrome (group 2), *J. Neurosurg.*, **29**:94, 1968.

Drake, C. G., Vanderlinden, R. G., and Amacher, A. L.: Carotid-choroidal aneurysms, *J. Neurosurg.*, **29**:32, 1968.

Law, W. R., and Nelson, E. R.: Internal carotid aneurysm as a cause of Raeder's paratrigeminal syndrome, *Neurology*, **18**:43, 1968.

Lombardi, G., Passerini, A., and Migliavacca, F.: Intracavernous aneurysms of the internal carotid artery, *Am. J. Roentgenol.*, **89**:361, 1963.

Perria, L., Rivano, C., Rossi, G. F., and Viale, G.: Aneurysms of the bifurcation of the internal carotid artery, *Acta neurochir.*, **19**:51, 1968.

Webb, R. C., Jr., and Barker, W. F.: Aneurysms of the extracranial internal carotid artery, *Arch. Surg.*, **99**:501, 1969.

Ophthalmic Artery

Drake, C. G., Vanderlinden, R. G., and Amacher, A. L.: Carotid-ophthalmic aneurysms, *J. Neurosurg.*, **29**:24, 1968.

Kothandaram, P., Dawson, B. H., and Kruyt, R. C.: Carotid-ophthalmic aneurysms. A study of 19 patients, *J. Neurosurg.*, **34**:544, 1971.

Middle Cerebral Artery

Cantu, R. C., and LeMay, M.: A large middle cerebral aneurysm presenting as a bizarre vascular malformation, *Brit. J. Radiol.,* **39**:317, 1966.

Kamrin, R. P.: Temporal lobe epilepsy caused by unruptured middle cerebral artery aneurysms, *Arch. Neurol.,* **14**:421, 1966.

McKissock, W., Richardson, A., and Walsh, L.: Middle cerebral aneurysms: Further results in the controlled trial of conservative and surgical treatment of ruptured intracranial aneurysms, *Lancet,* **2**:417, 1962.

Anterior Communicating Artery

Durston, J. H. J., and Parsons-Smith, B. G.: Blindness due to aneurysm of anterior communicating artery. With recovery following carotid ligation, *Brit. J. Ophthalmol.,* **54**:170, 1970.

McKissock, W., Richardson, A., and Walsh, L.: Anterior communicating aneurysms: A trial of conservative and surgical treatment, *Lancet,* **1**:873, 1965.

Pool, J. L., and Colton, R. P.: Anterior communicating aneurysms; A rebuttal, *J.A.M.A.,* **195**:115, 1966.

Richardson, A. E., Jane, J. A., and Payne, P. M.: Assessment of the natural history of anterior communicating aneurysms, *J. Neurosurg.,* **21**:266, 1964.

Talland, G. A., Sweet, W. H., and Ballantine, H. T., Jr.: Amnesic syndrome with anterior communicating artery aneurysms, *J. Nervous Mental Disease,* **145**:179, 1967.

Posterior Communicating Artery

McKissock, W., Richardson, A., and Walsh, L.: "Posterior-communicating" aneurysms, *Lancet,* **1**:1203, 1960.

Paterson, A.: Direct surgery in the treatment of posterior communicating artery aneurysms, *Lancet,* **2**:808, 1968.

Payne, J. W., and Adamkiewicz, J., Jr.: Unilateral internal ophthalmoplegia with intracranial aneurysm. Report of a case, *Am. J. Ophthalmol.,* **68**:349, 1969.

Posterior Cerebral Artery

Drake, C. G., and Amacher, A. L.: Aneurysms of the posterior cerebral artery, *J. Neurosurg.,* **30**:468, 1969.

Obrador, S., Dierssen, G., and Herrandez, J. R.: Giant aneurysm of the posterior cerebral artery. Case report, *J. Neurosurg.,* **26**:413, 1967.

Basilar Artery

Harel, D., Lavy, S., and Schwartz, A.: Aneurysm of basilar artery simulating a cerebellopontine angle tumor, *Confinia neurol.,* **29**:360, 1967.

Jamieson, K. G.: Aneurysms of the vertebrobasilar system. Further experience with nine cases, *J. Neurosurg.,* **28**:544, 1968.

Vertebral Artery

Morley, J. B.: Unruptured vertebro-basilar aneurysms, *Med. J. Australia,* **2**:1024, 1967.

Pericallosal Artery

Laitinen, L., and Snellman, A.: Aneurysms of the pericallosal artery: A study of 14 cases verified arteriographically and treated mainly by direct surgical attack, *J. Neurosurg.,* **17**:447, 1960.

Posterior Fossa Aneurysms

Arseni, C., Ghitescu, N., Cristescu, A., and Mihăilă, Gh.: The pseudotumoral form of aneurysms of the posterior cranial fossa, *Neurochirurgia,* **12**:123, 1969.

Pribram, H. F. W., Hudson, J. D., and Joynt, R. J.: Posterior fossa aneurysms presenting as mass lesions, *Am. J. Roentgenol.,* **105**:334, 1969.

Sachs, M., Hirsh, J. F., and David, M.: Anevrismes sacculaires rompus du système vertebro-basalaire. Revue de 19 cas personnels et de 88 cas publiés, *Acta neurochir,* **20**:105, 1969.

Troupp, H.: The natural history of aneurysms of the basilar bifurcation, *Acta neurol. scand.,* **47**:350, 1971.

Course of the Disease

Björkesten, G., and Troupp, H.: Changes in size of intracranial arterial aneurysms, *J. Neurosurg.,* **19**:583, 1962.

Crompton, M. R.: Cerebral infarction following the rupture of cerebral berry aneurysms, *Brain,* **87**:263, 1964.

———: Hypothalamic lesions following the rupture of cerebral berry aneurysms, *Brain,* **86**:301, 1963.

———: Intracerebral haematoma complicating ruptured cerebral berry aneurysm, *J. Neurol. Neurosurg. Psychiat.,* **25**:378, 1962.

————: The natural history of cerebral berry aneurysms, *Am. Heart J.,* **73**:568, 1967.

————: Recurrent haemorrhage from cerebral aneurysms and its prevention by surgery, *J. Neurol. Neurosurg, Psychiat.,* **29**:164, 1966.

du Boulay, G. H.: Some observations on the natural history of intracranial aneurysms, *Brit. J. Radiol.,* **38**:721, 1965.

Ellington, E., and Margolis, G.: Block of arachnoid villus by subarachnoid hemorrhage, *J. Neurosurg.,* **30**:651, 1969.

Galera, R., and Greitz, T.: Hydrocephalus in the adult secondary to rupture of intracranial arterial aneurysms, *J. Neurosurg.,* **32**:634, 1970.

Goldstein, S. L.: Ventricular opacification secondary to rupture of intracranial aneurysm during angiography. Case report, *J. Neurosurg.,* **27**:265, 1967.

Graf, C. J., and Hamby, W. B.: Report of a case of cerebral aneurysm in an adult developing apparently *de novo, J. Neurol. Neurosurg. Psychiat.,* **27**:153, 1964.

Jain, K. K.: Mechanism of rupture of intracranial saccular aneurysms, *Surgery,* **54**:347, 1963.

Lin, J. P.: Thrombosis of aneurysm of anterior communicating artery. Case report, *Acta radiol. diagn.,* **8**:74, 1969.

Logue, V., Durward, M., Pratt, R. T. C., Piercy, M., and Nixon, W. L. B.: The quality of survival after rupture of an anterior cerebral aneurysm, *Brit. J. Psychiat.,* **114**:137, 1968.

Schunk, H.: Spontaneous thrombosis of intracranial aneurysms, *Am. J. Roentgenol.,* **91**:1327, 1964.

Strang, R. R., Tovi, D., and Hugosson, R.: Subdural hematomas resulting from the rupture of intracranial arterial aneurysms, *Acta chir. scand.,* **121**:345, 1961.

Roentgenologic Findings

Allcock, J. M., and Drake, C. G.: Postoperative angiography in cases of ruptured intracranial aneurysm, *J. Neurosurg.,* **20**:752, 1963.

Bull, J. W.: Contribution of radiology to the study of intracranial aneurysms, *Brit. Med. J.,* **2**:1701, 1962.

Ekbom, K., and Greitz, T.: Carotid angiography in cluster headache, *Acta radiol. diagn.,* **10**:177, 1970.

Epstein, F., Ransohoff, J., and Budzilovich, G. N.:

The clinical significance of junctional dilatation of the posterior communicating artery, *J. Neurosurg.,* **33**:529, 1970.

Fox, J. L., Baiz, T. C., and Jakoby, R. K.: Differentiation of aneurysm from infundibulum of the posterior communicating artery, *J. Neurosurg.,* **21**:135, 1964.

Hassler, O., and Saltzman, G. F.: Angiographic and histologic changes in infundibular widening of the posterior communicating artery, *Acta radiol. diagn.,* **1**:321, 1963.

Wilkins, R. H., Wilkinson, R. H., and Odom, G. L.: Abnormal brain scans in patients with cerebral arterial spasm, *J. Neurosurg.,* **36**:133, 1972.

Wood, E. H.: Angiographic identification of the ruptured lesion in patients with multiple cerebral aneurysm, *J. Neurosurg.,* **21**:182, 1964.

Electroencephalography

Beatty, R. A., and Richardson, A. E.: The value of electroencephalography in the management of multiple intracranial aneurysms, *J. Neurosurg.,* **30**:150, 1969.

Binnie, C. D., Margerison, J. H., and McCaul, I. R.: Electroencephalogic localization of ruptured intracranial aneurysms, *Brain,* **92**:679, 1969.

De Vlieger, M., and Depre, J. O.: Echo- and electroencephalography in ruptured cerebral arterial aneurysms, *Acta neurol. psychiat. belg.,* **71**:154, 1971.

Medical Management

Boba, A.: Hypothermia: Appraisal of risk in 110 consecutive patients, *J. Neurosurg.,* **19**:924, 1962.

Gibbs, J. R., and Corkill, A. G. L.: Use of an antifibrinolytic agent (tranexamic acid) in the management of ruptured intracranial aneurysms, *Postgrad. Med. J.,* **47**:199, 1971.

Graf, C. J.: Prognosis for patients with non-surgically treated aneurysms. Analysis of the cooperative study of intracranial aneurysms and subarachnoid hemorrhage, *J. Neurosurg.,* **35**:438, 1971.

Slosberg, P. S.: The current status of medical treatment of intracranial aneurysms, *Prog. Neurol. Surg.,* **3**:230, 1969.

Walsh, L.: Experience in the conservative and surgical treatment of ruptured intracranial aneurysm, *Res. Pub. Assoc. Nerv. Ment. Dis.,* **41**:169, 1966.

Surgical Therapy

Alksne, J. F.: Stereotactic thrombosis of intracranial aneurysms, *New Engl. J. Med.,* **284**:171, 1971.

Beatty, R. A., and Richardson, A. E.: Predicting intolerance to common carotid artery ligation by carotid angiography, *J. Neurosurg.,* **28**:9, 1968.

Cuatico, W., Cook, A. W., Tyshchenko, V., and Khatib, R.: Massive enlargement of intracranial aneurysms following carotid ligation, *Acta. Neurol.,* **17**:609, 1967.

Drake, C. G.: Further experience with surgical treatment of aneurysms of the basilar artery, *J. Neurosurg.,* **29**:372, 1968.

Dutton, J.: Acrylic investment of intracranial aneurysms. A report of 12 years' experience, *J. Neurosurg.,* **31**:652, 1969.

Gallagher, J. P.: Pilojection for intracranial aneurysms; report of progress, *J. Neurosurg.,* **21**:129, 1964.

Gibbs, J. R.: Effects of carotid ligation on the size of internal carotid aneurysms, *J. Neurol. Neurosurg. Psychiat.,* **28**:383, 1965.

Gross, S. W., and Holzman, A.: Aneurysm of common carotid artery in the neck following partial ligation for an intracranial aneurysm, *J. Neurosurg.,* **11**:209, 1954.

Holmes, A. E., James, I. M., and Wise, C. C.: Observations on distal intravascular pressure changes and cerebral blood flow after common carotid ligation in man, *J. Neurol. Neurosurg. Psychiat.,* **34**:78, 1971.

Hudson, C. H., and Raaf, J.: Timing of angiography and operation in patients with ruptured intracranial aneurysms, *J. Neurosurg.,* **29**:37, 1968.

Hunt, W. E., and Hess, R. M.: Surgical risk as related to time of intervention in the repair of intracranial aneurysms, *J. Neurosurg.,* **28**:14, 1968.

Jain, K. K.: Surgery of intracranial berry aneurysms: A review, *Can. J. Surg.,* **8**:172, 1965.

Klafta, L. A., Jr., and Hamby, W. B.: Significance of cerebrospinal fluid pressure in determining time for repair of intracranial aneurysms, *J. Neurosurg.,* **31**:217, 1969.

Landolt, A. M., and Millikan, C. H.: Pathogenesis of cerebral infarction secondary to mechanical carotid artery occlusion, *Stroke,* **1**:52, 1970.

Lindqvist, G., and Norlén, G.: Korsakoff's syndrome after operation on ruptured aneurysm of the anterior communicating artery, *Acta psychiat. scand.,* **42**:24, 1966.

MacCarty, C. S., Michenfelder, J. D., and Uihlein, A.: Treatment of intracranial vascular disorders with the aid of profound hypothermia and total circulatory arrest: Three years' experience, *J. Neurosurg.,* **21**:372, 1964.

McKissock, W.: Recurrence of an intracranial aneurysm after excision: Report of a case, *J. Neurosurg.,* **23**:547, 1965.

Moore, W. S., and Hall, A. D.: Carotid artery back pressure. A test of cerebral tolerance to temporary carotid occlusion, *J. Cardiovascular Surg.,* **11**:72, 1970.

Ransohoff, J., Guy, H. H., Mazzia, V. D. B., and Battista, A.: Deliberate hypotension in surgery of cerebral aneurysm and correlative animal studies, *New York State J. Med.,* **69**(part 1):913, 1969.

Raskind, R., and Doria, A.: Long term follow-up of intracranial aneurysms treated by cervical carotid artery ligation, *Angiology,* **19**:326, 1968.

Rossi, P., Rosenbaum, A. E., and Zingesser, L. H.: The fate of the carotid artery after occlusion for treatment of aneurysm, *Radiology,* **95**:567, 1970.

Somach, F. M., and Shenkin, H. A.: Angiographic end-results of carotid ligation in the treatment of carotid aneurysm, *J. Neurosurg.,* **24**:966, 1966.

Strenger, L.: Neurological deficits following therapeutic collapse of intracavernous carotid aneurysms. Report of two cases, *J. Neurosurg.,* **25**:215, 1966.

Tindall, G. T., Goree, J. A., Lee, J. F., and Odom, G. L.: Effect of common carotid ligation on size of internal carotid aneurysms and distal intracarotid and retinal artery pressures, *J. Neurosurg.,* **25**:503, 1966.

VanderArk, G. D., and Kempe, L. C.: Classification of anterior communicating aneurysms as a basis for surgical approach, *J. Neurosurg.,* **32**:300, 1970.

Wright, R. L.: Intraaneurysmal pressure reduction with carotid occlusion. Observations in three cases of middle cerebral aneurysms, *J. Neurosurg.,* **29**:139, 1968.

———, and Sweet, W. H.: Carotid or vertebral occlusion in the treatment of intracranial aneurysms; value of early and late readings of carotid and retinal artery pressures, *Clin. Neurosurg.,* **9**:163, 1963.

Multiple Intracranial Aneurysms

Heiskanen, O.: Multiple intracranial arterial aneurysms, *Acta neurol. scand.*, **41**:356, 1965.

———, and Marttila, I.: Risk of rupture of a second aneurysm in patients with multiple aneurysms, *J. Neurosurg.*, **32**:295, 1970.

McKissock, W., Richardson, A., Walsh, L., and Owen, E.: Multiple intracranial aneurysms, *Lancet*, **1**:623, 1964.

Overgaard, J., and Riishede, J.: Multiple cerebral saccular aneurysms, *Acta neurol. scand.*, **41**:363, 1965.

Other Forms of Aneurysm

Burton, C., and Johnston, J.: Multiple cerebral aneurysms and cardiac myxoma, *New Engl. J. Med.*, **282**:35, 1970.

Handa, J., Shimizu, Y., Matsuda, M., and Handa, H.: Traumatic aneurysm of the middle cerebral artery, *Am. J. Roentgenol.*, **109**:127, 1970.

Raimondi, A. J., Yashon, D., Reyes, C., and Yarzagaray, L.: Intracranial false aneurysms, *Neurochirurgica*, **11**:219, 1968.

Smith, K. R., Jr., and Bardenheier, J. A., III: Aneurysm of the pericallosal artery caused by closed cranial trauma, *J. Neurosurg.*, **29**:551, 1968.

Stehbens, W. E.: Atypical cerebral aneurysms, *Med. J. Australia,* **1**:765, 1965.

Wolman, L.: Cerebral dissecting aneurysms, *Brain,* **82**:276, 1959.

Arteriosclerotic (Fusiform) Aneurysms

Bull, J.: Massive aneurysms at the base of the brain, *Brain,* **92**:535, 1969.

Courville, C. B.: Arteriosclerotic aneurysms of the circle of Willis: Some notes on their morphology and pathogenesis, *Bull. Los Angeles Neurol. Soc.,* **27**:1, 1962.

Denny-Brown, D., and Foley, J. M.: The syndrome of basilar aneurysm, *Trans. Am. Neurol. Assoc.,* **77**:30, 1952.

Ekbom, K., Greitz, T., Kalmer, M., Lopez, J., and Ottosson, S.: Cerebrospinal fluid pulsations in occult hydrocephalus due to ectasia of basilar artery, *Acta neurochir.,* **20**:1, 1969.

Septic (Mycotic) Aneurysms

Bell, W. E., and Butler, C., II: Cerebral mycotic aneurysms in children. Two case reports, *Neurology,* **18**:81, 1968.

Cantu, R. C., LeMay, M., and Wilkinson, H. A.: The importance of repeated angiography in the treatment of mycotic-embolic intracranial aneurysm, *J. Neurosurg.,* **25**:189, 1966.

Hourihane, J. B.: Ruptured mycotic intracranial aneurysm. A report of three cases, *Vascular Surg.,* **4**:21, 1970.

Ojemann, R. G., New, P. F. J., and Fleming, T. C.: Intracranial aneurysms associated with bacterial meningitis, *Neurology,* **16**:1222, 1966.

Roach, M. R., and Drake, C. G.: Ruptured cerebral aneurysms caused by micro-organisms, *New Engl. J. Med.,* **273**:240, 1965.

Additional References

Alvord, E. C., Loeser, J. D., Bailey, W. L., and Copacs, M. K.: Subarachnoid hemorrhage due to ruptured aneurysm, *Arch. Neurol.,* **27**:273, 1972.

Nibbelink, D. W., and Sahs, A. L.: "Cooperative study of intracranial aneurysms and subarachnoid hemorrhage," in Cerebrovascular Disease, National Institute of Neurological Diseases and Stroke, and National Heart and Lung Institute, edited by R. G. Siekert, National Institutes of Health, Bethesda, Md., 1970, pp. 176-193.

Nystrom, S. H.: On factors related to spontaneous healing of ruptured intracranial aneurysms, *Acta Pathol. Microbiol. Scand.,* **80**:566, 1972.

Okawara, S.: Warning signs prior to rupture of an intracranial aneurysm. *J. Neurosurg.,* **38**:575, 1973.

Pickering, L. K., Hogan, G. R., and Gilbert, E. F.: Aneurysm of the posterior inferior cerebellar artery. Rupture in a newborn, *Am. J. Diseases Children,* **119**:155, 1970.

Troupp, H., and Af Björkesten, G.: Results of a controlled trial of late surgical versus conservative treatment of intracranial arterial aneurysms, *J. Neurosurg.,* **35**:20, 1971.

Vascular Malformations, Fistulae, and Encephalofacial Angiomatosis

By a strange human frailty, auscultation of the skull seems to be the one thing most likely to be neglected in a routine neurological examination.

H. Cushing and P. Bailey

ARTERIOVENOUS MALFORMATIONS

Arteriovenous malformations, also called *arteriovenous aneurysms* or *angiomata,* are not neoplasms but developmental abnormalities in which the normal separation of afferent from efferent vascular channels fails to occur. They may be primarily arterial, capillary (cavernous), arteriovenous, telangiectatic, or venous. Capillary telangiectasis is usually asymptomatic and is an incidental finding at autopsy.

Arteriovenous malformations can become symptomatic at any age, and of all intracranial vascular anomalies are second in frequency only to congenital saccular aneurysms. They may be located superficially on the surface of the cerebral hemispheres or deep in the basal ganglia, thalamus, brainstem, cerebellum, or spinal cord. They may be multiple, and they sometimes occur in widely separated locations. Rarely, they are associated with vascular anomalies in other viscera or on the body surface.

Pathologic Anatomy

Gross Appearance Arteriovenous malformations may be barely visible or large enough to replace an entire hemisphere. They most

314

commonly extend through the gray and white matter of a cerebral hemisphere in the shape of a cone, with the base on the cortex and the apex pointing toward the ventricle. The overlying leptomeninges are often thick with scar tissue and russet-colored from minute hemorrhages; the neighboring gyri and underlying parenchyma are atrophic and discolored. During life the abnormal vessels are markedly enlarged and tortuous, "angry-looking," and distended with blood, presenting the writhing appearance of coiled snakes. Because oxygenated blood is shunted directly to the veins without passing through a capillary bed, the veins are often large and contain bright red blood under relatively high pressure.

Microscopic Appearance Even microscopically, it is frequently impossible to differentiate clearly between arteries and arterialized veins. The walls of the feeding and draining vessels are often thin in one place and thickened by intimal hypertrophy sufficient to block the lumen in another. Atherosclerosis and thrombosis often develop within these malformations, perhaps because of the abnormal volume of flow, the unusual branching, and the tortuosity and angulation that may occur. The neighboring brain parenchyma may be atrophic and infarcted from chronic ischemia.

Pathophysiology

Small lesions do not shunt enough blood to cause ischemic symptoms. However, they may cause seizures by irritating the adjacent gray matter, and a few may bleed. Generally, though, the smaller the malformation, the less likely it is to do either. On the other hand, large malformations short-circuit so much blood from artery to vein that they may have both local and systemic effects.

The local consequence is a diversion of blood from normal arteries through the malformation because of its lower pressure (Fig. 26-1). The reduced peripheral resistance causes the diastolic pressure within the cranial arteries to be lowered, resulting in a wide intracranial arterial pulse pressure. This condition is analogous to the widening of systemic pulse pressure that may occur with arteriovenous fistulae in other organs. Cerebral blood flow may be increased as much as 50 to 100 percent above normal; despite this vastly increased flow, however, tissue perfusion is markedly reduced. As a consequence, chronic ischemia—manifested by seizures, signs and symptoms of cortical atrophy, and dementia—may result.

The systemic effect of large malformations is an increase in cardiac output secondary to the voluminous cerebral flow. In infants the shunt may rarely overtax the left ventricle and result in cardiac decompensation of the high-output type.

Some investigators believe that arteriovenous malformations are static; others suggest that channels enlarge, diverting more and more blood in the manner just described.

Clinical Features

Although tiny arteriovenous malformations are sometimes discovered as incidental findings at autopsy, most of the larger ones produce signs and symptoms during life. These include (1) intracerebral, subarachnoid, or subdural hemorrhage; (2) convulsions; (3) headaches; (4) focal neurologic signs (weakness, sensory loss, aphasia, hemianopia); (5) dementia; and (6) bruits audible to the patient.

Hemorrhage In about half the patients, most often between the ages of 20 and 30, the arteriovenous malformation lies silent until hemorrhage occurs. Bleeding usually occurs from surface vessels into the subarachnoid space, but at times deeply placed lesions may bleed solely into surrounding brain. If bleeding

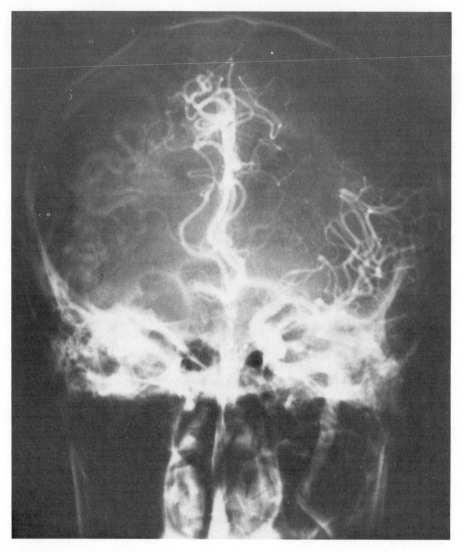

Figure 26-1 Left carotid arteriogram showing cross filling of a large arteriovenous malformation of the right hemisphere.

occurs in the brain parenchyma, the clinical picture is that of brain hemorrhage; with surface bleeding the patient experiences subarachnoid hemorrhage. Most often the bleeding is from a ruptured vein, so that hemorrhage is less intense than that from a saccular aneurysm or from rupture of the arterial portion of the malformation. When viewed at operation or autopsy, the

brain in the areas immediately adjacent to the lesion may show deposits of hemosiderin. This finding is proof that small and asymptomatic hemorrhages have occurred in the past.

Convulsions In 25 to 40 percent of patients, a convulsion is the initial symptom of arteriovenous malformation. In the majority of these patients symptoms begin with a focal or generalized seizure occurring first in adolescence or young adult life. The focal event may be overlooked if the spread to generalized activity is rapid. Because malformations often are located in the parietal or occipital regions, focal events may be sensory or visual in nature. Whenever a young person has episodic illusory or visual hallucinatory experiences, arteriovenous malformation should be a prime consideration.

Headaches Migraine-like cephalalgia is the initial symptom in about 15 percent of patients. When vascular headache and seizures occur in the same patient, the possibility of arteriovenous malformation should always be considered. At times the distinction between true migraine and vascular headache secondary to an arteriovenous malformation is quite difficult, but in a young person throbbing headaches always occurring in the same location should suggest intracranial vascular disease—most often an arteriovenous malformation. Only in very occasional cases is a saccular aneurysm responsible.

Local Neurologic Signs Hemiparesis, sensory loss, hypalgesia, homonymous hemianopia, or aphasia may occur transiently, as in an ischemic or postepileptic phenomenon (Todd's paralysis), and one or more of these conditions may be a permanent residuum of focal intracerebral hemorrhage or infarction. When the malformation diverts large quantities of blood before full growth has been attained, cortical atrophy may cause hypodevelopment of the opposite side of the body and of the same side of the skull. This peculiar asymmetry of the body and skull is a clue to disease of the cerebral hemisphere which began before maturation was complete.

Mental Changes Some investigators hold that about half the patients with large arteriovenous malformations eventually suffer intellec-

tual deterioration—at times only a subtle defect, but often progressive dementia. This change in personality and intellect is thought to be related to chronic diversion of blood from the cerebral tissues, since it is often found associated with cortical atrophy, either localized in the region of the malformation or generalized over one or both of the hemispheres. In some patients, subarachnoid bleeding produces adhesive arachnoiditis; the resultant obstruction to the cerebrospinal fluid pathways causes internal hydrocephalus, which also may contribute to intellectual deterioration.

Bruits Intracranial murmurs are found in 10 to 25 percent of the patients, the incidence being directly proportional to the diligence of the examiner. It is believed that the size rather than the location of the malformation determines the presence or absence of murmur. Such bruits are often absent during the acute phase of intracranial hemorrhage, their absence being due perhaps to the smallness of the offending lesion, but more probably to alterations in intracranial hemodynamics produced by vessel spasm. Since murmurs may come and go in the course of an intracranial hemorrhage, the skull and orbit should be auscultated frequently throughout the patient's illness.

A bruit over an occipital lobe angioma (cephalic bruit) may be heard only if blood supply to the occipital lobe is augmented, for example, during photic stimulation.

An arterial bruit in the neck may be heard in the appropriate location in cases where either the carotid or vertebral artery supplies the angioma. At times, the increased venous return may produce a venous hum over the internal jugular vein audible to the patient as well as the physician.

Examination of the Patient

General Examination Patients with large arteriovenous malformations may rarely have a widened brachial arterial pulse pressure. Occasionally intracranial malformations may communicate with extracranial arteries—usually those of the external carotid system—forming *cirsoid aneurysms.* Such malformations are accompanied by hyperpulsation of the external arteries, a palpable thrill, and often a loud bruit that can sometimes be heard by the patient himself. Rarely the first sign of a combined malformation is exophthalmos caused by intraorbital extension of the fistula or a nosebleed caused by bleeding vessels which communicate with those in the cranium. Infants with arteriovenous malformation, particularly of the vein of Galen, may be brought to the doctor because of hydrocephalus and signs of congestive cardiac failure. The hydrocephalus results from obstruction of the aqueduct of Sylvius by the abnormal vascular structures, and cardiac failure is produced by the large shunt of blood through the malformation. These complications are extremely rare in adults.

In youths and adults who have had large malformations since childhood, inspection of the face and skull may suggest atrophy of one hemisphere. On the side of the atrophy the cranial vault is small, the forehead low, and the malar bone high. The opposite side of the body, including the face, arm, leg, breast, and thorax, may be smaller than the normal side (Fig. 26-2).

Although cutaneous abnormalities such as nevi, neurofibromata, telangiectasis, and *café au lait* spots may suggest the presence of an associated congenital intracranial lesion, they are notoriously unreliable signs because they are found so commonly in the general population.

Neurologic Examination There may be focal neurologic abnormalities, such as visual field defects and hemiparesis, which suggest the anatomic location, but diagnosis depends on evidence of increased flow through the vessels feeding and draining the malformation.

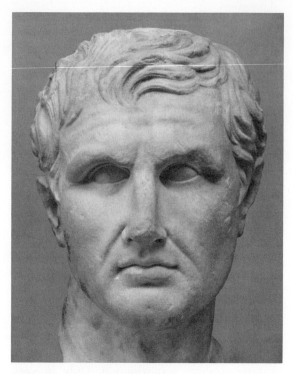

Figure 26-2 Bust of Menander showing right facial hemiatrophy, perhaps due to a left hemispheric lesion. *(Used with permission of the University Museum, University of Pennsylvania.)*

Bruits Abnormal patterns of pressure and flow may be manifest by a bruit over the carotid or vertebral arteries in the neck, or by cephalic or orbital murmurs alone. Such murmurs come and go, perhaps depending on changes in systemic blood pressure and/or cardiac output, and even on alterations in flow through the malformation itself. Increased flow through the draining jugular veins is sometimes accompanied by a venous hum, but this is a highly unreliable finding.

If a bruit is heard, it may be helpful to compress each carotid artery for about 10 sec while listening over the site where the murmur is loudest to determine if its characteristics can be altered. If the murmur is accentuated, one suspects that the artery compressed does *not* feed the malformation; if it disappears, perhaps the vessel is its major source of supply. Occasionally a bruit may be heard only in the orbit as a very soft souffle.

Eye Signs If the malformation involves the carotid arterial tree, diastolic pressure in the ophthalmic artery may be abnormally low. The wave of arterial blood transmitted into the venous system with each heartbeat is reflected by increased pulsations in the retinal veins on the side of the lesion, and the elevated venous pressure may prevent the blanching of the veins that normally occurs during systole.

The retinal vascular pattern may show angiomata either as part of or in addition to the intracranial malformation.

Venous Signs In most persons, the right jugular vein carries well over half the venous return from the two hemispheres. In some instances, however, the confluens sinuum is so constructed that the two hemispheres of the brain return their blood independently through the jugular veins. In such cases, flow through the jugular vein on the side of the malformation may be increased; and if both internal jugulars are gently compressed above the clavicles, the side with the increased venous return will fill first and become more prominent (Wadia's test). In patients with arteriovenous malformations, the jugular vein draining the side of the lesion contains mixed arterial blood with a high oxygen content. Consequently a P_{O_2} determination on a sample of blood from each jugular vein may provide evidence for detecting the site of the arteriovenous shunt.

Differential Diagnosis

The combination of a cutaneous nevus, focal motor seizures, a cephalic bruit, and an unequivocal venous sign in a young person suggests an intracranial arteriovenous malformation. The diagnosis is more difficult to make when intracranial hemorrhage is the sole manifestation.

The age of the patient sometimes helps to rule out hypertensive intracerebral hemorrhage, because this condition occurs most often in patients past middle age, while bleeding from a malformation usually occurs before. The greatest problem lies in differentiating between saccular aneurysm and arteriovenous malformation. Evidence for the latter diagnosis is (1) the presence of a bruit; (2) a previous history of seizures or of one-sided headaches; and (3) a history of previous subarachnoid hemorrhage, particularly if the hemorrhages have been "mild." Rupture of a saccular aneurysm is usually accompanied by massive arterial bleeding at the base of the brain and arterial spasm, whereas venous oozing from a malformation is less in volume and is usually located over the hemisphere, where it is less likely to involve the vital centers. Consequently the patient is often more seriously ill with bleeding from a saccular aneurysm than with bleeding from a malformation.

Both primary and metastatic neoplasms are occasionally associated with focal seizures, neurologic deficits, and an intracranial murmur which might suggest arteriovenous malformation. If bleeding from the abnormal vessels in the neoplasm produces subarachnoid hemorrhage as well, a distinction between the two conditions may not be possible on clinical grounds alone.

Natural History and Prognosis

It is probable that almost half the patients who have an intracranial arteriovenous malformation eventually have intracranial hemorrhage, with a mortality of about 6 percent. About a quarter are self-supporting despite symptoms, and invalidism occurs in about 10 percent. About two-thirds lead normal lives. It has been estimated that after recovery from the initial hemorrhage, there is a 6 percent risk of dying from subsequent hemorrhage. In one series, about a fourth of the patients with arteriovenous malformations survived more than 20 years, the majority with little or no disability. This prognosis is far better than that for saccular aneurysms.

Laboratory Findings

Skull X-rays At times, particularly in instances of cirsoid aneurysm, skull x-rays reveal widening of the grooves of the meningeal artery and the draining diploic veins in the calvarium. Usually, however, such venous grooves and arterial channel enlargements are of no help whatsoever. More useful are the occasional flecks of calcification which may be distributed in the walls of abnormal vessels or in the surrounding cortex.

Electroencephalogram Focal disturbances of brain wave activity may sometimes be found over areas adjacent to the malformation. These may consist of sporadic spike activity or of focal slow waves.

Radioactive Brain Scan Far more valuable than either skull x-ray or electroencephalography are brain scan and flow study using 99m$_{Tc}$. This is a rapid, safe method for localizing arteriovenous malformations within the substance of the brain. The uptake of radioactive material into the endothelium of the abnormal vessels or into the tissues immediately surrounding them is quite intense and gives surprisingly accurate localization of lesions 2 cm or more in size (Fig. 26-3).

Arteriography This is a procedure of choice for the definitive diagnosis and localization of arteriovenous malformations. Both carotid systems, and, at times, the vertebral-basilar system as well, must be studied in order to obtain the following information, which is essential for determining the feasibility of surgical extirpation:

1 Whether the malformation is fed by more than one arterial system (e.g., a malformation in the parietal or occipital lobes may be fed by the angular and temporal branches of the middle

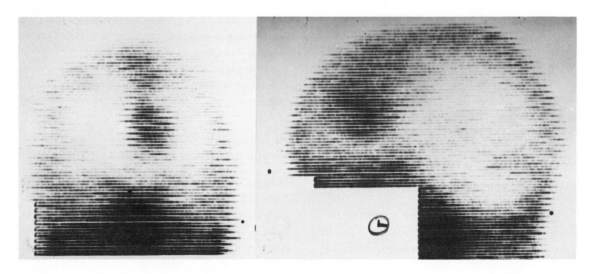

Figure 26-3 Technetium 99m brain scan in a patient with an arteriovenous malformation, also depicted in Figure 26-4.

cerebral artery as well as by the posterior choroidal branch of the posterior cerebral)

2 The precise limits of the malformation

3 Whether the patient has more than one arteriovenous malformation

4 Whether a hematoma has accumulated

The best angiographic evidence of arteriovenous malformation is the presence of large feeding arteries which lead to rapidly filling and draining veins. Signs suggestive of arteriovenous malformation are (1) a very short arterial phase in any or all of the arterial branches, (2) a tangle of opacified arteries and veins, and (3) unusually rapid filling of veins, which appear opacified during the "capillary" phase (Fig. 26-4*A* to *D*).

Unless rapid serial angiography is used, some small malformations with a rapid shunt will be missed completely. Occasionally, after subarachnoid hemorrhage, opacification of a malformation will not occur. Some investigators think this failure to fill may be due to spasm of the afferent arteries or compression by hematoma and that spasm or nonfilling of areas that normally are opacified should be regarded as a clue to the location of the lesion.

Air Study Pneumoencephalograms and/or ventriculograms are not indicated for patients suspected of having arteriovenous malformations, although such studies would reveal atrophy of the hemisphere containing the malformation and perhaps even a shift of the midline structures away from the side of the lesion if the patient has had a recent episode of cerebral bleeding. This combination of unilateral cerebral atrophy with shift of the brain to the opposite side is quite suggestive of a large arteriovenous malformation on the side of the enlarged ventricle.

Treatment

Treatment of these malformations has two goals: (1) to control the complications associated with the malformation and (2) to prevent its enlargement. Of the complications (focal seizures, cortical atrophy, the development of neurologic deficit, and rupture of vessels, producing intracerebral hematoma or subarachnoid hemorrhage), only focal seizures are amenable to medical therapy. Seizures per se are not an indication for surgery, since they can usually be controlled by anticonvulsant medication. If they are intractable, attempted removal of the malformation may be justified, even though the seizures may continue thereafter with lessened severity.

The other goals of surgery can be achieved only by total excision of the lesion; this is curative but, unfortunately, is not often feasible. Irradiation with x-ray has been of no avail and is not recommended, because the tolerance of neural tissue for radiation is about the same as that of the vessels. Ligation of jugular veins or of the carotid or vertebral arteries in the neck is fruitless and may even accelerate rather than retard development of the neurologic deficit. Plastic-ball emboli have been injected into the appropriate arterial tree in the hope that they will lodge in and occlude the arteries that feed the malformation. Such methods may prove useful in the future.

The decision to perform surgery in patients with arteriovenous malformations is dependent on the location of the lesion, its size, and the vessels that feed it. A small malformation in the medulla oblongata is inaccessible, whereas a large one in the nondominant frontal lobe might be removed. Generally, patients with lesions located in the frontal or temporal areas of the nondominant hemisphere are the best candidates for surgery.

CAROTICOCAVERNOUS FISTULA

Throughout its course through the cavernous plexus of veins, the internal carotid artery has the peculiar feature of being separated from venous blood only by the arterial wall and a thin

(A)   **(B)**

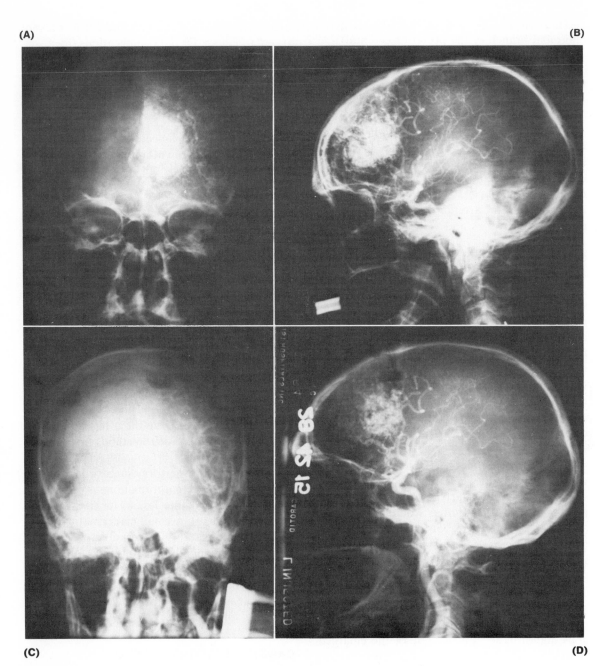

(C)   **(D)**

Figure 26-4   Left carotid arteriograms showing a large frontal arteriovenous malformation in the patient whose brain scan is illustrated in Figure 26-3. (C) Early phase.
(A) Late phase. (D) Early phase lateral projection. (B) Late phase.

venous endothelium. Any breach in the continuity of these walls results in a caroticocavernous fistula.

Etiology

About 75 percent of these fistulae develop after trauma; in many, fracture of the floor of the middle cranial fossa produces tension on the carotid siphon and ruptures it. Some caroticocavernous fistulae are due to rupture of saccular or arteriosclerotic aneurysms; in the remainder, no cause can be found. Traumatic fistulae are more common in men, whereas spontaneous fistulae develop more often in women.

The insertion of a catheter into the cavernous portion of the internal carotid artery sometimes perforates the artery and creates a fistula.

Clinical Features

Though not common, a history of unilateral migraine is sometimes obtained in cases of spontaneous caroticocavernous fistula. This relationship may be fortuitous, but in a few cases the headaches have ceased after rupture. The onset is usually abrupt, and the patient may feel or hear a "pop" inside his head.

The fistula is usually small at first, and little blood is detoured through it. It enlarges gradually as times goes on. In posttraumatic cases, symptoms and signs may appear within 24 hr after the injury but are occasionally delayed for weeks or months as the fistula slowly enlarges.

The onset may be painless or accompanied by severe pain in the distribution of the first division of the trigeminal nerve. The patient frequently begins to hear in his head a bruit which is synchronous with his heartbeat. His eyelids may become puffy and bluish, particularly on the side of the rupture. Pulsatile exophthalmos is usually noted and is best seen by observing the eye from above. There is often a continuous murmur with systolic accentuation and perhaps a thrill. The intensity of the murmur is variable

and may not be heard at all; hence repeated auscultation is advisable. The bruit can often be abolished by compressing the ipsilateral carotid artery. In other cases, external ophthalmoplegia develops.

Chemosis and injection limited to the bulbar conjunctiva are helpful differentiating features; in conjunctivitis both the palpebral and the bulbar conjunctive are edematous and injected. Although a caroticocavernous fistula usually produces ipsilateral exophthalmos, it may result in either contralateral or bilateral exophthalmos, and very rarely in none at all. This sign depends on the patency of the ophthalmic veins and the degree of cross circulation occurring at the circular sinus which connects the paired cavernous sinuses.

1 If the ipsilateral ophthalmic veins are not patent and the circular sinus is not functioning, there will be no exophthalmos on either side.

2 If the ophthalmic veins are patent only on the contralateral side and the circular sinus is adequate, a unilateral caroticocavernous fistula will result in contralateral exophthalmos only.

3 If the ophthalmic veins are patent on both sides and the circular sinus is functioning well, a unilateral caroticocavernous fistula will result in bilateral exophthalmos.

4 If all collaterals are open, exophthalmos may disappear spontaneously despite persistence of the fistula.

The retina is cyanotic, with distended hyperpulsatile veins which, unlike normal veins, expand during systole and contract in diastole. Diversion of blood from the arterial into the venous circulation may cause attenuation of the retinal arterioles on the side of the rupture. Papilledema and retinal hemorrhages may be present. Visual impairment may result from these or from secondary glaucoma, and all may either precede or follow surgical treatment. Ophthalmodynamometry may reveal a wide pulse pressure on the side of the fistula.

Some fistulae can divert huge quantities of blood from the brain and produce signs of cerebral ischemia. Consequently, if the fistula shows no signs of spontaneous regression, surgery should be considered.

Diagnosis and Angiographic Findings

The finding of pulsatile exophthalmos combined with a continuous bruit over the orbit is almost pathognomonic of a caroticocavernous fistula. Only the rare arteriovenous malformation in the orbit produces a similar picture. An unruptured aneurysm of the carotid siphon never produces a loud bruit or conjunctival injection of such extent. Endocrine exophthalmos

does not pulsate and is not associated with a bruit. In cases of cavernous sinus thrombosis there is no bruit; the patient is very ill, and signs of local infection are present.

Although carotid angiography is not essential for the diagnosis, it must be carried out before surgery is planned, so that possible contralateral aneurysm can be disclosed and the potential for flow from one to the other carotid can be determined. The degree of arterial filling above the fistula depends on the degree of diversion of blood into the vein (Fig. 26-5A and B). With a large defect, there is no filling of either the anterior or the middle cerebral artery, all the contrast material being diverted into the cavernous sinus and out through the venous systems.

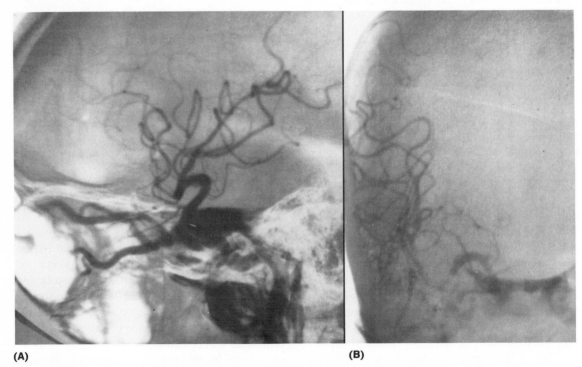

(A)   **(B)**

Figure 26-5 Carotid arteriogram shows filling of the cavernous sinus, pterygoid plexus, and ophthalmic and jugular veins during the early phases. (A) Lateral projection. (B) Towne projection. *(Courtesy of Dr. F. Farrell, Department of Radiology, Bowman Gray School of Medicine.)*

Treatment

About 10 percent of fistulae undergo thrombosis and close spontaneously, but before this happens they may cause ocular paralysis, blindness, or both. These conditions are usually permanent.

If surgery seems necessary, the choice of the best method presents a challenge. More operative procedures have been recommended for this condition than perhaps for any other intracranial lesion. Ligation of the internal or common carotid artery produces a cure in about 65 to 85 percent of the patients. In resistant cases ligation of the internal carotid artery in the neck is combined with ligation of the carotid above the cavernous sinus. Sometimes clipping of the ipsilateral ophthalmic artery, which may cause blindness, is also needed.

Recently pieces of muscle have been injected into the internal carotid artery. When fashioned in the correct size, these drift up the carotid and lodge in the fistula, leading to remission of symptoms.

ENCEPHALOFACIAL ANGIOMATOSIS

Known by various names, including Sturge-Weber-Dimitri syndrome, this condition is characterized by venous capillary hemangioma of the leptomeninges of one cerebral hemisphere and by a similar angioma (port-wine stain, nevus flammeus) of the face and scalp predominantly of the same side as the cerebral lesion. The cortex underlying the leptomeningeal hemangioma is almost always atrophic, and signs of neurologic deficit such as focal seizures, hemiparesis, and visual field defects may occur. Mental retardation, a prominent feature in the fully expressed syndrome, probably is a manifestation of a diffuse anomaly of brain development rather than of the focal damage beneath the angioma. At times the choroid of the homolateral eye is involved and glaucoma (buphthalmos) develops.

Because it characteristically involves the integument and the central nervous system, this congenital but nonhereditary syndrome is classified as belonging to the neurocutaneous disorders.

Pathology

Gross Appearance The capillary venous hemangioma usually lies in the piarachnoid of the parietooccipital region. The involved hemisphere is often smaller than the normal one. Associated angiomatosis elsewhere in the brain, dura, or skull is unusual. The vessels in the angioma may be calcified, and there is often calcification of the cortex of the adjacent brain, causing a gritty sensation when the brain is sliced with a knife.

Microscopic Findings Vessel calcification lies in the capillaries. The cortical neurons show evidence of ischemic damage in some cases. The nevus consists of dilated vessels engorged with blood and lined by a single layer of endothelial cells.

Pathogenesis

The distribution of the angiomata is explained on a developmental basis. During embryologic development the primordial vascular plexus splits into an inner layer supplying the brain and retina, and an outer layer supplying the meninges, choroid, and face. The common origin of the vessels of these structures explains why all may be affected simultaneously by persistence of primitive vessels. Because this plexus does not form in similar fashion in the hindbrain, hemangioma of the occipital region is not associated with angiomatosis of the structures lying in the posterior fossa.

Stenosis and thrombosis in the capillary-venous angioma of the leptomeninges leads to fibrosis, hyaline degeneration, and calcification. The results are a loss of neurons, gliosis, and secondary calcification in the subjacent gray and white matter. The epilepsy and mental retardation present in most cases are probably related not to the vascular anomaly per se but to some associated maldevelopment of the cerebrum which has not yet been defined.

Clinical Features

Nevus Flammeus A nevus flammeus is almost always found in the supraocular portion of the face on the same side as the intracranial abnormality. As best as we can determine, no case has been reported without involvement in this location, even though other portions of the face as well as the scalp, neck, mouth, nose, and conjunctivae may also be involved. At times the involvement of the face is bilateral, in which case the cortical abnormality usually lies on the side which is the more extensively involved. Many neuropathologists have erroneously considered the facial distribution to follow sensory divisions of the trigeminal nerve, but in reality the distribution is related to the layout of the fissures of the developing face.

The nevus flammeus is present at birth and does not show any postnatal growth, although its color may become more intense, giving the appearance of growth. It is usually flat but at times is associated with overgrowth of the soft tissues, and the skin may be nubbly. The angioma often involves episcleral vessels and sometimes the nasal and buccal mucosa. Rarely, it is bilateral, in which case it may be associated with bilateral glaucoma. Instances of nevus flammeus of the face without cerebral or meningeal involvement occur frequently. Whether these are *formes frustés* of the full-blown syndrome is unknown.

Epilepsy Convulsions, often with a focal onset, are seen in almost all cases. In the past,

status epilepticus has been a common cause of death in these patients.

Mental Retardation Impairment of intellect is a usual but not invariable accompaniment of this syndrome.

Focal Neurologic Deficit The hemispheric involvement frequently results in contralateral spastic hemiparesis, sensory loss, and homonymous hemianopia. Occasionally, growth of the limbs on the opposite side of the body is stunted.

Ocular Signs Various ocular phenomena may be observed on the same side as the facial and intracranial anomalies. The most frequent are congenital glaucoma (buphthalmos) and choroid angioma.

One of the most striking ocular signs is the presence of dilated, engorged, tortuous episcleral vessels.

In rare cases angiomatosis involves the iris on the side of the facial nevus, causing it to be darker than the other.

Angioma of the choroid, found most frequently between the optic disk and the macula, has a honeycomb pattern. It does not increase in size and at times may undergo spontaneous regression. Because it lacks pigment, it is lighter than the surrounding choroid, though it often merges imperceptibly with the normal choroid vasculature.

Diagnosis

A diagnosis of encephalofacial angiomatosis should be made only when a supraocular facial nevus and angiomatosis of the pia are present in the same patient. When present, intracranial calcification produces a characteristic, although not pathognomonic, radiologic picture, and the angiomata do not produce a bruit.

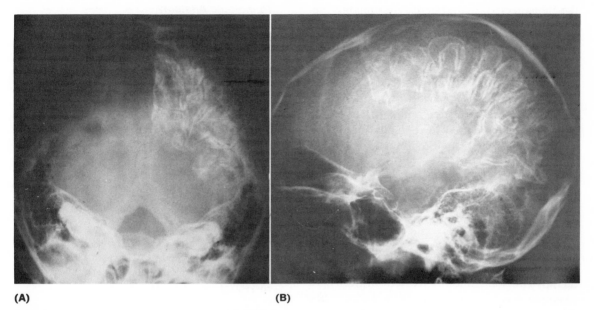

(A)   **(B)**

Figure 26-6 Characteristic tracklike calcification in the parietooccipital lobe of a patient with Sturge-Weber syndrome. (A) Towne view. (B) Lateral view. *(Courtesy of Dr. Carlos Gonzalez, Hahnemann Hospital, Philadelphia.)*

Laboratory Findings

Radiologic Features   After the first 2 years of life about two-thirds of the patients have the characteristic double-track or double-contoured calcification, visible on x-ray usually in the occipital or parietooccipital region because of calcification in adjacent gyri near their common sulcus (Fig. 26-6).

Thickening of the overlying skull is observed in some cases, but the vascular markings of the calvarium are normal.

Radioisotopic Brain Scan   This may show an increased area of uptake in the region of the abnormal vessels.

Angiography   About 5 percent of patients with Sturge-Weber syndrome are said to have associated vascular lesions (venous angiomata, thrombosis of intracranial arteries, anomalies of dural sinuses, or small arteriovenous malformations) demonstrable by carotid angiography. The angioma itself is reported to be visible in some cases as a diffuse increase in density of the contrast material. In a few cases, large veins are seen coursing through this area. There is no appreciable increase in the speed of circulation.

Pneumoencephalography   This reveals cortical atrophy and ventricular dilatation on the side of the angioma.

Electroencephalography   The most common pattern seen is unilateral depression or loss of the normal rhythms over a wide area on the side with cortical atrophy and angioma. Also seen are random theta or delta waves associated with focal spikes in patients with seizures. At times paroxysmal discharges are more prominent over the nonaffected hemisphere, presumably because bilateral discharge is suppressed on the side with cortical atrophy.

Course and Prognosis

Repeated seizures are the rule in the majority of patients, and death in status epilepticus may occur. Most of the patients eventually require institutional management because of their intellectual limitation.

Treatment

Therapy with the hydantoins, barbiturates, or diazepan (Valium) is usually effective in controlling the epilepsy. Frequent incapacitating seizures that are resistant to anticonvulsant therapy can sometimes be treated surgically. In some patients lobectomy can be performed, but if hemiplegia is present, a hemispherectomy often gives better results. Although excision of the diseased cerebral tissue may reduce the frequency of seizures, it does not necessarily improve the patient's mental status.

SUGGESTED READINGS

Arteriovenous Malformations

General

Feindel, W., and Perot, P.: Red cerebral veins: A report on arteriovenus shunts in tumors and cerebral scars, *J. Neurosurg.,* **22**:315, 1965.

Gold, A., Ransohoff, J., and Carter, S.: Vein of Galen malformation, *Acta neurol. scand.,* **40**(suppl. 11):1, 1964.

Paterson, J. H., and McKissock, W.: A clinical survey of intracranial angiomas with special reference to their mode of progression and surgical treatment: A report of 110 cases, *Brain,* **79**:233, 1956.

Pool, J. L., and Potts, D. G.: Aneurysms and Arteriovenous Anomalies of the Brain: Diagnosis and Treatment, Harper & Row, Publishers, Incorporated, New York, 1965.

Wyburn-Mason, R.: Arteriovenous aneurysm in midbrain and retina, facial naevi, and mental changes, *Brain,* **66**:163, 1943.

Pathologic Anatomy

McCormick, W. F.: The pathology of vascular ("arteriovenous") malformations, *J. Neurosurg.,* **24**:807, 1966.

Moyes, P. D.: Intracranial and intraspinal vascular anomalies in children, *J. Neurosurg.,* **3**:271, 1969.

Newton, T. H., and Cronqvist, S.: Involvement of dural arteries in intracranial arteriovenous malformations, *Radiology,* **93**:1071, 1969.

Rodda, R. A., and Calvert, G. D.: Post-mortem arteriography of cerebral arteriovenous malformations, *J. Neurol. Neurosurg. Psychiat.,* **32**:432, 1969.

Pathophysiology

Crawford, J. V., and Russell, D. S.: Cryptic arteriovenous and venous hamartomas of the brain, *J. Neurol. Neurosurg. Psychiat.,* **19**:1, 1956.

Wallace, J. M., Nashold, B. S., Jr., and Slewka, A. P.: Hemodynamic effects of cerebral arteriovenous aneurysms, *Circulation,* **31**:696, 1965.

Clinical Features

Boyd-Wilson, J. S.: The association of cerebral angiomas with intracranial aneurysms, *J. Neurol. Neurosurg. Psychiat.,* **22**:218, 1959.

Carroll, C. P. H., and Jakoby, R. K.: Neonatal congestive heart failure as the presenting symptom of cerebral arteriovenous malformation, *J. Neurosurg.,* **25**:159, 1966.

Dany, A., Vallat, J. N., Gaudin, H., and Valegeas, A.: Les anévrysmes cirsoïdes du corps calleux. A propos de 3 observations, *Neuro-Chirurgie,* **14**:489, 1968.

Deverall, P. B., Taylor, J. F., Sturrock, G. S., and Aberdeen, E.: Coarctation-like physiology with cerebral arteriovenous fistula, *Pediatrics,* **44**:1024, 1969.

Eckman, P. B., Kramer, R. A., and Altrocchi, P. H.: Hemifacial spasm, *Arch. Neurol.,* **25**:81, 1971.

Eisenbrey, A. B., and Hegarty, W. M.: Trigeminal neuralgia and arteriovenous aneurysm of the cerebellopontine angle, *J. Neurosurg.,* **13**:647, 1956.

Farrell, D. F., and Forno, L. S.: Symptomatic capillary telangiectasis of the brainstem without hemorrhage. Report of an unusual case, *Neurology,* **20**:341, 1970.

Fay, T.: "The Head": A neurosurgeon's analysis of a great stone portrait, *Expedition,* **2**(summer):12, 1959.

Johnson, M. C., and Salmon, J. H.: Arteriovenous malformation presenting as trigeminal neuralgia, *J. Neurosurg.,* **29**:287, 1968.

Lees, F.: The migrainous symptoms of cerebral angiomata, *J. Neurol. Neurosurg. Psychiat.,* **25**:45, 1962.

Malan, E., and Azzolini, A.: Congenital arteriovenous malformations of the face and scalp, *J. Cardiovascular Surg.,* **9**:109, 1968.

McConnell, T. H., and Leonard, J. S.: Microangiomatous malformations with intraventricular hemorrhage. Report of two unusual cases, *Neurology,* **17**:618, 1967.

McCormick, W. F., Hardman, J. M., and Boulter, T. R.: Vascular malformations ("angiomas") of the brain, with special reference to those occurring in the posterior fossa, *J. Neurosurg.,* **28**:241, 1968.

Moody, R. A., and Poppen, J. L.: Arteriovenous malformations, *J. Neurosurg.,* **32**:503, 1970.

Newton, T. H., Weidner, W., and Greitz, T.: Dural arteriovenous malformation in the posterior fossa, *Radiology,* **90**:27, 1968.

Robinson, J. L., Hall, C. J., and Sedzimir, C. B.: Subarachnoid hemorrhage in pregnancy, J. *Neurosurg.,* **36**:27, 1972.

Rockett, J. F., and Johnson, T. H., Jr.: Bilateral rete mirabile intracranial (vascular) anastomosis in man. A case report, *Radiology,* **90**:46, 1968.

Vitse, M., Mizon, J. P., and Silberberg, L.: Hémorragie méningèe au cours de la grossesse révélatrice d'une malformation vasculaire, *Bull. Fed. Gynec. Obstet. Franc.,* **18**:54, 1966.

Wadia, N. H.: Venous sign in cerebral angioma, *Brain,* **83**:425, 1960.

Wijngaarden, G. K. van, and Vinken, P. J.: A case of intradural arteriovenous aneurysm of the posterior fossa, *Neurology,* **16**:754, 1966.

Examination of the Patient

Danis, P.: Aspects ophthalmologiques des angiomatoses du système nerveus, *Acta neurol. psychiat. belg.,* **50**:615, 1950.

Hardison, J. E.: Cervical venous hum. A clue to the diagnosis of intracranial arteriovenous malformation, *New Engl. J. Med.,* **278**:587, 1968.

Differential Diagnosis

Boder, E., and Sedgwick, R. P.: Ataxia-telangiectasia. A familial syndrome of progressive cerebellar ataxia, oculocutaneous telangiectasia and frequent pulmonary infection, *Pediatrics,* **21**:526, 1958.

McCormick, W. F., and Nofzinger, J. D.: "Cryptic" vascular malformations of the central nervous system, *J. Neurosurg.,* **24**:865, 1966.

Natural History and Prognosis

Heiss, W. D., Kvicala, V., Prosenz, P., and Tschabitscher, H.: The importance of arterial shunting in areas of brain distant from an arteriovenous malformation, *Neurology,* **20**:376, 1970.

Kushner, J., and Alexander, E., Jr.: Partial spontaneous regressive arteriovenous malformation. Case report with angiographic evidence, *J. Neurosurg.,* **32**:360, 1970.

Porter, A. J., and Bull, J.: Some aspects of the natural history of cerebral arteriovenous malformation, *Brit. J. Radiol.,* **42**:667, 1969.

Schatz, S., and Botterell, H.: The natural history of arteriovenous malformations, *Res. Pub. Assoc. Nerv. Ment. Dis.,* **41**:180, 1966.

Svien, H. J., and McRae, J. A.: Arteriovenous anomalies of the brain: Fate of patients not having definitive surgery, *J. Neurosurg.,* **23**:23, 1965.

Troupp, H.: Arteriovenous malformations of the brain: Prognosis without operation, *Acta neurol. scand.,* **41**:39, 1965.

———, Marttila, I., and Halonen, V.: Arteriovenous malformations of the brain. Prognosis without operation, *Acta neurochir.,* **22**:125, 1970.

Laboratory Findings

Skull X-ray

Rumbaugh, C. L., and Potts, D. G.: Skull changes associated with intracranial arteriovenous malformations, *Am. J. Roentgenol.,* **98**:525, 1966.

Electroencephalography

Groethuysen, U. C., Bickford, R. G., and Svien, H. J.: Electroencephalogram in arteriovenous anomalies of the brain, *Arch. Neurol. Psychiat.,* **74**:506, 1955.

Radioisotopic Brain Scan

Kelly, D. L., Jr., Alexander, E., Jr., Davis, C. H., Jr., and Maynard, C. D.: Intracranial arteriovenous malformations: Clinical review and evaluation of brain scans, *J. Neurosurg.,* **31**:422, 1969.

Rosenthall, L.: Radionuclide diagnosis of arterial venous malformations with rapid sequence brain scans, *Radiology,* **91**:1185, 1968.

Arteriography

Kamrin, R. P., and Buchsbaum, H. W.: Large vascular malformations of the brain not visualized by serial angiography, *Arch. Neurol.,* **13**:413, 1965.

Olsson, O.: Vertebral angiography in cerebellar haemangioma, *Acta radiol.,* **40**:9, 1953.

Air Study

McRae, D. L., and Valentino, V.: Pneumographic findings in angiomata of the brain, *Acta radiol.,* **50**:18, 1958.

Morris, L.: Pneumoencephalographic findings in a case of vein of Galen aneurysm, *Brit. J. Radiol.,* **44**:798, 1971.

Treatment

Tönnis, W., and Walter, W.: Die Indikation zur Totalexstirpation der intrakraniellen arteriovenösen Angiome, *Deutsch Z. Nervenheilk.,* **186**:279, 1964.

Caroticocavernous Fistula

Bickerstaff, E. R.: Mechanisms of presentation of carotico-cavernous fistulae, *Brit. J. Ophthalmol.,* **54**:186, 1970.

Clemens, F., and Lodin, H.: Some viewpoints on the venous outflow pathways in cavernous sinus fistulas: Angiographic study of five traumatic cases, *Clin. Radiol.,* **19**:196, 1968.

Djindjian, R., Cophignon, J., Comoy, J., Rey, J., and Houdart, R.: Polymorphisme neuro-radiologique des fistules carotido-caverneuses, *Neuro-Chirurgie,* **14**:881, 1968.

Drift, J. H. A. Van der, Sparling, C. M., Berg, D. van den, and Magnus, O.: Spontaneous occlusion of a carotid-cavernous shunt, *Neurology,* **17**:187, 1967.

Gautier-Smith, P. C.: Bilateral pulsating exophthalmos due to metastases from carcinoma of prostate, *Brit. Med. J.,* **1**:330, 1960.

Gupta, P. D., Fort, M. L., Barron, K. D., Baron, J. K., and Sharp, J. T.: Cardiac hemodynamics in intracranial arteriovenous fistula, *Neurology,* **19**:198, 1969.

Hamby, W. B.: Carotid-cavernous fistula: Report of 32 surgically treated cases and suggestions for definitive operation, *J. Neurosurg.,* **21**:859, 1964.

Hayes, G. J.: External carotid-cavernous sinus fistulas, *J. Neurosurg.,* **20**:692, 1963.

Henderson, J. W., and Schneider, R. C.: The ocular findings in carotid-cavernous fistula in a series of 17 cases, *Am. J. Ophthalmol.,* **48**:585, 1959.

Lubow, M.: Carotid-cavernous fistula: Comments on ocular complications, *Am. J. Ophthalmol.,* **53**:121, 1962.

Stern, W. E., Brown, W. J., and Alksne, J. F.: The surgical challenge of carotid-cavernous fistula: The critical role of intracranial circulatory dynamics, *J. Neurosurg.,* **27**:298, 1967.

Taptas, J. N.: Les anéurysmes artério-veineux carotido-caverneux (étude pathogénique), *Neuro-Chirurgie,* **8**:385, 1962.

Wanissorn, R.: Mechanism of muscle embolization of carotid cavernous fistula and the fate of the emboli, *J. Neurosurg.,* **32**:344, 1970.

Encephalofacial Angiomatosis (Sturge-Weber-Dimitri Syndrome)

General

Alexander, G. L., and Norman, R. M.: Sturge-Weber Syndrome, John Wright & Sons, Ltd., Bristol, 1960.

Louis-Bar, D.: Les rapports entre les angiomatoses du type Sturge-Weber et les autres dysplasies (formes de passage), *Acta neurol. psychiat. belg.,* **50**:680, 1950.

Myle, G.: Sémiologie de l'angiomatose encéphalo-trigéminée ou encéphalo-cranio-faciale, *Acta neurol. psychiat. belg.,* **50**:713, 1950.

Peterman, A. F., Hayles, A. B., Dockerty, M. B., and Love, J. G.: Encephalotrigeminal angiomatosis (Sturge-Weber disease); clinical study of thirty-five cases, *J.A.M.A.,* **167**:2169, 1958.

Pathology and Pathophysiology

Roizin, L., Gold, G., Berman, H. H., and Bonafede, V. I.: Congenital vascular anomalies and their histopathology in Sturge-Weber-Dimitri syndrome (naevus flammeus with angiomatosis and encephalosis calcificans), *J. Neuropathol. Exptl. Neurol.,* **18**:75, 1959.

Wohlwill, F. J., and Yakovlev, P. I.: Histopathology of meningofacial angiomatosis (Sturge-Weber's disease): Report of four cases, *J. Neuropathol. Exptl. Neurol.*, **16**:341, 1957.

Ophthalmology

Jones, I. S., and Cleasby, G. W.: Hemangioma of the choroid: A clinicopathologic analysis, *Am. J. Ophthalmol.*, **48**:612, 1959.

Radiology

Bentson, J. R., Wilson, G. H., and Newton, T. H.: Cerebral venous drainage pattern of the Sturge-Weber syndrome, *Radiology*, **101**:111, 1971.

Chang, J. C., Jackson, G. L., and Baltz, R.: Isotopic cisternography in Sturge-Weber syndrome, *J. Nucl. Med.*, **11**:551, 1970.

Kuhl, D. E., Bevilacqua, J. E., Mishkin, M. M., and Sanders, T. P.: The brain scan in Sturge-Weber syndrome, *Radiology*, **103**:621, 1972.

O'Brien, M. S., and Schechter, M. M.: Arteriovenous malformations involving the Galenic system, *Am. J. Roentgenol.*, **110**:50, 1970.

Electroencephalography

Hellman, C. D., and Dickerson, W. W.: Études électroencéphalographiques de sept malades présentant un syndrome de Sturge-Weber, *Rev. neurol.*, **87**:211, 1952.

Rohmer, F., Gastaut, Y., and Dell, M. B.: L'EEG dans la pathologie vasculaire du cerveau, *Rev. neurol.*, **87**:93, 1952.

Surgery

Falconer, M. A., and Rushworth, R. G.: Treatment of encephalotrigeminal angiomatosis (Sturge-Weber disease) by hemispherectomy, *Arch. Disease Childhood*, **35**:433, 1960.

Norlen, G.: The surgical treatment in Sturge-Weber's disease, *Neurochirurgia*, **1**:242, 1959.

Brain Hemorrhage

It is impossible to remove a strong attack of apoplexy, and not easy to remove a weak attack.

Hippocrates

Previous chapters have dealt with the cerebral effects secondary to hemorrhage originating in the subarachnoid space and with arteriovenous malformations which usually lie, at least in part, on the surface of the brain.

In this chapter we will consider those hemorrhages which begin in the cerebral hemispheres (about 80 percent of the total) and those originating in the brainstem or cerebellum (about 20 percent).

Hemorrhage that originates within the substance of the brain results from the rupture of an artery, capillary, or vein in the parenchyma. Bleeding may follow injury or may be nontrau-matic (primary or spontaneous). Blood vessels which burst spontaneously may have been weakened by diseases such as hypertension and arteriosclerosis. Infiltrating brain tumors and systemic diseases such as blood dyscrasias may cause intracerebral hemorrhage by weakening vessels from within or eroding them from without.

INTRACEREBRAL HEMORRHAGE

Etiology and Pathogenesis

Primary Intracerebral Hemorrhage These hemorrhages represent about 10 percent of all areas coalesce, obstructing venules and producing hemorrhages. Hypertensive encephalopathy and eclampsia are examples of conditions in which arteriolar spasm plays a leading role.

3 The high incidence of hemorrhages in the brain, compared with their rarity in viscera, may perhaps be explained by the scanty adventitia and the frequent medial defects in cerebral arteries.

4 Hyalinosis (fibroid necrosis) tends to weaken the arterial intima, which is the best developed coat of the cerebral arteries. Hypertension may then trigger intimal rupture of small arteries and arterioles, leading to small dissecting aneurysms which may then cause confluent brain hemorrhage.

Less commonly, cerebral hemorrhage may be produced by one of the following mechanisms:

1 The rupture of small intracerebral arteriovenous malformations or aneurysms may cause continued oozing of blood and hematoma formation. These malformations and aneurysms are presumably destroyed in the process of rupture and are seldom found at autopsy.

2 Polyarteritis nodosa, as well as viral and rickettsial diseases, may cause inflammation of an artery, leading to necrosis of the arterial wall with subsequent rupture.

3 Toxins such as arsenic or deficiencies of vitamin B_1 and vitamin C may produce endothelial death. The resulting intracerebral hemorrhage is usually petechial rather than massive (coalescent hematoma).

4 Anticoagulants, even in doses below the toxic level, may cause massive intracerebral bleeding, presumably by altering normal clotting mechanisms.

5 Blood dyscrasias such as hemophilia, leukemia, thrombocytopenic purpura, polycythemia, and sickle-cell disease may lead to massive cerebral hemorrhage.

6 Neoplasms may cause bleeding, presumably from the erosion of normal cerebral vessels or from rupture of abnormal new vessels contained within the tumor. This complication occurs in about 3 to 5 percent of glioblastomas, in

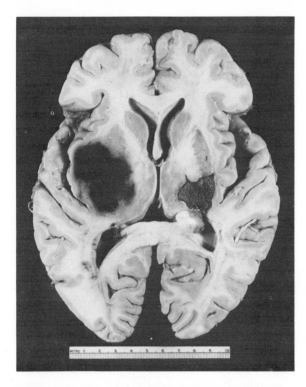

Figure 27-1 Transverse section of a brain showing two hemorrhages in the corpora striata, one new and the other old.

"strokes" (Fig. 27-1). It is believed that fulminant cerebral hemorrhages with rapid progression are due to arterial rupture, whereas more slowly evolving hemorrhages are venous in origin. This belief is actually a guess, because it is impossible for the pathologist to locate the site of the initial rupture. Although the relationship between hypertension and intracerebral hemorrhage is well established, the mechanism causing the hemorrhage is the subject of continuing debate. Some of the possibilities are as follows:

1 Hypertension causes tiny aneurysms to form in the walls of the arterioles. These aneurysms of Charcot-Bouchard may eventually rupture and bleed.

2 Arteriolar spasm produced by hypertension may cause distal hypoxia and necrosis, petechial hemorrhages, and cerebral edema. These melanotic melanoma, and occasionally in metastatic tumors, particularly hypernephroma, chorionepithelioma, and carcinomas of the lung and breast.

7 Hypersensitivity or Shwartzman's phenomenon can cause petechiae.

8 Thrombosis of a cerebral vein, especially when secondary to dehydration or septicemia, may result in cerebral hemorrhage.

Traumatic Intracerebral Hemorrhage One can be sure that trauma is a causative factor in the production of intracerebral hemorrhage only when the hemorrhage immediately follows a severe head injury. However, even though the relationship cannot be proved, there are, without doubt, three mechanisms by which trauma may cause delayed hemorrhage:

1 A vessel weakened by trauma may burst within a few weeks.

2 The initial trauma may cause an encephalomalacic cyst to form, and hemorrhage may develop in its wall.

3 A chronic intracerebral hematoma, present from the time of injury, may grow so slowly that it produces no symptoms or signs until days or weeks have passed.

Pathology

Most intracerebral hemorrhages begin in the region of the putamen and expand, pressing on adjacent structures such as the internal capsule and the insula (Fig. 27-2).

Arterial blood under high pressure forms a liquid hematoma which dissects along fiber pathways, compressing surrounding tissue while tearing traversing venules and capillaries. The vessels ruptured by the accumulating clot add their complement of blood, and the process tends to perpetuate itself. The brain swells, normal tissue is compressed, and secondary events (infarcts, cerebral edema, and tentorial herniation) begin; these may cause death, or bleeding may stop if vessels go into spasm or if the clot acts as a tampon. In patients who survive, the

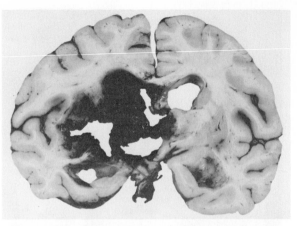

Figure 27-2 Coronal section of a brain showing striatal, capsular, and intraventricular hemorrhage. (Courtesy of John Moossy, M.D., Department of Pathology, Bowman Gray School of Medicine.)

blood eventually resorbs, leaving a cavity or fibrous tissue that may calcify.

When cerebral bleeding is venous in origin or when arterial bleeding ceases soon after onset, tissue is separated to accommodate a local hematoma. Progressive enlargement of this hematoma and increasing cerebral edema may simulate a neoplasm. In some cases, especially those with a small lesion, the hemorrhage is resorbed, leaving chocolate-colored fluid surrounded by a fibroglial wall. Laminated clots, some with calcification in the wall, are indicative of repeated hemorrhages, perhaps of venous origin.

Most of the large intracerebral hemorrhages are fatal, death being caused by flooding of the ventricular system or by swelling of such degree that it causes herniation of the mesial portions of the temporal lobes through the incisura of the tentorium cerebelli. The resultant displacement and compression of the brainstem ruptures veins and small arterioles in its upper portion, leading to hemorrhages, swelling of the midbrain and pons, and death.

Clinical Features

Spontaneous cerebral hemorrhage usually occurs between the ages of 50 and 75 and is slightly more frequent in men than in women. Some of the patients have had previous episodes of infarction or hemorrhage. Almost all are hypertensive, and the blood pressure is usually at a high level at the time the bleeding occurs. The ictus strikes most often during activity but occasionally occurs during sleep. Prodromata which may occur in the hours or days preceding hemorrhage (all probably related to elevated blood pressure) include headaches, syncope, mental deterioration, transient motor or sensory phenomena, retinal hemorrhages, and epistaxis.

In typical cases a hypertensive individual, during active work or in a fit of anger, suddenly complains of light-headedness and headache. He appears bewildered and alarmed and becomes insensible within the hour. Coma is deep, and hemiplegia is profound. Breathing is slow and stertorous; the respiratory cycle, Cheyne-Stokes; the pulse, slow and full. The paralyzed cheek puffs out with each expiration, and saliva drools from the corner of the mouth.

The clinical features of hypertensive cerebral hemorrhage are summarized in the following list:

1 Onset during activity
2 Rapid progression
3 75 percent mortality
4 Residual deficit in patients who survive
5 No neck murmurs (though intracranial murmurs may be present)
6 Retinal hemorrhages and exudates in many patients: papilledema frequent
7 Findings in the cerebrospinal fluid
   a Elevated pressure
   b Bloodstained cerebrospinal fluid (80 percent)
8 Roentgenologic findings
   a Skull film: shift of the pineal gland
   b Arteriogram: shift of the arteries and veins
   c Brain scan may be abnormal

Deep reflexes are absent on one side or both sides in the acute stage, and increased reflexes are rare until hours or days have passed. All four extremities are flaccid, those on the paralyzed side falling limply when dropped. At times the only lateralizing sign is absence of the corneal reflex on one side or a difference in the response to painful stimuli around the mouth. Initially the patient's head and/or eyes are deviated away from the side of the lesion because of cortical irritation. Later the direction of turning is toward the cortical defect so that the patient "is looking toward the lesion."

Pupils vary in size and in their response to light, but if increasing intracranial pressure involves the third nerve, one pupil may become large and fixed to light. Ophthalmoscopy may reveal retinal hemorrhages of all types. Papilledema is a frequent sign, sometimes developing in less than 12 hr.

Fever may be high, especially when the ventricular system is flooded. Vomiting and convulsions are common. *Many intracerebral hemorrhages do not rupture into the subarachnoid space; hence neck resistance and Kernig's sign may not be found.*

If bleeding continues, the patient may reach the terminal stage within hours. If the process becomes stabilized, a vegetative state ensues, and only diligent nursing care can keep the patient alive. A few patients make a remarkable recovery from this state, but the vast majority are never restored to a useful life after prolonged coma has occurred. If the hemorrhage ceases before coma develops, the patient has a better chance for eventual recovery.

In some patients there is a slowly progressive picture evolving over 5 to 10 days.

SPONTANEOUS HEMORRHAGE INTO OTHER PARTS OF THE BRAIN

Thalamic Hemorrhage

Hemorrhage in the thalamus produces contralateral hemisensory loss. If the adjacent internal capsule is involved, there is contralateral hemiparesis. The pupils are small but react to light, and if the subthalamic-diencephalic regions are

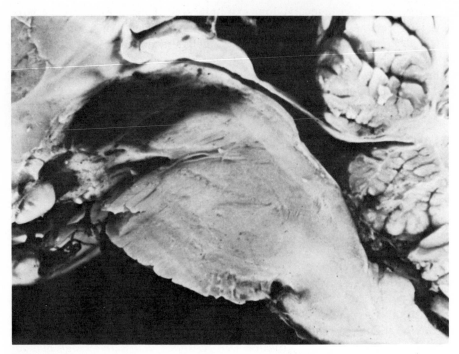

Figure 27-3 Hemorrhage in the midbrain.

involved, there is downward and inward deviation of the eyes.

Hemorrhage into the Brainstem

Midbrain This uncommon occurrence results in ipsilateral oculomotor paralysis and contralateral long-tract signs (Weber's syndrome). If the hemorrhage enlarges, these signs become bilateral and obstruction of the aqueduct of Sylvius leads to loss of consciousness and acute elevation of intracranial pressure (Fig. 27-3).

Pons Varolii With pontine hemorrhage, sudden deep coma without premonitory warning or headache is the rule, and death may occur within hours (Fig. 27-4). Bilateral long-tract signs and decerebrate rigidity are frequent. In earlier stages, contralateral hemiplegia may be

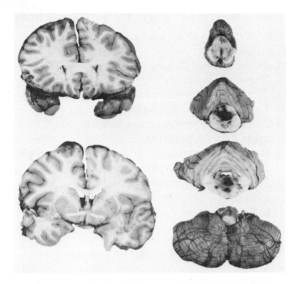

Figure 27-4 Coronal sections of edematous cerebral hemispheres which resulted in herniation of the hippocampal formation. Note the hemorrhage in the pons resulting from venous congestion secondary to the transtentorial herniation.

accompanied by homolateral facial paralysis. In contrast to hemispheric lesions, pontile hemorrhage is usually characterized by permanent deviation of the eyes and head away from the side of the lesion. In bilateral horizontal ocular paralysis, vertical ocular bobbing may occur either spontaneously or following caloric stimulation. In the late stages, a pentad of poor prognostic "P's" persists: paralysis, pulsus parvus, pinpoint pupils, pyrexia, and periodic respiration. These signs are so characteristic of a pontile lesion that the only conditions which need to be considered in the differential diagnosis are narcotic overdosage and ventricular hemorrhage.

Pontine hemorrhages secondary to pressure from supratentorial tumors are common but are usually small and multiple. The neural deficit which they would ordinarily cause is overshadowed by signs of the neoplasm.

Medulla Oblongata This type of hemorrhage is very rare and is rapidly fatal.

Cerebellar Hemorrhage

Clinical recognition of hemorrhage into the cerebellum is essential because this condition is often amenable to surgery (Fig. 27-5). Although death sometimes occurs rapidly, the clinical picture is more often that of an acutely expanding tumor in the posterior fossa with bilateral corticospinal tract signs and evidence of increased intracranial pressure. Oculomotor disturbances, nystagmus, persistent intractable vomiting, or hiccups are clues. Cerebellar signs are frequently absent, and the spinal fluid is often clear. The diagnosis depends primarily on a high index of suspicion, leading to vertebral angiography, air study, and surgery.

Intraventricular Hemorrhage

Primary intraventricular hemorrhage, resulting from rupture of vessels in the choroid plexus, is quite rare. Intraventricular hemorrhage is usu-

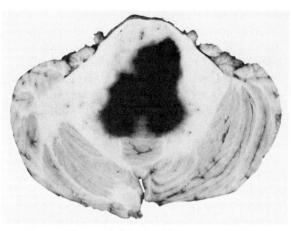

Figure 27-5 Coronal section of a brain showing hypertensive cerebellar hemorrhage with extension into the fourth ventricle. *(Courtesy of John Moossy, M.D., Department of Pathology, Bowman Gray School of Medicine.)*

ally secondary to intracerebral hemorrhage which ruptures into the ventricle. When the intracerebral hemorrhage stops, a clot may develop in the ventricle, obstructing the ventricular pathways and causing rapid increase in pressure. These rare cases can occasionally be cured surgically, but hemorrhage into the ventricle is usually a terminal event associated with deep coma, bilateral corticospinal tract signs, decerebrate rigidity, and hyperthermia.

DIFFERENTIAL DIAGNOSIS

The entities that may be confused with brain hemorrhage are subarachnoid hemorrhage, infarction, hypertensive encephalopathy, and possibly fulminating meningitis or brain abscess.

Because the use of anticoagulants is sometimes advocated as an emergency measure in patients with infarction, the differentiation between infarction and hemorrhage is of great importance. It is also a most difficult one to make. Infarction, like hemorrhage, begins with an acute deficit of normal function; and if the infarct is in the brainstem, coma may ensue rapidly. If the hemorrhage remains encapsulated in the brain, as it does in 15 to 20 percent of large cerebral hemorrhages, no signs of subarachnoid blood will be present, and the differentiation of hemorrhage from infarction may be impossible. Infarction tends to occur during repose, often after a series of premonitory transient ischemic attacks; cerebral hemorrhage, on the other hand, strikes without warning, usually during activity. Patients with infarction may not be hypertensive, although hypertension almost invariably precedes hemorrhage. If papilledema, retinal hemorrhages, or signs of meningeal irritation are present, hemorrhage is almost certain. Kernig's sign is never positive in patients with infarction, and resistance to neck flexion is rare, although it may be found in patients with an incipient cerebellar herniation secondary to brain edema during infarction. The presence of minimal localizing signs, despite deep coma, favors a diagnosis of cerebral hemorrhage over infarction. Initial transient unconsciousness, followed by progressive deterioration of the sensorium, is more in keeping with intracranial hematoma (either extradural, subdural, or intracerebral) than with cerebral infarction.

Although the spinal fluid is usually clear following cerebral infarction, the two conditions cannot always be differentiated on this basis. Hemorrhagic infarcts may cause xanthochromic or slightly bloodstained fluid, while *the spinal fluid remains clear following hemorrhages that remain encapsulated within the brain.* Even angiography may not solve the problem, because infarction can cause cerebral edema which displaces vessels and simulates encapsulated hemorrhage. Enzyme studies on samples of spinal fluid have not proved reliable in the differentiation of the two conditions. Brain scans may prove to be helpful in the differential diagnosis of this problem, but as yet no statistics have been published.

Subarachnoid hemorrhage, unlike cerebral hemorrhage, does not usually produce signs of brain damage as an initial manifestation. If destruction of tissue occurs later on, however, the clinical picture and laboratory findings may be much the same in both. Differentiation is based on the clinical history and on the fact that hypertension is usually less in patients with ruptured aneurysms.

Hypertensive encephalopathy may produce headache, focal neurologic signs, papilledema, and retinal hemorrhages. In the early stages, however, signs of subarachnoid blood are absent and the spinal fluid is clear.

COURSE OF THE DISEASE

Although brain hemorrhage does not produce immediate death, the mortality rate approaches 90 percent, even with the best management.

Petechiae, of course, are tolerated without major disability. Encapsulated hematomas of large size, situated either in the white matter or in the putamen or external capsule, are compatible with recovery and long survival, usually with some neurologic deficit. At times old intracerebral hematomas may cause symptoms suggestive of a slowly expanding intracranial lesion. On skull films, these may appear as calcified tumors, and they can often be removed successfully.

LABORATORY FINDINGS

Primary hemorrhage into the brain may cause leukocytosis, with white blood cell counts ranging from 15,000 to 20,000 per cu mm. Albuminuria, glycosuria, and hyperglycemia may occur as transient phenomena.

Although a lumbar puncture is essential for definitive diagnosis, it is best to forego it when papilledema or third-nerve paresis suggests incipient herniation of the uncus of the temporal lobe, and in cases where a hemorrhage into the posterior fossa is suspected. Lumbar puncture in such cases may precipitate fatal temporal lobe or cerebellar herniation. In most cases of brain hemorrhage, however, a lumbar puncture can be performed safely and the cerebrospinal fluid will be found to be bloodstained and under increased pressure. It must be emphasized, however, that clear fluid is found in 15 to 20 percent of cerebral hemorrhages, because blood has not entered the ventricular system or the subarachnoid space. The protein content of the fluid is often increased; sugar content is variable.

Roentgenograms of the skull may reveal lateral displacement of a calcified pineal gland.

The echoencephalogram is a valuable tool in detecting a lateral shift of the brain when the pineal gland is not calcified.

In comatose patients, electroencephalogram may show diffuse low-voltage slow waves due to pressure, with superimposed focal high-voltage delta activity overlying the hematoma.

A brain scan utilizing technetium ($99m_{Tc}$) at times demonstrates a lesion which may be a hematoma, an arteriovenous malformation, or a neoplasm.

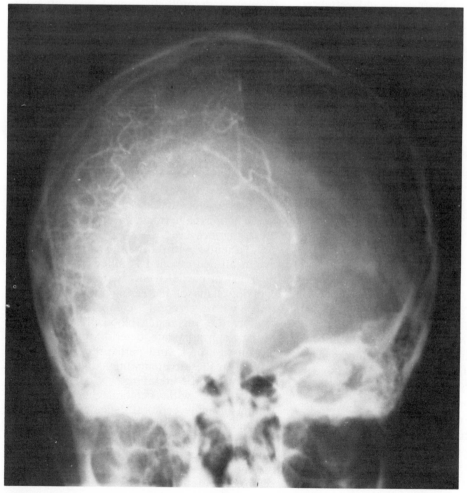

Figure 27-6 Right carotid arteriogram showing displacement of the anterior cerebral artery and its branches by hematoma of the right frontal lobe.

For visualization of a vascular lesion, angiography is necessary. The superficially placed leptomeningeal arteries, such as the anterior and middle cerebral, and the midline cerebral veins, or both may be displaced (Fig. 27-6). An intracerebral hematoma appears as an avascular area surrounded by stretched and displaced cerebral arteries and veins. At times angiography also shows the cause of the hemorrhage by revealing an arteriovenous malformation, an aneurysm, or abnormal vessels in a neoplasm.

Posterior views on brain scan and vertebral angiography may reveal the site of a cerebellar hematoma. When this condition is suspected, however, many prefer ventriculography, since it provides a quicker and more definitive anatomic diagnosis.

MANAGEMENT

The most successful treatment of brain hemorrhage is to prevent it by controlling hypertension. Once bleeding begins, medical treatment cannot stop it; the purpose of therapy is to keep the patient alive and as quiet as possible, in the hope that the hemorrhage will stop (see also Chap. 19).

Medical

General supportive measures, such as parenteral feedings, tracheostomy, anticonvulsant therapy, and the prevention of decubitus ulcers, will be discussed in Chap. 30 on general management. If the patient has been hypertensive in the past, elevated blood pressure should be lowered rapidly to about 140 to 160 mm Hg systolic, 80 to 100 mm Hg diastolic by means of parenteral hypotensive agents. If the hypertension is thought to be the result of elevated intracranial pressure, steroid therapy and surgical intervention must be considered.

The limbs should be exercised, passively or actively, several times daily in bed. Although no data are available to support the impression that strict bed rest should be enforced for at least a month following the ictus, this precaution seems wise. Thereafter gradual ambulation, careful attention to keeping hypertension under control, and a quiet life should be encouraged.

Surgical

For cerebral hemorrhage, removal of blood through a bur hole or evacuation of a clot through a craniotomy should be confined to otherwise healthy individuals whose hypertension is controlled, who are not comatose, and whose lesion lies in the nondominant hemisphere or in the poles of the dominant hemisphere. Evacuation of superficially located intracerebral hematoma may produce dramatic improvement, but those involving the internal capsule or thalamus are best left alone.

There are three groups of patients for whom surgery should be considered:

1 Those with cerebellar hemorrhage. Once this diagnosis is established, prompt evacuation of the hemorrhage is mandatory, for it may be a lifesaving measure.
2 Patients with cerebral hemorrhage in whom an acute deficit is followed by a "lucid interval" of partial recovery, then by gradually evolving signs of increasing intracranial pressure with cerebral compression—namely, bradycardia, increasing blood pressure, diminishing respiratory rate, deterioration in the level of consciousness, and perhaps third-nerve paralysis. In these patients immediate evacuation of a clot may be lifesaving.
3 Patients with cerebral hemorrhage in whom an acute cerebral deficit is followed by gradual recovery. Surgical intervention in such cases is warranted if a mass is demonstrated by contrast studies. It is often difficult, however, to distinguish a hematoma from a hemorrhagic cerebral infarction, in which surgical intervention is not indicated.

SUGGESTED READINGS

Intracerebral Hemorrhage

Etiology and Pathogenesis

Anttinen, E. E.: On the apoplectic conditions occurring among brain injured veterans: Especially regarding the causal relationship between the injury and the vascular accident, *Acta psychiat. neurol. scand.*, **143**(suppl.):1, 1960.

Crompton, M. R.: Intracerebral haematoma complicating ruptured cerebral berry aneurysm, *J. Neurol. Neurosurg. Psychiat.*, **25**:378, 1962.

De Villiers, J. C.: Intracranial haemorrhage in patients treated with monoamine oxidase inhibitors, *Brit. J. Psychiat.*, **112**:109, 1966.

Fisher, C. M.: "The pathology and pathogenesis of intracerebral hemorrhage," in Pathogenesis and Treatment of Cerebrovascular Disease, edited by W. S. Fields, Charles C Thomas, Publisher, Springfield, Ill., 1961, pp. 295-317.

Goodman, S. J., and Becker, D. P.: Intracranial hemorrhage associated with amphetamine abuse, *J.A.M.A.*, **212**:480, 1970.

Gray, O. P., Ackerman, A., and Fraser, A. J.: Intracranial haemorrhage and clotting defects in low-birth-weight infants, *Lancet*, **1**:545, 1968.

Hyland, H. H.: Nonaneurysmal intracranial hemorrhage, *Neurology*, **11**:165, 1961.

Johansson, S. H., and Melin, H. S.: Spontaneous cerebral hemorrhage and encephalomalacia: A clinico-pathological study of 263 cases with special reference to cardiovascular diseases and cerebral atherosclerosis, *Acta psychiat. neurol. scand.*, **35**:457, 1960.

Krayenbühl, H., and Siebenmann, R.: Small vascular malformations as a cause of primary intracerebral hemorrhage, *J. Neurosurg.*, **22**:7, 1965.

Mutlu, N., Berry, R. G., and Alpers, B. J.: Massive cerebral hemorrhage: Clinical and pathological correlations, *Arch. Neurol.*, **8**:644, 1963.

Russell, R. W. R.: Observations on intracerebral aneurysms, *Brain*, **86**:425, 1963.

Silverstein, A.: Intracranial hemorrhage in patients with bleeding tendencies, *Neurology*, 11(part 1):310, 1961.

Symonds, C. P.: Delayed traumatic intracerebral haemorrhage, *Brit. Med. J.*, **1**:1048, 1940.

Pathology

Cole, F. M., and Yates, P. O.: Comparative incidence of cerebrovascular lesions in normotensive and hypertensive patients, *Neurology*, **18**:255, 1968.

————, and ————: The occurrence and significance of intracerebral micro-aneurysms, *J. Pathol. Bacteriol.*, **93**:393, 1967.

————, and ————: Pseudo-aneurysms in relationship to massive cerebral haemorrhage, *J. Neurol. Neurosurg. Psychiat.*, **30**:61, 1967.

Freytag, E.: Fatal hypertensive intracerebral haematomas: A survey of the pathological anatomy of 393 cases, *J. Neurol. Neurosurg. Psychiat.*, **31**:616, 1968.

Clinical Features

Arseni, C., Ionescu, S., Maretsis, M., and Ghitescu, M.: Primary intraparenchymatous hematomas, *J. Neurosurg.*, **27**:207, 1967.

Ciemins, V. A.: Localized thalamic hemorrhage. A cause of aphasia, *Neurology*, **20**:776, 1970.

Goutelle, A., Lapras, C., Trillet, M., Rambaud, G., and Leger, G.: Les hématomes intra-cérébraux revelateurs d'une tumeur cérébrale, *Neurochirurgica*, **12**:218, 1969.

Spontaneous Hemorrhage into Other Parts of the Brain

Hemorrhage into the Brainstem

Chase, T. N., Moretti, L., and Prensky, A. L.: Clinical and electroencephalographic manifestations of vascular lesions of the pons, *Neurology*, **18**:357, 1968.

Cohen, S. I., and Aronson, S. M.: Secondary brain stem hemorrhages. Predisposing and modifying factors, *Arch. Neurol.*, **19**:257, 1968.

Dinsdale, H. B.: Spontaneous hemorrhage in the posterior fossa: A study of primary cerebellar and pontine hemorrhages with observations on their pathogenesis, *Arch. Neurol.*, **10**:200, 1964.

Epstein, A. W.: Primary massive pontine hemorrhage; A clinicopathological study, *J. Neuropathol. Exptl. Neurol.*, **10**:426, 1951.

Klintworth, G. K.: Paratentorial grooving of human brains with particular reference to transtentorial herniation and the pathogenesis of secondary brain stem hemorrhages, *Am. J. Pathol.,* **53**:391, 1968.

Koos, W. T., and Bock, F.: Spontaneous multiple intramedullary hemorrhages. Case report, *J. Neurosurg.,* **32**:581, 1970.

Koos, W. T., Sunder-Plassmann, M., and Salah, S.: Successful removal of a large intrapontine hematoma; case report, *J. Neurosurg.,* **31**:690, 1969.

Martin, P., and Noterman, J.: L'hématome bulbo-protubérantiel opérable, *Acta neurol. psychiat. belg.,* **71**:261, 1971.

Mastaglia, F. L., Edis, B., and Kakulas, B. A.: Medullary haemorrhage: A report of two cases, *J. Neurol. Neurosurg. Psychiat.,* **32**:221, 1969.

Silverstein, A.: Primary pontile hemorrhage—A review of 50 cases, *Confina neurol.,* **29**:33, 1967.

Cerebellar Hemorrhage

Chawla, J. C.: Spontaneous intracerebellar haemorrhage, *Brit. Med. J.,* **1**:93, 1970.

Fairburn, B., and Oliver, L. C.: Cerebellar softening; a surgical emergency, *Brit. Med. J.,* **1**:1335, 1956.

Fisher, C. M., Picard, E. H., Polak, A., Dalal, P., and Ojemann, R. G.: Acute hypertensive cerebellar hemorrhage: Diagnosis and surgical treatment, *J. Nervous Mental Disease,* **140**:38, 1965.

Lichtenstein, R. S.: Spontaneous cerebellar hematomas. A report of three operated cases and review of the literature, *Johns Hopkins Med. J.,* **122**:319, 1968.

McKissock, W., Richardson, A., and Walsh, L.: Spontaneous cerebellar hemorrhage: A study of 34 consecutive cases treated surgically, *Brain,* **83**:1, 1960.

Norris, J. W., Eisen, A. A., and Branch, C. L.: Problems in cerebellar hemorrhage and infarction, *Neurology,* **19**:1043, 1969.

Intraventricular Hemorrhage

Pia, H. W.: "The diagnosis and treatment of intraventricular haemorrhages," in Progress in Brain Research, vol. 30, Cerebral Circulation, edited by W. Luyendijk, Elsevier Publishing Company, Amsterdam, 1968, pp. 463–470.

Loeser, J. D., Stuntz, J. T., and Kelly, W. A.: Sponta-

neous remission of an intraventricular hemorrhage. Case report, *J. Neurosurg.,* **28**:277, 1968.

McConnell, T. H., and Leonard, J. S.: Microangiomatous malformations with intraventricular hemorrhage. Report of two unusual cases, *Neurology,* **17**:618, 1967.

Schurmann, K., Brock, M., and Samii, M.: Circumscribed hematoma of the lateral ventricle following rupture of an intraventricular saccular arterial aneurysm, *J. Neurosurg.,* **29**:195, 1968.

Differential Diagnosis

Achar, V. S., Coe, R. P. K., and Marshall, J.: Echo-encephalography in the differential diagnosis of cerebral haemorrhage and infarction, *Lancet,* **1**:161, 1966.

Aring, C. D., and Merritt, H. H.: Differential diagnosis between cerebral hemorrhage and cerebral thrombosis: A clinical and pathologic study of 245 cases, *Arch. Internal Med.,* **56**:435, 1935.

Kanaya, H., Yamasaki, H., Saiki, I., and Furukawa, K.: The use of echoencephalography to differentiate intracerebral hemorrhage and brain softening, *J. Neurosurg.,* **28**:539, 1968.

McCormick, W. F., and Ugajin, K.: Fatal hemorrhage into a medulloblastoma. Case report, *J. Neurosurg.,* **26**:78, 1967.

Stern, S., Lavy, S., Carmon, A., and Herishianu, Y.: Electrocardiographic patterns in haemorrhagic stroke, *J. Neurol. Sci.,* **8**:61, 1969.

Course of the Disease

Grantham, E. G., and Smolik, E. A.: Calcified intracerebral hematoma, *Ann. Surg.,* **115**:465, 1942.

Margolis, G.: The vascular changes and pathogenesis of hypertensive intracerebral hemorrhage, *Res. Pub. Assoc. Nerv. Ment. Dis.,* **41**:73, 1966.

Merrett, J. D., and Adams, G. F.: Comparison of mortality rates in elderly hypertensive and normotensive hemiplegic patients, *Brit. Med. J.,* **2**:802, 1966.

Mitsuno, T., Kanaya, H., Shirakata, S., Ohsawa, K., and Ishikawa, Y.: Surgical treatment of hypertensive intracerebral hemorrhage, *J. Neurosurg.,* **24**(part 1):70, 1966.

Laboratory Findings

Andersen, P. E.: Angiographic localization of small intracerebral hematomas, *Acta radiol. diagn.,* 1:173, 1963.

Baker, H. L., Jr.: Intracerebral hemorrhage masquerading as a neoplasm: A difficult neuro-radiologic problem, *Radiology,* 78:914, 1962.

Gargano, F. P., Flaten, P. A., and Meringoff, B. N.: The angiographic criteria for the diagnosis of basal ganglionic hemorrhages and their extensions, *Radiology,* 91:1119, 1968.

Guy, G., Simon, J., Javalet, A., Faivre, J., and Pecker, J.: Aspects artériographiques des hématomes intra-cérébraux spontanés. A propos d'une série de 305 cas, *Neuro-Chirurgie,* 15:461, 1969.

Huckman, M. S., Weinberg, P. E., Kim, K. S., and Davis, D. O.: Angiographic and clinico-pathologic correlates in basal ganglionic hemorrhage, *Radiology,* 95:79, 1970.

Leeds, N. E., and Goldberg, H. I.: Lenticulostriate artery abnormalities. Value of direct serial magnification, *Radiology,* 97:377, 1970.

Management

Aurell, M., and Hood, B.: Cerebral hemorrhage in a population after a decade of active antihypertensive treatment, *Acta med. scand.,* 176:377, 1964.

Cook, A. W., Plaut, M., and Browder, J.: Spontaneous intracerebral hemorrhage: Factors related to surgical results, *Arch. Neurol.,* 13:25, 1965.

Cuatico, W., Adib, S., and Gaston, P.: Spontaneous intracerebral hematomas: A surgical appraisal, *J. Neurosurg.,* 22:569, 1965.

Davies, S. H., Turner, J. W., Cumming, R. A., Gillingham, F. J., Girdwood, R. H., and Draig, A.: Management of intracranial hemorrhage in hemophilia, *Brit. Med. J.,* 2:1627, 1966.

Dooley, D. M., and Perlmutter, I.: Spontaneous intracranial hematomas in patients receiving anticoagulation therapy: Surgical treatment, *J.A.M.A.,* 187:396, 1964.

McKissock, W., Richardson, A., and Taylor, J.: Primary intracerebral haemorrhage: A controlled trial of surgical and conservative treatment in 180 unselected cases, *Lancet,* 2:221, 1961.

Meyer, J. S., and Bauer, R. B.: Medical treatment of spontaneous intracranial hemorrhage by use of hypotensive drugs, *Neurology,* 12:36, 1962.

Odom, G. L., Tindall, G. T., Cupp, H. B., Jr., and Woodhall, B.: Neurosurgical approach to intracerebral hemorrhage, *Res. Pub. Assoc. Nerv. Ment. Dis.,* 41:145, 1966.

Olsen, E. R.: Intracranial surgery in hemophiliacs. Report of a case and review of the literature, *Arch. Neurol.,* 21:401, 1969.

Ratnoff, O. D. (ed.): Treatment of Hemorrhagic Disorders, Harper & Row, Publishers, Incorporated, Hoeber Medical Division, New York, 1968.

Additional References

Beevers, D. G., Fairman, M. J., Hamilton, M., and Harpur, J. E.: Antihypertensive treatment and the course of established cerebral vascular disease, *Lancet,* 1:1407, 1973.

Bulter, A. B., Partsan, R. A., and Netsky, M. G.: Primary intraventricular hemorrhage. A mild and remedial form, *Neurology,* 22:675, 1972.

Fisher, C. M.: Pathological observations in hypertensive cerebral hemorrhage, *J. Neuropathol. Exptl. Neurol.,* 30:536, 1971.

Ito, A., Omae, T., and Katsuki, S.: Acute changes in blood pressure following vascular diseases in the brain stem, *Stroke,* 4:80, 1973.

Milhorat, T. H.: Intracerebral hemorrhage, acute hydrocephalus, and systemic hypertension, *J.A.M.A.,* 218:221, 1971.

Morin, M. A., and Pitts, F. W.: Delayed apoplexy following head injury ("traumatische Spät-Apoplexie"), *J. Neurosurg.,* 33:542, 1970.

Richardson, A.: Surgical therapy of spontaneous intracerebral haemorrhage, *Prog. Neurol. Surg.,* 3:397, 1969.

Sharma, S. M. and Quinn, J. L., III: Brain scans in autopsy proved cases of intracerebral hemorrhage, *Arch. Neurol.,* 28:270, 1973.

Yamaguchi, K., Uemura, K., Takahashi, H., Kowada, M., and Kutsuzawa, T.: Intracerebral leakage of contrast medium in apoplexy, *Brit. J. Radiol.,* 44:689, 1971.

Inflammatory Angiopathies

Never attempt to cover up gaps in your knowledge by even the most daring conjectures and hypotheses. No matter how the colorings of this bubble may please your eye, it will inevitably burst leaving you nothing but confusion.

I. P. Pavlov

Although there is evidence to support the belief that the collagen vascular diseases represent autoimmune disorders, the exact causes of the diseases to be discussed in the subsequent pages are not known. Some of them affect the arteries near their origins from the arch of the aorta (Takayasu's disease); others, the medium-sized and small arteries (polyarteritis nodosa); and some, the arterioles, capillaries, and venules (disseminated lupus erythematosus and noninfectious granulomatous angiitis). Even though the clinical features differ, many authorities postulate that the common denominators of all are a genetic predisposition, a challenging stress, and a pathologic reaction of blood vessels. Vessels of a certain location and size presumably contain protein moieties or enzyme systems unique to that type of vessel, and these react in abnormal fashion to antibodies circulating in the blood. Similar necrotizing inflammatory lesions have been produced in the blood vessels of some species of animals who have been sensitized to various agents. These reactions have been the subject of much investigation over the years. Sulfonamides, foreign proteins, hydralazine, broad-spectrum antibiotics, and high doses of desoxycorticosterone acetate can under certain circumstances cause arteritis. Without question other as yet unknown sensitizing agents exist, and perhaps sensitization to one's own body proteins may be the underlying cause in many of these reactions.

The inflammatory vascular diseases can be grouped in a continuum which relates the collagen disorders to the angiitides and even in some instances to the demyelinating diseases. One can begin by considering polyarteritis nodosa, which affects only the small and medium-sized arteries of the central nervous system. Closely related to this is disseminated lupus erythematosus, which affects not only arterioles but also capillaries and venules. This condition resembles acute hemorrhagic leukoencephalopathy, in which there is perivascular demyelinization as well as vasculitis. Other hypersensitivity reactions affect the perivascular myelin primarily, but in some (experimental allergic encephalomyelitis, for example), venules may be involved as well. The appearance of the lesions in different patients ranges from angiitis with minimal involvement of the brain parenchyma to parenchymatous reaction with minimal vasculitis. Therefore, some of these disorders present mixed forms which cannot be classified.

TAKAYASU'S DISEASE

This disease, named for the Japanese ophthalmologist who vividly described the ocular changes that may occur, is known also as *pulseless disease, obliterative brachiocephalic arteritis, the arteritis of young females, aortic arch syndrome, Martorell's syndrome,* and *reversed coarctation syndrome.* The disease is often confined to the aortic arch and great vessels, but at times involves the entire length of the aorta. Takayasu's disease has a strong predilection for women; it is not, as was once believed, restricted to the Orient but has been reported from many parts of the world, almost always in patients between the ages of 15 and 40 years.

Among the conditions that have been considered but not proved to be causes are nutritional deficiency, tuberculosis, syphilis, collagen disease, nonspecific allergic reaction, rheumatic fever, and autoimmune diseases.

Pathologic Findings

Most commonly involved are the aortic arch and the brachiocephalic, common carotid, and subclavian arteries, but the intracranial segments of these arteries and their branches are spared. The disease may also affect the celiac, superior mesenteric, and renal arteries or the aortic bifurcation.

The vascular lesion is characterized by patchy intimal thickening, longitudinal scarring, and segmental changes that produce narrowing of the lumen or aneurysmal dilatation. Thrombosis of the vessel is common, and evidence of recanalization is often present. Microscopically, one sees a chronic inflammatory process involving all three coats of the artery. Active lesions show edema; fragmentation of the tunica elastica; and focal or diffuse collections of lymphocytes, plasma cells, macrophages, and Langhans' giant cells. Follicles containing these elements are common, but there is no caseation (Fig. 28-1). The endarteritis and perivascular cuffing of syphilis are never seen. Common sequelae of the arteritis are weakening of the artery with aneurysm formation or progressive stenosis of the artery culminating in occlusion with infarction of distal tissue.

In contrast to other arteritides, to be described in subsequent sections of this chapter, Takayasu's disease spares the smaller arteries and arterioles.

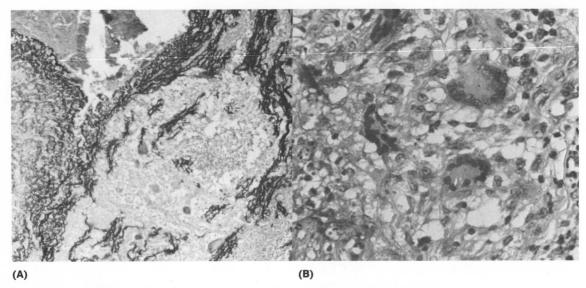

(A)   **(B)**

Figure 28-1 Histologic appearance of an artery in Takayasu's disease. (A) Destruction of the arterial wall. (B) Granulomatous changes with giant cells. (magnification × 100) *(Courtesy of Professor K. Sano.)*

Clinical Features

Three aortic syndromes, occurring singly or in combination, have been distinguished:

1 The aortic arch (Takayasu's) syndrome, involving the arch and the great vessels and resulting in neurologic and ophthalmic abnormalities.
2 The middle aortic syndrome, involving the celiac, superior mesenteric, and renal arteries and resulting in abdominal angina, malabsorption syndrome, and renal hypertension.
3 The aortic bifurcation (Leriche's) syndrome, involving the terminal aorta and the iliac arteries, and producing intermittent claudication of the hips and lower limbs and, in males, impotence secondary to failure of tumescence.

In this section only the aortic arch syndrome is discussed; the reader should bear in mind, however, that the other two syndromes may also occur in the same individual.

The classic picture of a young Oriental girl with head-low posture, alopecia, conjunctival injection, and frequent attacks of syncope, vertigo, and visual disturbances is seldom seen. Some cases have their onset with constitutional symptoms such as asthenia, lassitude, fatigue, vague musculoskeletal pain, arthralgias, anorexia, anemia, and weight loss, or with recurring headaches or pain over the region of the involved arteries. More commonly, however, the presenting symptoms are those due to carotid or subclavian-vertebral disease manifested by cerebrovascular insufficiency or infarction. Some of the patients have such low blood pressures and flow in the retinal and cerebral arteries that they assume a head-low posture to increase flow and improve vision.

Examination may reveal absence of the subclavian, brachial, and radial pulses; or the brachial blood pressure may be reduced or absent, and pulsations in the carotid arteries may be absent or impaired. The carotid sinuses are often hypersensitive. Pulsations, thrills, and bruits in the collateral vessels of the head, neck, or chest suggest an obstructive lesion of the aortic

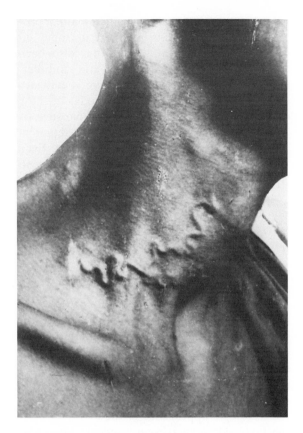

Figure 28-2 Dilated arterial collaterals in a patient with Takayasu's disease. *(Courtesy of Dr. M. S. Hirsch; reprinted from Bull. Johns Hopkins Hosp., 115:35, 1964.)*

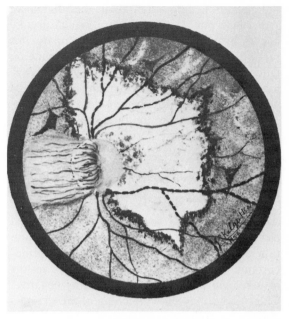

Figure 28-3 Funduscopic appearance in Takayasu's disease, showing segmentation of the blood column ("cattle-tracking" or "boxcar" appearance) and neovascularization. *(Courtesy of Dean, G. S. Medical College, Bombay, India.)*

arch and its major branches, but they are not specific for this syndrome (Fig. 28-2). Trophic changes such as perforation of the nasal septum, alopecia, and ulceration of the oral mucous membranes sometimes develop when blood flow to the head has been severely jeopardized.

About 50 percent of patients have systemic hypertension. This incidence would probably be higher if the blood pressure were recorded routinely in the lower extremities.

Funduscopic examination may show evidence of stasis of the blood column, with segmentation of the retinal arterioles and veins (the so-called "cattle-tracking" or "boxcar" appear- ance) (Fig. 28-3). Characteristic peripapillary neovascularization and arteriovenous anastomoses may also be present. Cataracts are common. If the carotid is involved on one side or both sides, the pressure in one or both of the ophthalmic arteries may be low or unrecordable.

Differential Diagnosis

The triad of findings on which a diagnosis of Takayasu's disease may be based are (1) stenosis or occlusion of more than one of the aortocranial arteries in a young woman; (2) hypersensitive carotid sinuses; and (3) ophthalmoangiopathy (including hyperemia of the bulbar conjunctivae or rubeosis oculi, neovascularization and anastomoses of the retinal arterioles, and cataracts). Low-grade fever and an elevated sedimentation rate strengthen the diagnosis. Atherosclerotic vascular disease, which usually occurs in older individuals, can simulate this picture. Differentiation can usually be made on clinical grounds. However, diabetes mellitus, hypothyroidism, or oophorectomy in a young woman will accelerate atherosclerosis and, except for the sedimentation rate, cause an identical picture. Syphilitic aortitis can be diagnosed by a previous history, other manifestations of syphilis, and positive serologic reactions.

Laboratory Findings

Almost all patients have moderate to marked elevation of their erythrocyte sedimentation rate, and about half show a normocytic, normochromic anemia with leukocytosis. The results of serologic studies for syphilis are negative. Chest x-rays may show notching of the ribs secondary to collateral circulation. Aortography demonstrates various degrees of stenosis or occlusion of the subclavian, brachiocephalic, carotid, and vertebral arteries. In some patients obstruction of the proximal subclavian or brachiocephalic artery produces reversal of blood flow in the vertebral artery, resulting in symptoms and signs of vertebral-basilar artery insufficiency (subclavian steal). Biopsy of an involved artery may be necessary for definitive diagnosis.

Course and Prognosis

This disease, protean in its manifestations, is unpredictable in its course. In the majority of cases, the course is one of progressive, relentless compromise of cerebral blood flow, leading eventually to permanent crippling. Though the process sometimes seems to be arrested, it may flare up at any time.

Treatment

Although there is no specific treatment for Takayasu's disease, corticosteroids in high doses have been used to halt the inflammatory process, with good results reported in some instances. Anticoagulant therapy has also been employed with equivocal results, and antituberculous therapy is given when there is evidence of tuberculosis elsewhere in the body. In those patients who have surgically accessible stenotic lesions, the most effective measure is repair of the affected artery or bypass of the lesion. Even in patients with fairly extensive involvement, bypass grafts have functioned well for some years. The long-range prognosis in such cases is not known, however, and lesions situated elsewhere in the body may become symptomatic at any time.

CRANIAL ARTERITIS

Known also as *giant-cell* or *temporal arteritis*, this inflammatory form of cerebrovascular disease is one of the causes of headache in people older than 50 years and may be responsible for sudden visual loss and brain infarction. Though it is usually classified as a collagen disorder, the only evidences supporting this classification are the histologic appearance of the artery or arteries involved, an increase in concentration of alpha$_2$-globulins and the dramatic response to corticosteroids. No serum factor similar to that found in rheumatoid arthritis or diagnostic cell, such as that for systemic lupus erythematosus, has been demonstrated. It is said to be a rare disease in tropical climates.

Pathologic Findings

This disorder almost always affects the branches of the external and/or internal carotids, but it may occasionally involve the vertebral-basilar system, the arteries of the upper and lower extremities, the aorta, and rarely the coronary arteries as well. Probably no part of any large or medium-sized artery is exempt. The arteritis is patchy in distribution, with normal segments of artery lying between severely affected areas.

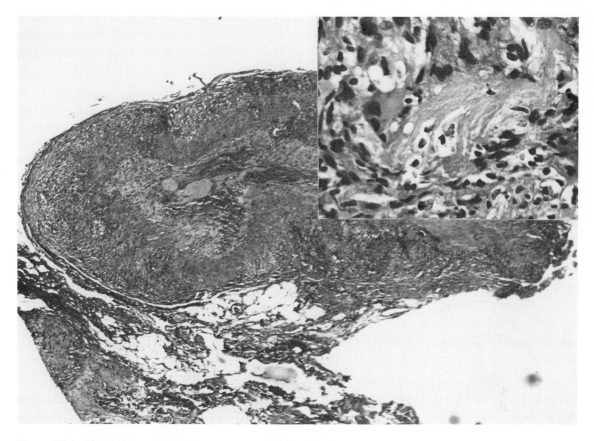

Figure 28-4 Photomicrograph of temporal artery biopsy. *Insert:* detail of giant cells. *(Reprinted from D. C. Mann and J. F. Toole, Cranial arteritis with liver involvement, Stroke, **3**: 131, 1972; by permission of The American Heart Association, Inc.)*

Histologically, changes are seen in the intima and media (Fig. 28-4), the internal elastic membrane being degenerated and infiltrated with lymphocytes, plasma cells, macrophages, and giant cells of the foreign-body type. Neutrophils are usually absent. Fibroblastic proliferation results in thickening of the wall and narrowing or obliteration of the vessel lumen, and granulomatous panarteritis develops. Damage to the intima may lead to mural thrombosis and arterial occlusion.

A few investigators believe that the histopathologic changes cannot be differentiated from those of polyarteritis nodosa and would classify the two diseases as variants of the same condition. Syphilitic arteritis has also been shown to mimic cranial arteritis. Muscle and skin biopsies of patients suffering with cranial arteritis are uniformly normal.

Clinical Features

Cranial arteritis affects both men and women over the age of 60 about equally. Peak incidence occurs between 65 and 75 years of age. Almost any segment of the cranial arterial tree may be affected, but symptoms are most frequently related to involvement of the temporal, ophthalmic, and occipital arteries, one of which is almost always involved at some stage of the disease. Most commonly affected are the superficial temporal arteries.

The most frequent clinical picture is that of a middle-aged or elderly individual with fever, vague myalgia, constitutional symptoms, and a tender temporal artery. He is suffering with a severe headache, is unable to sleep, and is completely incapacitated by the illness. The involved artery, which is exquisitely tender to touch, is thickened like a cord and difficult to compress. It is hypopulsatile and in advanced cases may have no pulse whatsoever (Fig. 28-5). The overlying skin is sometimes normal but

may be red, hot, and edematous. Ischemia of the skin with resultant areas of necrosis is rare. The following symptoms and signs are characteristic:

Head and Face Pain Cranial arteritis usually produces an intense, unremitting pain over the affected artery. The patient often distinguishes it from headache and characterizes it as a pain. It may be so severe that brushing the hair and lying down to sleep are impossible. Chewing may aggravate the pain by irritating the tender, narrowed temporal arteries that lie atop the contracting temporalis muscles, or by causing muscle ischemia with claudication. The discom-

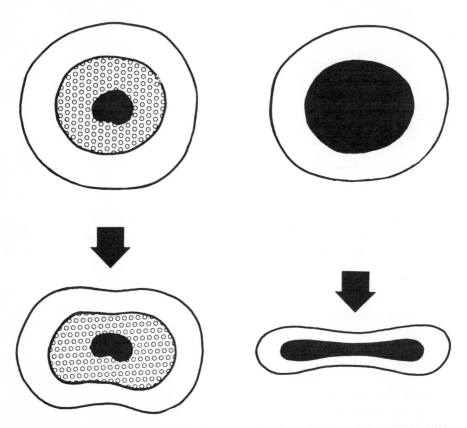

Figure 28-5 Palpation of superficial temporal artery. The artery on the right is normally compressible. The one on the left depicts a thickened artery with decreased compressibility.

fort may involve the face as well or the face alone.

Visual Phenomena   At times headache is of minor degree or even absent, and the clinical picture is dominated by visual or systemic manifestations which are due to involvement of the carotid, ophthalmic, or retinal arteries. In one series this situation was found in 40 percent of patients who complained primarily of visual abnormality and only secondarily of head or face pain. The usual manifestation is sudden loss of vision in one eye—either a scotoma or amaurosis. This is caused by occlusion of a branch of the central artery of the retina or of the ophthalmic artery itself. If the ophthalmic or other intracranial branches of the internal carotid artery are involved, conjunctival edema, periorbital swelling, photophobia, blurred vision, diplopia, ocular palsy, homonymous field defect, and amaurosis fugax occur.

Funduscopic examination in patients who have suffered occlusion of the central retinal artery shows attenuated arterioles and veins which are at least partially exsanguinated. The optic nerve is pale due to ischemia. Although the retina itself is pale and edematous, the macula appears normally red. Within 24 to 48 hr of occlusion, exudates and hemorrhages appear and a mild degree of papillitis may develop. If only a branch of the central retinal artery has been occluded, this sequence of events is produced in the area supplied by the occluded arteriole.

Visual impairment occurs in slightly less than half the cases of cranial arteritis, and may be altitudinal in nature if retinal arteriolar branch occlusion has occurred. If the ophthalmic artery or central retinal artery is affected, the eye is blind. This unfortunate condition is permanent in 15 to 20 percent of patients in whom it occurs. Unfortunately, involvement of one eye is a prelude to involvement of the other in almost 10 percent of the cases.

Systemic Manifestations   Symptoms such as malaise, lassitude, asthenia, and weight loss are frequent. Some patients have fever (100 to 101°F) and night sweats. In rare cases the predominant feature is mental change (depression, confusion, and mood disorders) secondary to brain infarction and edema caused by arteritis. A few patients have cerebral or myocardial infarction as the initial manifestation.

Polymyalgia Rheumatica   This systemic process is closely associated with cranial arteritis and may in fact be a part of the same disease process. It is characterized by myalgias of a migratory nature, possibly accompanied by arthralgia or neuralgia as well. The patient feels ill and has an elevated erythrocyte sedimentation rate and may have a low-grade fever. Neuromuscular examination is normal, as are electromyography, creatine phosphokinase, serum glutamic-oxalacetic transaminase, and aldolase. Muscle biopsy is normal.

Laboratory Findings

The erythrocyte sedimentation rate is almost invariably elevated, sometimes to as much as 100 mm in an hour. It reaches a peak during the acute inflammatory phase and may continue to be elevated for more than a year. In patients with a normal sedimentation rate, the diagnosis of active cranial arteritis is very unlikely.

About 50 percent of the patients have mild leukocytosis and a normocytic, normochromic anemia. There may be an increase in the $alpha_2$- or beta-globulins, as is found in collagen disorders.

Biopsy of the affected artery shows the characteristic inflammatory response and, depending on the stage of the illness, a varying degree of occlusion of the lumen by fibrosis and thrombosis. It is important to recognize that segmental distribution of the arteritis may lead to false-negative biopsies. Removal of a specimen for diagnosis occasionally relieves local pain by severing the adventitial nerves surrounding the inflamed artery.

Rarely, removal of an arterial segment results in cerebral infarction if that artery served as a source for the collateral blood supply to the brain. Biopsy of the involved artery is considered essential only in atypical cases or in patients who have visual disturbances alone. In typical instances, the diagnosis can be made on the basis of the clinical picture, the elevated sedimentation rate, and the response to steroid therapy.

Course and Prognosis

If untreated, cranial arteritis usually persists for many months before subsiding. For some patients the illness is completely debilitating. About 50 percent are left with partial or total blindness, and about 20 percent die from cerebral or myocardial infarction. The remainder, however, regain their former health and vigor.

The course of cranial arteritis is dramatically shortened and the prognosis vastly improved by steroid therapy. Fever may subside within hours, and local pain and constitutional signs resolve completely within 1 or 2 days. Appetite returns and, along with it, the patient's feeling of well-being.

Treatment

It is important to make the diagnosis of cranial arteritis and begin treatment before the inflammation spreads to the arteries supplying the retina. Once visual symptoms begin, the prognosis for recovery of vision is poor. It is extremely unusual for visual loss to occur after the initiation of steroid therapy, and a daily dose of 4 to 6 mg dexamethasone or 40 to 60 mg prednisone in divided doses should be initiated as soon as the diagnosis is made. In patients with visual loss, 40 units ACTH daily in an intravenous drip should be given during the first week, in addition to the oral steroids.

When symptoms have disappeared and the patient has been afebrile and without headache for about 1 week, the daily dose of steroids is gradually reduced to a maintenance level of 2½ mg (for dexamethasone) or 5 mg (for prednisone). After the sedimentation rate has been normal for some months, therapy is gradually withdrawn; if symptoms recur, however, steroids should be resumed promptly.

POLYARTERITIS NODOSA

The cause of polyarteritis nodosa is not known, but there is evidence to suggest that an infection such as Australia antigen may trigger an autoimmune reaction involving the medium-sized and small arteries which contain a well-developed muscularis. The classical descriptions of the disease note the systemic nature of the arteritis but stress that the pulmonary circulation is usually spared. The peripheral nervous system is usually affected and at times may be the only neurological manifestation of the disease.

Pathologic Findings

There is a widespread misconception that polyarteritis nodosa seldom affects the central nervous system, yet 8 to 46 percent of cases seen at autopsy show involvement of the arteries of the brain. The intracranial lesions may cause subarachnoid or intracerebral hemorrhage, hemorrhagic infarction, or multiple small hemorrhages distributed throughout the hemispheres. The brain is swollen, and on cut section, multiple infarctions of various sizes and in various distributions may be seen. The picture is therefore variable, and there is no characteristic appearance to the brain. There is inflammation of the adventitia and muscularis of the arteries, which are infiltrated with polymorphonuclear cells, lymphocytes, eosinophils, and reactive fibroblastic proliferation. The arterioles are thickened, and the lumen of the vessel is small and eccentrically placed, and may be occluded with thrombus. There may be infarction of tissue normally perfused by the diseased artery.

Clinical Features

This disease is more common in men than in women, by a ratio of 4:1, and usually has its onset between the ages of 20 and 40. Symptoms and signs secondary to involvement of the central nervous system are seldom the initial manifestations of polyarteritis nodosa. Myalgia, polymyositis, anemia, and fever almost always precede symptoms of central nervous system involvement by months or years. Renal disease with secondary hypertension is another frequent initial manifestation. Peripheral nerves are involved in about 50 percent of patients, with either a generalized symmetrical polyneuropathy or mononeuritis multiplex.

Of the symptoms referable to the central nervous system, headaches of variable severity, duration, and location are the most common presenting manifestations. Headache is not necessarily due to the disease itself but may be related to the hypertension. Signs of an organic psychosis and dementia such as confusion, disorientation, and behavior disorders are particularly prominent features of central nervous system involvement. Convulsions, either focal or generalized, are frequent.

In addition to the above symptoms and signs of diffuse involvement of the brain, a variable constellation of neurologic phenomena may occur as the result of obstruction of any of the intracranial arteries. These may be surface arteries or perforating branches. Obstruction of a major artery, such as the basilar, results in sudden disastrous neurologic deficit. If the wall of a surface artery is weakened, aneurysmal dilatation can result and rupture may occur. Parenchymal vessels may rupture and produce an intracerebral or intracerebellar hemorrhage. These hemorrhages are, at least in part, related to the hypertension which almost always accompanies the illness.

Cranial nerves may be affected selectively, and at times the initial neurologic manifestation may be related to paralysis of one of them. Facial palsy, deafness, and paralysis of one or more of the ocular nerves may be found.

It is to be emphasized that the neurologic manifestations are only a feature of the more generalized illness, which is accompanied by fever, anorexia with weight loss, pain in the joints and muscles, cutaneous eruption with purpura or ecchymoses, and subcutaneous nodules of erythema nodosum. At times involved arteries themselves may be seen over the dorsum of the hand, and they may be tender to palpation. Renal involvement occurs early and is manifested by flank pain, hematuria, azotemia, and hypertension.

Changes in the optic fundus are commonly seen. Some, such as spasm of the arterioles and hemorrhages and exudates, are secondary to hypertension; others, such as papilledema, are the result of increased intracranial pressure and brain swelling. Occlusion of the central retinal artery or its branches may result in sudden loss of vision.

Many pathologists would differentiate from this characteristic picture of polyarteritis a separate syndrome, *Wegener's granulomatosis*, which preferentially involves the respiratory tract, kidneys, and central nervous system. The distinguishing feature of Wegener's granulomatosis is involvement of the upper and lower parts of the respiratory tract characterized by recurrent sinusitis and ulceration of the mucous membranes, with concomitant bronchopulmonary involvement secondary to arteritis. The histologic changes in the arteries are indistinguishable from those of polyarteritis, and the neurologic complications which occur are similar to it.

Laboratory Findings

Anemia, leukocytosis with eosinophilia, and an elevated erythrocyte sedimentation rate are seen in almost all cases. The urine frequently contains protein, red blood cells, and very characteristic red blood cell casts, which are highly suggestive of the illness. The total protein level in the blood may be elevated, normal, or low, with a relatively increased proportion of globulin. Lumbar puncture usually reveals spinal fluid pressure to be normal; the spinal fluid often contains an increased amount of protein, and at times abnormal numbers of lymphocytes and polymorphonuclear cells. In the rare patient with subarachnoid hemorrhage, blood-stained fluid may be seen.

The electroencephalogram is often abnormal, showing focal slow waves of a nonspecific nature. The skull x-ray is normal, as is the brain scan.

Tissue diagnosis is obtained by performing a biopsy of involved tissue, such as skeletal muscle, skin, kidney, or testicle.

Course and Treatment

Polyarteritis nodosa usually has an explosive onset in middle age, and the course is often rapidly downhill. About 50 percent of affected individuals have a remission up to several years in duration, appearing usually in the first year. Renal impairment develops early and is accompanied by intractable hypertension. Death is frequently caused by renal decompensation or effects secondary to the hypertension, such as intracerebral hemorrhage or myocardial infarction. All medications which could possibly precipitate or aggravate the disorder must be stopped. Among these are hydralazine, the sulfonamides, and certain antibiotics.

Treatment with corticosteroids is effective as a temporary measure and may slow the course of the illness but does not affect the end result, which usually occurs within a few years. Steroids may control inflammation but not progressive narrowing of vessels, which may ultimately become occluded, producing infarction.

DISSEMINATED LUPUS ERYTHEMATOSUS

The cause of disseminated lupus erythematosus (DLE) is not known, although myxovirus particles have been isolated in some instances. Any of the collagen tissues or vascular beds of the body may be affected, but certain organs are usually involved more extensively than others. In some patients it is the skin; in others, the kidneys, spleen, liver, or lungs. Although peripheral neuropathy is the most common neurologic complication, involvement of the central nervous system does occur. Rarely it may be the presenting manifestation of DLE.

Pathologic Findings

The peritoneal, pleural, and pericardial surfaces are usually involved with inflammatory reaction, adhesions, and effusion. The heart is often enlarged, and the mitral and aortic valves may show verrucous vegetations, but the great vessels are not affected. When the central nervous system is affected, the brain or spinal cord may be edematous, with thickened meninges, and one or more of the large arteries at the base of the brain may be stenotic or even occluded. When the brain is cut, areas of ischemic infarction and petechial hemorrhages may be seen scattered in the hemispheres and brainstem.

The arterioles, capillaries, and venules of the gray and white matter are diffusely involved with an inflammatory reaction. Many are occluded by thrombus consisting of blood clot, fibrinoid material, or aggregations of platelets which cause microinfarctions in the brain parenchyma.

Clinical Features

Whereas polyarteritis nodosa predominantly affects men, DLE affects women between the ages of 15 and 40 years, with a sex ratio of 4:1.

Malar eruption (butterfly rash), arthralgia, myalgia, and neuralgia are its hallmarks. In some patients the arthritic manifestations predominate; in others, symmetric peripheral neuropathy or a proximal myopathy takes precedence. The most frequent neurologic manifestation is that of a symmetric peripheral neuropathy. In at least 2 percent of patients, seizures may be the first symptom, and as many as 30 percent have seizures during the course of the disease. Further signs of central nervous system disorder, such as psychosis or infarctions, develop later in many more.

The presenting picture may be that of an acute organic psychosis with convulsions, mental confusion, delirium, and increased intracranial pressure. Acute brainstem infarction or transverse myelitis is a rare manifestation of the illness.

Funduscopic examination may reveal vascular retinopathy and cytoid bodies.

An occasional patient may have hepatitis with secondary hepatic encephalopathy or signs of hypersplenism, thrombocytopenic purpura, and intracranial bleeding. Thrombotic thrombocytopenic purpura *(Moschcowitz disease)*, in which platelet thrombi plug arterioles and capillaries, particularly in the vessels of the central nervous system, is thought by many to be a variant of disseminated lupus erythematosus.

Laboratory Findings

Fever, anemia (normochromic, hypochromic, or hemolytic), increased sedimentation rate, a false-positive serology, and at times thrombocytopenia are nonspecific findings which may suggest the illness. The specific test for diagnosis of the disease is the presence of the lupus erythematosus cell and fluorescent antibodies in the blood or bone marrow. Most clinicians agree that this cell must be found before the diagnosis can be made with confidence (Fig. 28-6).

Chest x-rays may show nonspecific increase in bronchovascular markings with evidence of pulmonary fibrosis. Skull x-ray is normal. Elec-

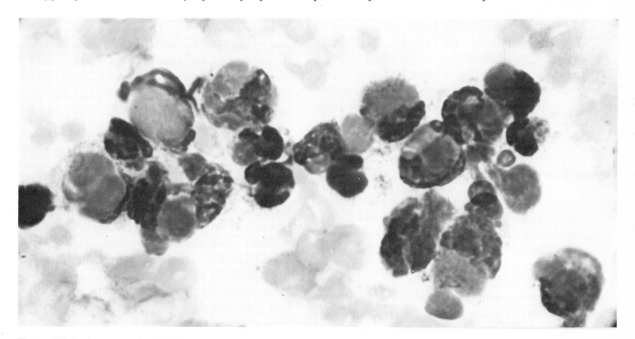

Figure 28-6 Lupus erythematosus cells in a peripheral blood smear.

troencephalograms are frequently abnormal, showing both focal and generalized dysrhythmia.

If tissue diagnosis is needed, muscle or renal biopsy or both may reveal characteristic vascular changes. Examination of the cerebrospinal fluid reveals no abnormality unless the patient has symmetric peripheral neuropathy or myelopathy, in which case the protein in the spinal fluid may be increased and there may be pleocytosis with abnormal colloidal-gold-curve reactions.

Differential Diagnosis

The differentiation of the systemic manifestations of disseminated lupus erythematosus is not germane to this text. Rarely the patient who has had no other symptoms or signs of the disease may present a clinical picture of increased intracranial pressure, mental change, and convulsions, which suggests encephalitis. In other patients elevated pressure causes headache and papilledema simulating a brain tumor.

When convulsions are the neurologic manifestation, the diagnosis of lupus erythematosus depends on the finding of other signs and symptoms of disseminated lesions. The diagnosis of multiple sclerosis might be entertained in some patients until the lupus erythematosus cells are found in the peripheral blood.

Course and Treatment

The course of the untreated disease is variable, with about three-fourths of the patients surviving more than 1 year but only one-fifth surviving more than 5 years. Spontaneous remission, which occurs in 40 percent, may be repeated in 20 percent.

The most common mode of death in patients with chronic lupus erythematosus is an intercurrent infection with renal failure.

Corticosteroid therapy slows the progression of the illness and in some patients may keep it under control for years.

NONINFECTIOUS GRANULOMATOUS ANGIITIS

Noninfectious granulomatous angiitis involves leptomeningeal arteries and veins, as well as their penetrating branches, in a manner similar to that of disseminated lupus erythematosus. However, it does not affect other organs of the body. No etiologic agent has been found, although some investigators suspect hypersensitivity or autoimmune reaction.

Pathologic Findings

The intima of small cerebral arteries and veins is thickened and infiltrated with lymphocytes, mononuclear cells, fibroblasts, and occasional giant cells. Proliferation narrows the vessel lumen, and the brain parenchyma shows small areas of rarefaction with loss of neurons and occasional small infarcts distributed throughout the cerebrum, brainstem, and cerebellum.

Clinical Features

The disease affects adults of both sexes equally and runs a fatal course which varies in duration from a few days to about 2 years. It is characterized by headache and convulsions, rapid mental deterioration with stupor and coma, and multifocal signs of neurologic deficit. Temporary remissions may occur.

Laboratory Findings

Low-grade fever and elevated sedimentation rate are found. Skull x-rays and results of contrast studies and blood cultures are normal, and lupus erythematosus cells are never found. Electroencephalograms show diffuse high-voltage slow-wave activity. Cerebrospinal fluid may be under slightly increased pressure and often contains minimally increased amounts of protein and lymphocytes.

Diagnosis and Treatment

The disease is said to be difficult to distinguish from viral or fungal meningoencephalitis; yet the differentiation is not academic. In a patient whose cerebrospinal fluid shows no characteristic changes and in whom appropriate x-rays for intracranial tumor or studies for collagen vascular disease are not diagnostic, brain biopsy may be performed. If inflammatory angiitis is found, corticosteroids should probably be given.

SUGGESTED READINGS

General

Adams, R. D., and Michelsen, J. J.: "Inflammatory lesions of the blood vessels of the brain," in Proceedings of the First International Congress of Neuropathology, vol. 1, Rome, 1952, Rosenberg & Sellier, Torino, 1954, pp. 347-351.

D'Cruz, I. A., Kulkarni, T. P., Gandhi, M. J., Juthani, V. J., and Murti, P. K.: Aortitis of unknown etiology, *Angiology,* **21**:49, 1970.

Glaser, G. H.: Collagen diseases and the nervous system, *Med. Clin. N. Am.,* **47**:1475, 1963.

Hedges, T. R.: The aortic arch syndromes, *Arch. Ophthalmol.,* **71**:28, 1964.

Kampmeier, R. H.: Collagen diseases—Unanswered questions on pathogenesis and etiology, *Arch. Internal Med.,* **106**:753, 1960.

Lee, J. E., and Haynes, J. M.: Carotid arteritis and cerebral infarction due to scleroderma, *Neurology,* **17**:18, 1967.

Torvik, A., and Berntzen, A. E.: Necrotizing vasculitis without visceral involvement. Postmortem examination of three cases with affection of skeletal muscles and peripheral nerves, *Acta med. scand.,* **184**:69, 1968.

Takayasu's Disease

General

Broadbent, W. H.: Absence of pulsation in both radial arteries, vessels being full of blood, *Trans. Clin. Soc. London,* **8**:165, 1875.

Martorell, F.: The syndrome of occlusion of the supra-aortic trunks, *J. Cardiovascular Surg.,* **2**:291, 1961.

Sen, P. K., Kinare, S. G., Engineer, S. D., and Parulkar, G. B.: The middle aortic syndrome, *Brit. Heart J.,* **25**:610, 1963.

Shimizu, K., and Sano, K.: Pulseless disease, *J. Neuropathol. Clin. Neurol.,* **1**:37, 1951.

Takayasu, M.: Case with peculiar changes of the central retinal vessels, *Acta Soc. Ophthalmol. Jap.,* **12**:554, 1908.

Etiology

Ask-Upmark, E.: Case of Takayasu's syndrome accelerated (initiated?) by oral contraceptives, *Acta med. scand.,* **185**:119, 1969.

Asherson, R. A., Asherson, G. L., and Schrire, V.: Immunological studies in arteritis of the aorta and the great vessels, *Brit. Med. J.,* **3**:589, 1968.

Hirsch, M. S., Aikat, B. K., and Basu, A. K.: Takayasu's arteritis: Report of five cases with immunologic studies, *Bull. Johns Hopkins Hosp.,* **115**:29, 1964.

Kinare, S. G.: Aortitis in early life in India and its association with tuberculosis, *J. Pathol.,* **100**:69, 1970.

Nakao, K., Ikeda, M., Kimata, S., Niitani, H., Miyahara, M., Ishimi, Z., Hashiba, K., Takeda, Y., Ozawa, T., Matsushita, S., and Kuramochi, M.: Takayasu's arteritis. Clinical report of eighty-four cases and immunological studies of seven cases, *Circulation,* **35**:1141, 1967.

Riehl, J. L., and Brown, W. J.: Takayasu's arteritis: An autoimmune disease, *Arch. Neurol.,* **12**:92, 1965.

Pathology

Nasu, T.: Pathology of pulseless disease: A systematic study and critical review of twenty-one autopsy cases reported in Japan, *Angiology,* **14**:225, 1963.

Clinical Features

Currier, R. D., DeJong, R. N., and Bole, G. C.: Pulseless disease: Central nervous system manifestations, *Neurology,* **4**:818, 1954.

Strachan, R. W.: The natural history of Takayasu's arteriopathy, *Quart. J. Med.,* **33**:57, 1964.

Ueda, H. S., Morooka, S., Ito, I., Yamaguchi, H., Takeda, T., and Saito, Y.: Clinical observations of 52 cases of aortitis syndrome, *Jap. Heart J.,* **10**:277, 1969.

Roentgenology

Paloheimo, J. A.: Obstructive arteritis of Takayasu's type. Clinical, roentgenological and laboratory studies on 36 patients, *Acta med. scand.* **181**(suppl. 468), 1967.

Sano, K., Aiba, T., and Saito, I.: Angiography in pulseless disease, *Radiology,* **94**:69, 1970.

Treatment

Inada, K., Katsumura, T., Hirai, J., and Sunada, T.: Surgical treatment in the aortitis syndrome, *Arch. Surg.,* **100**:220, 1970.

Cranial Arteritis

Bevan, A. T., Dunnill, M. S., and Harrison, M. J. G.: Clinical and biopsy findings in temporal arteritis, *Ann. Rheum. Dis.,* **27**:271, 1968.

Birkhead, N. C., Wagener, H. P., and Shick, R. M.: Treatment of temporal arteritis with adrenal corticosteroids; results in fifty-five cases in which lesion was proved at biopsy, *J.A.M.A.,* **163**:821, 1957.

Crompton, M. R.: The visual changes in temporal (giant-cell) arteritis: Report of a case with autopsy findings, *Brain,* **82**:377, 1959.

————: Giant-cell arteritis: General and neurologic aspects, *World Neurol.,* **2**:237, 1961.

Cullen, J.: Occult temporal arteritis. A common cause of blindness in old age, *Brit. J. Ophthalmol.,* **51**:513, 1967.

Desser, E. J.: Miosis, trismus, and dysphagia. An unusual presentation of temporal arteritis, *Ann. Internal Med.,* **71**:961, 1969.

Fisher, C. M.: Ocular palsy in temporal arteritis, *Minnesota Med.,* **42**:1258, 1959.

Gillanders, L. A.: Temporal arteriography, *Clin. Radiol.,* **20**:149, 1969.

Grahame, R., Bluestone, R., and Holt, P. J. L.: Recurrent blanching of the tongue due to giant cell arteritis, *Ann. Internal Med.,* **69**:781, 1968.

Greenhouse, A. H.: Cranial arteritis, *Current Concepts Cerebrovascular Dis.—Stroke,* **6**:11, 1971.

Hamilton, C. R., Jr., Shelley, W. M., and Tumulty, P. A.: Giant cell arteritis: Including temporal arteritis and polymyalgia rheumatica, *Medicine,* **50**:1, 1971.

Hamrin, B., Jonsson, N., and Hellsten, S.: "Polymyalgia arteritica," Further clinical and histopathological studies with a report of six autopsy cases, *Ann. Rheum. Dis.,* **27**:397, 1968.

Harrison, M. J. G., and Bevan, A. T.: Early symptoms of temporal arteritis, *Lancet,* **2**:638, 1967.

Hollenhorst, R. W.: Effect of posture on retinal ischemia from temporal arteritis, *Arch. Ophthalmol.,* **78**:569, 1967.

————, Brown, J. R., Wagener, H. P., and Shick, R. M.: Neurologic aspects of temporal arteritis, *Neurology,* **10**:490, 1960.

Horton, B. T.: Headache and intermittent claudication of the jaw in temporal arteritis, *Headache,* **2**:29, 1962.

————, Magath, T. B., and Brown, G. E.: An undescribed form of arteritis of the temporal vessels, *Proc. Staff Meetings Mayo Clinic,* **7**:700, 1932.

Hunder G. G., Disney, T. F., and Ward, L. E.: Polymyalgia rheumatica, *Mayo Clinic Proc.,* **44**:849, 1969.

Hutchinson J.: On a peculiar form of thrombotic arteritis of the aged which is sometimes productive of gangrene, *Arch. Surg. Lond.,* **1**:323, 1889/90.

Kjeldsen, M. H., and Reske-Nielsen, E.: Pathological changes of the central nervous system in giant-cell arteritis, *Acta ophthalmol.,* **46**:49, 1968.

Lamberg, S. I.: Temporal arteritis and sulfonamide therapy, *J.A.M.A.,* **201**:492, 1967.

Lie, J. T., Brown, A. L., Jr., and Carter, E. T.: Spectrum of aging changes in temporal arteries. Its significance in interpretation of biopsy of temporal artery, *Arch. Pathol.,* **90**:278, 1970.

Martin, T. H.: Pharyngeal edema associated with arteritis. A report of two cases, *Can. Med. Assoc. J.,* **101**:229, 1969.

Russell, R. W. R.: Giant-cell arteritis: A review of 35 cases, *Quart. J. Med.,* **28**:471, 1959.

————, and Earl, C. J.: Loss of vision from cranial arteritis without other symptoms, *Brit. J. Ophthalmol.,* **48**:619, 1964.

Schlezinger, N. S., and Schatz, N. J.: Giant cell arteritis (temporal arteritis), *Trans. Am. Neurol. Assoc.,* **96**:12, 1971.

Simmons, R. J., and Cogan, D. G.: Occult temporal arteritis, *Arch. Ophthalmol.,* **68**:8, 1962.

Smith, J. L., Israel, C. W., and Harner, R. E.: Syphilitic temporal arteritis, *Arch. Ophthalmol.,* **78**:284, 1967.

Warrell, D. A., Godfrey, S., and Olsen, E. G. J.:

Giant-cell arteritis with peripheral neuropathy, *Lancet,* **1**:1010, 1968.

Polyarteritis Nodosa

Aach, R., and Kissane, J. (eds.): Wegener's granulomatosis, *Am. J. Med.,* **48**:496, 1970.

Drachman, D. A.: Neurologic complications of Wegener's granulomatosis, *Arch. Neurol.,* **8**:145, 1963.

Fisher, C. M.: Ocular palsy in temporal arteritis: Part III. Neurologic manifestations of the arteritides other than temporal arteritis, *Minnesota Med.,* **42**:1617, 1959.

Ford, R. G., and Siekert, R. G.: Central nervous system manifestations of periarteritis nodosa, *Neurology,* **15**:114, 1965.

Gocke, D. J., Hsu, K., Morgan, C., Bonbardieri, S., Lockshin, M., and Christian, C. L.: Association between polyarteritis and Australia antigen, *Lancet,* **2**:1149, 1970.

Disseminated Lupus Erythematosus

Alpert, L. I.: Thrombotic thrombocytopenic purpura and systemic lupus erythematosus: Report of a case with immunofluorescence investigation of vascular lesions, *J. Mt. Sinai Hosp. N.Y.,* **35**:165, 1968.

Brandsma, M., Sternberg, T. H., and Davis, J. H.: Systemic lupus erythematosus, *Angiology,* **21**:172, 1970.

Burch, P. R., and Rowell, N. R.: Systemic lupus erythematosus: Etiological aspects, *Am. J. Med.,* **38**:793, 1965.

Dubois, E. L. (ed.): Lupus Erythematosus: A Review of the Current Status of Discoid and Systemic Lupus Erythematosus and Their Variants, McGraw-Hill Book Company, New York, 1966.

Estes, D., and Christian, C. L.: The natural history of systemic lupus erythematosus by prospective analysis, *Medicine,* **50**:85, 1971.

Granger, D. P.: Transverse myelitis with recovery: The only manifestation of systemic lupus erythematosus, *Neurology,* **10**:325, 1960.

Györkey, F., Min, K.-W., Sincovics, J. G., and Györkey, P.: Systemic lupus erythematosus and myxovirus, *New Engl. J. Med.,* **280**:333, 1969.

Johnson, R. T., and Richardson, E. P.: The neurological manifestations of systemic lupus erythematosus. A clinical-pathological study of 24 cases and review of the literature, *Medicine,* **47**:337, 1968.

Leading article: Drug-induced lupus syndromes, *Brit. Med. J.,* **2**:192, 1970.

Leading article: Virus-like structures in lupus erythematosus, *Brit. Med. J.,* **1**:643, 1970.

Meagher, J. N., McCoy, F., and Rossel, C.: Disseminated lupus erythematosus simulating intracranial mass lesion: Report of an unusual case, *Neurology,* **11**:862, 1961.

O'Brien, J. L., and Sibley, W. A.: Neurologic manifestations of thrombotic thrombocytopenic purpura, *Neurology,* **8**:55, 1958.

O'Connor, J. F.: Psychoses associated with systemic lupus erythematosus, *Ann. Internal Med.,* **51**:526, 1959.

Roberts, A. H.: Neurological complications of systemic diseases—II, *Brit. Med. J.,* **1**:95, 1970.

Schur, P. H.: Antinuclear antibodies (A.N.A.), *New Engl. J. Med.,* **282**:1205, 1970.

Wilske, K. R., Shalit, I. E., Willkens, R. F., and Decker, J. L.: Findings suggestive of systemic lupus erythematosus in subjects on chronic anticonvulsant therapy, *Arthritis Rheumat.,* **8**:260, 1965.

Noninfectious Granulomatous Angiitis

Citron, B. P., Halpern, M., McCarron, M., Lundberg, G. D., McCormick, R., Pincus, I. J., Tatter, D., and Haverback, B. J.: Necrotizing angiitis associated with drug abuse, *New Engl. J. Med.,* **283**:1003, 1970.

———, ———, ———, McCormick, R., and Haverback, B. J.: Necrotizing angiitis in young adult drug addicts, *J. Clin. Invest.,* **49**:19a, 1970.

Hughes, J. T., and Brownell, B.: Granulomatous giant-celled angiitis of the central nervous system, *Neurology,* **16**:293, 1966.

Kolodny, E. H., Rebeiz, J. J., Caviness, V. S., Jr., and Richardson, E. P., Jr.: Granulomatous angiitis of the central nervous system, *Arch. Neurol.,* **19**:510, 1968.

Liliequist, B., and Link, H.: Wegener's granulomatosis. Report of a case, *Angiology,* **19**:215, 1968.

McCombs, R. P.: Systemic "allergic" vasculitis: Clinical and pathological relationships, *J.A.M.A.,* **194**:1059, 1965.

Torvik, A., and Hognestad, J.: "Cerebral thromboangiitis obliterans": Report of a case with discussion of pathogenesis, *Acta pathol. microbiol. scand.,* **63**:522, 1965.

Wise, G. R., and Farmer, T.: Bacterial cerebral vasculitis, *Neurology,* **20**:387, 1970.

Additional References

Chynoweth, R., and Foley, J.: Pre-senile dementia responding to steroid therapy, *Brit. J. Psychiat.,* **115**:703, 1969.

Dalal, P. M., Deshpande, C. K., and Daftary, S. G.: Aortic arch syndrome, *Neurology (India),* **19**:155, 1971.

Mann, D. C., and Toole, J. F.: Cranial arteritis and liver involvement, *Stroke,* **3**:131, 1972.

Morooka, S., Ito, I., Yamaguchi, H., Takeda, T., and Sato, Y.: Follow-up observation of aortitis syndrome, *Japan. Heart J.,* **13**:201, 1972.

Torvik, A., Endresen, G., Abrahamsen, A., and Godal, H.: Progressive dementia caused by an unusual type of generalized small vessel thrombosis, *Acta neurol. scand.,* **47**:137, 1971.

Wilkinson, M. S., and Russell, R. W. R.: Arteries of the head and neck in giant-cell arteritis, *Arch. Neurol.,* **27**:378, 1972.

Rare and Unusual Vascular Diseases

The study of exceptional cases, gentlemen, is not to be disdained. They are not always mere baits for vain curiosity. Many a time, indeed, they supply the solution of difficult problems. In that respect they may be compared to the lost or erratic species which the naturalist anxiously seeks for, because they show the mode of transition between different zoological families, or enable him to unravel some knotty point of comparative anatomy or physiology.

J. M. Charcot

EHLERS-DANLOS SYNDROME

Ehlers-Danlos syndrome is a rare connective tissue disorder that is usually transmitted in an autosomal dominant manner. It is characterized by cutaneous hyperelasticity and fragility, hypermobility of joints due to the elasticity of joint capsules, and a bleeding tendency (Fig. 29-1).

Pathologic Findings

The basic cause is unknown, but a commonly held hypothesis is that it may lie in the cross-linking of the collagen fibers. Histological examination of the abnormal skin frequently shows a relative increase in the quantity of elastic tissue without any morphological alteration, either elastic or collagen.

Arteries may have reduction in the amount of the elastic fibers with fragmentation of the internal elastic membrane, leading to aneurysmal dilatations or dissection.

Clinical Features

From the patient's point of view, the cutaneous and joint characteristics are of primary concern,

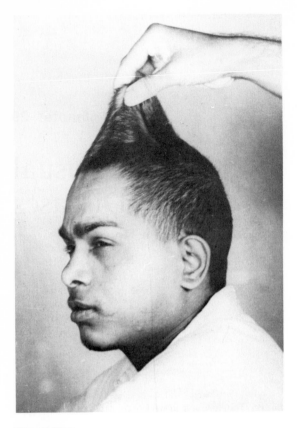

Figure 29-1

but it is the easy bruising and tissue fragility that may lead to serious consequences.

Cerebrovascular manifestations are a common cause of death in patients with Ehlers-Danlos syndrome. Intracranial aneurysms, both single and multiple, with subarachnoid hemorrhage have been reported. Caroticocavernous fistula occurring spontaneously is seen, and both of these conditions (aneurysms and caroticocavernous fistula) may have a familial incidence.

Course and Prognosis

This disorder varies in its degree of expression among individuals of a single kinship. While perhaps the majority of the patients are able to

live with minimal discomfort and disability, some are afflicted by grave and often fatal complications such as dissecting aneurysm of the aorta and intracranial or visceral hemorrhage.

Treatment

The excessive tissue fragility and the inherent hemorrhagic tendency in this disease make angiography and intracranial surgery risky.

Surgical management of patients presenting with hemorrhage poses special problems (with tissues "tearing like blotting paper"). This abnormal fragility of tissue, including that of the blood vessels, leading to multiple lesions, combines with delayed wound healing and seriously challenges the skill of the surgeon; hence a conservative approach by both the physician and the surgeon is preferred in the management of the vascular crisis.

PSEUDOXANTHOMA ELASTICUM

Pseudoxanthoma elasticum is an autosomal recessive disorder in which degeneration and secondary calcification of the elastic tissue leads to cutaneous lesions, angioid streaks of the retina, and vascular disturbances in many organs of the body.

Pathologic Findings

The arteries show marked thinning and destruction of the muscularis with deposition of calcium and bone, and the intima shows irregular thickening due to deposition of collagen. There is thickening and fragmentation of the elastic fibers in the deep layers of the skin. In the retina there is fragmentation of Bruch's membrane which is visible on ophthalmoscopic examination as angioid streaks.

Clinical Features

Yellowish papules forming plaques are found on the skin covering the neck, face, axilla, inguinal region, and the periumbilical area ("plucked chicken" appearance), and are due to fragmentation of the elastic fibers in the deep layers of the dermis. Because of the appearance of the skin lesions, this disorder was originally thought to be related to xanthomatosis, but because the lipid metabolism is normal, it is termed pseudoxanthomatosis.

Chorioretinitis with macular involvement results in progressive bilateral visual deterioration. Arterial degeneration results in hypertension, angina pectoris, gastrointestinal bleeding, unequal radial pulses, and calcification of peripheral arteries.

The cerebrovascular manifestations that have been reported are cerebral infarction, intracerebral hemorrhage, and subarachnoid hemorrhage due to ruptured cerebral aneurysm. Stenosis of components of the aortic arch may cause cerebrovascular insufficiency.

Treatment

No specific treatment is available other than repair of stenotic arteries and control of related hypertension. No preventive measures are known.

THROMBOANGIITIS OBLITERANS (CEREBRAL FORM)

First described by Buerger in 1924, thromboangiitis obliterans is an inflammatory and obliterative vascular disease of the arms and legs primarily, although in extremely rare instances involvement of the intracranial arteries has been reported. Some authorities vehemently deny its very existence as a separate entity, ascribing the clinical and pathologic findings to atherosclerosis. A few maintain that it is a vasculitis affecting not only arteries, but veins and peripheral nerves in the neurovascular bundles which supply the extremities, and they attribute the pathologic changes in these structures to intense and prolonged vasospasm in the vasa vasorum and vasa nervorum.

Pathologic Findings

The characteristic features of the cerebral form of this disease are believed to be:

1 The appearance of the terminal arteries on the exposed surface of the cerebral and cerebellar cortex as "whitish, shrunken, bloodless cords," which can be recognized readily at exploratory craniotomy.

2 A conglomeration of tiny cortical scars in the shape of a ring—often located between the areas supplied by the anterior, middle, and posterior cerebral arteries—which gives a granular atrophic appearance.

3 The presence of well-developed meningeal vascular anastomoses.

4 The involvement of small arteries, between 250 and 750 μ in diameter (atherosclerosis does *not* involve arteries of this size), showing severe narrowing of the lumen by loose connective tissue and thrombus; often one or more secondary smaller lumens is associated. The remainder of the artery shows no pathologic change.

Clinical Features

The disorder occurs primarily in young men who are heavy smokers. The clinical picture may be that of a fixed focal neurologic deficit or a "stuttering" stroke. In the past, quite a few patients were misdiagnosed as having brain tumor, and exploratory craniotomies were performed.

Differential Diagnosis

The clinical features are not particularly reliable in differentiating this disorder from atherosclerosis; however, the occurrence of an acute focal cerebrovascular deficit in a young man who has evidence of thromboangiitis obliterans elsewhere may be a helpful clue.

Laboratory Findings

It has been suggested that the angiographic appearance of blockage in most of the middle-sized branches of the middle cerebral artery and the visualization of the annular meningeal anastomoses might prove to be of diagnostic significance. Air studies have shown dilated lateral ventricles with puddling of air over the widened cortical subarachnoid space.

Course, Prognosis, and Treatment

Because of the scarcity of case reports of this disease, it has not been possible either to prognosticate or to attempt specific therapy.

FIBROMUSCULAR HYPERPLASIA (MEDIAL DYSPLASIA)

Fibromuscular hyperplasia is a nonatherosclerotic, noninflammatory lesion of unknown etiology. It involves the elastic, muscular, and fibrous elements of the intima and media of large arteries and produces hyperplastic changes of a segmental nature. It causes stenosis of the lumen and occasionally aneurysmal dilatation.

Clinical Features

The disorder occurs most commonly in young women but has no characteristic clinical features. The first examples were found in angiograms of the renal arteries. More recently, similar arteriographic appearances have been seen in the internal carotid arteries as a "string of beads," resulting from alternating areas of stenosis and aneurysmal dilatation, or from standing waves in a turbulent stream.

Although there have been one or two reports of involvement of the vertebral artery in the neck, in the majority of cases the midportion of the cervical internal carotid artery is involved. Patients may be asymptomatic or may have focal neurologic symptoms and signs due to ischemia of the area of distribution of the involved artery. In some of these there has been an associated intracranial, congenital saccular aneurysm. It is not known whether this association has a common pathology in both extracranial and intracranial arteries or whether systemic ar-

terial hypertension has resulted in aneurysmal dilatation.

In some patients ergot and its closely related congeners have been implicated. There is no malaise, fever, or involvement of other organ systems to suggest systemic illness.

Course and Prognosis

Because it has been recognized so recently, the natural history is not known; however, some have found the arterial lesions to be either static or very slowly progressive.

Treatment

Operative procedures such as excision of the lesion, saphenous venous grafting, or arteriotomy followed by dilatation and excision of the redundant coils and constricted segments have been tried. Corticosteroids have not proved to be of any value.

"MOYAMOYA" DISEASE (SPONTANEOUS OCCLUSION OF THE CIRCLE OF WILLIS)

In the early 1960s, an apparently new form of cerebrovascular disease was described in Japan. It is characterized by a combination of cerebral ischemia due to vascular occlusion, and hemorrhages from an abnormal net of vessels at the base of the brain. It is the angiographic appearance of this net of vessels that gives the disease the name "moyamoya" (Japanese for hazy, like a puff of cigarette smoke drifting in the air).

Etiology

This disease is confined almost exclusively to the Japanese.

Its cause is not known, although some consider the net-like vessels to be congenital vascular malformations; and others believe that occlusion of the arteries of the circle of Willis is the primary defect, with the net-like collateral circulation developing secondarily. There is no evidence to suggest that the disease is inflamma-

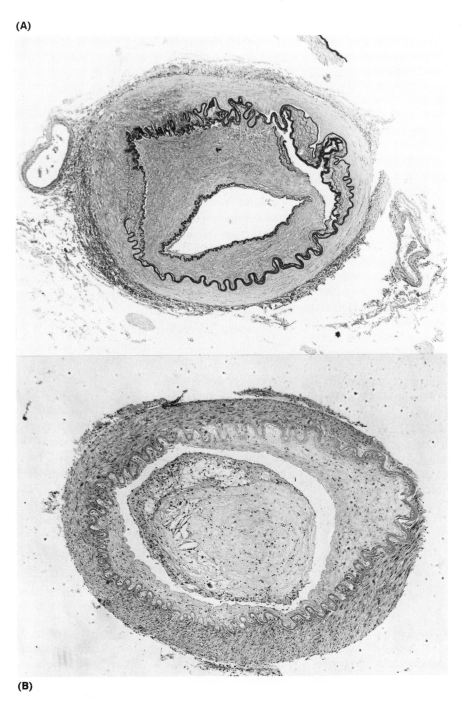

Figure 29-2 Histopathologic specimens. (A) Distal end of right internal carotid artery in a 24-year-old woman showing clot with recanalization. (B) Distal end of occluded left internal carotid artery in a 6-year-old girl. *(Courtesy of Dr. T. Kudo, Department of Surgery, Keio University, Tokyo.)*

tory or infectious; nor is it suggestive of Taka-yasu's disease. Angiographic evidence of intra-cranial multiple arterial occlusions, however, in association with a moyamoya-like vascular net have also been described in children with tuber-culous meningitis.

Pathologic Findings

Reports available on two patients have shown marked narrowing of the lumens of the distal segments of the internal carotid arteries with in-timal thickening and thrombus formation ex-tending into the proximal portions of both ante-rior and middle cerebral arteries (Fig. 29-2A and B). There is no evidence of atheroma or inflammation. The vessel walls of the anastomo-tic network are described as being very thin, reminiscent of the findings in encephalofacial angiomatosis (Sturge-Weber syndrome).

Clinical Features

Moyamoya is somewhat more common in women; depending upon the age of the patient, the signs and symptoms differ.

In juveniles the presenting manifestations are focal neurologic deficit, mental impairment, headaches, and convulsions. The deficit is mild but recurrent, and the residual signs persist.

In adults the headache, convulsions, and fo-cal neurologic signs also occur, but many pa-tients suffer *subarachnoid hemorrhage* as well. Except for occasional papilledema as seen asso-ciated with subarachnoid hemorrhage, exami-nation shows the fundus to be normal.

Laboratory Findings

The angiographic appearance of moyamoya is similar to that of the retinal neovascularization and the characteristic peripapillary arteriove-nous anastomoses which one sees in Takayasu's disease. However, no ocular abnormalities have been described in moyamoya disease. Angiogra-phy shows the disease to be confined to supra-tentorial arteries. All cases show occlusion of the main branches of the circle of Willis, espe-cially the carotid bifurcation, with extensive de-velopment of meningeal collateral circulation— the so-called "rete mirabile." The process may be unilateral or bilateral.

Serial angiography in children with this dis-ease has shown that narrowing of the carotid bifurcation is the first stage, followed by devel-opment of the anastomotic network (Fig. 29-3). In some young patients, collateral circulation has been shown to disappear later on, but the obstruction of the carotid siphon persists and presumably blood supply to the hemisphere is maintained through the vertebral-basilar sys-tem. At times, especially in juveniles, angiogra-phy reveals moyamoya disease of the ethmoidal and nasal vessels.

Standard laboratory studies have failed to show any evidence of an underlying infectious, metabolic, or immunological disorder.

Course and Prognosis

The natural history of this disorder differs, de-pending upon the patient's age at the onset. In juveniles mild but recurrent attacks of focal neurologic deficit occur with variable degrees of residual neural impairment. In adults, on the other hand, focal neurologic deficit from sub-arachnoid hemorrhage (presumably due to the moyamoya) occurs but with remarkable recov-ery and no recurrence. It has not been deter-mined how many of the juvenile cases progress into the adult form.

Treatment

No specific treatment for this perplexing disor-der is available; however, some surgeons are at-tempting perivascular sympathectomy of the cervical carotid artery and excision of the supe-rior cervical ganglion.

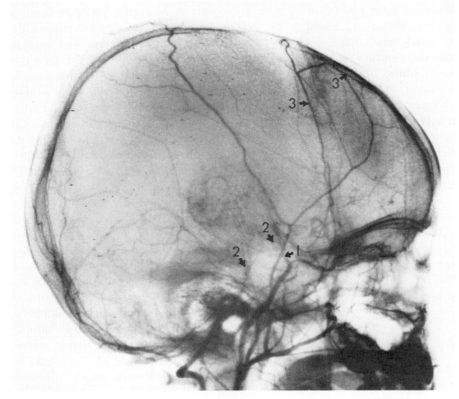

Figure 29-3 Arteriogram showing occluded internal carotid artery with profuse external carotid and leptomeningeal anastomoses. *(Courtesy of Dr. T. Kudo, Department of Surgery, Keio University, Tokyo.)*

VASCULAR DISEASE OF THE PITUITARY GLAND

Infarction

Acute pituitary necrosis can be caused by infarction into a normal pituitary gland or an adenoma; however, it usually occurs in a woman in whom the gland has hypertrophied during pregnancy or in whom obstetric complications such as massive hemorrhage with shock develop. Although the patient survives the acute episode, she may develop hypopituitarism with atrophy of the breasts, inability to lactate, amenorrhea, and lack of regrowth of pubic hair (Sheehan's syndrome).

An unusual cause of pituitary necrosis is insidious pressure atrophy as the result of aneurysm or dilatation of the internal carotid arteries where they lie adjacent to the gland.

Hemorrhage

Persons with pituitary adenomas may have bleeding into the tumor, causing pituitary apoplexy. The hemorrhage may occur spontaneously in the neoplasm, or it may be triggered by the use of anticoagulant or irradiation therapy to the adenoma.

If the hemorrhage is confined, the patient has severe headache and may become blind when the hematoma compresses the optic chiasm or nerves. If there is rupture into the subarachnoid space, signs of subarachnoid hemorrhage develop. In other instances, the clinical picture is one of ocular palsies or blindness due to compression of the adjoining cavernous sinus or optic chiasm. Some patients may have acute pituitary insufficiency with hypotension.

Diagnosis rests on the knowledge or suspicion that the patient has been harboring a pituitary adenoma. Neither the acromegalic features nor the clinical evidence of hypopituitarism are found invariably. Skull x-rays show an enlarged sella turcica. Lumbar puncture may reveal bloodstained cerebrospinal fluid, polymorphonuclear pleocytosis, and at times necrotic tumor tissue. Carotid angiogram demonstrates the suprasellar extension of an intrasellar tumor and also helps in excluding a diagnosis of ruptured aneurysm.

Treatment

Endocrine replacement and supportive therapy may be sufficient. However, if vision is impaired, craniotomy is necessary for removal of blood clot and necrotic tissues which cause pressure on the visual pathways.

DISSECTING HEMATOMAS OF THE AORTOCRANIAL ARTERIES

When the force of the blood column flowing through an artery separates the intima from the media, a *dissecting hematoma* is formed. Most dissection does not result in dilatation of the walls of an artery; if it does, it is called a *dissecting aneurysm.*

Etiology and Pathogenesis

Dissections that result from primary disease of the artery are called "spontaneous"; those secondary to injury, "traumatic." The nontraumatic varieties are most frequently associated with atherosclerosis or cystic necrosis of the media. Cystic necrosis occurs more often in patients

with myxedema or Marfan's syndrome than in the average population. In some individuals hypertension seems to play a part, and in rare cases syphilis may contribute to the development of a dissecting hematoma. Sudden stretching of the artery as a result of trauma or strenuous exertion may lead to tearing of its intima, but perhaps the most common cause of a local dissection is trauma to the arch or its branches by catheters and needles introduced for arteriography. Experimentally, chronic ingestion of *Lathyrus odoratus* (sweet peas) has resulted in dissection of the arch in animals. No similar cases have been reported in human beings.

Even a small tear in the intima can enlarge as the bloodstream burrows circumferentially, proximally, and distally beneath the flap. If dissection occurs, blood beneath the intima reduces the lumen of the artery progressively and may eventually cause obstruction. When it reaches branches of the artery, it may continue along them as well as along the parent artery. Some dissections reenter the main channel to create a so-called double-barreled artery. Others perforate through the media into the surrounding adventitia, continue to dissect, and eventually rupture into the mediastinum or into the pericardial, pleural, or abdominal cavity.

The cervical segments of the carotids, the brachiocephalic artery itself, or at times the left subclavian proximal to the origin of the vertebral artery may also be the sites of spontaneous or traumatic dissection. These may be iatrogenic, following needle puncture or the introduction of a catheter by a physician. Rarely, a tear in the subclavian artery may be initiated by hyperextending and wrenching the arm, and there are reports of dissection of the carotid artery following sudden blows to the neck which do not damage the skin.

Intrathoracic Dissection

Aortic Arch and Its Branches Spontaneous dissection occurs most frequently in hypertensive men over the age of 50 and usually begins in the ascending aorta. Most often the intimal tear is a spontaneous occurrence not related to exertion; it may be painless, but more often the initial symptom of the tear is excruciating substernal pain which may radiate into the shoulders, back, neck, or jaw, depending on which vessels are involved. The dissection causes stenosis or occlusion, first in the brachiocephalic, then in the left carotid, and finally in the left subclavian artery. The signs produced by the acute obstruction of one or more of these arteries are similar to those of the slowly progressive forms of arterial obstruction but are often more devastating—not only because the blockage is acute, but also because it occurs at the origin of the vessel, so that there is no opportunity for collateral circulation to develop in its distal branches.

In addition to the loss of neural function caused by occlusion of the aortocranial arteries, there may be transverse myelopathy resulting from obliteration of the segmental arteries that spring from the thoracic aorta to supply the spinal cord. Depending on the site of the initial tear in the aorta, one or more of the great vessels may be spared. At times the dissection bypasses them all and involves only the smallest segmental arteries, to produce transverse myelopathy as the initial neurologic deficit.

About half the patients with acute dissection of the aortic arch are extremely ill and in shock. Others evidently have no symptoms at the onset and come to the physician with signs secondary to obstruction of the aortic branches. In some of these patients, peripheral pulses may disappear only to reappear once more when stripping of the adventitia by the column of blood destroys sympathetic nerves and peripheral vasodilatation occurs.

Differential Diagnosis No other illness produces a picture similar to that of acute dissection of the aortic arch. A combination of substernal pain and loss of the subclavian or carotid pulses on one side or both sides with preservation of the femoral pulses is almost pathognomonic of this syndrome. When pulses are not obliterated, stenosis of an artery may be suggested by murmurs and by a difference in blood pressure between the two arms or in ophthalmic artery pressures.

Even if all pulses and pressures are equal, the diagnosis may still be suspected in patients with a clinical picture suggesting an acute vascular catastrophe. The chief consideration in the differential diagnosis is myocardial infarction, but stenosis or occlusion of coronary arteries by the hematoma may produce the electrocardiographic signs of acute myocardial infarction, and distortion of the aortic ring may cause aortic insufficiency. Other conditions to be considered in the differential diagnosis are acute pancreatitis, perforation of an abdominal viscus, and acute transverse myelopathy of any cause. Rarely the only manifestations are those of loss of blood supply to peripheral nerve roots or the brachial plexus.

Laboratory Findings The leukocyte count shows a mild to moderate elevation. Hemoglobin concentration is usually normal but may be low if dissection into the surrounding tissues has resulted in significant loss of blood. Chest x-ray may show the mediastinum to be slightly widened from a collection of blood or an aneurysm, and fluid (blood) may be seen in the left pleural cavity. Angiograms may reveal occlusion of arteries at their origins and sometimes demonstrate separation of the column of contrast material from the external wall of the artery.

Prognosis and Treatment In one series of more than 50 cases, over half the patients were dead within 1 week and more than 80 percent were dead within 1 year. The most frequent cause of death is rupture of the dissecting hematoma into the pericardium, the thorax, or the peritoneal cavity. At times death is caused by cardiac decompensation leading to pulmonary edema and pneumonia.

Although some advocate conservative management with hypotensive medications, the only definitive treatment is surgery. In some patients the diseased segment of the vessel can be successfully replaced by graft, or it can be opened and the torn segment of the intima reattached.

Intracranial Dissecting Hematoma

For a century it has been recognized that injuries to the head can cause hemorrhage into the brain or a rupture of the veins bridging the subdural space. Attention has only recently been given to the fact that trauma can also stretch the arteries at the base of the brain sufficiently to rupture their intima. The basilar and the internal carotid arteries above the clinoid pro-

cesses are particularly susceptible to this type of injury. The middle cerebral artery has also been the site of dissecting hematoma.

Occlusion of a cerebral artery hours or even weeks after trauma to the head may be secondary to dissecting hematoma or may result from the disruption of an atheromatous plaque.

DRUG-INDUCED CEREBROVASCULAR DISORDERS

Drugs taken by an individual, whether prescribed by a physician or not, often produce side reactions which at times may be detrimental to the individual's health (Fig. 29-4). When

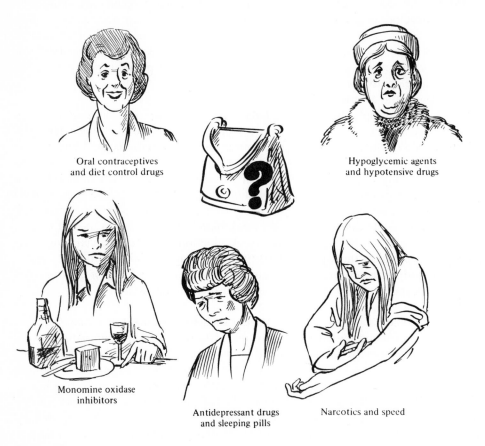

Oral contraceptives
and diet control drugs

Hypoglycemic agents
and hypotensive drugs

Monomine oxidase
inhibitors

Antidepressant drugs
and sleeping pills

Narcotics and speed

Figure 29-4

faced with a patient with symptoms and signs suggestive of a cerebrovascular disorder, a physician should always consider the possibility of a drug-induced disorder such as those which are listed below:

Orthostatic hypotension produced by antihypertensive medications, sedatives, antidepressants, and tranquilizers may precipitate transient ischemic attacks and cerebral or spinal cord infarcts.

A *hypertensive crisis* may result when people receiving monoamine oxidase inhibitors consume tyramine-rich products, such as wine or cheese, and may produce hypertensive encephalopathy, intracerebral hemorrhage, or subarachnoid hemorrhage.

A *hypocoagulable state* may exist in patients with poorly controlled anticoagulant therapy or in those who use large doses of salicylates, alcohol, and anticonvulsants, and may result in subdural hemorrhage, intracerebral hemorrhage, or spinal epidural hemorrhage.

Oral contraceptives containing estrogen and progesterone in various combinations produce a variety of complications. Depending variously upon genetic, racial, serum lipid, and unknown factors, a very small percentage of these women develop malignant hypertension, acute migraine, cerebral arterial or venous infarcts, pseudotumor cerebri, or retinal vascular occlusions.

Patients on digitalis therapy may develop a *hypersensitive carotid sinus reflex* with resultant hypotension, bradycardia, and cerebrovascular insufficiency. Digitalis-induced paroxysmal atrial tachycardia may result in *transient ischemic attacks.*

Antidiabetic drugs may produce *hypoglycemia,* clinically simulating a "stroke."

A gamut of drugs ranging from sulfonamides, procainamide, anticonvulsants, and corticosteroids have been held responsible for the production of *collagen vascular disorders* and *allergic angiitis.*

Intravenously administered amphetamines have been shown to produce *acute necrotizing angiitis,* both cerebral and systemic, and this has resulted in cerebral ischemia, cerebral infarct, and subarachnoid hemorrhage.

Intravenously administered heroin or opium have on occasion resulted in *acute transverse myelopathy.*

Lysergic acid diethylamide (LSD), due to its methysergide(Sansert)-like action, has been suspected of producing *internal carotid artery obstruction.*

SUGGESTED READING

Ehlers-Danlos Syndrome

Bannerman, R. M., Graf, C. J., and Upson, J. F.: Ehlers-Danlos syndrome, *Brit. Med. J.,* **3**:558, 1967.

Beighton, P.: The Ehlers-Danlos Syndrome, William Heinemann Ltd., London, 1970.

Imahori, S., Bannerman, R. M., Graf, C. J., and Brennan, J. C.: Ehlers-Danlos syndrome with multiple arterial lesions, *Am. J. Med.,* **47**:967, 1969.

Rubinstein, M. K., and Cohen, N. H.: Ehlers-Danlos syndrome associated with multiple intracranial aneurysms, *Neurology,* **14**:125, 1964.

Schoolman, A., and Kepes, J. J.: Bilateral spontaneous carotid-cavernous fistulae in Ehlers-Danlos syndrome. Case report, *J. Neurosurg.,* **26**:82, 1967.

Pseudoxanthoma Elasticum

Connor, P. J., Juergens, J. L., Perry, H. O., Hollenhorst, R. W., and Edwards, J. E.: Pseudoxanthoma elasticum and angioid streaks. A review of 106 cases, *Am. J. Med.,* **30**:537, 1961.

Goodman, R. M., Smith, E. W., Paton, D., Bergman, R. A., Siegel, C. L., Ottesen, O. E., Shelley, W. M., Pusch, A. L., and McKusick, V. A.: Pseudoxanthoma elasticum: A clinical and histopathological study, *Medicine,* **42**:297, 1963.

Huang, S.-N., Steele, H. D., Kumar, G., and Parker, J. O.: Ultrastructural changes in the elastic fibers in pseudoxanthoma elasticum, *Arch. Pathol.,* **83**:108, 1967.

Messis, C. P., and Budzilovich, G. N.: Pseudoxanthoma elasticum. Report of an autopsied case with cerebral involvement, *Neurology*, **20**:703, 1970.

Thromboangiitis Obliterans (Cerebral Form)

Buerger, I.: Thromboangiitis obliterans. Concepts of pathogenesis and pathology, *J. Internat. Chir.*, **4**:339, 1939.

Davis, L., and Davis, R. A.: "Cerebral thromboangiitis obliterans" in Principles of Neurological Surgery, W. B. Saunders, Philadelphia, 1963, pp. 202–208.

Fisher, C. M.: Cerebral thromboangiitis obliterans, *Medicine*, **36**:169, 1957.

Torvik, A., and Hognestad, J.: "Cerebral thromboangiitis obliterans." Report of a case with discussion of pathogenesis, *Acta pathol. microbiol. scand.*, **63**:522, 1965.

Zülch, K. J.: The cerebral form of von Winiwarter-Buerger's disease: Does it exist? *Angiology*, **20**:61, 1969.

Fibromuscular Hyperplasia (Medial Dysplasia)

Adams, D. F., and Lebowitz, R. L.: Corrugated arteries. Fixed pathology or functional alteration, *Arch. Surg.*, **104**:18, 1972.

Andersen, P. E.: Fibromuscular hyperplasia of the carotid arteries, *Acta radiol. diagn.*, **10**:90, 1970.

Bergan, J. J., and MacDonald, J. R.: Recognition of cerebrovascular fibromuscular hyperplasia, *Arch. Surg.*, **98**:332, 1969.

Ehrenfeld, W. K., Stoney, R. J., and Wylie, E. J.: Fibromuscular hyperplasia of the internal carotid artery, *Arch. Surg.*, **95**:284, 1967.

Elias, W. S.: Intracranial fibromuscular hyperplasia, *J.A.M.A.*, **218**:254, 1971.

Hartman, J. D., Young, I., Bank, A. A., and Rosenblatt, S. A.: Fibromuscular hyperplasia of internal carotid arteries. Stroke in a young adult complicated by oral contraceptives, *Arch. Neurol.*, **25**:295, 1971.

Houser, O. W., and Baker, H. L., Jr.: Fibromuscular dysplasia and other uncommon diseases of the cervical carotid artery: Angiographic aspects, *Am. J. Roentgenol.*, **104**:201, 1968.

———, ———, Sandok, B. A., and Holley, K. E.: Cephalic arterial fibromuscular dysplasia, *Radiology*, **101**:605, 1971.

Morris, G. C., Jr., Lechter, A., and DeBakey, M. E.: Surgical treatment of fibromuscular disease of the carotid arteries, *Arch. Surg.*, **96**:636, 1968.

Ranier, W. G., Cramer, G. G., Newby, J. P., and Clarke, J. P.: Fibromuscular hyperplasia of the carotid artery causing positional cerebral ischemia, *Ann. Surg.*, **167**:444, 1968.

Sandok, B. A., Houser, O. W., Baker, H. L., Jr., and Holley, K. E.: Fibromuscular dysplasia. Neurologic disorders associated with disease involving the great vessels in the neck, *Arch. Neurol.*, **24**:462, 1971.

Moyamoya Disease

Galligioni, F., Andrioli, G. C., Marin, G., Briani, S., and Iraci, G.: Hypoplasia of the internal carotid artery associated with cerebral pseudoangiomatosis. Report of 4 cases, *Am. J. Roentgenol.*, **112**:251, 1971.

Kudo, T.: Spontaneous occlusion of the circle of Willis. A disease apparently confined to Japanese, *Neurology*, **18**:485, 1968.

Mathew, N. T., Abraham, J., and Chandy, J.: Cerebral angiographic features in tuberculous meningitis, *Neurology*, **20**:1015, 1970.

Nishimoto, A., and Takeuchi, S.: Abnormal cerebrovascular network related to the internal carotid arteries, *J. Neurosurg.*, **29**:255, 1968.

Simon, J., Sabouraud, O., Guy, G., and Turpin, J.: Un cas de maladie de Nishimoto. A propos d'une maladie rare et bilaterale de la carotide interne, *Rev. neurol.*, **119**:376, 1968.

Suzuki, J., and Takaku, A.: Cerebrovascular "Moyamoya" disease. Disease showing abnormal net-like vessels in base of brain, *Arch. Neurol.*, **20**:288, 1969.

———, and Kodama, N.: Cerebrovascular "Moyamoya" disease. Second report: Collateral routes to forebrain via ethmoid and superior nasal meatus, *Angiology*, **22**:223, 1971.

Taveras, J. M.: Multiple progressive intracranial arterial occlusions: A syndrome of children and young adults, *Am. J. Roentgenol.*, **106**:235, 1969.

Vuia, O., Alexianu, M., and Gabor, S.: Hypoplasia and obstruction of the circle of Willis in a case of atypical cerebral hemorrhage and its relationship to Nishimoto's disease, *Neurology*, **20**:361, 1970.

Zappia, R. J., Winkelman, J. Z., Roberson, G. H., Rosenbaum, H. E., and Gay, A. J.: Progressive intracranial arterial occlusion syndrome. Report of a case with unusually high ophthalmodynamometry (ODM) values, *Arch. Ophthalmol.,* **86**:455, 1971.

Vascular Disease of the Pituitary Gland

Dastur, H. M., and Pandya, S. K.: Haemorrhagic adenomas of the pituitary gland: Their clinical and radiological presentations and treatment, *Neurology (India),* **19**:4, 1971.

Epstein, S., Pimstone, B. L., de Villiers, J. C., and Jackson, W. P.: Pituitary apoplexy in five patients, *Brit. J. Med.,* **2**:267, 1971.

Locke, S., and Tyler, H. R.: Pituitary apoplexy. Report of two cases, with pathological verification, *Am. J. Med.,* **30**:643, 1961.

Nourizadeh, A. R., and Pitts, F. W.: Hemorrhage into pituitary adenoma during anticoagulant therapy, *J.A.M.A.,* **193**:623, 1965.

Sheehan, H. L., and Davis, J. C.: Pituitary necrosis, *Brit. Med. Bull.,* **24**:59, 1968.

Dissecting Hematoma of the Aortocranial Arteries

General

Frantzen, E., Jacobsen, H. H., and Therkelsen, J.: Cerebral artery occlusions in children due to trauma to the head and neck. A report of 6 cases verified by cerebral angiography, *Neurology,* **11**:695, 1961.

Gherardi, G. J., and Lee, H. Y.: Localized dissecting hemorrhage and arteritis, *J.A.M.A.,* **199**:187, 1967.

Etiology and Pathogenesis

Collins, J. J., Jr.: Dissecting aneurysms in turkeys and man, *Arch. Surg.,* **102**:159, 1971.

Lewin, W.: Vascular lesions in head injuries, *Brit. J. Surg.,* **55**:321, 1968.

Dissecting Hematoma of the Aortic Arch

Austen, W. G., and DeSanctis, R. W.: Surgical treatment of dissecting aneurysm of the thoracic aorta, *New Engl. J. Med.,* **272**:1314, 1965.

Braunstein, H.: Pathogenesis of dissecting aneurysm, *Circulation,* **28**:1071, 1963.

Chase, T. N., Rosman, N. P., and Price, D. L.: The cerebral syndromes associated with dissecting aneurysm of the aorta. A clinicopathological study, *Brain,* **91**:173, 1968.

Daily, P. O., Trueblood, H. W., Stinson, E. B., Wuer-

flein, A. D., and Shumway, N. E.: Management of acute aortic dissections, *Ann. Thoracic Surg.,* **10**:237, 1970.

DeBakey, M. E., Henly, W. S., Cooley, D. A., Morris, G. C., Jr., Crawford, E. S., and Beall, A. C., Jr.: Surgical management of dissecting aneurysms of the aorta, *J. Thoracic Cardiovascular Surg.,* **49**:130, 1965.

Hirst, A. E., Jr., Johns, V. J., Jr., and Kime, S. W., Jr.: Dissecting aneurysms of the aorta: A review of 505 cases, *Medicine,* **37**:217, 1958.

McCloy, R. M., Spittell, J. A., Jr., and McGoon, D. C.: The prognosis in aortic dissection (dissecting aortic hematoma or aneurysm), *Circulation,* **31**:665, 1965.

Spittell, J. A., Jr.: Dissecting aneurysm (dissecting hematoma) of the aorta, *Mod. Concepts Cardiovascular Dis.,* **33**:837, 1964.

Thompson, G. B.: Dissecting aortic aneurysm with infarction of spinal cord, *Brain,* **79**:111, 1956.

Weisman, A. D., and Adams, R. D.: The neurological complications of dissecting aortic aneurysm, *Brain,* **67**:69, 1944.

Wheat, M. W., Jr., Harris, P. D., Malm, J. R., Kaiser, G., Bowman, F. O., Jr., and Palmer, R. F.: Acute dissecting aneurysms of the aorta. Treatment and results in 64 patients, *J. Thoracic Cardiovascular Surg.,* **58**:344, 1969.

———, and Palmer, R. F.: Dissecting aneurysms of the aorta, *Current Problems Surg.,* July 1971.

Dissection of Cervical Arteries

Boström, K., and Lilliequist, B.: Primary dissecting aneurysm of the extracranial part of the internal carotid and vertebral arteries. A report of three cases, *Neurology,* **17**:179, 1967.

Boyd-Wilson, J. S.: Iatrogenic carotid occlusion: Medial dissection complicating arteriography, *World Neurol.,* **3**:507, 1962.

Brice, J. G., and Crompton, M. R.: Spontaneous dissecting aneurysms of the cervical internal carotid artery, *Brit. Med. J.,* **2**:790, 1964.

Hockaday, T. D.: Traumatic thrombosis of the internal carotid artery, *J. Neurol. Neurosurg. Psychiat.,* **12**:229, 1959.

Houck, W. S., Jackson, J. R., Odom, G. L., and Young, W. G.: Occlusion of the internal carotid artery in the neck secondary to closed trauma to the head and neck: A report of two cases, *Ann. Surg.,* **159**:219, 1964.

Thapedi, I. M., Ashenhurst, E. M., and Rozdilsky, B.: Spontaneous dissecting aneurysm of the internal carotid artery in the neck. Report of a case and review of the literature, *Arch. Neurol.,* **23**:549, 1970.

Intracranial Dissecting Hematomas

Attar, S., Fardin, R., Ayella, R., and McLaughlin, J. S.: Medical vs. surgical treatment of acute dissecting aneurysms, *Arch. Surg.,* **103**:568, 1971.

Duman, S., and Stephens, J. W.: Post-traumatic middle cerebral artery occlusion, *Neurology,* **13**:613, 1963.

Editorial: Treatment of dissecting aortic aneurysm, *Lancet,* **1**:525, 1972.

Hayman, J. A., and Anderson, R. McD.: Dissecting aneurysm of the basilar artery, *Med. J. Australia,* **2**:360, 1966.

Spudis, E. V., Scharyj, M., Alexander, E., and Martin, J. F.: Dissecting aneurysms in the neck and head, *Neurology,* **12**:867, 1962.

Wolman, L.: Cerebral dissecting aneurysms, *Brain,* **82**:276, 1959.

Drug-induced Cerebrovascular Disorders

AtLee, W. E., Jr.: Talc and cornstarch emboli in eyes of drug users, *J.A.M.A.,* **219**:49, 1972.

Bergeron, R. T., and Wood, E. H.: Oral contraceptives and cerebrovascular complications, *Radiology,* **92**:231, 1969.

Blackwell, B., Marley, E., Price, J., and Taylor, D.: Hypertensive interactions between monoamine oxidase inhibitors and foodstuffs, *Brit. J. Psychiat.,* **113**:349, 1967.

Citron, B. P., Halpern, M., McCarron, M., Lundberg, G. D., McCormick, R., Pincus, I. J., Tatter, D., and Haverback, B. J.: Necrotizing angiitis associated with drug abuse, *New Engl. J. Med.,* **283**:1003, 1970.

Collaborative Group for the Study of Stroke in Young Women: Oral contraception and increased risk of cerebral ischemia or thrombosis, *New Engl. J. Med.,* **288**:87, 1973.

Goodman, S. J., and Becker, D. P.: Intracranial hemorrhage associated with amphetamine abuse, *J.A.M.A.,* **212**:480, 1970.

Irey, N. S., Manion, W. C., and Taylor, H. B.: Vascu-

lar lesions in women taking oral contraceptives, *Arch. Pathol.,* **89**:1, 1970.

Kazmier, F. J., and Spittell, J. A., Jr.: Coumarin drug interactions, *Mayo Clinic Proc.,* **45**:249, 1970.

Lamy, P. P., and Kitler, M. E.: Untoward effects of drugs (including non-prescription drugs) (in two parts), *Dis. Nervous System,* **32**:18 and **32**:105, 1971.

Leading article: Drug-induced lupus syndromes, *Brit. Med. J.,* **2**:192, 1970.

Masi, A. T., and Dugdale, M.: Cerebrovascular diseases associated with the use of oral contraceptives. A review of the English-language literature, *Ann. Internal Med.,* **72**:111, 1970.

Montgomery, B. M., and Pinner, C. A.: Transient hypoglycemic hemiplegia, *Arch. Internal Med.,* **114**:680, 1964.

Patel, A. N.: Self-inflicted strokes (editorial), *Ann. Internal Med.,* **76**:823, 1972.

Richter, R. W., and Rosenberg, R. N.: Transverse myelitis associated with heroin addiction, *J.A.M.A.,* **206**:1255, 1968.

Rumbaugh, C. L., Bergeron, R. T., Fang, H. C. H., and McCormick, R.: Cerebral angiographic changes in the drug abuse patient, *Radiology,* **101**:335, 1971.

——, ——, Scanlan, R. L., Teal, J. S., Segall, H. D., Fang, H. C. H., and McCormick, R.: Cerebral vascular changes secondary to amphetamine abuse in the experimental animal, *Radiology,* **101**:345, 1971.

Salmon, M. L., Winkelman, J. Z., and Gay, A. J.: Neuro-ophthalmic sequelae in users of oral contraceptives, *J.A.M.A.,* **206**:85, 1968.

Schein, P. S., Yessayan, L., and Mayman, C. I.: Acute transverse myelitis associated with intravenous opium, *Neurology,* **21**:101, 1971.

Sobel, J., Espinas, O. E., and Friedman, S. A.: Carotid artery obstruction following LSD capsule ingestion, *Arch. Internal Med.,* **127**:290, 1971.

Weiss, S. R., Raskind, R., Morganstern, N. L., Pytlyk, P. J., and Baiz, T. C.: Intracerebral and subarachnoid hemorrhage following use of methamphetamine ("speed"), *Internat. Surg.,* **53**:123, 1970.

Wells, C. E., and Urrea, D.: Cerebrovascular accidents in patients receiving anticoagulant drugs, *Arch. Neurol.,* **3**:553, 1960.

General Principles of Management and Rehabilitation

A little neglect may breed mischief.

Benjamin Franklin
Poor Richard's Almanac, 1758

GENERAL PRINCIPLES OF MANAGEMENT

Patients suffering acute cerebrovascular episodes sometimes require emergency lifesaving measures. At other times, the ictus seems so minor that the physician may be tempted to advise the patient to ignore the symptoms. Each patient poses a singular problem whose management must be tailored to suit the circumstances. The principles of therapy outlined in the following pages are general enough to be applicable to many varieties of neurovascular disorders.

The decision whether to treat the patient at home or in the hospital is affected by such considerations as socioeconomic conditions, the availability of a hospital bed, the desires of the patient and his family, and the gravity of the illness. Because seemingly minor attacks often give warning of more serious difficulties to come, it is usually advisable to place the patient in the hospital for observation. Patients in coma or status epilepticus and those suffering intracranial hemorrhages must be hospitalized immediately; but the occasional patient who is first seen a week or so after the onset of what has become a well-established, nonprogressive cerebral infarction need not be admitted to the hospital if arrangements for ambulation and rehabilitation can be made at home.

Respiratory System

Maintenance of the Airway   The most essential step in the management of any neurologic emergency is the maintenance of an adequate airway. This problem is present during the acute phase of any illness complicated by convulsions or coma. Later, difficulty in swallowing may cause tracheal obstruction due to the aspiration of food or secretions.

The comatose patient must be kept in the lateral decubitus or head-low position, and an oral airway or tongue-holding forceps must be used to keep the tongue from obstructing the pharynx. These devices, however, can be used for 24 to 48 hr only; if the mouth is kept open for longer periods, the mucous membranes become excessively dry and dried secretions accumulate in the hypopharynx. For these reasons, constant surveillance is essential and frequent aspiration of nasopharyngeal secretions is vital. A soft polyethylene catheter must be passed into the nasopharynx and oropharynx, the hypopharynx, and possibly even the upper trachea several times daily. Many nurses are hesitant to perform this necessary task, fearing that the paroxysms of coughing sometimes induced may tip the balance against a patient whose condition is already precarious. Although coughing is certainly undesirable in a comatose patient with intracranial bleeding, it is less harmful than an airway partially obstructed by secretions which could be removed by suction or by making the patient cough. Vigorous probing with the catheter must be avoided, however; it may cause mucosal ulceration and resultant bleeding.

Tracheostomy, once a maneuver of desperation for patients *in extremis,* is now generally recommended for any patient who is likely to be in prolonged coma. Elective tracheostomy eliminates the possibility of aspiration, reduces the respiratory dead space, and facilitates cleansing of the tracheobronchial tree. Most important of all, there is no need for minute-by-minute nursing care to prevent acute respiratory obstruction.

When death from cerebrovascular disorder seems to be imminent and unavoidable, the performance of a tracheostomy to prolong life hardly seems justifiable. The grounds on which this decision is made are so empirical that consultation with another physician experienced in the field is usually advisable in such cases. See section on Brain Death later in this chapter.

Gas Inhalation   Some administer 90 to 100 percent oxygen by nasal catheter, mask, or tent to patients with acute neurovascular disorders. In patients with emphysema or other chronic pulmonary disease causing carbon dioxide retention, oxygen administration, by depressing respiration, can produce further accumulation of CO_2 and lead to narcosis and rarely to death. Because oxygen produces vasoconstriction in normal cerebral vessels, 5 to 7 percent carbon dioxide is frequently added in order to induce arteriolar dilatation. However, the advisability of administering this mixture is debatable because it may dilate healthy arterioles while not affecting those supplying the infarcted or ischemic region which are already maximally dilated from locally accumulated products of tissue metabolism. When this occurs, the administration of CO_2 will divert blood from the ischemic region to healthy tissue—so-called "intracerebral steal." To prevent this from happening, others have advocated hypocarbia induced by forced hyperventilation in order to constrict healthy arterioles and force more blood through the vasoparalytic ischemic area—the Robin Hood effect (phenomenon of stealing from the rich to pay the poor). Both of these are seen to be of more theoretical than practical benefit, and their efficacy must await further study.

Though the administration of oxygen, with or without carbon dioxide, may give the family and the physician a feeling of therapeutic activity, it probably has little effect on cerebrovascular resistance and tissue oxygenation in patients with cerebral atherosclerosis unless there is superimposed cardiopulmonary disease. The administration of oxygen at 2 or 3 atm, on the other hand, increases the volume of oxygen dissolved in blood as much as 6 vol percent and, theroretically at least, could increase oxygenation in ischemic cerebral tissue. However, hyperbaric oxygen therapy for cerebral ischemia has not proved to be practical.

Pulmonary Atelectasis and Bronchopneumonia Because bronchopneumonia is the most frequent cause of death following cerebrovascular episodes, its prevention is particularly important. Both bronchopneumonia and the segmental atelectasis which often precedes it can usually be prevented by changing the position of the patient frequently, by using suction or tapotage, and by deep-breathing exercises. If the patient is unable to breathe deeply, intermittent positive-pressure breathing exercises, administered several times daily, are of immense value. If this therapy is not available, inhalation of a mixture containing 10 percent carbon dioxide and 90 percent oxygen will often induce hyperventilation.

The prophylactic administration of antibiotics is probably not justified unless the patient is comatose or cannot cough. Fever, unexplained tachycardia, tachypnea, productive cough, and physical or roentgenologic evidence of pulmonary infection are indications for the immediate initiation of antibiotic therapy given orally, if possible, to avoid disruption of the skin by needles. Sputum cultures should be taken if the patient does not respond within 24 hr. Antibiotic therapy should then be altered, depending on growth of organisms and the results of sensitivity tests.

Pulmonary Edema Left-sided heart failure secondary to systemic hypertension or acute myocardial infarction is the most common cause of pulmonary edema in patients with acute cerebrovascular disorders. Occasionally the overenthusiastic administration of intravenous fluids may be a contributory factor, and at times the intracranial lesion itself may cause pulmonary edema, either by initiating the inappropriate secretion of pituitary antidiuretic hormone (ADH) or by activating reflex mechanisms as yet poorly understood.

Oversecretion of antidiuretic hormone lowers urinary output and causes elevation of the specific gravity despite adequate fluid intake. This oliguria is not usually a problem in patients suspected of having cerebral edema, because they are purposely kept somewhat dehydrated. In patients with cerebral infarction, on the other hand, adequate hydration is desirable to reduce hemoconcentration and sludging. In the presence of chronic oliguria, the administration of even 2 or 3 liters of fluid daily may eventually result in overhydration and the development of pulmonary edema. In all patients with acute cerebrovascular disorders, careful attention must be paid to the fluid intake and urinary output. If urinary volume remains low and specific gravity high despite adequate intake, and if the concentration of serum electrolytes, particularly sodium, begins to fall, inappropriate excretion of ADH is probable. The daily fluid intake should be restricted to less than 1,000 ml.

Pulmonary Embolism Embolus to the pulmonary artery or one of its major branches results immediately in right-sided heart strain, dyspnea, cyanosis, and shock. When recognized early and if the patient's condition will tolerate major surgery, the clot can be removed. Diagnosis is made by clinical signs and use of radioisotopic lung scan.

Emboli lodging more distally in the smaller branches of the pulmonary arterial system may cause symptoms ranging from dyspnea to no symptoms whatsoever, depending upon size of the occluded artery and whether there is concomitant pleural irritation and infarction of lung tissue.

Signs of embolus include tachypnea, tachycardia, fever, leukocytosis, pleural friction rub, and sometimes characteristic changes on plain chest x-ray. Radioisotopic lung scans can be diagnostic. Treatment is supportive and generally directed at prevention of recurrence by use of anticoagulants or by ligation of the vena cava or femoral veins.

Cardiovascular System

Heart Patients with symptomatic cerebrovascular disease frequently have concomitant cardiac abnormalities. Previously asymptomatic hypertension may announce itself with an acute intracranial episode and cardiac decompensation. Cerebral infarction may be secondary to the hypotension caused by myocardial infarction, or cardiac dysrhythmia. A good clinician, therefore, always considers the cerebral vessels, the heart, and the cervical vessels as a unit and treats all three in every patient who has a stroke of any kind.

Every patient who presents the slightest evidence of heart failure following an ictus must be digitalized to ensure good cardiac output and adequate oxygenation of the blood, and to prevent pulmonary congestion.

Phlebothrombosis In patients confined to bed, phlebothrombosis usually lies silently until it strikes with pulmonary embolus. Occasionally painless edema of the leg, prominent veins with minimal heat, positive Homans' sign, unexplained tachycardia, or a low-grade fever can be clues. Rarely, phlegmasia cerulea dolens is the initial indication of thrombosis.

Active and passive exercise beginning on the day of the ictus, frequent change of posture, elastic stockings, and rapid ambulation are the best preventives. Some clinicians advocate that anticoagulants be used for all patients confined to bed for a prolonged period unless other diseases make their use too risky.

Systemic Blood Pressure

Hypertension The practitioner must occasionally solve the question of whether elevated blood pressure in a patient suffering with an acute neurovascular episode is a cause or an effect of the intracranial abnormality. Knowledge of several facts can be of great assistance in resolving this problem.

1 Primary intracranial processes seldom if ever cause hypertension in alert patients. However, in those who are stuporous or comatose, it may be very difficult to differentiate hypertension occurring as a result of intracranial disease from systemic hypertension with secondary encephalopathy.

2 Primary intracranial diseases sufficiently advanced to cause systemic hypertension are usually accompanied by increased intracranial pressure and papilledema. In contrast, patients with encephalopathy secondary to systemic hypertension generally have retinal hemorrhages, exudates, and minimal papilledema.

3 Blood pressure elevation of recent onset could mean malignant hypertension or hypertension due to an intracranial tumor. In malignant hypertension systolic and diastolic pressures are both greatly elevated, the diastolic level at times reaching 130 to 180 mm Hg. Blood pressure elevations caused by increased intracranial pressure are primarily systolic and out of proportion to the diastolic elevation, resulting in a wide pulse pressure. When intracranial tumors cause pressure on the brainstem sufficient to result in hypertension, other vegetative disturbances will be obvious to the examiner. There will be sinus bradycardia because of pressure on the vagal nuclei and respiration will be slow and deep because of respiratory center depression.

When moderate hypertension is found in a patient who has had a recent cerebral infarction, it is well to leave it uncontrolled for about 6 weeks. Transitory fluctuations in pressure may be managed by changing the patient to head-up or head-low positions in bed. Rauwolfia derivatives, if used at all, must be employed in very low doses, since some patients are unusually responsive to this medication after cerebral infarction. As a general rule, rauwolfia should be avoided and oral natriuretic drugs such as chlorothiazide and hydrochlorothiazide used instead. See page 232 for a detailed discussion of these medications.

If one suspects that intracranial bleeding is the result of hypertension, the blood pressure should be lowered with fast-acting agents such as hydralazine, guanethidine, intramuscular reserpine, alpha-methyldopa, trimethaphan camsylate (Arfonad), or diazoxide.

Hypotension It is extremely unusual for intracranial lesions to produce hypotension except for the rare pituitary apoplexy (Chap. 29). Consequently, when the blood pressure of a patient with an intracranial disorder falls, one should search for a systemic cause such as (1) acute loss of blood, (2) myocardial infarction, (3) pulmonary embolism, (4) gram-negative bacteremia, (5) an intraabdominal catastrophe (e.g., pancreatitis or a perforated bowel), (6) a reaction to some medication such as a psychomimetic or hypotensive drug, or (7) acute adrenal exhaustion or, rarely, pituitary insufficiency secondary to apoplexy. Specific therapy would depend on the cause; but until this can be determined, the patient must be in the Trendelenburg position and should be given oxygen. The administration of whole blood or vasopressor agents will help to keep the blood pressure at normotensive levels.

Intracranial Hypertension

Edema is a stereotyped response of the brain to a variety of acute insults. It results from the extravasation of fluid out of the bloodstream into the extracellular spaces or from a swelling of the neurons and glial elements themselves. Depending on its cause, it may be focal or generalized.

As the involved areas expand, they sometimes compress adjacent structures and interrupt their function. This process can be self-perpetuating if veins are compressed by the edema and capillary pressures are increased by backing up of venous blood.

Edema may follow any acute neurovascular disorder, but in the majority of patients it does not produce clinical manifestations. With some diseases, however, massive edema of a cerebral hemisphere causes the brain to shift to one side. The resultant pressure on the midbrain produces deterioration of consciousness, slowing of the heart rate and respiration, arterial hypertension, and even death. If incipient transtentorial herniation occurs as well, it will be evidenced by third-nerve palsy even though papilledema may not be present.

When cerebral edema is severe enough to cause pressure, it must be reduced by the measures to be described. Neurosurgical decompression may be necessary if the edema persists, but the medical regimens outlined in the following paragraphs can stabilize the patient's condition prior to surgery, facilitate neurosurgical procedures, and help control postoperative cerebral edema. Often they reduce pressure dramatically, only to be followed some hours later by recurrence of the edema and signs of increased pressure—the so-called "rebound effect."

Posture in Bed The simple maneuver of elevating the patient's head may reduce pressure somewhat by promoting venous drainage.

Dehydrating Agents A *retention enema* of concentrated magnesium sulfate held in the rectum for 15 to 30 min is an effective dehydrating agent. The patient should be given 120 to 180 ml of a 40 to 60 percent solution repeated every 6 to 8 hr.

Urea or *mannitol* may be given intravenously in doses of 2 mg per kg of body weight and may be repeated as often as required.

Glycerol may be given through a nasogastric

tube in doses of 1 to 2 mg per kg of body weight at intervals of 2 to 3 hr. Some authorities think that it does not cause "rebound effect."

Agents that promote diuresis by increasing the volume of fluid in the extracellular compartment also increase blood volume; hence they must be avoided in patients with unrelieved intracranial hemorrhage. Because of the rapid diuresis, unconscious patients must be catheterized to prevent bladder distention.

Adrenocorticosteroids These agents are sometimes dramatically effective in temporarily reversing the progress of brain edema. The means by which they act are unknown. An initial dose of dexamethasone 10 mg intravenously is followed by 6 to 10 mg intramuscularly three times a day for several days; the dosage is then gradually decreased over the next several days. This method of therapy produces remarkable improvement at times, and, together with fluid restriction to 1 liter daily, may prove to be the simplest means for medical management of cerebral edema.

Removal of Cerebrospinal Fluid Lumbar puncture for the withdrawal of large quantities of cerebrospinal fluid in an effort to relieve increased intracranial pressure secondary to cerebral edema is dangerous and is mentioned only to be condemned. After the surgeon has decompressed the brain by craniotomy, repeated ventricular taps may be helpful.

Skin

The prevention of decubitus ulcers is the responsibility of both the physician and the nurse, but most of the work falls on the nurse. Development of pressure sores is a sign of inadequate nursing care, not of the patient's poor resistance. If the patient is not able to change position, he must be turned every 1 to 2 hr. By using the supine, prone, and right- and left-lateral po-

sitions in rotation, pressure points are changed and the development of pressure sores may be retarded. Many authorities recommend an alternating-pressure air mattress; others, a soft mattress covered with lamb's wool or a water bed. If sheets are used, they must be clean, dry, and unwrinkled, and pressure points such as the occiput, the sacrum, and the heels must be protected.

Areas of persistent rubor over pressure points are the earliest sign of incipient breakdown and are a danger signal of great importance. The occurrence of ulceration is very serious; the best treatment is to keep the area dry, free of pressure, covered with sterile gauze, and scrupulously clean until it heals.

Genitourinary Tract

Urinary retention or incontinence occurs most commonly in patients with dementia, those whose level of consciousness is depressed, and those with lesions in the paracentral lobules or on the medial orbital surface of the frontal lobe.

Catheterization of incontinent patients should be avoided if possible because it is easier to change bedclothes than to treat urinary tract infection. A condom drain or a urinal will help the nurse keep the male patient dry; women can wear sanitary napkins and be put on a bedpan at intervals throughout the day. If continence does not return after 3 to 4 days, one may have to reconsider the situation and resort to a collection device.

Urinary incontinence in women may at times initiate vaginitis, for which douching is necessary; therefore a periodic examination of the vagina is necessary in all women in whom incontinence lasts for any length of time.

In men with retention due to prostatic obstruction, an indwelling catheter may be necessary. The collecting system should be closed to outside contamination and must be inserted using strict sterile precautions, thus avoiding urinary tract infections. Even so, urinalysis and culture should be made weekly and if pyuria or bacilluria develop, appropriate antibacterial agents should be initiated.

The catheter should be removed at least every 2 weeks and efforts made to establish normal micturition using encouragement and sometimes parasympathomimetic drugs.

Gastrointestinal Tract

Oral Hygiene Dentures must be removed from unconscious patients, and the mouth should be kept closed so that the mucous membranes do not become dehydrated and fissured.

Patients who are alert but apraxic may have difficulty in swallowing; they should not be given solids until liquids and puréed foods are well tolerated, because a cud or bolus may be retained in the mouth and later aspirated.

Vomiting After an acute cerebral vascular episode, some patients will vomit until the gastric contents are expelled. During this time, every precaution must be taken to prevent aspiration of the vomitus. Once the stomach is empty, retching is less dangerous, since aspiration cannot occur. Chlorpromazine (Thorazine), 50 to 100 mg, or trimethobenzamide hydrochloride (Tigan), 250 to 500 mg every 4 to 6 hr, may control the vomiting effectively but may also induce hypotension.

Persistent and intractable vomiting suggests a lesion in the posterior fossa or an intraabdominal difficulty unrelated to the neurologic problem.

Gastroduodenal Ulcers Acute peptic ulcers, called *stress* or *Cushing's ulcers,* occasionally develop in patients with intracranial lesions. They are most often associated with abnormalities of the hypothalamus but may occur in patients who have lesions in any part of the brain. Some

authorities attribute them to irritation of the esophageal and gastric mucosa caused by tube feeding; others believe that adrenocorticosteroids secreted in response to the stress of the cerebral episode may be responsible. Whatever the cause, Cushing's ulcers may lead to gastrointestinal bleeding which is particularly severe in patients who are being treated with anticoagulants. Fortunately, most of these ulcers are asymptomatic and do not bleed or perforate.

Singultus (Hiccup) Persistent hiccuping in a patient with a cerebrovascular disorder indicates dehydration, myocardial infarction, azotemia, phrenic nerve irritation by supra- or infradiaphragmatic disease, or a lesion in the posterior fossa which is affecting the medullary respiratory centers. It is an occasional occurrence in the lateral medullary artery syndrome (posterior inferior cerebellar). In most cases it ceases after about a week. In other cases, it is a very ominous sign and is often resistant to treatment. Trimethobenzamide hydrochloride (Tigan) or one of the phenothiazine derivatives may be helpful.

Bowels Fecal incontinence is hardly ever a problem, but impaction may become one. If the patient does not have spontaneous bowel movements, he should be given a gently cleansing enema every second day. A low-residue diet will help to reduce the bulk of the stool, and patients on liquid diets do not need bowel movements. If incontinence with repeated stools and diarrhea develops after an interval of constipation, one must consider impaction, perform a digital examination, and perhaps remove feces manually. A glycerine or olive-oil enema should be used to soften the stool and promote spontaneous movement. This situation should never develop, as it is a manifestation of inattention on the part of the physician. Persistent diarrhea should cause one to suspect excessive feeding of high-protein (concentrate) foods or, if the patient has been on antibiotics, a gastrointestinal disorder such as streptococcal or fungal enteritis.

Eyes

Because of lack of muscle tone, the eyelids of unconscious patients may not close spontaneously. Consequently, a rapid evaporation of tears with drying out of the globe, secondary infection, and corneal ulceration may occur. For this reason methylcellulose drops should be instilled every 4 hr and the eyelids must be sealed with cellophane tape. Conscious patients who have facial paralysis should be trained to close their paralyzed lid manually when they desire to sleep.

General Considerations

Nutrition If fluid balance and vitamin intake are maintained, the patient may be treated without feedings for a week or 10 days. Vitamins given orally in liquid form are easy to swallow and are preferable to injections, since perforation of the skin is to be avoided as much

as possible. A reducing diet is beneficial for patients who are overweight, especially as an aid to future ambulation, and should be started on the day of admission. After the patient has lost weight sufficient for one to see his ribs, he should be given a diet containing 40 Gm fat and 70 Gm protein, with sufficient carbohydrate to bring the total intake to 1200 to 1500 Cal daily. In order to avoid dehydration due to the use of hypertonic feedings (the hyperalimentation syndrome), 2 to 3 liters of fluid should be given daily.

Tube feeding should be avoided whenever possible by urging the patient to drink from a glass or with a straw, or if necessary by force-feeding him, using a syringe with a rubber tube attached.

Fluids and Electrolytes If the patient is unconscious, fluids and electrolytes are administered intravenously, by hypodermoclysis, or by nasogastric tube. For an average-sized adult, we recommend a program such as that listed in Table 30-1. When the BUN is elevated, the serum potassium level must be estimated daily and po-

Table 30-1   Intravenous Formula Providing Maintenance Nutrition for Patient Weighing 60 to 70 kg to Be Given over 24-hr Period

Formula	Provides daily				
	Protein, Gm	Calories	Na, mEq	K, mEq	H_2O, ml
1,000 ml of 5% protein hydrolysate in 5% dextrose and water	50	345	10	17	1,000
To 700 ml of 10% dextrose in water add 300 ml of 50% dextrose 50 mM NaCl (2.9 Gm in 50 ml) 20 mM KCl (1.5 Gm in 20 ml) Soluble vitamins		880	50	20	1,070
					125*
Total	50	1,225	60	37	2,195

* If completely utilized, 270 Gm of dextrose will yield 125 ml H_2O.
Source: G. D. Webster, Food and fluids for the stroke patient, *Current Concepts Cerebrovascular Dis.—Stroke,* **5**:25, 1970. By permission of The American Heart Association, Inc.

tassium administered only as necessary. If the patient is febrile, about 500 ml of 5 percent glucose in water should be added for each degree of fever and urinary output watched, making sure it is commensurate with the additional fluid intake.

Prolonged fluid loss caused by diarrhea, dehydrating agents, or enemas may lead to profound hypopotassemia with cardiac dysrhythmia, encephalopathy, abdominal distention, and loss of reflexes. If this occurs, intravenous potassium can be lifesaving. Electrolyte balance is disturbed by renal disease, diabetes mellitus, diabetes insipidus, inappropriate secretion of antidiuretic hormone, and the administration of corticosteroids or dehydrating agents. Frequent determinations of sodium, potassium, chloride, and carbon dioxide must be done on the patient's serum when any of these conditions is present.

Exercise For all patients who have had cerebral vascular episodes, active and passive exercises in bed should be initiated on the day the ictus occurs. For those with intracranial bleeding, exercise should be passive and confined to the limbs. The hemiplegic patient must be taught to move his own paralyzed limbs with his intact ones. Until he can, a nurse, a physical therapist, or a member of the family should move them through their full range of motion at least twice daily.

The most important joint in the upper extremity is the shoulder, since it is particularly vulnerable to subluxation, with resultant pain and rapid ankylosis. Sympathetic dystrophy then leads to trophic changes, pain, discoloration, and swelling in the hand and arm (shoulder-hand syndrome). If the patient has pain about the shoulder when the arm is raised, the limb must be elevated to the point at which pain occurs, then moved a bit higher before being lowered. With each exercise the arm should be

elevated just a bit more, until the full range of motion is finally achieved.

Putting the hip, knee, and ankle through the full range of motion is particularly important as a prophylaxis against the development of thrombosis in one of the deep veins of the leg.

The subject of rehabilitation is discussed more fully later in this chapter.

Pain and Restlessness For headache, 10 grains acetylsalicylic acid may be given every 3 hr by mouth. In order to prevent dyspepsia or gastric ulceration, milk or some other liquid demulcent should be given with the aspirin. If the patient is unable to take pills, the tablets can be crushed, or liquid aspirin can be used. If necessary, $\frac{1}{4}$ to $\frac{3}{4}$ grain codeine may be given for a short time, as well. Narcotics such as morphine and meperidine (Demerol) should not be used, since they may depress the respiratory center, particularly if the patient has a posterior fossa lesion or increased intracranial pressure.

Subarachnoid hemorrhage produces intractable and agonizing headaches, which can often be relieved temporarily by the careful removal of 10 to 20 ml of spinal fluid through lumbar puncture with manometric control.

Phenobarbital and chloral hydrate, which occasionally produce agitation, particularly in children and elderly patients, should not be used for pain or headache. Older patients often respond well to paraldehyde given in doses of 5 to 10 ml orally, rectally, or if necessary intramuscularly.

For agitation caused by organic psychosis and not by pain, diazepam (Valium) or chlorpromazine (Thorazine) is very helpful in calming the patient. The dosage must be individualized, but 10 mg diazepam or 25 mg chlorpromazine orally three or four times daily can be used for the first dose. Diazepam can be given intravenously if necessary. Often a reassuring member of the family or of the nursing staff will do more to quiet a restless patient than medications or restraints.

At times restlessness is due to bladder distention and can be relieved by catheterization.

Convulsions Convulsions may occur at any stage in the evolution of a cerebrovascular lesion. It is estimated that 10 to 20 percent of patients have a seizure during the acute ictus of stroke and that 5 to 10 percent have recurrent convulsions as a residual abnormality following recovery from the episode. Three or four daily doses of 32 to 60 mg phenobarbitol combined with 100 mg diphenylhydantoin are usually adequate to prevent convulsions, and some clinicians use these medications prophylactically in patients who have any deficit attributable to a lesion of the cerebral hemispheres because the incidence of convulsions as a sequela to cerebral hemorrhage or infarction varies from 10 to 20 percent in some series.

The first consideration for a patient in status epilepticus is to ensure an open airway. Paraldehyde, amobarbital (Amytal), phenobarbital, diphenylhydantoin (Dilantin), chlordiazepoxide (Librium), and diazepam (Valium) have all been recommended as the anticonvulsant of choice in an acute emergency. The best of the above medications is the one with which the physician is most familiar. If convulsions continue, additional doses of barbiturates are administered until seizures are controlled or respiratory depression is noted. Diphenylhydantoin is used by some, but it has been associated with cardiac arrest and probably should not be employed intravenously. We prefer to start therapy with diazepam (Valium), 10 to 20 mg, intravenously and repeat it as often as necessary because it quickly controls seizures without depressing respiration. If, as rarely happens, seizures continue unabated and are of focal onset, intracarotid medication can be considered.

Fever The most frequent causes of fever following ictus are bronchopneumonia and urinary tract infection. When fever develops in a patient with an indwelling catheter, cystitis, pyelitis, and bacteremia must be considered first. A very few patients may have "central" fever secondary to abnormalities in the upper part of the brainstem and hypothalamus. Thrombophlebitis may produce a low-grade fever. Some clinicians are convinced that fecal impaction is accompanied by fever, but this is debatable.

Chest x-rays and examinations of the blood and urine are essential for the diagnosis of any unexplained fever, and treatment depends on its cause.

Surgical Intervention

Intracranial surgery plays no role in the therapy of cerebral infarction and is seldom useful in massive brain hemorrhage or massive infarction. In patients with cerebellar hemorrhage or infarction, the posterior fossa should be explored as an emergency procedure, and in patients with subdural hematoma the blood clot must be evacuated as soon as possible. Immediate neurosurgical consultation is indicated for patients with intracranial hypertension and evidence of upper brainstem compression. In cases of subarachnoid hemorrhage, the difficult problems regarding management and the time of angiography call for immediate surgical consultation and group decision. Patients who are in good general health except for recurrent neurologic deficit due to vascular insufficiency may need arteriography of all four major vessels as a basis for determining the feasibility of reconstructive extracranial vascular surgery.

Brain Death

Patients with intracranial vascular catastrophes may develop the total loss of all brain function despite continuation of heartbeat and detectable blood pressure. If all the following conditions are met, then the patient can be declared dead by reason of brain death and all life-support systems can be stopped: the absence of all neural reflexes, including dilated pupils fixed to light stimulation; no deviation of the eyes in response to caloric testing; areflexia; no movement, either spontaneous or reflex; and no spontaneous respirations. In addition, there must be no detectable electrical activity on two successive electroencephalograms, several hours apart, and the patient must not be hypothermic or poisoned. In instances where electroencephalographic facilities are not available, the total and persistent absence of all clinically elicitable brainstem reflexes in a comatose person will have the same connotation.

REHABILITATION OF THE PATIENT WITH HEMIPLEGIA

Rehabilitation begins when a physician first sees his patient. Even before a definitive diagnosis has been reached, he must initiate a program designed to prevent complications and minimize neurologic deficit. The principles of management just described help to prevent the complications of immobilization. In this section, measures are outlined which may aid in the ambulation of the patient.

If recovery is to occur, spontaneous improvement is usually discernible within a few days of the ictus; as a rule, the more rapid the initial recovery, the more complete it will be eventually. If there has been no recovery of volitional activity after 6 to 12 weeks, it can be assumed with some confidence that little will occur. Recovery almost always occurs first in the proximal muscles of the torso, hip, and leg, followed by the distal leg, proximal arm, and lastly the hand. This return of function resembles the normal acquisition of skills in infants and children. Mass activity always appears before isolated joint movement is possible (Table 30–2).

Even after motor power begins to reappear, improvement may cease at any stage. Further recovery is dependent on many factors, one of the most important being motivation. Recovery may be hindered by associated dementia, aphasia and apraxia, cerebral disturbances, disorder of spatial relations caused by hemianopia and hemisensory defects, and poor family relationships.

Table 30–2   Return of Function in Patients with Hemiplegia

Average time after onset of ictus	Reflex	Movement
0 hr	1. Loss or diminution of tendon reflexes 2. Hypotonia	No voluntary or reflex movement
4–48 hr	1. Tendon reflexes more active 2. Minimal increase in muscle tone (seen first in palmar and plantar flexors)	Reflex withdrawal to painful stimuli
3 days–6 weeks	1. Finger-jerks brisk 2. Gradual increase in muscle tone, especially adductors and flexors of the upper limb and adductors and extensors of the lower limb 3. Appearance of clonus (first seen in plantar flexors) 4. Clasp-knife phenomenon elicited in knee extensors and/or elbow flexors	Movement of proximal muscles of leg followed in 7–10 days by movement of toes. Movement of shoulder

Acute Stage of the Illness

During the flaccid stage it is helpful for the patient with hemiplegia to have his feet placed firmly against a footboard to prevent shortening of his Achilles tendon and overstretching of his dorsiflexors. His feet should extend beyond the end of the mattress to avoid decubiti of the heels, and the weight of his bed covers should not rest on his feet. Soft wool socks also help to protect the heels from pressure. The affected leg must be supported on the lateral side to prevent muscle contracture of the hip in external rotation. A pillow should be put in the axilla of the affected arm to maintain abduction. Other pillows should be arranged so that the elbow is higher than the shoulder and the hand higher than the elbow, in order to prevent edema. As described earlier, the patient must be turned every hour during the day and every 2 hr at night. The involved joints must be carried through their range of motion at least twice daily beginning on the day of the ictus.

Subacute Stage

No patient should stay in bed a day longer than necessary. Bed rest, once the solace both of the sick and the healer, is now known to be a cause of bedsores, thrombophlebitis, bronchopneumonia, disuse atrophy of skeletal muscles, osteoporosis with renal calculi, and, most sinister of all, pulmonary embolism and a loss of the patient's will to be ambulatory.

Patients who have been kept in bed more than a week must begin ambulation slowly, first with elevation of the head of the bed for gradually lengthening times, then with dangling the feet over the bedside before being allowed to sit in a chair and to stand. When he is first helped to stand, the patient's blood pressures must be determined in the recumbent and erect positions to ascertain if he has developed postural hypotension. If so, tilt-table exercises are necessary to reestablish vasomotor tone.

The patient can soon be taught to place his normal foot underneath his affected knee, slide it down his paralyzed leg to the ankle and move the useless limb with his good one. Once this simple technique has been mastered, the patient must be taught to pull himself upright with his good arm. By combining these two procedures he learns to swing himself into a sitting position at the edge of the bed. In this position he should be taught to use his paretic arm for support. An overhead trapeze attached to the bed is a most useful device for allowing the patient to pull himself up.

Learning to Stand

After the patient has learned to sit up by himself, he is taught to stand. From a sitting position with legs dangling over the side, he slides off the bed, distributing his weight onto both legs with the therapist supporting the weak side. At this stage friendly reassurance is extremely helpful, since many patients with hemiplegia have a fear of falling when they stand. As soon as he is up, the patient balances on his good leg and should attempt to place as much weight as possible on the paretic one. After this, he should sit back on the bed and place his affected hand in his lap in order to prevent its dangling at the side. Some patients, especially those with parietal lobe lesions, are ambivalent about their affected extremities and tend to neglect them or to regard them as strange, unearthly, and unpleasant impediments, rather than as their own limbs. This attitude must be overcome by reeducation.

Once the patient learns to stand and sit, a portable commode should be substituted for the bedpan.

Learning to Walk

As soon as the patient can stand, he should be fitted with oxford shoes with broad, low heels. Exercises designed to promote weight distribution and balance in various positions are then carried out by the therapist or member of the family. Learning to walk is a very painstaking procedure, begun between parallel bars and progressing to a walker or a four-legged stick. The physical therapist should not support the patient but may help when necessary. Patients with cerebellar ataxia must use a four-legged walker.

In many hemiplegic patients the knee does not lock in extension or tends to collapse when bearing weight; these patients should be fitted with a long leg brace. In some, the knee supports weight adequately but the ankle does not; for them a short leg brace should be adequate.

From the beginning, the patient is encouraged to use his normal hand to dress, undress, use cutlery, and carry out various other everyday maneuvers. As soon as there is any function in his affected hand, he should be forced to use it for activities which normally involve both hands.

In later stages mechanical devices such as the stationary bicycle or rowing machine may be used to assist in strengthening muscles.

Driving a Car

Many patients who have recovered sufficiently to walk desire to drive an automobile. The decision to allow this is one that can be particularly difficult and should be made by the physician and family together; they must not let emotions interfere. Driving a car is one of the most complicated learned skills; it requires intact reflex responses as well as rapid decisions. If a cerebrovascular episode destroys one or more of the pathways involved in these activities, then driving should be forbidden, especially in instances of homonymous hemianopia, visual extinction, or uncontrolled seizures. For those cases where the only deficit is that of foot drop, ankle clonus, or lower limb ataxia, foot controls can be replaced. Ultimately the decision is dependent

not only on the neurologic evaluation but on the locally prevalent laws as well.

MANAGEMENT OF THE PATIENT WITH APHASIA

The plight of an aphasic hemiplegic patient is in many ways similar to that of a parachutist who breaks an arm and leg landing in a foreign country. He is helpless, and the people use a language which he can neither understand nor speak. The patient's dependent isolation, especially of the young who may not fully comprehend the situation, is often accentuated by the attitude of others.

This isolation can be unbearable for an extrovert. Therefore, the first aim in dealing with aphasics is to establish emotional contact. Relatives and nurses should be instructed to speak to the patient and to listen to his attempt at articulation. Even if he seems to understand nothing at all, they must compensate for the loss of verbal communication by friendly gestures or smiles. In some cases the patient may understand a word or two; thus, any discussion he should not hear must not be carried on in his presence.

Before commencing therapy it is essential to record the patient's defects. Aphasia is rarely, if ever, an isolated disturbance; reading, writing, understanding, speaking, counting, drawing, recognizing and appreciating music, and gesticulation are impaired, though in different degrees. In short, the entire process of symbolization is disturbed, making a global approach to the problem necessary. Psychologic problems of emotional lability, suppressed anger, hopeless frustration, and a morbid fear of the future compound this organic loss.

Speech therapy is a long process requiring months of hard work, and the goal is not words but communication. Language is used mainly not for factual communication but for human contact. If, by speech therapy, the patient regains the habit of contact, a major goal will have been attained.

Sometimes a patient will do well in a group of aphasic persons who relearn together with a speech therapist, but more often he will do better when individual attention is given. Usually the patient can comprehend gestures with less difficulty than the spoken or written word; if he is multilingual, he may find it simpler to comprehend his mother tongue.

The degree and rapidity with which individuals regain use of language varies considerably. As a general rule, a child with aphasia has a better prognosis than an adult. A left-handed aphasic has a better prognosis than one who is right-handed.

SUGGESTED READINGS

General Principles

Ford, A. B., and Katz, S.: Prognosis after strokes. Part I: A critical review, *Medicine,* **45**:223, 1966.

Hierons, R.: Vascular coma, *Internat. J. Neurol.,* **2**:375, 1961.

Hurwitz, L. J.: Management of major strokes, *Brit. Med. J.,* **3**:699, 1969.

McDowell, F. J.: Initial treatment of cerebrovascular diseases, *Mod. Treatment,* **2**:15, 1965.

Mead, S.: The doctor has a stroke, *Lancet,* **2**:574, 1963.

Merrett, J. D., and Adams, G. F.: Comparison of mortality rates in elderly hypertensive and normotensive hemiplegic patients, *Brit. Med. J.,* **2**:802, 1966.

Moore, F. D.: Changing minds about brains, *New Engl. J. Med.,* **282**:47, 1970.

Over, R. P., and Belknap, E. L.: Educating stroke patient families, *J. Chronic Diseases,* **20**:45, 1967.

Respiratory System

Dulfano, M. J., and Ishikawa, S.: Hypercapnia: Mental changes and extrapulmonary complications; an expanded concept of the "CO_2 intoxication" syndrome, *Ann. Internal Med.,* **63**:829, 1965.

Gregory, I. C.: Tracheostomy, *Brit. J. Hosp. Med.,* **3**:611, 1970.

Richards, P.: Pulmonary oedema and intracranial lesions, *Brit. Med. J.,* **2**:83, 1963.

Cardiovascular System

Burch, G. E., and Phillips, J. H.: The large upright T wave as an electrocardiographic manifestation of intracranial disease, *South Med. J.,* **61**:331, 1968.

Lavy, S., Stern, S., Herishianu, Y., and Carmon, A.: Electrocardiographic changes in ischaemic strokes, *J. Neurol. Sci.,* **7**:409, 1968.

Tomkin, G., Coe, R. P. K., and Marshall, J.: Electrocardiographic abnormalities in patients presenting with strokes, *J. Neurol. Neurosurg. Psychiat.,* **31**:250, 1968.

Systemic Blood Pressure

Illingsworth, G., and Jennett, W. B.: The shocked head injury, *Lancet,* **2**:511, 1965.

Montgomery, B. M.: The basilar artery hypertensive syndrome, *Arch. Internal Med.,* **108**:559, 1966.

Intracranial Hypertension

Bakay, L., and Lee, J. C.: Cerebral Edema, Charles C Thomas, Publisher, Springfield, Ill., 1965.

Buckell, M., and Walsh, L.: Effect of glycerol by mouth on raised intracranial pressure in man, *Lancet,* **2**:1151, 1964.

Dyken, M., and White, P. T.: Evaluation of cortisone in the treatment of cerebral infarction, *J.A.M.A.,* **162**:1531, 1956.

Gärde, A.: Experiences with dexamethasone treatment of intracranial pressure caused by brain tumors, *Acta neurol. scand.,* **41**(suppl. 13, part 2):439, 1965.

Matson, D. D.: Treatment of cerebral swelling, *New Engl. J. Med.,* **272**:626, 1965.

Plum, F.: Brain swelling and edema in cerebral vascular disease, *Res. Pub. Assoc. Nerv. Ment. Dis.,* **41**:318, 1966.

Richardson, A. E.: Some clinical aspects of cerebral oedema, *Proc. Roy. Soc. Med.,* **58**:604, 1965.

Shenkin, H. A., and Bouzarth, W. F.: Clinical methods of reducing intracranial pressure. Role of the cerebral circulation, *New Engl. J. Med.,* **282**:1465, 1970.

Skin

Bailey, B. N.: Bed sores, *Brit. J. Hosp. Med.,* **3**:223, 1970.

Elson, R. A.: Anatomical aspects of pressure sores and their treatment, *Lancet,* **1**:884, 1965.

Line, R. E.: Polyether urethane foam: A nursing tool in the prevention and treatment of decubitus ulcers, *Nurs. Clin. N. Amer.,* **1**:417, 1966.

Genitourinary Tract

Blandy, J. P.: Catheterization, *Brit. Med. J.,* **2**:1531, 1965.

Comarr, A. E.: Editorial: In defense of the intraurethral catheter, *Am. J. Surg.,* **111**:157, 1966.

Hardy, A. G.: Complications of the indwelling urethral catheter, *Paraplegia,* **6**:5, 1968.

Gastrointestinal Tract

Connell, A. M.: The physiology and pathophysiology of constipation, *Paraplegia,* **4**:244, 1966.

Dalgaard, J. B.: Cerebral vascular lesions and peptic ulceration, *Arch. Pathol.,* **69**:359, 1960.

McCrory, W. W.: Cerebral disease and gastrointestinal hemorrhage, *J.A.M.A.,* **197**:935, 1966.

Nutrition

Albanese, A. A., Lorenze, E. J., and Orto, L. A.: Effect of strokes on carbohydrate tolerance, *Geriatrics,* **23**:142, March 1968.

Dudrick, S. J., Long, J. M., Steiger, E., and Rhoads, J. E.: Intravenous hyperalimentation, *Med. Clin. N. Am.,* **54**(3):577, 1970.

Webster, G. D.: Food and fluids for the stroke patient, *Current Concepts Cerebrovascular Dis.—Stroke,* **5**:25, 1970.

Fluid and Electrolyte Disturbances

Bernard-Weil, E., David, M., and Pertuiset, B.: "Inappropriate" secretion of anti-diuretic hormone without corresponding hyponatraemia in cerebral pathology: Its therapeutic implications, *J. Neurol. Sci.,* **3**:300, 1966.

Blumentals, A. S. (ed.): Symposium on acid-base balance, *Arch. Internal Med.,* **116**:647, 1965.

Clift, G. V., Schletter, F. E., Moses, A. M., and Streeten, D. H. P.: Syndrome of inappropriate vasopressin secretion: Studies on the mechanism of the hyponatremia of a patient, *Arch. Internal Med.,* **118**:453, 1966.

Convulsions

Dodge, P. R., Richardson, E. P., Jr., and Victor, M.: Recurrent convulsive seizures as a sequel to cerebral infarction: Clinical and pathological study, *Brain,* **77**:610, 1954.

Gastaut, H., Naquet, R., Poire, R., and Tassinari, C. A.: Treatment of status epilepticus with diazepam (Valium), *Epilepsia,* **6**:167, 1965.

Leading article: Status epilepticus: A medical emergency, *Brit. Med. J.,* **3**:63, 1967.

Lombroso, C. T.: Treatment of status epilepticus with diazepam, *Neurology,* **16**:629, 1966.

Louis, S., and McDowell, F.: Epileptic seizures in nonembolic cerebral infarction, *Arch. Neurol.,* **17**:414, 1967.

Prensky, A. L., Raff, M. C., Moore, M. J., and Schwab, R. S.: Intravenous diazepam in the treatment of prolonged seizure activity, *New Engl. J. Med.,* **276**:779, 1967.

Richardson, E. P., Jr., and Dodge, P. R.: Epilepsy in cerebrovascular disease: A study of the incidence and nature of seizures in 104 consecutive autopsy-proven cases of cerebral infarction and hemorrhage, *Epilepsia,* **3**:49, 1954.

Surgical Intervention

Ojemann, R. G.: The surgical treatment of cerebrovascular disease, *New Engl. J. Med.,* **274**:440, 1966.

Brain Death

May, P. G., and Kaelbling, R.: Coma of over a year's duration with favorable outcome, *Diseases Nervous System,* **29**:837, 1968.

Silverman, D., Saunders, M. G., Schwab, R. S., and Masland, R. L.: Cerebral death and the electroencephalogram, *J.A.M.A.,* **209**:1505, 1969.

Rehabilitation of the Patient with Hemiplegia

Adams, G. F., and Hurwitz, L. J.: Mental barriers to recovery from strokes, *Lancet,* **2**:533, 1963.

Belmont, I., Benjamin, H., Ambrose, J., and Restuccia, R. D.: Effect of cerebral damage on motivation in rehabilitation, *Arch. Phys. Med. Rehabil.,* **50**:507, 1969.

Ben-Yishay, Y., Diller, L., Gerstman, L., and Haas, A.: The relationship between impersistence, intellectual function and outcome of rehabilitation in patients with left hemiplegia, *Neurology,* **18**:852, 1968.

Bourestom, N. C.: Predictors of long-term recovery in cerebrovascular disease, *Arch. Phys. Med. Rehabil.,* **48**:415, 1967.

DeCencio, D. V., Leshner, M., and Voron, D.: Verticality perception and ambulation in hemiplegia, *Arch. Phys. Med. Rehabil.,* **51**:105, 1970.

Fields, W. S., and Spencer, W. A. (eds.): Stroke Rehabilitation: Basic Concepts and Research Trends, Warren H. Green, Inc., St. Louis, 1967.

Hirschenfang, S., Shulman, L., and Benton, J. G.: Psychosocial factors influencing the rehabilitation of the hemiplegic patient, *Diseases Nervous System,* **29**:373, 1968.

Knapp, M. E.: The hemiplegic patient—Physical problems, *Postgrad. Med.,* **39**:A-125, 1966.

Rusk, H. A., and Taylor, E. J.: Living with a Disability, McGraw-Hill Book Company, New York, 1953.

Shanan, J., Cohen, M., and Adler, E.: Intellectual functioning in hemiplegic patients after cerebrovascular accidents, *J. Nervous Mental Disease,* **143**:181, 1966.

Wylie, C. M.: Age and the rehabilitative care of stroke, *J. Am. Geriat. Soc.,* **16**:428, 1968.

Acute Stage of the Illness

Atkinson, W. J.: Posture of the unconscious patient, *Lancet,* **1**:404, 1970.

Gordon, E. E.: Early application of physical medicine in stroke, *J. Rehabil.,* **29**:26, 1963.

Subacute Stage

Bobath, B.: Observations on adult hemiplegia and suggestions for treatment, *Physiotherapy,* **45**:279, 1959, and **46**:5, 1960.

Moskowitz, E.: Complications in the rehabilitation of hemiplegic patients, *Med. Clin. N. Am.,* **53**(3):541, 1969.

Moskowitz, H., Goodman, C. R., Smith, E., Balthazar, E., and Mellins, H. Z.: Hemiplegic shoulder, *New York State J. Med.,* **69**(1):548, 1969.

Rusk, H. A.: Rehabilitation Medicine: A Textbook in Physical Medicine and Rehabilitation, 2d ed., The C. V. Mosby Company, St. Louis, 1964.

United States Department of Health, Education, and Welfare: Strike Back at Stroke, Public Health Service, Division of Chronic Diseases, 1961.

Learning to Stand

American Heart Association: Do It Yourself Again: Self-help Devices for the Stroke Patient, New York, 1969.

Ekwall, B.: Method for evaluating indications for rehabilitation in chronic hemiplegia, *Acta med. scand. suppl.,* **450**:1, 1966.

Nickel, V. L.: Orthopedic rehabilitation—Challenges and opportunities, *Clin. Orthop.,* **63**:153, 1969.

United States Department of Health, Education, and Welfare: Up and Around (booklet to aid the stroke patient in activities of daily living), Public Health Service, Division of Chronic Diseases, Heart Disease Control Program, 1969.

Learning to Walk

Hastings, A. E.: Patterns of motor function in adult hemiplegia, *Arch. Phys. Med. Rehabil.,* **46**:255, 1965.

Peszczynski, M.: The rehabilitation of potential of the late adult hemiplegic, *Am. J. Nursing,* **63**:111, 1963.

Spiegler, J. H., and Goldberg, M. J.: The wheelchair as a permanent mode of mobility. A detailed guide to prescription (in 2 parts), *Am. J. Phys. Med.,* **47**:315, 1968, and **48**:25, 1969.

Stern, P. H., McDowell, F., Miller, J. M., and Elkin, R. D.: Quantitative testing of motility defects in patients after stroke, *Arch. Phys. Med. Rehabil.,* **50**:320, 1969.

Twitchell, T. E.: The restoration of motor function following hemiplegia in man, *Brain,* **74**:443, 1951.

Ullman, M.: Behavioral Changes in Patients Following Strokes, Charles C Thomas, Publisher, Springfield, Ill., 1962.

Williams, D.: Management of the chronic neurological patient, *Brit. Med. J.,* **2**:1554, 1964.

Autobiographies by Patients

Coates, A.: To whom it may concern; an experience in the North Carolina Memorial Hospital, Chapel

Hill, University of North Carolina, School of Medicine, 1972.

Hodgins, E.: Episode: Report on the Accident Inside My Skull, Atheneum Publishers, New York, 1964.

————: Listen: The patient, *New Engl. J. Med.,* **274**:657, 1966.

Ritchie, D. E.: Stroke: A Study of Recovery, Doubleday & Company, Inc., Garden City, N.Y., 1961.

Van Rosen, R. E.: Comeback: The Story of My Stroke, The Bobbs-Merrill Company, Inc., Indianapolis, 1962.

Management of the Patient with Aphasia

American Heart Association: Aphasia and the Family, New York, 1969.

Bloom, L. M.: A rationale for group treatment for aphasic patients, *J. Speech Hearing Disorders,* **27**:11, 1962.

Carson, D. H., Carson, F. E., and Tikofsky, R. S.: On learning characteristics of the adult aphasic, *Cortex,* **4**:92, 1968.

Cumming, W. J. K., Hurwitz, L. J., and Perl, N. T.: A study of a patient who had alexia without agraphia, *J. Neurol. Neurosurg. Psychiat.,* **33**:34, 1970.

Eagleson, H. M., Jr., Vaughn, G. R., and Knudson, A. B. C.: Hand signals for dysphasia, *Arch. Phys. Med. Rehabil.,* **51**:111, 1970.

Faglioni, P., Scotti, G., and Spinnler, H.: Impaired recognition of written letters following unilateral hemispheric damage, *Cortex,* **5**:120, 1969.

Horwitz, B.: An open letter to the family of an adult patient with aphasia, *Rehabil. Lit.,* **23**:141, 1962.

Longerich, M. C.: Manual for the Aphasic Patient, The Macmillan Company, New York, 1958.

Sarno, M. T., and Sands, E.: An objective method for the evaluation of speech therapy in aphasia, *Arch. Phys. Med. Rehabil.,* **51**:49, 1970.

Schuell, H., Carroll, V., and Street, B. S.: Clinical treatment of aphasia, *J. Speech Hearing Disorders,* **20**:43, 1955.

Additional References

Foley, W. J., McGinn, M. E., and Lindenauer, S. M.: Automobile drivers and cerebrovascular insufficiency, *J.A.M.A.,* **207**:749, 1969.

Meyer, J. S., Charney, J. Z., Rivera, V. M., and Mathew, N. T.: Treatment with glycerol of cerebral oedema due to acute cerebral infarction, *Lancet,* **2**:993, 1971.

Mooney, V., Perry, J., and Nickel, V. L.: Surgical and non-surgical orthopaedic care of stroke, *J. Bone Joint Surg.,* **49-A**:989, 1967.

Griffith, V. E.: Stroke in the Family: A Manual of Home Therapy, Delacorte, New York, 1970.

Korein, J.: On cerebral, brain, and systemic death, *Current Concepts Cerebrovascular Dis.–Stroke,* **8**:9, 1973.

Smith, G. W.: Care of the Patient with a Stroke. A Handbook for the Patient's Family and the Nurse, Springer Publishing Company, Inc., New York, 1959.

Solomon, G. E., Hilal, S. K., Gold, A. P., and Carter, S.: Natural history of acute hemiplegia of childhood, *Brain,* **93**:107, 1970.

Walsh, R. E., Michaelson, E. D., Harkleroad, L. E., Zighelboim, A., and Sackner, M. A.: Upper airway obstruction in obese patients with sleep disturbance and somnolence, *Ann. Internal Med.,* **76**:185, 1972.

Zankel, H. T.: Stroke Rehabilitation: A Guide to the Rehabilitation of an Adult Patient Following a Stroke, Charles C Thomas, Publisher, Springfield, Ill., 1971.

————, Cobb, J. B., and Huskey, F. E.: The rehabilitation of 500 stroke patients, *J. Am. Geriatric. Soc.,* **14**:1177, 1966.

Index

Index

Valsalva's maneuver:
hypertensive vascular disease aggravated by, 231
during patient examination, 87
ruptured aneurysms precipitated by, 281
Van den Bergh reaction, 285
Vascular plexus, evolution of, 5-6
Vasodepressor responses of carotid sinuses, 101, 103
Vasodilating agents, 201-202
Vasospasm:
arteriolar, 189-190
caused by blood clots, 218
cerebral embolism and, 219, 222, 223
intracranial aneurysm and, 302
in subarachnoid hemorrhage, 291
TIAs and, 188-189
Venography, 246
Venous anastomoses, 6
Venous angle (foramen of Monro), 40
Venous lacunae, 37
Venous plexus of internal carotid arteries, 17
Venous sinuses, diseases of, 243-248
laboratory findings on, 245-246
management of, 246-247
Venous spinovascular diseases, 253
Venous system, 35, 36, 37, 38, 39, 40-46
cavernous sinuses in, 43-44
thrombosis of, 245
deep, 35, 39, 40, 41
dural sinuses in: anatomy of, 41, 42-43
characteristics of, 63
occlusions of, 244-245
petrosal sinuses and, 44
role of, in cerebral circulation, 63-65
secondary, 45-46
superficial, 35, 37, 38, 39
superior petrosal sinuses in, 9
anatomy of, 44
thrombosis of, 245
(See also specific veins)
Ventral diencephalic veins, development of, 9
Ventral medullary syndrome, 251
Ventral pharyngeal arteries, development of, 6
Vertebral arteries, 81
anastomoses of, 2, 144
anastomotic channels between, 8
anatomy of, 23-25, 27, 28
anomalies of, 4
atherosclerosis of, 24, 112, 142
autonomic nerve fibers around, 61-62
brain infarction and, 7
development of, 2-3, 6
dissecting hematomas in, 368
internal carotid arteries compared with, 143-144
intracranial aneurysm in, 302
intracranial course of, 25
kinks of, 24, 143, 157
left, 144, 157
lesions in, as cause of spinal cord infarctions, 250
medial dysplasia in, 364

Vertebral arteries:
stenoses of, 24, 210
Takayasu's disease and, 348
(See also Vertebral-basilar artery syndrome; Vertebral-basilar system)
Vertebral-basilar artery syndrome, 75, 78, 141-152
etiology and pathogenesis of, 142-143
laboratory findings and differential diagnosis in, 148-149
pathologic findings and clinical features of, 144-147
pathophysiology of, 143-144
patient examination for, 147-148
symptoms and signs of, 146
Vertebral-basilar system, 25
anatomy of, 23-30
angiography of, 278
area supplied by, 144, 178
role in cerebral circulation, 134
atherosclerosis of, 161
branches of, 26, 27
in cerebral circulation, 134
collateral circulation provided by, 186
cranial arteritis in, 348
effects of syphilis on, 238
embolism in, 221
intracranial aneurysms in, 298
(See also Anterior inferior cerebellar arteries; Basilar arteries; Posterior cerebral arteries; Posterior inferior cerebellar arteries; Superior cerebellar arteries; Vertebral arteries)
Vertebral column (see Spinal cord)
Vertical nystagmus, 106
Vertigo:
brainstem lesions and, 29
infarctions and, 26
subclavian steal syndrome and, 155
as symptom of cerebrovascular disease, 78-79
as symptom of vertebral-basilar syndrome, 144, 146, 147
TIAs and, 193
Viral meningitis, 285
Virchow, R., 262
Virchow-Robin, spaces of, 162
Vision, loss of: from caroticocavernous fistulae, 325
from cerebrovascular insufficiency, 61
from cranial arteritis, 348, 351, 352
from encephalopathy, 231
from intracranial aneurysms, 301
from pituitary hemorrhage, 367-368
as symptom of vertebral-basilar syndrome, 144, 146
from TIAs, 193
(See also Amaurosis fugax)
Visual defects, 75, 77, 78
atherosclerosis of carotid arteries and, 128
from brainstem lesions, 29
from caroticocavernous fistulae, 323
from carotid artery syndrome, 128
from cavernous sinus thrombosis, 245

Visual defects:
from cerebral embolisms, 221
from encephalofacial angiomatosis, 325, 326
from extradural hematomas, 274
glaucoma as, 325
from internal carotid stenosis, 130
from intracranial aneurysms, 301
from intracranial vein diseases, 247
modes of progression of, 76
from polyarteritis nodosa, 353, 354
from pseudoxanthoma elasticum, 363
from subarachnoid hemorrhage, 283, 325, 336, 353
from Takayasu's disease, 347
in vertebral-basilar syndrome, 78, 148
(See also specific visual defects)
Vitamin B_1 deficiency, 333
Vitamin C deficiency, 333
Vomiting, general management of, 381

Wadia's test, 319
Walking, hemiplegic patients learning, 386-387
Wallenberg's syndrome, 26
Weber's syndrome, 336
Weiss, Soma, 101
Whiplash injuries:
as cause of spinovascular diseases, 252
effects of, 142
Willis, Sir Thomas, 122
Willis, circle of, 19, 28, 93
anastomotic connections in, 56
arterial pressure at, 54
atherosclerosis of, 112
blood flow regulation by, 161
calcification of, 167
cerebral infarction and, 178
collateral circulation through, 124-125
configurations in, 1, 6, 7
development of, 6
different patterns of, 30
effects of syphilis on, 238
effects of traction on, 287
inadequate crossover to, congenital anomalies and, 106
intracranial anastomoses in, 30
intracranial aneurysms in, 229, 298
Moyamoya disease of, 364, 365, 366, 367
as pressure equalizer, 56, 94
vasospasm in, 189
vessels supplying, 115
Women:
atherosclerosis among, 123, 348
carotid artery syndrome among, 123
cranial arteritis among, 349
disseminated lupus erythematosus among, 354
infraclinoid intracavernous aneurysm among, 300
intracerebral hemorrhage among, 335
intracranial aneurysm in, 298
medial dysplasia among, 364